CULTURE, BRAIN, AND ANALGESIA

CULTURE, BRAIN, AND ANALGESIA

Understanding and Managing Pain in Diverse Populations

Edited by

Mario Incayawar, MD, MSc, DESS

Director
Runajambi–Institute for the Study of Quichua Culture and Health
Otavalo, Ecuador

Knox H. Todd, MD, MPH

Professor and Chair
Department of Emergency Medicine
The University of Texas MD Anderson Cancer Center
Houston, Texas, USA

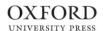

OXFORD
UNIVERSITY PRESS

OXFORD
UNIVERSITY PRESS

Oxford University Press is a department of the University of Oxford. It furthers the
University's objective of excellence in research, scholarship, and education by publishing
worldwide

Oxford   New York
Auckland   Cape Town   Dar es Salaam   Hong Kong   Karachi
Kuala Lumpur   Madrid   Melbourne   Mexico City   Nairobi
New Delhi   Shanghai   Taipei   Toronto

With offices in
Argentina   Austria   Brazil   Chile   Czech Republic   France   Greece
Guatemala   Hungary   Italy   Japan   Poland   Portugal   Singapore
South Korea   Switzerland   Thailand   Turkey   Ukraine   Vietnam

Oxford is a registered trademark of Oxford University Press in the UK and certain other
countries.

Published in the United States of America by
Oxford University Press
198 Madison Avenue, New York, NY 10016

Library of Congress Cataloging-in-Publication Data
Culture, brain, and analgesia: understanding and managing pain in diverse populations / edited by
   Mario Incayawar, Knox H. Todd.
      p.; cm.
   Includes bibliographical references and index.
   ISBN: 978-0-19-976887-5 (hardcover: alk. paper)
   I. Incayawar, Mario.   II. Todd, Knox H.
   [DNLM: 1. Pain—ethnology.   2. Analgesia—methods.   3. Analgesics—therapeutic use.
   4. Cultural Competency.   5. Cultural Diversity.   6. Pain Management—methods. WL 704]
   LC Classification not assigned
   616′.0472—dc23
   2012022943

9 8 7 6 5 4 3 2 1
Printed in the United States of America
on acid-free paper

CONTENTS

PART 2: CULTURE AND PAIN ASSESSMENT

PART 3: DISPARITIES AND INEQUITIES IN PAIN MANAGEMENT

PART 4: CROSS-CULTURAL MANAGEMENT OF PAIN

PART 5: PHARMACOGENOMICS AND ANALGESIC DRUGS

PART 6: CONTEXTUAL ISSUES IN PAIN MEDICINE

PART 7: THE FUTURE OF ANALGESIA IN DIVERSE POPULATIONS

FOREWORD

The publication of *Culture, Brain, and Analgesia* is a watershed moment in medical history. Never before has so much significant, high-quality, and universally relevant material on the topic been gathered in a single place. It marks an advance for the modern movement to recognize pain management as a human right, a movement that gained formal recognition when the World Health Organization and the European and International Associations for the Study of Pain announced a global "Day Against Pain" in 2004, and when the United States Congress declared 2001–2010 as "The Decade of Pain Control and Management."

Since the earliest days of our existence, pain and suffering have been regarded as humankind's constant companions. Because pain and suffering were such potent, inevitable, and essentially untamed forces, they stimulated much thought about their role in providing meaning to life. Unlike pleasure and happiness, which can be shared, pain and suffering are ultimately personal. In order to make then more endurable they came to be rationalized as profound, deep, and meaningful experiences that found a home in many religious traditions. Shamanism, for example, is the oldest spiritual healing tradition. Would-be shamans throughout the world had to endure horrible pain and suffering, such as bodily dismemberment, reduction of the body to a skeleton by scraping away the flesh, and substitution of their blood and viscera. Only then could they spend time in Hell to learn about healing from demons and the souls of dead shamans, followed by an ascent to heaven to be consecrated as healers by God. Although this ghastly process took place only in dreams and trance states, it was perceived to be very real. The pain and suffering of gruesome dismemberment and reassembly were the stepping stones to wisdom and the capacity to heal both oneself and others.

Hinduism has presented fertile ground for the pain of self-mortification as can be seen in the veneration of sadhus, especially in rural, traditional areas of India. Sadhus are spiritual ascetics who, at the extreme, appear wasted and who twist their bodies into odd, painful positions for years without surcease. Suffering is inherent to the tensions of the Hindu cosmos. Kali, the Dark Goddess, is a ferocious and bloodthirsty aspect of the god Siva who personifies the forces of destruction and evil in the universe. She wears a necklace of human skulls and a belt of amputated limbs. She demanded human sacrifices and rivers of blood to sustain her bottomless stomach and fertile womb, which gives birth forever to all things. The holiest icons of Hinduism are Shiva lingam stones, which are naturally found and which represent the phallus of Shiva who castrated himself.

In traditional Judaism, suffering represents just punishment for sins. In the biblical book of Deuteronomy, the Hebrew God threatened those who did not keep his commandments and fulfill his statutes with severe burning, fever, inflammation, mildew, boils, fever, scabs, untreatable rash, madness, blindness, and confusion. He declared, "I kill and I make alive I wound and I heal … I will render vengeance to my enemies." Jewish scripture clearly states that sinners suffer, but it also presents puzzling questions such as the prophet Jeremiah's query: "Why is it that the wicked live so prosperously? Why do scoundrels enjoy peace?" And there is still debate about why God allowed Satan to strike guiltless Job "with painful boils from the sole of his foot to the crown of his head." Although the Hebrews found nothing noble in personal suffering, they did contribute to the world the notion that collective suffering possesses a redemptive power and a promise of better things to come in this life.

Christianity comes in many shapes and forms but its one irreducible belief is that humankind was saved by Christ's suffering, crucifixion, and death. Christian scripture invites believers to share in Christ's sufferings, states that the Christian congregation is truly the body of Christ, and that suffering has redemptive value. We should, like Christ, endure bodily suffering, "for whoever has suffered in the flesh has ceased for sin ... those who suffer accordingly to God's will do right and entrust their souls to a faithful creator." Bodily decay renews our spiritual nature.

The redemptive value of suffering was poignantly expressed in the prophet Isaiah's description of the Suffering Servant [a metaphor for the people of Israel]: "Ours were the sufferings he bore, ours the sorrows he carried ... and through his wounds we are healed." Centuries later Christ became the Suffering Servant: "He himself bore our sins in his body that we might die to sin and live to righteousness. By his wounds you have been healed." This glorification of suffering influenced Christian attitudes towards illness for almost two thousand years and was aided by a mistranslation of a key word in the Bible. The early Church encouraged the healing of sickness but after the signing of the Edict of Milan in 313 the persecution of Christians by the Romans ended and the Church no longer needed to focus on bodily healing to recruit new members. For several centuries the text from the biblical book of James had served as a model for healing. James wrote that sick people should call the elders of the Church to pray at their bedside and to anoint them with oil in the name of the Lord. The sick should then confess their sins to one another and they will be "healed." In AD 400 St. Jerome translated the Bible into Latin but instead of translating "They will be healed," he wrote, "They will be saved." This alteration displaced the healing of illness by spiritual salvation.

The glorification of suffering has influenced Christian attitudes for almost two thousand years and, for many Christians became an avocation. Indeed, when Paul asked God to heal him of the infirmity he called a thorn in his flesh, God refused. Instead, God said, "My grace is sufficient for you, for my power is made perfect in weakness." This was a brilliant new idea: a handicap was rationalized into an asset by perceiving it so. Instead of regarding physical pain and suffering as a defect or liability, declare it an opportunity to receive the power of God and make the most of it.

Pain is central to many other religious traditions. This is perfectly understandable in that religion attempts to impose some meaning to life and, until fairly recently in human history, there was not much that could be done to alleviate pain and suffering. Religion has dealt with pain not by trying to stop it but rather by trying to transform it into an experience that leads to meaning, insight, and even salvation. Although religious and medical traditions have often been intertwined, physicians and healers throughout history have struggled to control pain by utilizing a host of substances such as coca leaves, opium, cannabis, scopolamine, atropine, and nitrous oxide. Then, in the mid-1800s, chloroform and ether became available. For the first time, the promise of pain control through the use of reliable agents became a reality. Even Queen Victoria allowed the use of chloroform to facilitate the birth of her eighth child and the social elite in London followed her lead. With experience and the development of safer medications the use of anesthesia for painless surgery and childbirth spread rapidly throughout Europe.

As might be expected, this innovation, which challenged attitudes established over thousands of years, met with both religious and even medical criticism. Painless childbirth was seen as antithetical to God's will as expressed in the biblical book of Genesis: "In pain you will bring forth children." Moreover, obstetric pain was thought to produce spiritual rewards and was a form of baptism that regenerated a woman's whole nature. The first President of the American Dental Association wrote: "I think anesthesia is of the devil … I do not think that men should be prevented from passing through what God intended them to endure." Leaders of the American temperance movement felt that anesthesia threatened the virtue of women because it was a form of intoxication and therefore was inherently immoral.

Many physicians were anti-anesthesia because of its perceived harmful effects, such as poisoning a person's blood and causing convulsions, asphyxia, bronchitis, pneumonia, and brain inflammation. Anesthesia was thought to slow the birthing process, change patients into corpses, and weaken the divinely given "life force" of the soul, which was manifested by consciousness. It took many decades for these objections to be dispelled. The process was propelled by the discovery of safer chemical agents that could be used for local, regional, general, and dissociative anesthesia. As the physiological mechanisms of pain were delineated, many new methods for pain control were developed, ranging from medications to electrical and other devices and surgery. These changes also came about because of changing attitudes towards illness and suffering that emerged at the turn of the 20th century. Theologians and faith healers reinterpreted the Bible with a new emphasis on healing as a central component of Christ's ministry. Attention was focused on the twenty percent of the Gospels that are devoted to Christ's healing encounters with sick persons. Books were published and sermons preached emphasizing every Christian's duty to pray for self-healing as well as the healing of others. Persons were no longer encouraged to share in Christ's suffering. The Second Vatican Council in the 1960s reaffirmed the religious healing practices of the early Church and the sacrament of Extreme Unction, which was traditionally administered to dying persons, was renamed Anointing of the Sick and called upon God to raise ill persons from their sick beds. The amazing rise and growth of the new megachurches has been based on a theology of hope and freedom from depression and illness.

The declaration that the control of pain and suffering is a basic human right is the natural outcome of the interaction between scientific advances in analgesia and cultural changes in our attitudes. In fact, cultural changes have provided a fertile environment for the development of scientific advances. Fortunately no groups in today's world extol the virtues of pain and suffering and, at least in this area, we have been spared the vitriolic clashes between the forces on conservatism and liberalism that bedevil the areas of stem cell research, contraception, the termination of pregnancy, and homosexuality.

Most of my professional career has been devoted to the study of persons who deliberately mutilate and injure themselves. Such behaviors have been present since the earliest days of humankind and were usually thought to be an attenuated form of suicide that was senseless and horrific. As recently as the mid-1980s a well-known American psychiatrist expressed the widely held belief that confronting patients who repeatedly cut and burned their skin left one "feeling a combination of helpless, hopeless, horrified, guilty, furious, disgusted, and sad." The publication of my book *Bodies under Siege* in 1987 (a third edition was published in 2011) helped to change this negative attitude. In it I showed that deliberate self-harm was the opposite of suicidal behavior and that its use of pain was novel in that it served to provide temporary relief from many insufferable symptoms such as mounting anxiety, depression, racing thoughts, fluctuating emotions, and depersonalization. Further, I showed that painful body modification rituals, some extending as far back as the Stone Age, often served the purposes of fostering spirituality, social orderliness, and physical healing. Thus, in a counterintuitive manner individuals and societies have discovered the therapeutic potential of deliberately created pain to reduce the suffering caused by pathological pain. These understandings have changed greatly both professional and lay attitudes towards self-injurers.

Culture, Brain, and Analgesia is a state-of-the-art book. Its diverse chapters teach us about the varieties and assessment of pain experiences and introduce us to a future in which pain management will be personalized. It is an entry into a brave new world of possibilities that was unimaginable until now. Drs. Incayawar and Todd are to be congratulated for conceiving such a book and bringing together a group of distinguished contributors. It is now the principal integrative document for establishing pain management as a basic human right that will be culturally sensitive, genomics-wise, and efficacious. Pain is a cruel master that saps the vitality of life. Julius Caesar even wrote, "It is easier to find men who will volunteer to die than to find men who are willing to endure pain with patience." Incayawar and Todd's impressive book presages a world in which the victims of debilitating pain will be unchained from their medical suffering and freed from enduring a life of pain with patience.

Armando Favazza, MD, MPH
Emeritus Professor of Psychiatry
University of Missouri-Columbia

PREFACE

At the dawn of the 21st century, the world is becoming smaller and human interactions more diverse. Widespread access to the Internet, a more global economy, and enhanced migration are contributing to this transformation. Tirelessly, and perhaps anxiously, the medical community is coping with this new world.

Worldwide patient-clinician encounters are less homogenous today and this diversity poses a particular challenge for pain medicine. Health professionals need to know more than just some elements of cultural variability in pain experiences. They also have a need to understand how pain experiences and treatment responses among patients from different ethnocultural groups could be modulated by neurobiological, pharmacogenetic, genetic, and epigenetic factors.

Pain is a clinical, public health, and fundamental human rights issue. According to the Institute of Medicine's 2011 report titled *Relieving Pain in America—A Blueprint for Transforming Prevention, Care, Education, and Research*, 116 million American adults suffer from chronic pain; more than the total affected by heart disease, cancer, and diabetes combined. Pain causes 40 million medical visits annually and costs the United States $635 billion each year in healthcare expenditures and lost productivity. Pain has been proposed as the fifth vital sign. It is widely present in clinical practice and healthcare workers from all over the world have daily encounters with patients in pain. It is the single most frequent complaint brought to the offices of physicians. Moreover, inadequate treatment of pain is highly prevalent and has been well-documented among specific social strata, age groups, and medical settings, and is particularly notorious among minority groups. Indeed, African-American and Latino patients in the United States seem two to three times more likely to receive inadequate pain treatment than Anglo-Americans.

Research literature in the field of culture and pain medicine is sparse and scholarship in this area is limited. Reflecting these deficiencies, medical trainees receive minimal training to manage pain among patients from diverse populations. Furthermore, health professionals including pain practitioners have limited knowledge of the role culture plays in pain assessment and management.

This volume focuses on the complex and striking relationships among culture, brain, pain, and analgesia and wants to respond to the above-mentioned gaps and unmet needs.

This book has its roots in the earlier clinical experiences of Mario Incayawar as a medical student responding to the calls of Quichua (Inca) patients in the Andean highlands of South America. Since he was the first Quichua medical student in the country, villagers enthusiastically considered him as their trusted doctor and consulted him for a variety of reasons including nonmedical ones. Seeing stoical patients who were affected by serious and painful clinical conditions deeply intrigued him. One example provides a vivid image of the diversity of pain responses in the Andes: Relatives asked Mario Incayawar to help a 50-year-old male patient who had been complaining of distended abdomen for the past eight days. He was in bed, unable to walk, sleepless, weak, and unable to eat. After a physical examination, it was suspected that the patient was suffering from peritonitis and urgent hospitalization was recommended. What was striking in this case was the patient's "indifference" and lack of pain expression during the abdominal physical examination. Incayawar also had the chance to see similar cases at the medical school in Quito, the capital of Ecuador, with Latino patients. The Latino patients were more expressive and defensive when they were subjected to the abdominal palpation. Since those days, his interest has grown for understanding how culture modulates pain and its biological underpinnings.

Like Mario, Knox Todd's motivation to pursue research on pain derived from his clinical experience. Early in his career, he was called to assist a 40-year-old man who had collapsed in the hallway outside his office, a few steps away from a busy county emergency department. As the episode unfolded, he found that the man had just been discharged from the department after receiving a diagnosis of three fractured ribs. Despite the incapacitating nature of the man's pain, his treating trauma surgeons had to be convinced that the patient deserved their attentions. This disconnect between a basic human need, the relief of pain, and the clinicians' attitudes was striking and drove Knox's career interest in the fascinating world of pain.

We made a significant effort to cover important regions of the world. The chapters are original contributions from recognized world experts in the field of culture, brain, and analgesia. The contributors came from Beirut, China, Denmark, Finland, India, Italy, Norway, Quebec (Canada), Quichua (Ecuador), Singapore, the United Kingdom, and the United States.

This book presents original research data, case vignettes, and pilot pain studies. It is hoped that the material in this volume will appeal to a broad cross-section of health practitioners, students, and academicians, including primary care physicians; pain medicine specialists; psychiatrists; psychologists; social workers; mental health, community, and public health workers; health policy makers; and health administrators.

Many colleagues and friends generously contributed to this book. Mario Incayawar is deeply grateful to Dr. Knox H. Todd for warmly welcoming the idea for this book and for his commitment with this challenging academic journey. Similarly, Knox Todd greatly appreciates Dr. Incayawar's introduction to pain scholars from the broad range of disciplines represented by the collected authors. The enthusiasm, encouragement, and support we received from Ms. Andrea L. Seils, Senior Editor, Clinical Medicine, and the reassuring and diligent management of Ms. Staci Hou, Assistant Editor, Medicine, both at Oxford University Press is greatly appreciated. With their flexible and highly professional assistance, they have greatly facilitated the successful completion of our book.

Mario Incayawar wants to express gratitude to the Government of Quebec, Fond FCAR doctoral award for conducting pain research among the Quichua (Inca) in the Andes, and the John Simon Guggenheim Memorial Foundation for its generous 2006 fellowship that helped him in the editing of this book. Knox Todd thanks The Mayday Fund of New York for their early and continuing support of pain researchers in emergency medicine.

Our heartfelt appreciation goes to our contributors. Without their outstanding and diligent work, this volume would not have seen the light.

This book will not respond to all your questions. Rather, it will provide you with a guidepost for understanding your patient in a multicultural setting, making an appropriate diagnosis, and preparing a good quality personalized treatment plan.

Our Quichua (Inca) pain patients from the most remote Andean communities in South America and the challenging cross-cultural doctors-patients interactions worldwide provided the motivation to prepare this book.

MARIO INCAYAWAR, MD, MSc, DESS
Director
Runajambi–Institute for the Study of Quichua Culture and Health
Otavalo, Ecuador.

KNOX H. TODD, MD, MPH
Professor and Chair
Department of Emergency Medicine
The University of Texas MD Anderson Cancer Center
Houston, Texas, USA.

February 11, 2012

CONTRIBUTORS

Huda Abu-Saad Huijer, RN, PhD, FEANS, FAAN
Professor of Nursing Science
Director, Hariri School of Nursing
American University of Beirut,
Beirut, Lebanon

Karen O. Anderson, PhD, MPH
Associate Professor
Department of Symptom Research
The University of Texas MD Anderson
    Cancer Center
Houston, Texas, USA

Fabrizio Benedetti, MD
Professor of Physiology
Department of Neuroscience
University of Turin Medical School
National Institute of Neuroscience
Turin, Italy

Dinesh Bhugra, MA, MSc, MBBS, FRCPsych, MPhil, PhD
Professor of Mental Health and Cultural
    Diversity
Institute of Psychiatry
King's College London
London, UK

Lise Bouchard, MA, PhD
Director of Research
Runajambi–Institute for the Study of
    Quichua Culture and Health
Otavalo, Ecuador

Lynn Clark Callister, RN, PhD, FAAN
Professor Emerita
Brigham Young University College of
    Nursing
Provo, Utah, USA

Evelyn Ruiz Calvillo, RN, DNSc
Professor Emeritus of Nursing
School of Health & Human Services
California State University, Los Angeles
Los Angeles, California, USA

Elisa Carlino, PhD
Post-Doctoral Fellow
Department of Neuroscience
University of Turin
Turin, Italy

Simon K. C. Chan, MBBS
Clinical Associate Professor (Honorary)
Department of Anaesthesia and
    Intensive Care
The Chinese University of Hong Kong
Shatin, NT, Hong Kong, China

Victor T. Chang, MD
Hematology/Oncology Service
New Jersey Veterans Affairs Health Care
    System East Orange
East Orange, New Jersey, USA

Mitchell J. M. Cohen, MD
Vice Chair for Education
Director, Pain Medicine Program
Department of Psychiatry
Jefferson Medical College
Philadelphia, Pennsylvania, USA

Lori E. Crosby, PsyD
Associate Professor of Clinical Pediatrics
University of Cincinnati College of Medicine
Division of Behavioral Medicine and
    Clinical Psychology
Cincinnati Children's Hospital Medical
    Center
Cincinnati, Ohio, USA

Stephen Dahmer, MD
Integrative Family Medicine Attending
Beth Israel Continuum Center for Health
    and Healing, New York
New York, USA

Lara Dhingra, PhD
Co-Chief, Research Division
Department of Pain Medicine and
    Palliative Care
Beth Israel Medical Center
New York, New York, USA
Assistant Professor
Departments of Neurology and Psychiatry
    and Behavioral Sciences
Albert Einstein College of Medicine
Bronx, New York, USA

Patrick A. Dion, PhD
Scientific Coordinator
Centre of Excellence in Neurosciences at
    University of Montréal
Centre Hospitalier de l'Université de
    Montréal
Assistant Researcher
Departments of Pathology and Cellular
    Biology
University of Montréal
Montréal, Québec, Canada

Armando Favazza, MD
Emeritus Professor of Psychiatry
Department of Psychiatry
University of Missouri
Columbia, Missouri, USA

Roger B. Fillingim, PhD
Professor
Department of Community Dentistry and
    Behavioral Sciences
University of Florida College
    of Dentistry
Gainesville, Florida, USA

Laura P. Gelfman, MD
Fellow in Palliative Medicine
Brookdale Department of Geriatrics and
    Palliative Medicine
Mount Sinai School of Medicine New York,
New York, USA

Tony Gin, MD
Professor and Chairman
Department of Anaesthesia and Intensive
    Care
The Chinese University of Hong Kong
Shatin, NT, Hong Kong, China

Burel R. Goodin, PhD
Post-Doctoral Fellow
Comprehensive Center for Pain Research
University of Florida College of Dentistry
Gainesville, Florida, USA

Alexander R. Green, MD, MPH
Associate Director
The Disparities Solutions Center
Massachusetts General Hospital
Assistant Professor of Medicine
Harvard Medical School
Boston, Massachusetts, USA

Carmen R. Green, MD
Professor of Anesthesiology, Obstetrics &
    Gynecology, and Health Management
    & Policy
Director, Health Disparities Research
    Program Michigan Institute for Clinical
    & Health Research
Ann Arbor, Michigan, USA

Susham Gupta, MBBS, MRCPsych
Consultant Psychiatrist
East London NHS Foundation Trust
Assertive Outreach Team—City &
    Hackney
London, UK

Mohammadreza Hojat, PhD
Research Professor of Psychiatry and
    Human Behavior
Director of Jefferson Longitudinal Study
Center for Research in Medical Education
    and Health Care
Jefferson Medical College
Philadelphia, Pennsylvania, USA

Inger Margrethe Holter, PhD, RN
Project Coordinator
Norwegian Nurses Association
Norway

He Hong-Gu, PhD, RN, MD
Assistant Professor
Alice Lee Centre for Nursing Studies
Yong Loo Lin School of Medicine
National University of Singapore
Singapore

Mario Incayawar, MD, MSc, DESS
Director, Runajambi–Institute for the
    Study of Quichua Culture and Health
Otavalo, Ecuador
Former Henry R. Luce Professor in Brain,
    Mind and Medicine, Cross-Cultural
    Perspectives
Claremont Colleges
Claremont, California, USA

**Oren K. Isacoff, BA, BSc, MD/MBA
    (student)**
University of Pennsylvania
Philadelphia, Pennsylvania, USA

Gurvinder S. Kalra, MD, DPM
Assistant Professor
Department of Psychiatry
Lokmanya Tilak Municipal Medical
    College & Sion General Hospital
Mumbai, Maharashtra, India

Hesook Suzie Kim, PhD, RN
Professor Emerita
College of Nursing
University of Rhode Island
Kingston, Rhode Island, USA
Project Director for Research Programs
Institutt for helsefag
Buskerud University College
Drammen, Norway

Cheryl Koopman, PhD
Associate Professor (Research)
Department of Psychiatry and Behavioral
    Sciences
Stanford University
Stanford, California, USA

Anna Lee, PhD
Professor
Department of Anaesthesia and Intensive
    Care
The Chinese University of Hong Kong
Prince of Wales Hospital
Shatin, NT, Hong Kong, China

Keh-Ming Lin, MD, MPH
Professor Emeritus of Psychiatry
University of California, Los Angeles
Los Angeles, California, USA
2008–2009 Fellow, Center for Advanced
    Study in the Behavioral Science at
    Stanford (CASBS)
Diplomate, American Board of Psychiatry
    and Neurology
Distinguished Life-Time Fellow, American
    Psychiatric Association

Graciete Lo, MA
Pre-Doctoral Fellow
Department of Pain Medicine and
    Palliative Care
Beth Israel Medical Center
New York, New York, USA
Department of Psychology
Fordham University
Bronx, New York, USA

**Sioui Maldonado-Bouchard, MSc, PhD
    (candidate)**
Research Assistant
Runajambi–Institute for the Study of
    Quichua Culture and Health
Otavalo, Ecuador
Doctoral Interdisciplinary Program in
    Neurosciences
Laboratory on Spinal Cord Injury
    Recovery
Texas A&M University
College Station, Texas, USA

Salimah H. Meghani, PhD, MBE, CRNP
Assistant Professor
Biobehavioral and Health Sciences
    Division
University of Pennsylvania School of
    Nursing
Philadelphia, Pennsylvania, USA

Nancy Merner, PhD
Post-Doctoral Fellow
Centre of Excellence in Neurosciences at
    University of Montréal
Centre Hospitalier de l'Université de
    Montréal
Montréal, Québec, Canada

Rod Moore, DDS, PhD, Dr Odont
Dental Anxiety Research and Treatment
    Center
Royal Dental College
Faculty of Health Sciences
Århus University
Århus, Denmark

R. Sean Morrison, MD
Professor, Geriatrics and Medicine
Department of Geriatrics and Palliative
    Medicine
Mount Sinai School of Medicine, New York
New York, USA

Bernardo Ng, MD, DFAPA
Clinical Assistant Professor
Department of Psychiatry
University of California, San Diego
La Jolla, California, USA
Medical Director
Sun Valley Behavioral Medical Center
Imperial, California, USA

Guadalupe R. Palos, DrPH
Office of Cancer Survivorship
The University of Texas MD Anderson
    Cancer Center
Houston, Texas, USA

Mark J. Pletcher, MD, MPH
Associate Professor, In Residence
Departments of Epidemiology &
    Biostatistics and Medicine
University of California,
    San Francisco
San Francisco, California, USA

Antonella Pollo, MD
Assistant Professor
Department of Neuroscience
University of Torino
Torino, Italy

Mythili Prabhu, MD
Department of Obstetrics and
    Gynecology
University of Michigan Medical
    School
Ann Arbor, Michigan, USA

Judy F. Pugh, PhD
Associate Professor
Department of Anthropology
Michigan State University
East Lansing, Michigan, USA

Cielito C. Reyes-Gibby, DrPH, MSN
Associate Professor
Department of Emergency Medicine
The University of Texas MD Anderson
    Cancer Center
Houston, Texas, USA

Fatima Rodriguez, MD, MPH
Brigham and Women's Hospital
Department of Medicine
Harvard Medical School
Boston, Massachusetts, USA

Guy A. Rouleau, MD, PhD, FRCPC
Director
Centre of Excellence in Neurosciences
University of Montréal
Centre Hospitalier de l'Université
    de Montréal
Director
Ste-Justine Hospital Research Center
Professor
Department of Medicine
University of Montréal
Montréal, Québec, Canada

Donna Schwartz-Barcott, PhD, RN
Professor
College of Nursing
University of Rhode Island
Kingston, Rhode Island, USA

Emilie Scott, MD
Department of Family Medicine
University of California, Irvine
South Orange, California, USA

Susan Sharp, MA, PsyD (student)
PGSP-Stanford PsyD Consortium
Palo Alto University
Stanford Psychology and Biobehavioral
    Sciences Laboratory
Stanford School of Medicine
Palo Alto, California, USA

Kimberly Sibille, PhD
Research Assistant Professor
Department of Community Dentistry and
　Behavioral Sciences
University of Florida
Gainesville, Florida, USA

Anna Szuto, MSc
Genetic Counsellor
Centre of Excellence in Neurosciences,
　University of Montréal
Centre Hospitalier de l'Université de
　Montréal
Montréal, Québec, Canada

Raymond C. Tait, PhD
Vice President, Research
Professor
Department of Psychiatry
Adjunct Professor, Center for Health Care
　Ethics
Saint Louis University
Saint Louis, Missouri, USA

Raymond Y. Teets, MD
Institute for Family Health
Beth Israel Residency in Urban Family
　Medicine
Department of Family and Social Medicine
Albert Einstein College of Medicine of
　Yeshiva University
New York, New York, USA

Joseph Telfair, DrPH, MSW, MPH
Professor
Public Health Research and Practice
Director, UNCG Center for Social,
　Community and Health Research and
　Evaluation
University of North Carolina at
　Greensboro
Greensboro, North Carolina, USA

Knox H. Todd, MD, MPH
Professor and Chair
Department of Emergency Medicine
The University of Texas MD Anderson
　Cancer Center
Houston, Texas, USA

John Tsoi, LMSW
Project Director
Asian Family Caregiver Program
Department of Pain Medicine and
　Palliative Care
Asian Services Center
Beth Israel Medical Center
New York, New York, USA

Katri Vehviläinen-Julkunen, RN, PhD
Professor
Department of Nursing Science
Faculty of Health Sciences
University of Eastern Finland
Kuopio, Finland

CULTURE, BRAIN, AND ANALGESIA

RELEVANCE OF PAIN AND ANALGESIA IN MULTICULTURAL SOCIETIES

KNOX H. TODD, MD, MPH
Professor and Chair, Department of Emergency Medicine,
The University of Texas MD Anderson Cancer Center,
Houston, Texas, USA

MARIO INCAYAWAR, MD, MSC, DESS
Director, Runajambi-Institute for the Study of Quichua Culture
and Health, Otavalo, Ecuador

Pain is the most common complaint bringing people to a physician's office.[1] In New Zealand, 82% of the population report a life-disrupting pain experience, while in a World Health Organization (WHO) international study, 22% of primary care patients in 14 countries reported persistent pain.[2,3] Almost two decades ago, the U.S. Department of Health and Human Services reported that pain caused 40 million medical visits per year, costing the country over $100 billion annually in healthcare expenditure and lost productivity.[4]

Today, according to the Institute of Medicine's 2011 report titled *Relieving Pain in America—A Blueprint for Transforming Prevention, Care, Education, and Research*, 116 million American adults suffer from chronic pain; more than the total affected by heart disease, cancer, and diabetes combined, and costing the country $635 billion each year.[5] Undoubtedly, pain is widespread around the world and its importance as a global public health problem has been recognized by the WHO.[3]

Moreover, inadequate treatment of pain is highly prevalent in the medical setting. This neglect has been documented among children, the elderly, those with cancer, surgical patients, and ethnic minority groups, among others.[6–10] Due in part to recognition of this worldwide neglect, pain has been declared a fundamental issue of human rights.[11]

THE NATURE OF PAIN

Beyond an enumeration of pain prevalence and its costs, we understand that pain is among the most universal of human experiences. With very rare exceptions, we have all

1

experienced the garden variety of acute aches and pains resulting from illness or injury. Acute pain often occurs as the result of an identifiable series of events, such as hitting one's thumb with a hammer, or breaking a wrist after tripping over the cat. Acute pain can also result from medical diseases involving inflammation and infection as in cases of appendicitis or meningitis. Acute pain brings to consciousness some very useful signals and is associated with behaviors that tend to remove painful stimuli or encourage healing, such as "take your hand out of the fire," "remain still so that your broken bone will heal," or "tell those around you that you require help." In fact, for those unable to sense pain due to hereditary sensory neuropathies (congenital absence of pain), life is short. The inability to sense pain impairs homeostatic protective responses, leading to recurrent injuries, infections, and death.

Chronic and persistent pain lasts longer than the expected time of healing after injury or disease, and may continue for months or years. In contrast to acute pain, it serves no useful purpose. In some cases, pain is related to clearly evident disease or nerve injury, as in cancer-related pain or traumatic limb injuries. In other cases, we have little understanding of the provenance of chronic pain, and it may appear without an obvious antecedent. Many theories attempt to explain chronic pain as a result of various disorders in peripheral and central nervous system function, and our understanding of the pathophysiology of chronic pain continues to evolve.

The International Association for the Study of Pain defines pain as "An unpleasant sensory and emotional experience associated with actual or potential tissue damage or described in terms of such damage."[12] Humans are driven to find meaning in their experience of both acute and chronic pain. This definition recognizes not only the emotional component of pain, but also that descriptions or narratives surrounding pain are essential to our understanding of the pain experience. Medical historian Roselyne Rey states that "Pain is a bio-psycho-social phenomenon. Nociception reflects anatomy and physiology, but cultural and social factors are the foundation for the expression and treatment of pain."[13] This description highlights the critical importance of beliefs and behaviors specific to the social, ethnic, age, or cultural group with which we identify. This cultural context is important to caregivers and healthcare professionals who attempt to ameliorate pain and suffering, as it assists both the understanding of pain's meaning to those who suffer it and helps interpret their pain-related behaviors.

UNDERSTANDING PAIN

Although humans share common anatomic and physiologic features related to pain, the pain experience is a private affair. Each of us experiences our own unique sensation of pain and we face the task of interpreting its meaning and expressing it to others. This is no mean feat. As Elaine Scarry notes, "To have pain is to have certainty; to hear about pain is to have doubt."[14]

Even among academicians who study and treat pain, pain-related communications can be challenging. The editors of this book first met in 2002 at Claremont Colleges in California, where Dr. Incayawar invited an interdisciplinary group of scholars to present their work on pain from a variety of different viewpoints at the Luce Faculty Seminar on Health Disparities in the United States. During the conference, it was evident that many of the words and phrases used to speak about pain had different and even conflicting meanings for different disciplines. The phrase, "natural history of disease" means very different things to a physician and historian, while "illness" may be interpreted very differently by a psychiatrist and cultural anthropologist.

One of the purposes of this book is to bring together a broad array of disciplines to present views of pain from contrasting vantage points. In fact, one of the difficulties faced by the editors was how much standard terminology should be emphasized over discipline-specific language. In the end, although we attempted to promote common terminology, discipline-specific terms and meanings are retained in many cases, with adequate explanations of how these words or phrases should be interpreted.

HISTORICITY OF ANALGESIA

Although pain perception is a private affair, pain-related behaviors, interpretation of pain's meaning by oneself and by others, and certainly pain treatment are public and play out in a specific time and place. To better understand the potential for plasticity in cultural and social norms related to pain and its treatment, it may be useful to review a limited example of historical changes in attitude related to the use of opioids, such as morphine, to treat pain in the United States and Great Britain over relatively short periods of time. We will consider two examples: the treatment of terminal cancer pain, and analgesic use for acute abdominal pain, as might be experienced in cases of appendicitis.

Regarding terminal malignancy, H. L. Snow wrote the following in 1893: "[T]he golden rule in cancer not amenable to cure by surgical eradication, is to initiate at the earliest moment the administration of opium or morphia in small, continued, gradually-increased doses.... Making certain local exceptions, the patient with an incurable malignant tumour should thus become permanently subject to the morphine habit, purposely induced."[15] Thus, physical dependency on opioids as the preferred outcome for terminal cancer pain treatment received general acceptance in the prevalent medical culture. By the mid 1900s, attitudes toward opioid use and dependency had changed remarkably. In the *Journal of the American Medical Association*, a leading practitioner wrote: "The use of narcotics in the terminal cancer [patient] is to be condemned ... Morphine usage is an unpleasant experience to the majority of human subjects because of undesirable side-effects. Dominant in the list of these unfortunate effects is addiction."[16]

For the treatment of pain lacking a definite diagnosis, medical attitudes again have shifted markedly over the years. J. K. Spender, writing in 1887 in the *British Medical Journal*, appeared to favor the generous use of analgesics when he noted the following: "Before we can relieve a given pain, says the philosopher, we must find out its cause. Wise and deep saying! Then if we fail to know the cause, is the pain to go on unhindered? ... If we see a man bleeding to death, must we refuse to stop the living tide until we know for certain where the blood comes from?"[17] A quarter of a century later, Sir Vincent Zachary Cope, in a classic treatise on abdominal pain, wrote: "In order to diagnose acute abdomen successfully, all clinical signs must be present in their unaltered state. Administration of analgesia would delay diagnosis and result in increased mortality."[18] The latter surgical dictum was remarkably persistent. Only after a large number of rigorously conducted clinical trials demonstrated the safety of intravenous opioid administration for severe acute abdominal pain did our surgical colleagues relent (in the 20th edition of this surgical classic) from what increasingly appeared (to our eyes) a barbarous practice.[19,20]

MULTIDISCIPLINARY AND INTEGRATIVE PAIN MEDICINE

While the above example illustrates how specific historical and cultural contexts modify acute and cancer pain treatment, it should be recognized that pain has exceedingly complex influences on a variety of human functions. Pain impairs our ability to communicate, disconnects us from loved ones and family, and erects barriers to playing our accustomed roles in society. To understand and optimally treat this multitude of pain effects, there is increasing recognition of the value of cross-disciplinary investigation and collaboration in managing those with pain. While unidisciplinary approaches may be adequate for treating acute pain, chronic pain, in particular, requires a multidisciplinary approach. Collaborating specialists in occupational therapy, social work, nursing, psychiatry, psychology, medicine, and pharmacology may be required to provide superior pain treatment. For each of these specialties, the ability to communicate with other members of an interdisciplinary team is important, as is an understanding of the intricate interactions between culture and pain.

Given increases in global mobility and migration, we live in worlds that are more ethnically diverse than ever before. Particularly for pain sufferers and healthcare providers who lack a common culture and language, disparate assumptions about causes of pain and its appropriate treatment complicate the doctor/patient relationship immensely.

As Sir William Osler told us, "It is much more important to know what sort of a patient has a disease, than what sort of a disease a patient has." Given the increasing ethnic and cultural diversity we experience in almost all parts of the world, this statement is as pertinent as ever. In many locales, no single ethnic group constitutes a majority. Ethnic groups may speak different languages entirely, and certainly have different conceptions of disease and health, and particularly in the meanings they ascribe to pain.

Competent medical practice requires at least a general idea of how culture influences pain experience and expression and how communication styles differ by culture. At the same time, practitioners must understand that intraethnic variations are common, and a general understanding of cultural norms for an ethnic group is only a beginning to understanding the specific meaning of pain to an individual.

A broad need for education in both cultural competency and pain exists in undergraduate and graduate school of study.[21,22] For those who study or treat pain, *Culture, Brain and Analgesia* provides information and tools from a broad range of disciplines that will improve our understanding of the complex relationships among pain, culture, and pain treatment. Our contributors represent a broad array of disciplines, including anthropology, sociology, epidemiology, linguistics, psychology, nursing, dentistry, medicine, and philosophy. The text begins with a number of chapters addressing cultural modulation of pain experiences, followed by discussions of culture and pain assessment. Next, we examine disparities and inequities in pain management, and the cross-cultural management of pain. Finally, our contributors consider pharmacogenomics and analgesic drugs as well as contextual issues in pain medicine.

This text provides a broad exposure to issues of pain and culture. We hope that students of pain who read these chapters find it of use in enhancing their cultural fluency. Our goal is to promote a more thorough understanding of pain and prevent the many misunderstandings that color our current approaches to pain assessment and treatment. Ultimately, our aim is to reduce unnecessary pain and suffering. There is no higher goal.

REFERENCES

1. Osterweis M, Kleinman A, Mechanic D. *Pain and disability: Clinical, behavioral, and public policy perspectives.* Washington, DC: National Academy Press; 1987.
2. James FR, Large RG, Bushnell JA, Wells JE. Epidemiology of pain in New Zealand. *Pain.* Mar 1991;44(3):279–283.
3. Gureje O, Von Korff M, Simon GE, Gater R. Persistent pain and well-being: a World Health Organization Study in Primary Care. *JAMA.* Jul 8 1998;280(2):147–151.

4. U.S. Department of Health and Human Services, Management of Cancer Pain Guideline Panel, United States, Agency for Health Care Policy and Research . *Management of cancer pain. no. 94–0592.* Rockville, MD: U.S. Dept. of Health and Human Services, Public Health Service, Agency for Health Care Policy and Research; 1994.

5. IOM (Institute of Medicine). *Relieving Pain in America: A Blueprint for Transforming Prevention, Care, Education, and Research.* Washington, DC: The National Academies Press; 2011.

6. Todd KH, Samaroo N, Hoffman JR. Ethnicity as a risk factor for inadequate emergency department analgesia. *JAMA.* Mar 24–31 1993;269(12):1537–1539.

7. Bonham VL. Race, ethnicity, and pain treatment: striving to understand the causes and solutions to the disparities in pain treatment. *J Law Med Ethics.* Spring 2001;29(1):52–68.

8. Cleeland CS, Gonin R, Hatfield AK, et al. Pain and its treatment in outpatients with metastatic cancer. *N Engl J Med.* Mar 3 1994;330(9):592–596.

9. Ng B, Dimsdale JE, Rollnik JD, Shapiro H. The effect of ethnicity on prescriptions for patient-controlled analgesia for post-operative pain. *Pain.* Jul 1996;66(1):9–12.

10. Todd KH, Deaton C, D'Adamo AP, Goe L. Ethnicity and analgesic practice. *Ann Emerg Med.* Jan 2000;35(1):11–16.

11. Brennan F, Carr DB, Cousins M. Pain management: a fundamental human right. *Anesth Analg.* Jul 2007;105(1):205–221.

12. International Association for the Study of Pain. Available at: http://www.iasp-pain.org/AM/Template.cfm?Section=Pain_Definitions#Pain. Accessed 2/9/2012.

13. Rey R. *The History of Pain.* Cambridge, MA: Harvard University Press; 1998.

14. Scarry E. *The Body in Pain: The Making and Unmaking of the World.* New York: Oxford University Press; 1985.

15. Snow HL. *The Path of Improvement in Cancer Treatment.* London: Morton and Burt; 1893.

16. Lee L. Medication in the control of pain in terminal cancer with reference to study of newer synthetic analgesics. *JAMA.* 1941;116(3):216–220.

17. Spender J. Remarks on "Analgesics." *BMJ.* 1887;1(1372):819–822.

18. Cope Z. *Early Diagnosis of the Acute Abdomen.* New York: Oxford University Press; 1921.

19. Silen W. *Cope's Early Diagnosis of the Acute Abdomen* New York: Oxford University Press; 2000.

20. Thomas SH, Silen W, Cheema F, et al. Effects of morphine analgesia on diagnostic accuracy in Emergency Department patients with abdominal pain: a prospective, randomized trial. *J Am Coll Surg.* Jan 2003;196(1):18–31.

21. Champaneria MC, Axtell S. Cultural competence training in US medical schools. *JAMA.* May 5 2004;291(17):2142.

22. Mezei L, Murinson BB. Pain education in North American medical schools. *J Pain.* Dec 2011;12(12):1199–1208.

Cultural Modulation of Pain Experiences

2

A LINGUISTIC APPROACH FOR UNDERSTANDING PAIN IN THE MEDICAL ENCOUNTER

LISE BOUCHARD, MA, PHD
Director of Research, Runajambi–Institute for the Study
of Quichua Culture and Health, Otavalo, Ecuador

Key Points

- Pain is a private experience that can be made public through gestures, mimics, and language.
- Subjective reporting still dominates much patient-doctor communication about pain.
- There are four levels of linguistic representations of pain: (1) cries and moans; (2) pain interjections specific to each language; (3) lay descriptions; and (4) professional descriptions.
- Pain interjections and lay descriptions of pain by patients can vary greatly across languages, due to the specifics of their phonetics, grammar, semantics, and lexicon.
- Miscommunication can arise from subtle linguistic differences, even between people who speak the same language.
- Health professionals' awareness of potential linguistic discrepancies, self-monitoring, as well as familiarity with the patients' linguistic expressions and cultural beliefs can improve doctor-patient communication, diagnosis, and treatment outcome.

Physicians are confronted daily with the task of interpreting their patients' narration, making pain-related speech a recurrent concern in the medical encounter. Yet, despite the important role of language and culture in the representation of pain, few studies have tackled the topic. In this chapter we examine pain through a linguistic-anthropological lens. We discuss the pain experience, its expression and description across cultures. Using examples from different regions of the world, we illustrate how linguistic factors interfering in doctor-patient communication can lead to problems of interpretation and unfavorable clinical outcomes. Finally, we suggest actions that can be taken in the clinical setting to optimize the understanding of patients' pain description using basic linguistic tools and in so doing improve the quality of care.

THE DEFINITION OF PAIN

Across the years, scholars have suggested different definitions of pain. Notably, Melzack and Torgerson[1] questioned the then widely accepted concept that pain is a sensation varying only in intensity. They, instead, stated that: "The word 'pain' represents a category of experiences, signifying a multitude of different, unique events having different causes, and characterized by different qualities varying along a number of sensory and affective dimensions." That definition provided the basis for the elaboration of an innovative instrument to describe and measure pain: the McGill Pain Questionnaire. Since 1979, the International Association for the Study of Pain has proposed the following definition of pain: "An unpleasant sensory and emotional experience associated with actual or potential tissue damage, or described in terms of such damage." Some authors also proposed definitions of pain from an anthropological and linguistic point of view.

PAIN FROM A LINGUISTIC PERSPECTIVE

Fabrega and Tyma[2] suggested that pain has three components: (1) internal condition (mental, neurological, and bodily dimensions); (2) external accompaniments (behavioral dimension including nonverbal and linguistic); and (3) theoretical attributes shaped by the culture of an individual (conceptual dimension). In other words, pain is a private experience that can be made public through gestures, mimics, and language within a particular cultural frame.

Three decades ago Diller[3] noted that subjective pain reporting dominated much patient-doctor communication. This remains true today despite technological advances such as fMRI, which allow researchers to see the activation of the pain-related areas in the brain. Of course, fMRI is not currently used in clinical settings, and pain professionals must rely on patients' pain narration (and thus on the linguistic dimension) for assessing the expression of pain and interpreting their patients' pain.

We can perceive others' pain only when it is made public, and we are able to better understand the experience of pain if we share the same language and culture. However, health professionals working in a multicultural setting often see patients of distinct linguistic and cultural backgrounds, and thus experience difficulties in achieving clear communication. They may sometimes be unaware of the linguistic discrepancy and assume that there is mutual understanding with their patient. Such miscommunication between ethnically and culturally discordant doctors and patients can result in poor-quality health care.

THE REPRESENTATION OF PAIN ACROSS LANGUAGES AND CULTURES

Levels of linguistic representation

According to Diller[3], there are four levels of linguistic representation of pain: 1) cries and moans; 2) pain interjections specific to each language (e.g., "ouch" in English); 3) lay descriptions (such as "terrible stinging pain"); and 4) professional descriptions (such as "referred pain in the arm"). A representation of pain may include more than one of these levels. Interestingly, Diller[3] points out that adding adjectives, such as Melzack did in his McGill Pain Questionnaire, may facilitate connecting lay descriptions and professional descriptions and help associate the linguistic descriptions given by the patients with the quantitative clinical measurements. The pain interjections and lay descriptions of pain can vary greatly across languages, due to the specifics of their phonetics, grammar, semantics, and lexicon.

Phonetic variation

The common interjections used spontaneously to express pain, such as the pain experienced when we hit our toe on a table, differ from one language to another. While English speakers will say "ouch," French speakers from Québec will say "ayoy." In Spanish it will be "ayay," in Singalese "aba," and in Arabic "uwa." Papen[4] points out that these differences appear for two reasons. First, not all the sounds are present in all languages. For instance, the sound "ch" in the English interjection "ouch" does not exist in French. Therefore, it cannot be used in the formation of words or onomatopoeias in this language. Secondly, these interjections are learned and transmitted culturally; thus, an English speaking child learns from his parents and at school to say "ouch." The fact that the same phenomenon can be observed with the linguistic representation of animal sounds supports this analysis. For example, the sound emitted by a duck has acoustically specific characteristics, but the onomatopoeias representing it are not universal. In English it is "quack-quack" but in Chinese it is "wang-wang," and in Persian "maag-maag." Differences linked to specificities of a particular language's grammar may be more subtle and difficult to perceive.

Variations due to grammatical differences

Through an analysis of pain's construal in the English language, Halliday[5] has shown that it can be linguistically categorized as a thing, a process, and a quality. For example, in English, in the clause "I have a headache," the word "headache" is a composite thing: *head+ache*. In contrast, in the clause "My head aches," the word "aches" is a process, not a thing and the subject of that process is "my head." Pain may also be a quality, such as in the word "sore." According to its specific grammar, each language will favor one way of expressing pain over another. In the case of English, all of the preceding clauses are grammatically correct; however, "I have a headache" is preferred because in the grammar of this language, the first position in the clause has a particular meaning. This is what is called the *theme* of the sentence (i.e., the setting for the information presented in the rest of the clause). In the sentence "My head aches," the theme is "my head." However, because the speaker thinks of his headache as something that affects him as a whole, he wants to put emphasis on himself, rather than on his head. The speaker uses the wording "I have a headache" so that the word "I" is the theme of the clause. Languages with a grammar similar to English will do the same, while others will use different formulations. Because of this linguistic characteristic of English, the expectations of a health professional who is an English speaker will be that the patient will put the most important element first in the clause. Therefore, the English speaking health professional will focus his attention on the beginning of the narration. However, in many cultures it is inappropriate to talk without providing an introduction and contextualizing the topic. In Ecuador, for instance, when Spanish speaking people visit a doctor, they first give details about how things are going in their life, how their family members treat them, etc., before talking about their symptoms. This is just one example illustrating the subtle differences in speech about pain from one language to another and how these can render the communication between two people difficult.

Lexical and semantic variations

Lexical variations may seem obvious when we examine words used to describe pain in several languages (see Tables 2.1 and 2.2). However, in some cases, speakers of the same language who belong to different linguistic communities (or sociocultural subgroups) will assign different meanings to certain words. Diller[3] points out that speakers of different Thai dialects use the same vocabulary but define certain words differently. For instance, the word for pain " čhèp" both in Standard Bangkok Thai and in the Thai dialect of rural Southern Thailand has a superordinate taxonomic function. In other words, it is a cover term for a

TABLE 2.1 The Word Pain in Several Languages

Language	Word for Pain
Arabic:	Alam
Catalan:	Dolor
Chinese:	Tong
French:	Douleur
Haitian Creole:	Doulè
Japanese:	Itami
Persian:	Dard (physical pain), ranj (psychological suffering)
Russian:	Bol'
Swahili:	Maumivu
Tamil:	Vali
Taiwanese:	Thia^n
Thai:	Čhèp
Vietnamese:	Đau

For more pain terms, please see Table 1 of Chapter 30.

TABLE 2.2 The Word Pain in several Amerindian Languages

Language	Word for Pain
Aymara:	Ch'isiña (burning pain, piercing pain), k'amiña (toothache), k'ichi (stomach ache), Makhurkha (muscle pain)
Cree:	Wesukāyètumoowin, wesukūpināwin
Diidiitidq:	Ṗiṗx̣ic̣p (earache), qatqabx̣ (headache)
Gitsenimx̱:	Kujax̱ (severe pain), siip hak'oo' (back ache)
Innu:	Nenekātshun
Lakota:	Ksuyeya
Maya:	Kuxuc
Nahuatl:	Tēcocohcāyó-tl
Nisga'a:	Siip
Quichua:	Nanay
Shuar:	Najam

A constantly growing glossary of pain words with recorded pronunciations is available on this book's website at: www.runajambi.org/analgesia/glossary.html

series of words related to pain. However, in the rural Southern Thai dialect, "chèp" is also used to express thermal-diffuse internal aching, whereas the Standard Bangkok Thai uses "pùat" to express this. This semantic divergence may be attributable to a separate diachronic development from a common form. This occurs as a consequence of isolation, due to either geographical or political reasons. Below are some examples of the representation of pain in different regions of the world. For a detailed linguistic study of pain in Greek, please see Lascaratou.[6]

Northern India

Adopting an anthropological approach, Pugh[7] examined pain in the context of North Indian culture and medicine, more specifically in Unani Tibb and Greco-Arab medicine.

According to this study, pain is omnipresent in popular North Indian culture. Metaphors on pain are found profusely in everyday speech, popular mythology, love songs, classical poetry, and modern novels. They are used to describe the sensory qualities of pain including location, intensity, quantity, weight, temperature, and patterns of movement.

Interestingly, in this culture, distinctive sensory expressions are associated with pain in particular parts of the body. For instance, *splitting and bursting pains* is considered to affect primarily the head while a *pinching pain* is related to the stomach, more precisely to the feeling of hunger. Another expression, *shooting pain*, is used to talk about a warm, sharp, radiating pain that quickly pervades the affected body areas; for example, the eyes, nerves, heart, and limbs. It is often accompanied by throbbing and considered a heated condition present not only in pain but also in fever and emotional states such as anger and passion. This affective dimension of pain tallies with the integrated mind-body system of Indian culture.

Pugh[7] points out that in India, appropriate pain behavior styles vary according to specific categories of persons, situations, and types of pain. Differences related to gender are the most marked. Men are perceived as capable of expressing their pain discreetly, while women are seen as less able to tolerate pain. However, in public settings and in company of men, women often stay silent because of the social code of conduct based on sexual taboos. This can even extend to avoiding talking about pain related to the sexual reproductive system in the presence of elderly women of the same household. Consequently, in the medical encounter, people from North India may refrain from expressing their pain and this may affect communication and mislead the health professional in his diagnosis.

Mohawk

The case of the Mohawk nation in Canada and the United States is striking. Most members of this Amerindian nation are native English speakers. At first glance they seem to speak the same language as the English speaking Canadian and American physicians who treat them. However, a study conducted by Woolfson, Hood, Secker-Walker, and Macaulay[8] sheds new light on the intricacies of Mohawk English and the potential for miscommunication during the medical interview due to sociolinguistic differences.

In speech, some words or phrases, called metalinguistic cues, are placed before a remark to express the speaker's attitude toward what is being said. Phrases such as "*It seems to me,*" "*maybe,*" and "*in my opinion*" are very common in many varieties of English; however, in Mohawk English, they are metalinguistic cues that take on subtly different meanings. They tell the listener whether the speaker views the statement as a fact, belief, opinion, or memory. Cues in Mohawk English may also be used to show respect to the listener or to reflect religious beliefs such as the belief that health is under the Creator's control and thus statements about health must concede human limitations.

Mohawk English speakers use metalinguistic cues much more frequently than speakers of Standard English. In fact, as Woolfson and his collaborators point out: "[Mohawk English speaking] Informants do not make a statement without qualifying whether it is a belief, opinion, or unproved fact."[8] This peculiar usage of metalinguistic cues is due to the influence of Mohawk language grammar. Although many individuals are native English speakers and do not speak the Mohawk language, they do understand it. The presence of a Mohawk grammar substrate is noticeable. In other words, some of the grammatical rules they follow when they speak English come from the grammar of a language they do not speak but do understand: Mohawk. This Amerindian language uses evidential particles, that is, words that do not belong to any of the inflected grammatical word classes such as nouns, pronouns, verbs, or articles, to indicate whether a statement is a belief, opinion, or unproven fact. Mohawk English speakers use English metalinguistic cues as they would use Mohawk evidential particles. This type of phenomena is common in situations in which two languages are in daily contact within a society. To illustrate this, consider the following example: If a doctor asks "How do you feel now, after taking the new medication I gave you last time?" The Mohawk patient may answer "*I don't know, I think* it may be helpful. *I suppose … It seems* that it made me feel better." The patient uses metalinguistic cues (in italics) to convey an opinion, because according to Mohawk culture, to be polite he has to inform the doctor about the validity of what is being said— whether it is a fact, a belief, or an opinion. However, as Schiffrin[9] pointed out, the use of *I think* and *It seems* at the beginning of a statement indicates that a speaker is not confident about the reliability of what he is saying. Therefore, this abundant use of metalinguistic cues may appear to the non-Mohawk English-speaking physician as equivocation, indecision, and waffling. This linguistic divergence may jeopardize the quality of the communication in the medical encounter. Although the health professional and the patient speak the same language, they may make erroneous assumptions about what is being said because they use different grammars or sociolinguistic norms.

In addition, Woolfson and his collaborators[8] report that Mohawk people, along with many other Amerindians, view direct questions as rude and prefer to speak impersonally. This constitutes another linguistic phenomenon that can contribute to distorted communication in the clinical setting; after all, the medical interview is usually based on a series of direct questions.

Somali women

Studies conducted among Somali women living in the United States and Sweden give us some insight into beliefs about pain and how it is expressed in that culture. According to Ness,[10] the immigrant Somali women she interviewed in Minnesota shared a strong belief that Allah knows all about their experience of pain and that he is the only one who can help. They also think that when it comes to pain, everybody is the same. They added that Somali people experience fear of dying when they are told they need surgery.

As for the expression of pain, they feel that talking about pain in their own language is important and more natural. They declare they can express their pain freely to anybody, man or woman, and that they do not see it as a private matter.

In their study of Somali women in Sweden, Finnström and Söderhamn[11] point out that possible physical sources of pain for their informants included childbirth, cuts and sores, infections, and food poisoning, as well as allergies and fever. According to the interpreter who contributed to the research, the inclusion of allergies and fever to the list is due to the fact that the word *xanuun* ("pain" in the Somali language) also means discomfort and illness. Pain was also seen as having emotional sources, including discrimination, family problems, sadness, worries, stress, and anger. These findings agree with those of a study conducted in Finland,[12] according to which pain may be a way of communicating about psychological suffering among Somalis.

Interestingly, even if all the informants said they were familiar with the concept of evil eye or evil spirits (jinns) as traditional explanations of pain, they declared that they did not believe in these anymore. This change in their notion of pain causation may be a result of acculturation due to immigration, or the pressure to perform in front of the interviewers.

The Somali women interviewed in Sweden acknowledged that language barriers limited how they explained symptoms to doctors and nurses. They also believed interpreters were not helpful because of their lack of knowledge of medical terminology. They believed that women are better able than men to express pain, although they considered themselves stoic. They believed they were more tolerant of pain than men, and considered moaning and crying to be signs of weakness. They also viewed pain as a natural part of life and thought that religion could help those who suffer. Despite their stoical attitude, the women valued analgesics and requested them. The interviewees said that pain can be expressed through body language, by talking to friends or family members, or by resting. However, crying and wailing are not acceptable ways of expressing pain in Somali culture and withdrawing when in pain is uncommon. On the contrary, Somalis enjoy having family members around for support. Consulting a psychologist is stigmatized and associated with mental illness. Thus, it is not culturally well accepted to see a psychologist or psychiatrist to relieve pain.

Isan, northeastern Thailand

A study was conducted in northeastern Thailand among Isan people.[13] The Isan are closely related to a majority ethnic group in Laos and speak a language of the Thai-Lao family. The aim of the study was to explore the meanings attributed to pain by children living with pain in that culture. It included 17 children who had experienced pain from gastroenteritis or who had a motorcycle accident, and 32 chronically ill children at a hospital hematological ward.

The children provided somewhat surprising responses. According to the authors, the main definition of pain given by the children was distress and torture. However, they also found that parents influence their children`s pain-related behavior as well as the language they use to describe pain. Parents encourage their children to endure pain and to avoid taking analgesics. Besides possible concerns about developing medication dependence, there may be a culturally based explanation for this. Buddhist teachings extol the virtues of avoiding confrontation, aiming for reconciliation, and refraining from expressing emotions. They advise people to accept their conditions. The researchers point out that in accordance with these beliefs, Thai people do not usually express their pain, sorrow, and anger because it could be unpleasant for their parents and others, and be socially unacceptable. They are inculcated not to bother others, especially more senior people. Children are likely then to refrain from expressing their pain to healthcare professionals. This lack of expression of pain to healthcare professionals in order to avoid distracting them or being a nuisance may prevent timely treatment. This is even more common in the case of Isan children because their families encourage them to avoid analgesic medications. These children try to endure pain until it becomes unbearable before expressing it to their parents.

Quichuas (Inca People)

The Quichua once made up a large proportion of the Tahuantinsuyu (Inca confederation). Nowadays, they constitute the most numerous group of indigenous people in the Americas, with a conservative estimate of over 15 million individuals living mostly in the Andean countries of Bolivia, Ecuador, Peru, and parts of Colombia and Argentina. Despite their large number, there are very few Quichua physicians and culturally sensitive medical care is almost inexistent. In Ecuador, for instance, services are offered in Spanish only. Consequently, Quichua people must turn to *mishu* (as the mestizo or latino dominant group is called in Quichua) physicians who do not speak their language and do not receive any special training to serve this large part of the population (at least 40%) whose language and culture are not Hispanic. This is one of the reasons many prefer to seek help from traditional Quichua healers and avoid hospitals.[14] When they decide to consult a physician, however, they are confronted with a situation of miscommunication combined with bigotry and racial discrimination. They are often treated like unwelcome foreigners in the land they have inhabited for thousands of years.

Pain and mental disorders in the Andes

The examples we have seen until now have illustrated how miscommunication due to linguistic and cultural factors can prevent health professionals from making an accurate evaluation of patients' pain and can lead to its inadequate treatment. Although this obviously remains a concern, another kind of problem can also arise; the patient's comments on pain may hide psychological suffering. During fieldwork in northern Ecuador, I observed that Quichua patients who were suffering from depression discussed physical pains exclusively with the physician. During the clinical interview, they would not talk about psychological suffering at all, even when asked to do so. Only when the physician, Quichua himself, used a very specific Quichua expression did they start to talk about their feelings of sadness, despair, sorrow, etc.

This Quichua physician was aware that Quichua people usually talk overtly about psychological suffering with family members. He also knew that Quichua people distinguish two categories of illnesses: Quichua illnesses, treatable by a *yachactaita* (Quichua healer); and serious injuries and chronic or acute diseases treatable by a physician (with some illnesses treatable by both).[15] The Quichua physician rapidly understood that the patients were focusing on physical pains because they thought that as a physician, he was there to cure physical ailments and talking to him about feelings and emotions would not have been appropriate. He thus used a Quichua expression likely to elicit speech about sadness, preoccupation, anxiety, and other psychological suffering: *"Pinsamintuta charinguichu?"* ("Do you have sad thoughts, worries?"). This was the key to a vault of worries and concerns. These words triggered ample disclosure of emotional concerns.

This example shows that pain can be a psychological marker for psychiatric disorders. It also illustrates how valuable linguistic and cultural knowledge are for making a more accurate diagnosis, providing a more adequate treatment, and obtaining a better clinical outcome.

PROBLEMS OF INTERPRETERS

The lack of services in the patient's language creates linguistic barriers that may prevent access to care altogether or affect treatment outcome. Potential miscommunication due to differences in ethnomedical systems, beliefs, and expectations also exists.[16]

Seeking the help of an interpreter is sometimes viewed as the viable solution for overcoming language barriers in the clinical setting. Although access to professional interpreters may contribute to improving patients' health, respect for traditional health beliefs is also important for delivery of culturally sensitive healthcare services.[14,17] However, lay interpreters, such as patients' bilingual family members, may not be as helpful as they may appear at first. Their translation may not be reliable. Given the doctor-patient sociolinguistic gap, they may modify the patient's comments in an effort to adjust it to the health professional's speech register. Due to a lack of appropriate medical knowledge, they may also inaccurately report the doctor's speech to the patient.[14,16] This is a complaint expressed, for instance, by Somali women in Sweden.[11] The problems of working with interpreters have also been documented in the Canadian Eastern Arctic by Penney.[18] She mentions that a lack of training within a medical setting of Inuktitut-English interpreters leads to physician frustration and inadequate treatment. For example, she points out that interpreters are sometimes confronted by the dilemma of either conveying the exact meaning of the physician`s message or rephrasing it when it may be culturally inappropriate. Also, because Western medicine is unfamiliar to Inuit culture, traditional Inuktitut does not have technical-medical term equivalents. They must be created. Unfortunately, interpreters, who are bilingual residents of the communities, may have little formal education and English may be a second language for them. They may misunderstand certain medical concepts, making it difficult to develop an appropriate term in Inuktitut.

CONCLUSION

Language is at the heart of the expression and description of pain. The experience of pain is an internal condition that can be made public through four levels of linguistic representations, including cries and moans, interjections, lay description, and professional description.

Interjections and lay descriptions of pain made by patients vary according to cultures and languages. Health professionals rely on patients' subjective reporting in the assessment of pain and do not always share the same cultural and linguistic background. Consequently, miscommunication may occur due to linguistic differences in phonetics, grammar, semantics, and lexicon. Problems may even arise when the doctor and the patient speak the same language but do not follow the same grammar rules or do not share the same sociolinguistic norms. It is therefore crucial for health professionals working in multicultural clinical settings to be aware of the "intangible" linguistic elements that may render communication erratic. This goes beyond translation, language proficiency of patients, or skills of interpreters and is essential for facilitating communication and ultimately improving diagnostic and therapeutic interventions.

Healthcare and health education institutions should include the study of linguistic factors in doctor-patient communication training. This would improve health professionals' clinical skills and the quality of care.

Table 2.3 provides some recommendations to help achieve a successful doctor–patient communication.

ACKNOWLEDGMENT

I would like to thank Sioui Maldonado Bouchard, M.Sc. for her assistance in reviewing the English usage.

TABLE 2.3 Linguistic Clinical Pearls

1. Health professionals should keep in mind that even subtle linguistic factors can interfere in the communication between doctors and their patients.
2. They should stay alert and self-monitor during the medical encounter, while remaining aware of their own conversational expectations based on their own grammars and sociolinguistic norms.
3. They should become aware of the linguistic expressions and cultural health beliefs of their patients. (Basic familiarity with at least major ethnocultural groups is desirable.)
4. With patients of other ethnocultural groups, health professionals should ask supplementary questions and rephrase patients' statements to confirm mutual understanding.
5. They should be cautious when using information obtained from ad-lib interpreters without any formal training in medical terminology.
6. To assure understanding, they should avoid highly technical jargon when talking to their patients.

REFERENCES

1. Melzack R, Torgerson WS. On the language of pain. *Anesthesiology.* Jan 1971;34(1):50–59.
2. Fabrega H Jr., Tyma S. Language and cultural influences in the description of pain. *Br J Med Psychol.* Dec 1976;49(4):349–371.
3. Diller A. Cross-cultural pain semantics. *Pain.* Aug 1980;9(1):9–26.
4. Papen RA. *Ouch! The Language of Pain* [sound recording]. Washington, DC: All Things Considered/ National Public Radio; 2003.
5. Halliday MAK. On the Grammar of Pain. *Studies in English Language.* London; New York: Continuum; 2005:306–337.
6. Lascaratou C. *The Language of Pain.* Amsterdam: John Benjamins; 2007.
7. Pugh JF. The semantics of pain in Indian culture and medicine. *Cult Med Psychiatry.* Mar 1991;15(1):19–43.
8. Woolfson P, Hood V, Secker-Walker R, Macaulay AC. Mohawk English in the medical interview. *Med Anthropol Q.* 1995;9(4):503–509.
9. Schiffrin D. The management of a co-operative self during argument: the role of opinion and stories. In: Grimshaw AD, ed.. *Conflict Talk.* Cambridge: Cambridge University Press; 1990:241–259.
10. Ness SM. Pain expression in the perioperative period: insights from a focus group of Somali women. *Pain Manag Nurs.* Jun 2009;10(2):65–75.
11. Finnstrom B, Soderhamn O. Conceptions of pain among Somali women. *J Adv Nurs* May 2006;54(4):418–425.
12. Tiilikainen M. Suffering and symptoms: aspects of everyday life of Somali refugee women. In: Lilius MS, ed. *Variations on the Theme of Somaliness.* Turku, Finland: Centre for Continuing Education of Abo Akademi University; 2001:309–317.
13. Jongudomkarn D, Aungsupakorn N, Camfield L. The meanings of pain: A qualitative study of the perspectives of children living with pain in north-eastern Thailand. *Nurs Health Sci.* Sep 2006;8(3):156–163.
14. Incayawar M, Bouchard L, Maldonado-Bouchard S. Living without psychiatrists in the Andes: plight and resilience of the Quichua (Inca) People. *Asia Pac Psychiatry.* 2010;2:119–125.
15. Bouchard L. The awakening of collaboration between Quichua healers and psychiatrists in the Andes. In: Incayawar M, Wintrob R, Bouchard L, eds. *Psychiatrists and Traditional Healers: Unwitting Partners in Global Mental Health.* Chichester, England: Wiley-Blackwell; 2009:79–91.

16. Diaz-Duque OF. Communication barriers in medical settings: Hispanics in the United States. *Int J Sociol Lang.* 1989;79:93–102.
17. Ngo-Metzger Q, Massagli MP, Clarridge BR et al. Linguistic and cultural barriers to care. *J Gen Intern Med.* Jan 2003;18(1):44–52.
18. Penney CA. Interpretation for Inuit patients: essential element of health care in eastern Arctic. *CMAJ.* Jun 1 1994;150(11):1860–1861.

3

CULTURE, PLACEBO, AND ANALGESIA

Clinical and Ethical Considerations

ANTONELLA POLLO, MD
Assistant Professor, Department of Neuroscience,
University of Torino, Torino, Italy

ELISA CARLINO, PHD
Post-Doctoral Fellow, Department of Neuroscience,
University of Turin, Turin, Italy

FABRIZIO BENEDETTI, MD
Professor of Physiology, Department of Neuroscience,
University of Turin Medical School, National Institute
of Neuroscience, Turin, Italy

Key Points
- Experimental studies on placebo analgesia provide the best model to study the placebo response.
- Neurochemical, pharmacological, and neuroimaging studies are elucidating the mechanisms by which the activation of identifiable neural pathways, such as the descending pain inhibitory system, produce analgesia following treatments devoid of specific activity.
- Conditioning, expectation, anxiety reduction, and reward are the main mechanism by which placebo analgesia is generated.
- Knowledge on placebo mechanisms gained in the research setting can be transferred to the clinic, to ameliorate the design of clinical trials and to improve therapy.
- To administer a placebo does not necessarily mean to give an inert treatment; rather, it means to optimize the context surrounding the therapeutic act, in order to maximize patient expectations of improvement.

INTRODUCTION

In developing human societies across the world, the use of drugs containing active ingredients has been preceded by long centuries of ritual practices revolving around the hieratic figure of the shaman. Although many active ingredients of today's medications are chemically derived from herbal extracts and balms known to traditional healers, the prehistoric emergence of medication was more attributable to psychology than chemistry. Thus, social ceremonies such as dancing, chanting, praying, and performing symbolic actions helped induce analgesia, because of the efficacy of these functions in convincing the ailing patient that the pain would diminish. We now refer to such practices with the term *placebo*, a word which entered the medical vocabulary only in the nineteenth century, to denote the intention of pleasing the patient by giving him a therapy, even if pharmacologically inactive. The cultural meaning and acceptance of the practice of administering placebos has evolved in parallel with our ability to understand its physiological basis, and the availability of alternative and more effective remedies.

This chapter will offer a brief outline of our current knowledge of the neurobiological mechanisms of the placebo response, followed by some clinical and ethical considerations on its exploitation in medical use, such as treatment evaluation in clinical trials and therapy. More comprehensive coverage of these topics can be found in a number of recent reviews and books[1-9].

THE MECHANISMS OF PLACEBO ANALGESIA

External darts for internal targets

Basic research over the last couple of decades in the fields of physiology, pharmacology, and neurobiology has elucidated several mechanisms underlying the placebo response. With the largest number of studies, our best understanding of placebo response is in the area of placebo analgesia. This area is the most promising for transferring our acquired theoretical knowledge to the bedside. Most data on placebo analgesia come from experimental studies, rather than clinical studies, although in some cases clinical studies are performed with the exclusive aim of investigating the placebo effect. Different mechanisms can be at play, alone or in combination, in generating placebo analgesia:

Classical conditioning: the repeated contingency between a salient response-provoking stimulus and a neutral one can induce the same response after the neutral stimulus alone. Thus, a placebo pill devoid of active principle (salient stimulus) but retaining external aspect and taste (neutral stimuli) of the original drug can induce the therapeutic response.[10]

Expectation: anticipation of a future outcome triggers internal changes resulting in specific experiences (e.g., analgesia). The anticipation is generated as the product of cognitive engagement, initiated by factors such as verbal instructions, environmental clues, emotional arousal, previous experience, and the interaction with care-providers.[11]

Anxiety reduction: the awareness that a therapy has begun (independent of its efficacy) changes the interpretation of ambiguous sensations from harmful and threatening to benign and unworthy of attention. Closely related mechanisms are self-efficacy (the belief in one's ability to manage the disease) and self-reinforcing feedback (a positive loop whereby the subject attends selectively to signs of improvement, taking them as evidence that the placebo treatment has been successful)[12].

Reward: placebos have reward properties, associated with the beneficial outcomes they provide. In other words, the expected clinical benefit is a form of reward, which triggers the placebo response through the activation of dopamininergic, mesolimbic. and mesocortical pathways. This is analogous to what happens during life-sustaining functions, such as eating, drinking, or sex.[13]

Common to all these mechanisms is the presence of something in the context surrounding the patient, be it a conditioned stimulus, or an object or event triggering expectation, reducing anxiety, or activating reward mechanisms. Thus, environmental entities act on the organism like darts targeting specific neural pathways, selected during evolution for the advantage they provide in enabling positive reactions to illness.

Activation of the descending antinociceptive system

The most significant achievement of placebo analgesia research was the landmark demonstration of the release of endogenous opioids.[14] Its importance is twofold: first, it provided the first evidence that tangible changes occurred inside the human nervous system following the administration of sham treatments. Second, it spurred intense scientific interest in a field that is now among the most fertile in neuroscience research.

Following the demonstration that naloxone reduced the placebo response in dental postoperative pain,[14] many studies independently and with different approaches confirmed the role of the descending antinociceptive system. Pharmacological evidence was offered by Amanzio and Benedetti[15] who could, with the opioid antagonist naloxone, completely reverse placebo analgesia induced in experimental ischemic arm pain. Subsequently, neuroimaging techniques such as positron emission tomography (PET), functional magnetic resonance imaging (fMRI), magneto-electroencephalography (MEG) and electro-encephalography (EEG) allowed characterization of the spatial and temporal domains of placebo analgesia, both during analgesia and in its anticipatory phase.[16–18]

During placebo analgesia, reduced pain-related brain activation has been reported in strict correlation with psychophysical pain measures, supporting the view that what is altered is not the evaluation of unchanged incoming pain information, but rather direct modulation of nociceptive afferent signals.[19–23] Areas of the pain matrix showing decreased activation include the thalamus, insula, rostral anterior cingulate cortex (rACC), primary somatosensory cortex, supramarginal gyrus, and left inferior parietal lobule. Modulation extends to the spinal cord level, where responses to painful heat stimulation in the ipsilateral dorsal horn are reduced under placebo analgesia.[24] Direct evidence of endogenous opioid release in the course of a placebo analgesic experiment was obtained by Zubieta et al.[25] in a PET study employing a μ-opioid receptor-selective radiotracer, with binding changes in the pregenual rACC, insula, nucleus accumbens and dorsolateral prefrontal cortex (DLPFC).

Changes in activity in many brain areas have also been reported during the pain anticipatory phase, that is, the time lag between display of a cue signaling the impending pain stimulus and delivery of the stimulus. For example, Wager et al[20] observed an increase in DLPFC activity, negatively correlated with signal reductions in the thalamus, ACC, and insula, and with reported pain intensity; but positively correlated with increases in a midbrain region containing the grey (PAG). Further support for a link between limbic areas and the PAG came from a connectivity analysis showing correlation between the activation of the rACC and that of the PAG and bilateral amygdalae.[22] In a recent paper, the same authors also demonstrated strict opioid-specificity of this coupling, which was abolished by naloxone administration.[26] By piecing together these results, a central role for cognitive and evaluative processes emerges, whereby the prefrontal cortex (namely, the DLPFC) could drive activation of the descending antinociceptive system just before the onset of placebo analgesia. In an fMRI study, Watson et al[27] specifically compared anticipatory brain activity preceding a painful stimulus in two conditions: during placebo conditioning (a situation where the subject learns the association between a cue and placebo analgesia, with the painful stimulation surreptitiously reduced) and during placebo analgesia (with stimulus intensity restored to the initial painful level). Based on their findings of similar activity modulation in the DLPFC, medial frontal cortex, and anterior mid-cingulate cortex (aMCC), they speculated that the main effect of placebo arises from reduction of pain anticipation during placebo conditioning that is subsequently maintained during placebo analgesia. In other words, in conditioning, altered activity in the cingulate cortex during anticipation leads to learning of the association via activation of the prefrontal cortex; during the anticipation phase of the post-conditioning phase (placebo analgesia), activation of prefrontal cortex may represent retrieval from memory of the effectiveness of the sham treatment. In agreement with this hypothesis, comparable findings were recently obtained by Lui et al,[28] who described an overlap of anticipation of analgesia-related activity in the frontal cortex, during the conditioning and post-conditioning sessions, and also detected a build-up over time of fMRI signal changes related to anticipation of analgesia during conditioning.

It can be hypothesized that if prefrontal cognitive functions are impaired, placebo analgesia would be disrupted. Indeed, in Alzheimer patients, a loss of placebo responses on one hand and reduction of connectivity between the prefrontal lobes and the rest of the brain on the other, appear to progress in parallel.[29] Transitory inhibition of excitability in the prefrontal cortex, as can be obtained by repetitive transcranial magnetic stimulation (rTMS), was equally effective in producing abolition of placebo analgesia.[30]

THE CLINICAL USE OF PLACEBOS

Although in ancient times the use of placebos was pervasive in medical practice, and probably inescapable due to the paucity of effective treatments, the advent of the antibiotic age and of the randomized clinical trial to assess the value of new drugs drew a sharp line between what was to be considered an effective treatment and its negative placebo counterpart. Suddenly, the availability of active molecules, chemically engineered in the laboratory, made the good old remedy not only obsolete, but despicable on ethical grounds. Placebos were still deceptively administered, with the aim of discerning malingering or avoid real drug side effects, but this practice was gradually condemned, and for the most part, remains so today. However, recent advances in our understanding of the neurobiological mechanisms of placebo effects are ushering in a new shift in our views of placebos. As we acknowledge that placebos alter the physical substrate of our nervous tissue and recognize their ability to affect its functions and modulate its output, we come to realize that the difference between the mechanism of action of an analgesic and that of a sham treatment is much less than expected. Although placebos deserve a higher ranking than that of "treatments devoid of activity for the condition being treated," it is nonetheless important to reach a consensus as to what extent they can be used in medical practice, differentiating between appropriate limits to their use in clinical trials and in daily pain management.

Placebos in clinical trials

In clinical trials, the desired goal is to limit and reduce placebo effects as much as possible, in order to isolate the specific effect of the active molecule under scrutiny. In doing this, many different factors are grouped together under the same label, and collectively evaluated in the placebo arm of a trial. In addition to biological phenomena, other factors can potentially contribute to symptom amelioration, such as natural history (the time course of a symptom or disease in the absence of any external intervention), regression to the mean (a statistical phenomenon whereby the second measurement of a symptom is likely to yield a value nearer to the average, i.e., an improvement), biases, and errors of judgement. Data from the placebo arm of trials must therefore be used with caution to evaluate the pure placebo effect (e.g., to estimate the proportion of placebo-responders), and careful dissection should be made by the use of a natural history group and by ruling out other biases.[18]

The ethical problem of placebo use in clinical trials is addressed in the Declaration of Helsinki by the World Medical Association (WMA), which states that a placebo control may be ethically acceptable only when there is a scientifically sound methodological reason or the study involves a minor condition with no additional risk of serious harm.[31] Deception is never allowed as it conflicts with the patient's right to consent or refuse treatment, and participation in a placebo-controlled trial must include an informed consent. Much controversy arises as to how this general principle should be applied in practice, with a lively debate on the superiority of placebo- vs active-controlled trials.[32-33] Knowledge derived from placebo research may be helpful in the development of trial methodology circumventing the need for a placebo arm. An example is offered by the "open/hidden" protocol, where two groups of patients receive the same treatment, one overtly, the other covertly (for instance by a computer-controlled infusion pump, unbeknown to the patient). The covert administration deprives the patient of expectations about the treatment, which are crucial in the genesis of the placebo response; as a consequence, the placebo component of the treatment is abolished. Thus, the placebo component stands out as the difference between the two kinds of administration, with no patients receiving a sham treatment. The application of the open/hidden protocol also helps solve another theoretical problem. In fact, any drug has the potential to interact directly with patient expectation mechanisms. Thus, the ascribing of its effect to the pharmacodynamic or the placebo component can be difficult, if not impossible. In other words, a secondary effect of any drug can be to interfere with one or more expectation-activated biochemical mechanisms (e.g., the opioid system), with no possibility for the experimenter to know if the observed effect derives from activation of a nonspecific placebo pathway or from the specific action of a drug (uncertainty principle)[34].

The influence of patients' expectations on placebo analgesia magnitude has at least another significant consequence for the interpretation of clinical trial results. In fact, patient expectations are not usually among the controlled variables, but they have the potential to differentially influence improvement in both control (placebo) and drug arms, thus weakening the attempt to separate out pharmacodynamic effects. For example, a study on acupuncture showed that results could be drastically reversed by redistributing the subjects according to what they believed to be their group of assignment. In other words, no differences were found with the standard grouping, but the subjects expecting real acupuncture reported significantly less pain than those believing themselves to be in the sham group, regardless of the real assignment.[35] Similar results were obtained in another study, analyzing four randomized controlled trials in which real acupuncture was compared to sham acupuncture for four different painful conditions (migraine, tension-type headache, chronic low back pain, and osteoarthritis of the knee). Here too, the crucial factor was not the treatment received but whether patients believed in acupuncture and expected a benefit from it.[36]

Finally, an issue of great interest is the understanding of what makes a patient a placebo-responder. Efforts to identify personality traits or other characteristics in persons who react to placebos have thus far failed, although first steps are being taken in genetic research, which seem to point to the existence of specific alleles associated with some types of placebo responses, at least in psychiatric disorders.[37–38] It may be possible to create placebo responders and nonresponders in the laboratory setting by manipulating placebo responses in either positive or negative directions, using pharmacology, learning, or physical means (e.g., rTMS).[39] It remains an open question, however, whether such techniques could be useful in clinical trials. In fact, a trial without placebo-responders would show reduced effects not only in the placebo, but also in the active treatment arm, with little change on the difference between the two. Moreover, the trial would not be representative of the general population.

Placebos in clinical use

If the need in clinical trials is for minimization of placebo effects, the opposite is true in clinical practice, where the potential for therapeutic benefit of a placebo procedure is to be exploited. In spite of firm opposition on ethical grounds to the deceptive use of placebo, because of its inadequacy as a pain treatment or as a means to discredit the patient's pain report,[40] the general practice of placebo administration appears widespread. A high percentage of physicians surveyed in two recent reports acknowledged using placebos, usually to calm patients, avert requests for unnecessary medication, or as a supplemental treatment.[41–43] It can be argued that deception is not necessarily involved in the use of a placebo or that it can represent an effective treatment, which it would be unethical to withdraw.[44,45] A recent trial among patients with irritable bowel syndrome (IBS) investigated the effect of placebo administered without deception. Surprisingly, open-label placebo was superior to no-treatment control, as assessed by IBS Global Improvement Scale and other secondary measures. However, the placebo was presented to patients as "placebo pills made of an inert substance, like sugar pills, that have been shown in clinical studies to produce significant improvement in IBS symptoms through mind-body self-healing processes." While this is a totally honest statement, it is not neutral; it certainly raises expectations of improvement, because it is presented as effective, no matter by what mechanism.[46]

Once again, we are confronted with the importance of expectations. By grading the degree of expectation, proportional responses can be obtained in the clinical setting. For example, changing the symbolic meaning of a basal physiological infusion in postoperative patients resulted in different additional painkiller requests. While all patients received a physiological solution, those who believed that they would receive an analgesic drug demanded significantly less pain reliever than those who believed that they would receive no analgesic at all. An intermediate level of certainty, in those believing they had a 50% chance to receive the active drug, resulted in an intermediate request.[47]

While it remains unethical to administer placebos *per se*, there is ample space for less direct use, by exploiting the expectation mechanism. As expectations can be elicited by any aspect of the therapeutic context, it is in optimizing these expectations that the knowledge of placebo mechanisms can both fruitfully and ethically be applied. To the extreme, total elimination of context-induced expectations can be achieved with hidden drug administration. In this case, dose requirement for the achievement of a given level of analgesia are invariably higher than in the open condition.[48]

The first and foremost aspect of the psychosocial context is the patient-provider interaction (Table 3.1). Indeed, the placebo effect has recently been defined as a form of interpersonal healing.[49] A list of eight specific clinical actions has been proposed, including the following: speak positively about treatments, provide encouragement, develop trust, provide reassurance, support relationships, respect uniqueness, explore values,

TABLE 3.1 Factors affecting placebo response in the patient/provider interaction

Patient	Attitude and personality
	(e.g., optimistic/pessimistic, extroversion/introversion)
	Past experience with the treatment
	Desire for relief
	General expectations (towards healthcare)
	Specific expectations (toward treatment and provider)
Provider	Ability to raise positive expectation
	Communication skills
	Trust in the treatment
	Empathic interaction

and create ceremony.[50] Nonverbal clues intentionally or unintentionally conveyed by the therapist also are important. Deceiving clinicians as to the substance (placebo or drug) being administered to two groups of patients, when in fact both groups received a placebo, resulted in a bigger effect in the group believed by the clinicians to receive a drug.[51] In a study comparing the effect of sham acupuncture for IBS patients accompanied by either warm empathic or neutral-limited interpersonal interaction between patients and practitioner, better scores on a combined outcome measure were obtained for the augmented group.[52]

Another important aspect is what the context can teach us about other patients' experiences. Just by watching others, it is possible to obtain useful information (so-called social observational learning). Just like other forms of learning (prior experience, conditioning, expectation induced by verbal communication), social observational learning can induce placebo responses. For example, healthy volunteers observing the beneficial effect of a placebo in a demonstrator, displayed placebo responses that were comparable to those induced by directly experiencing the benefit through a conditioning procedure. Verbal suggestions alone produced significantly smaller effects.[53]

CULTURE AND PLACEBO

A key aspect to be addressed in order to optimize the application of placebo knowledge in the clinical setting is the relationship between placebo effects and culture. In spite of the scarcity of studies on this topic, there are suggestions from clinical trials that placebo rates of healing vary widely among different countries.[54] For instance, in evaluation studies on antacid treatment of peptic ulcer, placebo rates were found to range from zero to 100%, with a mean of 35.3%.[54] Among others, nationality was suggested as a reason for variation. While the placebo rate was very low in Brazil (about 7%), it was very high in Germany (about 59%). Interestingly, such discrepancy cannot be ascribed purely to ethnic susceptibility to the placebo effect, because if different medical conditions are examined, placebo rates change. For example, Germans showed the least improvement in placebo treatment of hypertension.[54] On a different line of enquiry, cultural variations have been found in examining death rates among Chinese and white Americans. It was found that Chinese, but not whites, die significantly earlier if they have a combination of disease and birth year that Chinese astrology and medicine consider ill-fated.[55] Although this is a negative outcome, it exemplifies how the same context factors can have varying influence due to the different meaning ascribed to them by different cultures.

CONCLUSION

Shifts in medical culture and moral views regarding placebo use have changed rapidly, with definitions of placebo, in turn, connected to: a magic realm, suggestibility and power of the mind, a diagnosis of malingering, research instruments allowing a focus on specific drug effects, and finally, reaching the modern concept of the broader context surrounding the patient-clinician interaction and its influence on specific pharmacologic effects. Medical education should keep pace with this evolution of our knowledge and our views regarding placebo. Currently, placebo effects receive little attention in the course of medical training.[56] This knowledge gap should be filled, to allow the next generation of clinicians to better exploit the placebo effect to their patients' advantage.

REFERENCES

1. Benedetti F. Placebo and endogenous mechanisms of analgesia. *Handb Exp Pharmacol.* 2007;177:393–413.
2. Benedetti F. Mechanisms of placebo and placebo-related effects across diseases and treatments. *Annu Rev Pharmacol Toxicol.* 2008;48:33–60.
3. Benedetti F. *Placebo effects: understanding the mechanisms in health and disease.* Oxford: Oxford University Press; 2008.
4. Enck P, Benedetti F, Schedlowski M. New insights into the placebo and nocebo responses. *Neuron.* 2008;59(2):195–206.
5. Price DD, Finniss DG, Benedetti F. A comprehensive review of the placebo effects: recent advances and current thought. *Annu Rev Psychol.* 2008;59:565–590.
6. Zubieta JK, Stohler CS. Neurobiological mechanisms of placebo responses. *Ann NY Acad Sci.* 2009;1156:198–210.
7. Benedetti F. *The patient's brain: the neuroscience behind the doctor-patient relationship.* Oxford: Oxford University Press; 2010.
8. Tracey I. Getting the pain you expect: mechanisms of placebo, nocebo and reappraisal effects in humans. *Nat Med.* 2010;16(11):1277–1283.
9. Benedetti F, Carlino E, Pollo A. How placebos change the patient's brain. *Neuropsychopharmacology.* 2011;36(1):339–354.
10. Wickramasekera I. A conditioned response model of the placebo effect: predictions of the model. In: White L, Tursky B, Schwartz GE, eds. *Placebo: Theory, Research and Mechanisms.* New York: Guilford Press; 1985.
11. Kirsch I, Lynn SJ. Automaticity in clinical psychology. *Am Psychol.* 1999;54(7):504–515.
12. Price DD, Milling LS, Kirsch I, Duff A, Montgomery GH, Nicholls SS. An analysis of factors that contribute to the magnitude of placebo analgesia in an experimental paradigm. *Pain.* 1999;83(2):147–156.
13. de la Fuente-Fernández R. The placebo-reward hypothesis: dopamine and the placebo effect. *Parkinsonism and Related Disorders.* 2010;15:S3:S72–S74.
14. Levine JD, Gordon NC, Fields HL. The mechanisms of placebo analgesia. *Lancet.* 1978;2:654–657.
15. Amanzio M, Benedetti F. Neuropharmacological dissection of placebo analgesia: expectation-activated opioid systems versus conditioning-activated specific sub-systems. *J Neurosci.* 1999;19(1):484–494.
16. Rainville P, Duncan GH. Functional brain imaging of placebo analgesia: methodological challenges and recommendations. *Pain.* 2006;121(3):177–180.
17. Kong J, Kaptchuk TJ, Polich G, Kirsch I, Gollub RL. Placebo analgesia: findings from brain imaging studies and emerging hypothesis. *Rev Neurosci.* 2007;18(3–4):173–190.
18. Colloca L, Benedetti F, Porro CA. Experimental designs and brain mapping approaches for studying the placebo analgesic effect. *Eur J Appl Physiol.* 2008;102(4):371–380.
19. Lieberman MD, Jarcho JM, Beman S, et al. The neural correlates of placebo effects: a disruption account. *Neuroimage.* 2004;22(1):447–455.

20. Wager TD, Rilling JK, Smith EE, et al. Placebo-induced changes in fMRI in the anticipation and experience of pain. *Science.* 2004;303(5661):1162–1167.

21. Koyama T, McHaffie JG, Laurienti PJ, Coghill RC. The subjective experience of pain: where expectations become reality. *Proc Nat Acad Sci.* 2005;102(36):12950–12955.

22. Bingel U, Lorenz J, Schoell E, Weiller C, Buchel C. Mechanisms of placebo analgesia: rACC recruitment of a subcortical antinociceptive network. *Pain.* 2006;120(1–2):8–15.

23. Kong J, Gollub RL, Rosman IS, et al. Brain activity associated with expectancy-enhanced placebo analgesia as measured by functional magnetic resonance imaging. *J Neurosci.* 2006;26(2):381–388.

24. Eippert F, Finsterbusch J, Bingel U, Buchel C. Direct evidence for spinal cord involvement in placebo analgesia. *Science.* 2009;326(5951):404.

25. Zubieta JK, Bueller JA, Jackson LR, et al. Placebo effects mediated by endogenous opioid activity on μ-opioid receptors. *J Neurosci.* 2005;25(34):7754–7762.

26. Eippert F, Bingel U, Schoell ED, et al. Activation of the opioidergic descending pain control system underlies placebo analgesia. *Neuron.* 2009;63(4):533–543.

27. Watson A, El-Deredy W, Iannetti GD, et al. Placebo conditioning and placebo analgesia modulate a common brain network during pain anticipation and perception. *Pain.* 2009;145(1–2):24–30.

28. Lui C, Colloca L, Duzzi D, Anchisi D, Benedetti F, Porro CA. Neural bases of conditioned placebo analgesia. *Pain.* 2010;151(3):816–824.

29. Benedetti F, Arduino C, Costa S, et al. Loss of expectation-related mechanisms in Alzheimer's disease makes analgesic therapies less effective. *Pain.* 2006;121(1–2):133–144.

30. Krummenacher P, Candia V, Folkers G, Schedlowski M, Schonbachler G. Prefrontal cortex modulates placebo analgesia. *Pain.* 2010;148(3):368–374.

31. World Medical Association Declaration of Helsinki—Ethical Principles for Medical Research Involving Human Subjects. 59th WMA General Assembly, Seoul, October 2008. URL: http://www.wma.net/en/30publications/10policies/b3/index.html. Accessed June 29, 2012.

32. Howick J. Questioning the methodologic superiority of "placebo" over "active" controlled trials. *Am J Bioethics.* 2009;9(9):34–38.

33. Miller FG. The rationale for placebo-controlled trials: methodology and policy considerations. *Am J Bioethics.* 2009;9(9):49–50.

34. Colloca L and Benedetti F. Placebos and painkillers: is mind as real as matter? *Nature Reviews Neuroscience.* 2005;6(7):545–552.

35. Bausell RB, Lao L, Bergman S, Lee WL, Berman BM. Is acupuncture analgesia an expectancy effect? *Eval Health Prof.* 2005;28(1):9–26.

36. Linde K, Witt CM, Streng A, et al.The impact of patient expectations on outcomes in four randomized controlled trials of acupuncture in patients with chronic pain. *Pain.* 2007;128(3):264–271.

37. Furmark T, Appel L, Henningsson S, et al. A link between serotonin-related gene polymorphisms, amygdala activity, and placebo induced relief from social anxiety. *J Neurosci.* 2008;28(49):13066–13074.

38. Leuchter AF, McCracken JT, Hunter AM, Cook IA, Alpert JE. Monoamine oxidase a and catechol-o-methyltransferase functional polymorphisms and the placebo response in major depressive disorder. *J Clin Psychopharmacol.* 2009;29(4):372–377.

39. Carlino E, Pollo A, Benedetti F. Can we create placebo responders and non-responders in the lab? In: Wells CD, ed. *Proceeding of the 3rd International Congress on Neuropathic Pain.* Medimond International Proceedings, Bologna, Italy, Monduzzi Editore; 2010:5–9.

40. Sullivan M, Gregory W. Terman, et al. APS position statement on the use of placebos in pain management. *J Pain.* 2005;6(4):215–217.

41. Sherman R, Hickner J. Academic physicians use placebos in clinical practice and believe in the mind-body connection. *J Gen Intern Med.* 2007;23(1):7–10.

42. Nitzan U, Lichtenberg P. Questionnaire survey on use of placebo. *BMJ* 2008;329(7472):944–946

43. Fässler M, Meissner K, Schneider A, Linde K. Frequency and circumstances of placebo use in clinical practice—a systematic review of empirical studies. *BMC Med* 2010;23;8:15.

44. Lichtenberg P, Heresco-Levy U, Nitzan U. The ethics of the placebo in clinical practice. *J Med Ethics.* 2004;30:551–554.

45. Miller FG, Colloca L. The legitimacy of placebo treatments in clinical practice: evidence and ethics. *Am J Bioethics.* 2009;9(12):39–47.

46. Kaptchuk TJ, Friedlander E, Kelley JM, et al. Placebos without deception: a randomized controlled trial in irritable bowel syndrome. *PLoS One* 2010;5(12):e15591.

47. Pollo A, Amanzio M, Arslanian A, Casadio C, Maggi G, Benedetti F. Response expectancies in placebo analgesia and their clinical relevance. *Pain.* 2001;93(1):77–83.

48. Amanzio M, Pollo A, Maggi G, Benedetti F. Response variability to analgesics: a role for non-specific activation of endogenous opioids. *Pain.* 2001;90(3):205–215.

49. Miller FG, Colloca L. The placebo effect. Illness and interpersonal healing. *Persp Biol Med.* 2009;52(4):518–539.

50. Barrett B, Muller D, Rakel D, Radago D, Marchand L, Scheder JC. Placebo, meaning and health. *Perspect Biol Med.* 2006;49(2):178–198.

51. Gracely RH, Dubner R, Deeter WD, Wolskee PJ. Clinician's expectations influence placebo analgesia. *Lancet.* 1985;1(8419):43.

52. Kelley JM, Lembo AJ, Ablon JS, et al. Patient and practitioner influences on the placebo effect in irritable bowel syndrome. *Psychosom Med.* 2009;71(7):789–797.

53. Colloca L, Benedetti F. Placebo analgesia induced by social observational learning. *Pain.* 2009;144(1–2):28–34.

54. Moerman DE. Cultural variations in the placebo effect: ulcers, anxiety, and blood pressure. *Medical Anthropology Quarterly* 2000;14(1):51–72.

55. Phillips DP, Ruth TE, Wagner LM. Psychology and Survival. *Lancet.* 1993;342(8880):1142–1145.

56. Raz A, Guindi D. Placebos and medical education. *McGill J Med.* 2008;11(2):223–226.

4

PAIN IN CHILDREN ACROSS CULTURES

HUDA ABU-SAAD HUIJER, RN, PHD, FEANS, FAAN
Professor of Nursing Science, Director, Hariri School
of Nursing, American University of Beirut,
Beirut, Lebanon

Key Points

- The expression of pain is directly related to culture.
- Accurate assessment of pain is essential for a proper and successful management of pain in children.
- Pain is private, subjective, and multidimensional in nature.
- A patient's self-report is the most reliable and valid indicator of the perceived pain intensity, quality, and meaning of the pain experience.
- Culture influences all aspects of a painful episode, including its meaning, perception, tolerance, threshold, behaviors, beliefs, and coping strategies.

INTRODUCTION

Culture, however imprecise the definition, is an important influence on the experience and response to pain. The definition of culture is complex and might include concepts such as ethnicity, race, skin color, religion, language, among others.[1] Psychosocial perspectives on cultural diversity in pain among adults have been addressed by several authors since the early 1950s.[2,3] The importance of similar work in children remains warranted. Pain expression, assessment, and reporting, in addition to pain management, may be greatly influenced by the culture of the child, parents, or caregivers.[4-6] This chapter will examine the influence of culture on pain in children.

PAIN EXPRESSION IN DIFFERENT CULTURES

It has been hypothesized that the expression of pain is directly related to culture. Two children from different cultures having the same degree of pain might communicate their pain in different ways. Culture and religion play significant roles in the meaning of pain and the expression of pain.

In 1972, Mechanic[3] identified a social-learning perspective regarding pain expression and specifically bodily complaints in humans. Mechanic considered that children learn how to react and respond to different symptoms and feelings by observing the behaviors of others and by social expectations in general. Mechanic raised the question at that time of whether cultural differences identified in the literature are "a result of the fact that children with particular prior experiences and upbringing come to have more symptoms, interpret the same symptoms differently, express their concerns and seek help with greater willingness, or use a different vocabulary for expressing distress?" Later, several authors raised the linkage between culture and pain expression, which is based on the principle that children's behavior related to pain and illness is a learned response from parents and the surrounding culture.[6]

A few examples of pain expression variability around the world will illustrate our topic. A qualitative study explored the expression of pain among 49 north-eastern Thai-Isan children aged 4 to 18.[7] Pain was defined by the children as distress and torture; one 14-year-old child with brain tumor described his headache as "I think of many big pieces of stone in my head and I want to get them out of my head … .If only I could die so that I don't have to be in such anguish."

Patience and endurance have great significance to pain expression in the Thai-Isan culture. Parents in the study were noted to encourage their children to be patient and enduring when experiencing pain and to show dislike whenever a child openly complained of pain. Thai-Isan children believe they can express pain to their parents only and not to a healthcare provider until the pain becomes unbearable, which necessarily reduces the effectiveness of pain management. The authors compared the expression of pain in the Thai-Isan culture to Buddhist settings in which people tend to avoid confrontation, aim for settlement and resolution, and refrain from expressing emotion. Children are taught that distress such as pain is managed by endeavor and effort, by calming the mind, and by accepting one's own condition, given that it is beyond human control.

Similarly, in Arab-Muslim cultures, Arabs believe that health and illness are the will of God and humans have no control over their health or illness.[8] Arab children are taught to live within the expectations of the culture, which include obeying parents, respecting the elders, showing faithfulness, and parental devotion. They are also taught that the expression of symptoms, particularly pain, is not appropriate in the presence of strangers. Similarly, Arab men are less willing to show pain than Arab women. Perhaps as a result of this repression, in Arab culture emotional and psychological problems are often expressed in the form of generalized pain and other physical symptoms.

Abu-Saad[5] conducted a qualitative study with Arab-American children to examine how they perceive, describe, and cope with pain. The author found gender differences in the expression of pain and attributed these to the cultural expectations that girls are more emotional, sensitive, and expressive than boys regarding behavioral expressions.

Stafford, Trohab, and Gueldner[9] reported the case of a 6-year old Somali Muslim girl living in the United States who presented several times to the emergency room with recurrent abdominal pain, ultimately diagnosed as the culturally influenced presentation of an obsessive compulsive disorder. The authors emphasized the need for pediatric healthcare providers to understand the unique psychosocial presentations of distress, and the role of normative cultural values in health-seeking behaviors.

In Taiwanese culture children express pain differently. A qualitative study conducted on 90 Taiwanese children, aged 5 to 14 years, reported that most defined pain as "uncomfortable or feeling bad or lots of pain."[10] In the study, vocalization of the crying was considered inappropriate for Taiwanese children; parents tended to educate children not to cry with a vocal sound; rather they are allowed to use only a crying expression and tears. Thus, for Taiwanese children, crying is observed through changes in facial expressions and not vocalizations.

In India, Raval, Martini, and Raval[11] studied how acceptable it is for children to express feelings of sadness, anger, and physical pain in front of others. Of the children studied, 6.25% reported that they would definitely or probably not show their pain to their mother, 15% indicated they would not show it to their father, and 8.75% would not show it to a peer. The most frequently cited reason for not expressing pain in the presence of their mother or father was a desire to avoid scolding. In the presence of a peer, however, the most frequently cited reason for not expressing pain was a desire to maintain self-esteem. The most common method of controlling pain in front of parents or friends was to manipulate facial expressions.

PAIN ASSESSMENT

Assessment of pain in the pediatric population is very challenging. Inadequate pain assessment in children may lead to an underestimation of pain and consequent undertreatment in this population. An accurate assessment is essential for proper and successful pain management. Pain in children is difficult to quantify and qualify, however, due to the great variability in children's cognitive abilities, medical conditions, and responses to pain and treatment.[11]

Pain is also private, subjective, and multidimensional in nature. It cannot always be rated accurately and objectively. Its existence and sensation can only be evaluated by the person suffering from it,[12,13] and this evaluation can only be derived from the person's verbal and nonverbal behaviors.

Three pain assessment methods are reported in the literature: self-report, behavioral measures,[14,15] and physiological measures.[15] Behavioral and physiological measures are used mainly with preverbal children. Behavioral measures such as motor responses, facial expressions, and crying, require a change in the behavior of the child as a result of harmful stimuli.[15] Behavioral cues may be at times misleading.[14] Therefore, combining behavioral and physiological assessment methods might render more accurate results. Physiological variables, such as blood pressure and heart rate changes, in addition to the measurement of palm sweating,[15,16] may be seen to indicate the presence of pain in children; however, these measures are not specific to pain and may not change if pain persists. As such, they are not reliable indicators of the presence of pain and are recommended for use in conjunction with other measures.

Self-report measures such as direct questioning using self-rating scales and pain adjective descriptors are used when children are able to verbally communicate.[14,15] Self-report is considered the "Gold Standard" for pain assessment in children.[17] A patient's self-report is the most reliable and valid indicator of the perceived intensity, quality, and meaning of the pain experience,[18] and is usually based on the child's own report of his or her actual subjective pain experience. Although self-report measures are considered the first choice for the assessment of pain in children, they cannot be used by preverbal and cognitively impaired children who have limited cognitive and linguistic abilities. Self-report scales are also susceptible to substantial bias.[19,20]

The most wildly used self-report scales are the Oucher Scale, the Abu-Saad Pediatric Pain Assessment tool (PPAT), the Poker Chip Tool, the visual analog scale, and the Wong-Baker FACES scale, the latter being the most commonly used.[14, 21, 22] Despite the availability of several validated tools to assess pain in children, a number of concerns, namely cognitive or cultural, remain regarding the ability of children to report their pain. Badr Kurdahi, Puzantian, Abboud, Abdallah, and Chahine[23] reported on the development of the DOLLS tool to assess pain in 45 children with cancer in Beirut, Lebanon. The rationale for developing the tool was based on the fact that several nurses noted that for some Lebanese children it was difficult to assess their pain using the Wong and Baker FACES scale (made of 6 one-dimensional faces), and it could be easier to manipulate 3-dimensional dolls. The results of the study showed good psychometric properties of the tool. In addition to being easy and comfortable to use, it is culturally sensitive for use by both the child and the nurse.

Many studies validating pediatric pain assessment tools in specific cultures have been conducted over the last decade—a necessary step before use in actual practice. Gharaibeh and Abu-Saad[24] validated three assessment tools: the Poker Chip, Faces, and Word Description Scales in 95 Jordanian children and found them valid, reliable, and useful in the pediatric Jordanian population. Madi, Al-Mayouf, Grainger, and Bahabri[25] reported on the feasibility, reliability, and validity of the childhood health assessment questionnaire, containing one module related to pain assessment, which they modified for Arab children. They concluded that the questionnaire was an adequate tool for use among children from Saudi Arabia suffering from juvenile rheumatoid arthritis. The Childhood Health Assessment Questionnaire and Child Health Questionnaire was validated cross-culturally as well in 32 different countries by Ruperto et al.[26] The instrument assesses quality of life, health-related quality of life, disability, and pain in children diagnosed with juvenile idiopathic arthritis. The investigators found that cross-cultural adaptation is a valid process to obtain reliable instruments to be used across countries with different socio-economic and socio-demographic conditions.

In Thailand, a study was conducted to assess the validity of a newly constructed pediatric pain assessment tool. Seventeen nurses, 150 postoperative children, and 150 family caregivers participated in the study comparing the tool with the standard Faces Scale and Numeric Rating Scale. There was no difference in children's pain scores and no statistical difference in children's pain score ratings between the three groups, suggesting the new tool is appropriate for Isan children in northeast Thailand.[27] Another study conducted in the same country on 122 Thai children compared three pain scales: the visual analogue scale (VAS), the Wong-Baker Faces Pain Rating Scale (WBFPS), and the Faces Pain Scale–Revised, and found significant correlations between the three pain scales. In addition, the pain scales demonstrated sufficient convergent validity and agreement for clinical use in Thai children.[28]

These studies illustrate the importance of cultural validation of pain assessment tools across all pediatric age groups and patient populations in order to assess pain properly, thereby promoting more effective management.

PAIN MEANING AND REPORTING

The meaning of pain and the methods children use to report pain have been thought to be somewhat similar across cultures. Culture, however, helps children develop their own meaning of pain and pain behavior and the methods to communicate these, thus shaping their overall perspective of health and illness. Culture influences all aspects of a painful episode, including pain meaning, perception, tolerance, threshold, behaviors, beliefs, and coping strategies, as well as shaping the conditions under which some pain responses are reinforced and others discouraged.[29]

A cross-sectional study[30] conducted in Kuwait among Arabic-speaking children aged 6–12 to evaluate their expression of pain and its assessment, reported that the most frequently used words to describe pain were: "it hurts," and "it hurts a lot," followed by "a burning sensation."

In the northeast of Thailand, children described their experience of pain as "disheartening," "suffering," and "torturing"; pain was defined as "distress and torture."[27] Spanish-speaking children with cancer described their pain to be "annoying," "aching," and "awful."[31] Similar descriptions of pain have been reported in American children with cancer in Texas, where the most frequently used words were "annoying," "uncomfortable," "hurting," and "comes and goes."[32]

In the Netherlands, hospitalized children 7–17 years of age most frequently chose sensory words to describe their pain, such as "cutting," "beating," "burning," "hurting," and "stinging." The number of words selected increased with age, reflecting cognitive development and pain experience. Girls, in general, chose more words than boys to describe pain.[21] In another study, Dutch children 7–12 years of age with juvenile rheumatoid arthritis described their arthritis pain as "hurting," "stinging," "warm," and "uncomfortable." Children were found also to use different strategies, such as rest and distraction, to relieve pain.. Medications were not commonly used, reflecting the cultural value of avoiding the use of pharmacological measures until absolutely necessary.[33]

In the study done by Abu-Saad,[4] when Asian-American children aged 9–12 years experienced pain, they reported feeling embarrassed and afraid, as well as like crying and being alone. Girls more than boys identified psychological causes for the pain and more often chose affective and evaluative words to describe pain compared to boys, who chose sensory word descriptors. Strategies for relieving pain included Chinese medicine and household remedies. In contrast, within Jordanian culture,[24] children preferred reporting pain using the Poker Chip Scale followed by the Faces Scale, and least preferred the Word Description Scale.

THE CAREGIVER PERCEPTION

Healthcare providers and parents learn about pain, pain expression, and pain management in childhood. Cultural background modulates their ability to assess pain in children and manage it. There is almost always a tendency to feel that one's own cultural norms are correct and to evaluate others' beliefs in light of them; thus, when a child perceives, expresses, or reacts to pain in a way that doesn't conform to a healthcare provider's beliefs or expectations, the healthcare provider may consider the behavior inappropriate or frustrating. Healthcare providers should remember that patients' diverse cultural patterns are not necessarily right or wrong, or normal or abnormal, and are better thought of as different. Providers should examine first their own cultural beliefs about pain.[34]

Several factors help explain inadequate pain assessment and management when the child and healthcare provider are from different cultures,[34] namely: language and interpretation problems, nonverbal communication styles, culturally or linguistically inappropriate pain assessment tools, underreporting, reluctance to use pain medications, lack of access to pain medications, providers' fears of drug abuse, and, finally, prejudice and discrimination.

A study conducted in Morocco[35] to identify issues in managing pain in children with cancer concluded that certain cultural beliefs were obstacles to adequate pain management. Moroccan physicians who participated in this study reported that illness-related pain was considered inevitable for some Moroccans: "In some settings, suffering is normal. It has to be endured, especially by boys, otherwise they don't measure up." Medical staff reported that even though barriers to the use of morphine for treating pain still exist, families and healthcare providers are beginning to understand better its importance in pain management.

Some parents in Morocco still refuse morphine for their children because of fears the child will become addicted; some physicians share this point of view as well.

In a systematic review of cross-cultural studies in procedural pain among children and their caregivers,[29] five studies[36-40] compared health professionals' administration of pain medication for procedural pain according to children's cultural backgrounds. Only one study[37] found significant differences in health professionals' administration of pain medication associated with the children's cultural backgrounds. Being a child, African-American, or covered by Medicaid insurance were factors that were found to significantly increase the risk for undertreatment for pain. Another study,[39] using the same data set as the research referred above, reported no significant difference in pain medication administration based on children's cultural backgrounds. According to Kristjánsdóttir, Unruh, McAlpine, and McGrath[29] the contradictory findings between these two studies may be due to differences in the type of pain medications and/or the specific type of orthopedic injuries explored in each study.

In a research conducted by Badr Kurdahi et al[23] to describe the relationship between the different types of pain reporting (child, nurses, and parents), the results suggested that children's self-reports were correlated to both observed behavioral measures by parents and nurses and to physiological measures. The authors concluded that although the accuracy of children's ratings of their pain is considered to be the gold standard in pain assessment, nurses and parents play a major role in pain assessment, particularly after painful procedures or after surgery, when self-reports may not be possible. Parental involvement is crucial, more so in developing countries, where pain management remains a neglected area of practice and where nurses do not offer children the opportunity to express or report their pain using culturally reliable and valid tools.[24,41] Thus, the value of assessments performed by nurses or parents who are often well aware of the child's reactions and behavioral responses to pain must be taken into consideration, especially in younger children and in children who cannot complete a self-report because of physical or mental disability.

In contrast, Alwugyan, Alroumi, and Zureiqi[30] reported major discrepancies between Kuwaiti children and their parents when describing, localizing, and assessing the intensity of pain. The authors concluded that if there is poor agreement between children and parents' pain ratings, making it unclear which assessment is the better estimate of the correct level of pain the child is experiencing, the child's pain assessment should be used.

Significant variations in reporting pain between different caregivers (parents, physicians, and nurses) as observers' of a child in pain have been reported. Pillai Riddell and Craig[42] examined whether caregiver judgments of infant pain would vary with different infant caregiver groups and infant age; older infants were attributed significantly more pain than younger infants, pediatricians reported significantly lower levels of pain than parents, while nurses fell midway when compared to the other groups.

An earlier study reported on the cultural difference in the perception and expression of pain and anxiety in Anglo and Hispanic children with cancer and their parents.[43] Children had surprisingly similar behavioral responses. Hispanic parents, however, reported significantly higher levels of anxiety than Anglo parents. The study did not provide comparison of behavioral responses to pain between parents and children.

The systematic review conducted by Kristjánsdóttir, Unruh, McAlpine, and McGrath[29] also examined studies comparing parents' response to their child's procedural pain. Out of the fourteen studies reviewed, three compared parents' responses. In one study,[44] Black parents were significantly more likely to agree to be present for their child's hypothetical medical procedure than White or Hispanic parents. In the second study,[45] English-speaking Hispanic parents, compared to Spanish-speaking Hispanic parents, Black parents and

White parents were significantly less likely to choose to remain present during highly invasive procedures. Compared to the other cultural groups, Black parents were significantly less likely, and English-speaking Hispanic parents were more likely, to want the physician to decide if they should stay during some of the medical procedures. The authors suggested that there may be larger differences among minority groups (Black and Hispanic parents) than between minority groups and White parents.[45] The two studies used different measures, which may have impacted their findings.

CONCLUSION

In the systematic review, Kristjánsdóttir, Unruh, McAlpine, and McGrath[29] reported discrepancies in the results of the studies reviewed regarding the influence of culture on procedural pain with regard to the child, the parents, or the healthcare professionals. Disagreements have been reported regarding the development of culturally specific self-report pain intensity measures for children. Despite the fact that parents have a significant influence on their children's experiences around painful procedures, there is limited and contradictory research on cultural differences in parental reactions related to children's procedures. The authors argue that the research design in most studies is primarily descriptive and exploratory, rather than analytical; that most of the cultural comparisons used subcultural groups within a single country; that finding homogeneous samples in a country with a heterogeneous population, such as the United States, is a challenge; and that parents and children's ethnicity/culture may not be identical for comparison purposes, especially if the child does not live in a traditional family structure. In addition, children may identify with several cultures, especially if the family has immigrated to a country with a different dominant culture.

Despite all the evidence provided, cultural recommendations for pain assessment in children remain hard to define. Most studies compare differences and similarities among diverse cultures and ethnic groups; very few have provided recommendations to develop adequate skills needed for the care of a child in pain regardless of the cultural background. Narayan[34] presented some general principles related to patients in pain as a foundation for meeting patients' cultural needs and preferences. A major principle is to understand the patient as a unique person and to explore the patient's own experience of illness and pain. Caregivers are to perceive pain management from the patient's perspective and to promote shared decision making, as well as adapt care to meet the patient's needs and expectations. Last but not least, caregivers of a child in pain should be cognizant of their culturally acquired attitudes about pain before taking care of others.

REFERENCES

1. Finley GA, Kristjánsdóttir Ó, Forgeron PA. Cultural influences on the assessment of children's pain. *Pain Res Manag.* 2009;14(1):33–37.
2. Zborowski M. Cultural components in responses to pain. *J Nurs Issues.* 1952;8:16–30.
3. Mechanic D. Social psychologic factors affecting the presentation of bodily complaints. *N Engl J Med.* 1972;286:1132–1139.
4. Abu-Saad H. Cultural group indicators of pain in children. *Matern Child* Nurs J. 1984;13:187–196.
5. Abu-Saad H. Cultural components of pain: The Arab-American child. *Issues Compr Pediatr Nurs.* 1984;7:91–99
6. Beyer J, Knott C. Construct validity estimation for the African-American and Hispanic versions of the Oucher Scale. *J Pediatr Nurs.* 1998:1320–31.

7. Jongudomkarn D, Aungsupakorn N, Camfield L. The meanings of pain: A qualitative study of the perspectives of children living with pain in north-eastern Thailand. *Nurs Health Sc.,* 2006;8:156–163.

8. Zahr L, Hatter-Pollara M. Nursing care of Arab children: Consideration of cultural factors. *J Pediatr Nurs.* 1998;13:349–355.

9. Stafford B, Trohab C, Gueldner BA. Intermittent abdominal pain in a 6-year-old child: the psycho-social-cultural evaluation. *Curr Opin Pediatr.* 2009;21:675–677.

10. Cheng S, Foster RL, Hester NO, Huang C. A qualitative inquiry of Taiwanese children's pain experience. *J Nurs Res.* 2003;11:241–249.

11. Raval VV, Martini TS, Raval PH. "Would others think it is okay to express my feelings?" Regulation of anger, sadness and physical pain in Gujarati children in India. *Soc Dev.* 2007;6:79–105.

12. Merkel S, Malviya S. Pediatric pain, tools, and assessment. *J Perianesth Nurs.* 2000;15(6):408–414.

13. Waddie NA. Language and pain expression. *J Adv Nurs.* 1996;23:868–872.

14. Cohen LL, Lemanek K, Blount RL, et al. Evidence-based assessment of pediatric pain. *J Pediatr Psychol.* 2007;33:939–955.

15. Twycross A. Assessing pain in children. *Anaesth Intensive Care Med.* 2003;4:401–403.

16. McGrath PA, Seifert CE, Speechley KN, Booth JC, Stitt L, Gibson MC. A new analogue scale for assessing children's pain: an initial validation study. *Pain.* 1996; 64:435–443.

17. Finley GA, McGrath PJ. Introduction: The roles of measurement in pain management and research. In: GA Finley, PJ McGrath, eds., *Measurement of Pain in Infants and Children.* Seattle, WA: IASP Press; 1998:1–4.

18. Abu-Saad H. Assessing children's responses to pain. *Pain,* 1984;19:163–171.

19. Liossi C. Management of paediatric procedure-related cancer pain. *Pain Reviews.* 1999;6:279–302.

20. Pain Management in Children with Cancer of Texas Cancer Council. http://www.childcancerpain.org/. Accessed August 20, 2010.

21. Abu-Saad HH, Kroonen E, Halfens R. On the development of a multidimensional Dutch pain assessment tool for children. *Pain.* 1990; 43:249–256.

22. Wong D, Baker C. Pain in children: comparison of assessment scales. *Pediatr Nurs.* 1988;14(1):9–17.

23. Badr Kurdahi L, Puzantian H, Abboud M, Abdallah A, Chahine R. Assessing procedural pain in children with cancer in Beirut, Lebanon. *J Pediatr Oncol Nurs.* 2006;23:311–320.

24. Gharaibeh M, Abu-Saad H. Cultural validation in pediatric pain assessment tools: Jordanian perspective. *J Transcult Nurs.* 2002;13:12–18.

25. Madi MS, Al-Mayouf MS, Grainger CG, Bahabri SA. The Arabic version of childhood health assessment questionnaire modified for Arabic children. *Saudi Medical Journal.* 2004;25:83–87.

26. Ruperto N, Ravelli A, Pistorio A, et al. Cross-cultural adaptation and psychometric evaluation of the Childhood Health Assessment Questionnaire (CHAQ) and the Child Health Questionnaire (CHQ) in 32 countries. Review of the general methodology. *Clinical Experimental Rheumatology.* 2001;19:S1–S9.

27. Jongudomkarn D, Angsupakorn N, Siripul P. The Development and Validation of the Khon Kaen University Pediatric Pain Assessment Tool for School-Aged Isaan Children in Thailand. *J Transcult Nurs.* 2005;19:213–222.

28. Newman CJ, Lolekha R, Limkittikul K, Luangxay K, Chotpitayasunondh T Chanthavanich P. A comparison of pain scales in Thai children. *Arch Dis Child.* 2005;90:269–270

29. Kristjansdottir O, Unruh AM, McAlpine L, McGrath PJ. Cross-cultural studies in procedural pain in children and their caregivers: a systematic review. *J Pain.* 2012;13(3):207–219.

30. Alwugyan D, Alroumi F, Zureiqi M. Expression of pain by children and its assessment in Kuwait. *Medical Principles and Practices.* 2007;16(suppl 1):21–26.

31. Jacob E, Sambuco G, McCarthy KS, Hockenberry M. Intensity, location, and quality of pain in Spanish-speaking children with cancer. *Pediatr Nurs.* 2008; 34:45–52.

32. Jacob E, Hesselgrave J, Sambucco G, Hockenberry MJ. Variations in pain, sleep, and activity during hospitalization in children with cancer. *J Pediatr Oncol Nurs.* 2007;24:208–219.

33. Abu-Saad HH, Uiterwijk M. Pain in children with juvenile rheumatoid arthritis; a descriptive study. *Pediatr Res.* 1995;38(2):194–197.

34. Narayan MC. Culture's effect on pain assessment and management. Cultural patterns influence nurses' and their patients' responses to pain. *Am J Nurs.* 2010;110:38–47.

35. McCarthy P, Chammas G, Wilimas J, Msefer Alaoui F, Harif M. Managing children's cancer pain in Morocco. *J Nurs Scholarsh.* 2004;36:11–15.

36. Bohannon AS. *Physiological, Self Report and Behavioral Ratings of Pain in Three to Seven Year Old African American and Anglo American Children* [dissertation]. Coral Gables, FL: University of Miami;. 1995.

37. Hostetler MA, Auinger P, Szilagyi PG. Parenteral analgesic and sedative use among ED patients in the United States: combined results from the National Hospital Ambulatory Medical Care Survey (NHAMCS) 1992–1997. *Am J Emerg Med.* 2002;20:139–143.

38. Karpman RR, Del Mar N, Bay C. Analgesia for emergency centers' orthopaedic patients: does an ethnic bias exist? *Clin Orthop Relat Res.* 1997;334:270–275.

39. Yen K, Kim M, Stremski ES, Gorelick MH. Effect of ethnicity and race on the use of pain medications in children with long bone fractures in the emergency department. *Ann Emerg Med.* 2003;42:41–47.

40. VanderBeek B, Mehlman C, Foad S, Wall E, Crawford A. The use of conscious sedation for pain control during forearm fracture reduction in children: does race matter? *J Pediatr Orthop.* 2006;26:53–57.

41. Finley GA, Forgeron PA, Arnaout M. Action research: Pediatric pain service development in Jordan. *J Pain Symptom Manage.* 2008;35:447–454.

42. Pillai Riddell RR, Craig KD. Judgments of infant pain: The impact of caregiver identity and infant age. *J Pediatr Psychol.* 2007;32:501–511.

43. Pfefferbaum B, Adams J, Aceves J. The influence of culture on pain in Anglo and Hispanic children with cancer. *J Am Acad Child Adolesc Psychiatry,* 1990;29:642–647.

44. Bauchner H, Vinci R, Waring C. Pediatric procedures: do parents want to watch? *Pediatrics.* 1989; 84:907–909.

45. Jones M, Qazi M, Young KD. Ethnic differences in parent preference to be present for painful medical procedures. *Pediatrics.* 2005:116:e191–e197.

5

PAIN IN INDIAN CULTURE

Conceptual and Clinical Perspectives

JUDY F. PUGH, PHD
Associate Professor, Department of Anthropology,
Michigan State University, East Lansing, Michigan, USA

Key Points
- Concepts of pain in Indian culture are influenced by religion, traditional medicine, and biomedicine.
- Traditional medicine embeds important everyday ideas about hot/cold, diet, and weather.
- Indian expressions of pain involve somatic, affective, and social components.
- Indians in diaspora communities frequently present with pain complaints expressed in somatic terms and involving widespread "body pain."
- The clinical interpretation of pain's relationship to mental disorders requires awareness of cultural ideas and sensitivities about "mental distress."
- There are a number of culturally salient approaches to pain management.

India is a complex, dynamic country and an increasingly important player in the global world and its transnational arenas. Indians, together with other South Asian groups such as Pakistanis and Bangladeshis, constitute prominent ethnic minorities in the United States, the United Kingdom, and Canada. Many Indians have been born and raised in the West, and many others now arrive as immigrants, students and scholars, business travelers, and family members on visits. They display wide social and economic diversities and range occupationally from highly educated professionals to working-class families and individuals. The cultural frameworks that interconnect India with its diaspora communities continue to shape people's lives and inform their perspectives on family, livelihood, spirituality, health, and other core aspects of human existence. Exploring these cultural frameworks provides special insight into Indian and other South Asian understandings of pain and suffering and the ways in which they accommodate the fluid relationship between tradition and modernity.

INTRODUCTION AND GUIDEPOSTS

This chapter examines the culture of pain by exploring frameworks and patterns that span India and Indian communities in the West. It has four components: (1) a discussion of the key themes from religion, traditional medicine, and biomedicine that constitute a broad Indian perspective on pain, its causes, and its meanings; (2) a description of Indian styles of pain presentation and a consideration of the problematic issue of widespread "body pain"; (3) an identification of culturally salient approaches to pain treatment, a subject that has been neglected in the literature on pain management in India and overseas Indian communities; (4) a recommendation for practical guidelines for healthcare practitioners in their interactions with Indian and other South Asian pain patients in clinical settings in the West.

The anthropological orientation in the paper emphasizes the interpretation of key cultural themes and concepts. Cultural analysis in anthropology and other fields involves the explication of central ideas held by various social groups, such as religious and ethnic communities, occupational groups, regional collectivities, and even nation-states.[1] The present account of basic pain concepts in Indian culture builds on several types of materials. The discussion of pain-related concepts and practices in India is based on the medical anthropological literature, including the author's long-term study and ethnographic field research with various healing traditions and religious practices in India's Hindu and Muslim communities. The description of pain concepts in diaspora settings draws on the medical and social scientific literature on health, illness, and pain among Indian and other South Asian patients in the United States, Canada, and the United Kingdom.

An appreciation of the Indian cultural construction of pain recognizes that its key meanings and practices have their own variations in the context of social diversities and individual circumstances and experiences. Indian society both in the home country and abroad displays many forms of diversity based on class, caste, occupation, education, religion, region, and language. People's life-outlooks, including their healthcare ideas and practices, typically refract widespread cultural concepts into the socially and economically situated contexts of their lives, livelihoods, and families.

CULTURAL FRAMEWORKS OF PAIN: MEANINGS AND CAUSES

Indian culture's complex configuration of health-related concepts is built on multiple sources of influence and legitimacy, specifically religion, traditional medicine, and biomedicine. Religion and traditional healing have profoundly shaped fundamental concepts and attitudes related to illness and pain, inculcating often deep-seated notions of the body and the mind/body relationship, ideas about etiology, and notions of effective treatment. For decades, Western biomedicine, with its aura of science and modernity, has had a strong institutional presence in India. Its conceptual framework and its therapeutic practices, however, have been subject to cultural interpretations among the Indian populace, giving rise to commonly held perceptions of its strengths, weaknesses, and dangers. Moreover, it often intermingles with religious and traditional medical sensibilities and practices, forming a network of ideas that Indians and other South Asians may tap selectively in dealing with various kinds of illnesses and pain-related conditions.

Religious perspectives

India has been one of the world's great crucibles of the spiritual, and it is home to many religious traditions. Hindus comprise 80.5%, Muslims 13.4%, and Sikhs, Jains, Christians,

Buddhists, and Parsis together about 6% of the population.[2] The present discussion concentrates on cultural perspectives among Hindus and Muslims, but these views may also hold meaning for members of other Indian faiths that have shared a long historical interaction with Hinduism and Islam in the subcontinent.

Indian religions lend to understandings of life the foundational idea that pain is integral to the very texture of existence. Pain and suffering are an inevitable part of life and the life-world. *Dukh* and *dard*, the most common Hindi-Urdu words for pain, recur in Indian life and its religious and traditional medical discourses. These terms communicate pain in its interconnections with bodily distress, emotional and mental anguish, spiritual crisis, and familial and social conflict. Their networks of meanings may embed ideas of imbalance and disconnection, distress and difficulty, and sadness and anxiety, which contribute to perceptions of severe or chronic pain and suffering as a heavy weight or burden.[3] Interestingly, in traditional medical and religious settings, people sometimes refer to chronic pain as "old pain" (*purana dard*), which conveys not simply the fact that the pain has been continuous, but that it has continued for a long time and has become embedded in a person's life-situation.

Ideas of divine will, along with notions of fate or destiny, are important elements in Indian views of pain. Hindus and Muslims may see their suffering as reflecting divine will, and some may interpret their pain as punishment for their misdeeds. The notion of fate or destiny, which is expressed in the Hindu concept of *karma* and the Muslim concept of *qismat*, registers a sense that particular episodes of suffering are part of a person's "lot" in life.[4] In India, people often apply ideas of fate or destiny to serious illness and chronic or disabling pain, but they also make personal efforts to manage their circumstances, a stance supported by Indian religious values. Moreover, for many Indians, the idea of fate expresses a basic awareness of the limitations inherent in all situations and a recognition that spiritual forces may play an often incomprehensible role in the vicissitudes of human distress and well being.

Other spiritual beliefs may also be invoked in times of suffering. Notions related to the evil eye, spirit affliction, planetary and other astrological influences, and malefic magic are held by some South Asians in their home countries and in Western diaspora settings.

Traditional medical perspectives

The humoral medical traditions of Ayurveda and Unani have had a pronounced influence on Indian concepts of person, body, and illness.[5] Ayurveda is the ancient Hindu tradition, Unani the classic Greco-Arab tradition elaborated under Islamic regimes in the Middle East and brought by the Muslims to South Asia. These two traditions have undergone considerable expansion in the last half-century. They have their own colleges, practitioners, and supervisory councils within the Government of India's Ministry of Health and Family Welfare, and hundreds of ethno-pharmaceutical companies manufacture traditional medicines as shiny packaged products with a growing appeal in India's rising middle classes[6] and an expanding availability in diaspora communities.

Ayurveda and Unani conceptualize person and body as dynamic systems with a network of internal processes and external interactions with the surrounding environment. These traditions circulate ideas about the influence of climate, diet, behavior, emotion, and social relationships on pain and illness.[7] They emphasize the hot/cold qualities of illnesses, foods, causal forces, and remedies, and they define the role of humors in bodily processes. Wind, bile, and phlegm are the three humors of Ayurveda, and phlegm, yellow bile, black bile, and blood are the four humors of Unani, and imbalances among them are causes and indications of illness. These humoral ideas may inform the perceptions and conduct of Indians and other South Asians without being explicitly acknowledged or directly identified as part of Ayurveda or Unani.

Humoral theories apply to pain as well. The body is vulnerable to pain generated by heat and cold, wind, dampness and dryness, and other factors from both external and internal sources. External heat may contribute to headache, and heating foods, hard work, and exercise can also produce excess heat in the body, which in turn may bring on a headache or cause stomach upsets. Phlegm, which is cold, underlies head colds and other congestive pains. External cold, including the wind, which is often considered cooling even in hot weather, may exacerbate rheumatism, arthritis, and muscle pain. Cold, windy foods, along with external cold, can disturb proper digestion and elimination, which are essential to bodily health and comfort. Indigestion and constipation can degrade bodily substances and produce noxious matter that circulates throughout the body and collects in various sites, giving rise to numerous forms of pain, including stomach ache, intestinal cramps, muscle and joint pain, backache, and earache, along with other illnesses.[8] Ayurveda and Unani have detailed theories of mental illness,[9] and these theories suggest that emotional factors such as distress, nerves, worries, anger, and fear contribute to bodily imbalances that make a person more vulnerable to chronic pain and illness. And lastly, traditional medicine recognizes the influence of manual labor and physical strain on the body and the production of pain.[3,8]

Other cultural factors may impact illness and pain, particularly through dietary customs. For example, values of vegetarianism may restrict the intake of meat, fish, and sometimes milk, which may lead to certain nutritional deficiencies. For instance, research has found that low Vitamin D levels were common among young UK South Asian women with complaints of widespread body pain.[10]

Traditional medical diagnosis and treatment aim to identify and manage the underlying causes of pain and illness, while also facilitating symptom relief. Serious and chronic pain, however, opens up multiple lines of causality that are often recognized and addressed in traditional medical settings. Cases of chronic pain are particularly likely to raise questions of deeper somatic, affective, social, dietary, environmental, and spiritual causes.

Biomedical perspectives

Secularism and science have a strong place in Indian society. The government's policies and programs have given massive support to biomedical institutions in order to improve health care and social services, and various types of biomedical healthcare professions have long been part of the country's medical landscape, though based mostly in cities and towns.[11–12] Biomedicine's standard features in India are its usual hallmarks, including laboratory diagnostics; etiologies based on structural, biochemical, and genetic factors; treatments with powerful drugs and surgery; and a specialized focus on individual organs or regions of the body. Many Indians consider biomedical care effective for acute and life-threatening illnesses that require technical laboratory diagnosis, potent, quick-acting medicines, and possibly surgery. Biomedical ideas circulate freely in the general populace, but like other traditions, these ideas are interpreted within the contexts of people's diverse outlooks and situations.

STYLES OF PAIN PRESENTATION AND THEIR INTERPRETATION IN BIOMEDICAL SETTINGS

Culture's impact on pain experience and on patients' ways of presenting pain is evident across all types of therapeutic settings. Several issues related to styles of pain presentation among Indian patients in biomedical settings in the West offer a context in which to examine the multifaceted role of culture in influencing these important interactions. These issues have arisen from reports that South Asians, specifically in the United Kingdom, frequently consult general practitioners with complaints of widespread pain.

Several studies highlight the point that Indian and other South Asian patients present pain complaints to general practitioners more frequently than members of other ethnic groups in the United Kingdom, and that they complain more frequently of widespread pain.[13-17] Complaints of "body pain," "pain everywhere," "pain in the whole body," and "pain on one side" appear to be more common among South Asians than complaints of localized pain.[17] Moreover, studies in the United Kingdom report that South Asian patients with "body pain" complaints are often reticent to discuss possible underlying psychological contributors.[13-17] A study based on interviews with South Asian women in the United States indicates that they often mention widespread pain in discussing their experiences of well-being and distress, and that they appear to find physical symptoms more relevant than psychological symptoms.[18]

These styles of symptom presentation and discussion have raised the question of somatization, or the expression of psychological distress or mental disorder in the idiom of somatic discomfort. A study of a group of general practitioners in the United Kingdom revealed their concerns about South Asian patients' complaints of widespread pain, specifically the difficulty of reaching a diagnosis in the absence of localized complaints, and the dilemma of interpreting patients' pain complaints as somatic expressions of psychological distress, especially depression, when patients do not readily engage in discussions about mental factors.[17] This debate has raised questions about the nature and role of physical versus affective distress in Indian and other South Asian diaspora communities, as well as questions about attitudes toward the expression of mental distress and mental illness and their relationship to chronic pain.

A broad perspective based on continuities between India and overseas Indian communities suggests the following points as relevant considerations for the clinical understanding of Indian and other South Asian patients' pain presentations in Western biomedical settings: (1) patients' presentations of widespread pain in India and in diaspora settings often display an experiential and conceptual emphasis on pain as physical distress; (2) patients widely consider somatic pain to have emotional or psychological accompaniments, which are embedded in a rich heritage of affective expressions and a close mind/body relationship;[3,19] (3) pain patients may not spontaneously identify these emotional components, but they may do so if a physician asks, and they may refer specifically to "physical" (*sharirik*) or "mental" (*mansik*) pain; (4) pain (and other) patients have detailed notions of mental distress and may see pain as part of a syndrome of mental distress and even mental disorder;[19-20] (5) pain patients typically do not interpret these syndromes as "depression,"[19] and they may lack familiarity with the biomedical category of depression;[15,19] (6) patients may downplay the presentation of emotional accompaniments of pain in their interactions with medical practitioners because they may not consider biomedicine an appropriate arena for this kind of personal or family-related discussion,[19] or because they are concerned about the social stigma of mental illness;[21-22] (7) pain patients may sidestep practitioners' references to depression because they may not believe biomedicine offers effective treatments for psychological or mental distress.[15,19]

PATIENT-PHYSICIAN INTERACTIONS IN INDIA

Many Indians in diaspora settings will have had experiences with the varied styles of practitioner-patient interactions in India. In India, patients across a variety of therapeutic traditions may present with a site-specific pain, several site-specific pains, and diffuse pain spread across the body. Complaints of "body pain" are common, but complaints of localized pain also occur. Depending on the setting, patients may mention other bodily symptoms, such as stiffness, swelling, fever, weakness, indigestion, constipation, itching, and heart palpitations, as well as emotional distresses such as worry, nervousness, unhappiness, and family conflict. It should be noted that across biomedical and traditional therapeutic settings in India, some practitioners spend time talking with pain-afflicted patients and perhaps family members as well, eliciting additional symptoms, and discussing personal situations, while other practitioners diagnose quickly and with little discussion. The presentation of pain varies in these settings, often in ways that are determined by the practitioner and not by the patients.

CULTURAL PERSPECTIVES ON THE TREATMENT OF PAIN

South Asian families, including those in diaspora communities, usually play pivotal roles in dealing with a family member's pain and illness and in deciding on treatments.[21-24] Many families have a hierarchical structure in which men may have more authority over major health-related decisions than women, but women may also play an important role depending on the particular family and the situation. Patients' decisions about treatments for serious illness and chronic pain are commonly made in consultation with the family, and while healthcare practitioners' advice is noted, the family's views often have the stronger influence in selecting therapeutic strategies.

Numerous approaches to pain management are recognized in Indian culture and society (Table 5.1).

Biomedical drugs for pain, including aspirin, ibuprofen, and narcotic-based analgesics, are sold in pharmacies and all-purpose stores in India. Like modern pharmaceuticals more generally, they are considered to be quick-acting medications focused on symptom relief, but many Indians and other South Asians have strong concerns about their side effects. In India, people may note the "heating" or "drying" effects of modern drugs or express concern about potentially unknown side effects. These same kinds of observations and apprehensions appear in Indian and other South Asian communities in the United Kingdom, United States, and Canada.[22-23] In the United Kingdom, South Asians with musculoskeletal pain are more likely than members of other ethnic groups to discontinue disease-modifying antirheumatic drugs,[25] and while the reasons are not fully understood, the patients' expressed worries about side effects are certainly part of the picture. In addition, biomedicine's use of surgery to treat various types of chronic pain taps into many Indians' pronounced anxiety and frequent resistance to "going under the knife."

Ayurveda and Unani treat pain with traditional medicines, diet, and massage. Prepackaged medicines are widely sold in pharmacies and general stores in India, and hand-prepared compounds are still dispensed by some traditional practitioners. These medications are often available in ethnic shops and groceries in the United Kingdom, United States, Canada, and other countries and through Internet sites, and they may be recommended by local Ayurvedic *vaids* and Unani *hakims,* who can be found in some diaspora communities. The fact that sales of Ayurvedic medications by India's ethno-pharmaceutical companies have rapidly increased in the last 20 years is a mark of their growing popularity.[6] The attraction lies primarily in the idea that they are free of side effects and that they work slowly and thoroughly to correct the systemic imbalances underlying many pain and illness conditions. Their similarity to home remedies and family treatments also enhances their appeal.

TABLE 5.1 Therapeutic Strategies for Managing Pain in Indian Culture

Type of therapy	Specific therapeutic actions
Biomedical	use aspirin, ibuprofen, and other analgesics
	use over-the-counter balms for massage
Traditional medicinal	use traditional oral medications
	use traditional balms and liniments for massage
Traditional dietary	avoid windy foods such as legumes
	avoid hard-to-digest foods such as ripe bananas
	avoid constipating foods
	avoid foods to which individuals have personal sensitivities
Behavioral	make various appropriate adjustments to posture and movement
Environmental	for "cold" conditions, particularly musculoskeletal problems: keep warm, especially in cold, damp weather; wear warm clothing
	eat "warm" or "hot" foods to support proper digestion
	avoid rapid shifts between hot and cold places
Emotional and Social	reduce family stresses and disagreements
	avoid conflicts in work settings
	seek family support in managing treatment
	talk with supportive family members and friends
Spiritual	Hindus: perform prayers, vows, and fasts for particular deities
	Muslims: offer prayers
	Sikhs: offer prayers
	Hindus, Muslims, Sikhs: visit saints' tombs
	Hindus, Muslims, Sikhs: use amulets
	Hindus, and occasionally Muslims and Sikhs: seek astrological advice and wear gemstone rings for afflicting planets

Many Ayurvedic and Unani medications are available for pain, including joint and muscle pain, back pain, headache, stomach and intestinal pain, menstrual cramps, earache, toothache, and kidney and liver pain. These medications, usually as pills, tablets, or syrups, typically contain carminatives, digestives, laxatives, and other alteratives believed to restore bodily balance, rid the system of noxious substances, and remove blockages that underlie or contribute to various pain conditions. They may contain analgesic substances for immediate symptom relief, but their broader pain-relieving effect lies in their capacity to correct internal imbalances—to treat the cause rather than the symptoms, as people like to say. Side effects and other problems with biomedical analgesics lead some patients to turn more exclusively to traditional medicines. A recent report indicates, for instance, that in India Ayurvedic medicines are becoming the treatment of choice for rheumatism and arthritis.[26]

Medicated oils and balms are popular in India in the form of home remedies and packaged Ayurvedic and Unani products. Massage has great cultural cachet in South Asian society: it marks and enacts relationships of respect and care within the family, and its therapeutic use builds on these customs. Ayurvedic and Unani companies produce dozens of medicated oils and balms recommended for joint and muscle pain, backache, and headache. They are typically formulated to disperse noxious substances and congested matter beneath the skin and within muscles, joints, and tissues. They often contain anodynes as well, much like over-the-counter ointments and balms in the West. They may be used alone or in tandem with oral medications and diet.

Given the importance of systemic balance in the maintenance of health and the overall prevention of pain, diet often remains an important part of treatment regimens in diaspora settings. As noted earlier, foods may be classified as hot or cold, and they are selected for use in treating various kinds of illnesses.[22–23] "Hot" foods, for example, are recommended to help relieve "cold" conditions, such as muscle pain, arthritis, and head colds with congestion. Windy or hard-to-digest foods such as legumes or ripe bananas should be avoided by people afflicted with rheumatism, and foods that promote digestion should be favored.[8]

Religious healing is important for many South Asians in times of illness and suffering. Hindu temples, Islamic mosques, and Sikh *gurdwaras* are present in or near many communities in the West, and Hindus, Muslims, and Sikhs alike may also offer prayers at home. Hindus may undertake vows and fasts for particular deities. People may also seek explanations for their suffering, as well as relief from pain and other afflictions, by consulting spiritual guides, astrologers, religious saints, and amulet-writers.[21–22] In some cases, notions of the evil eye and magical powers may be assessed in these settings and appropriate amulets and other remedies recommended.

SUGGESTIONS FOR PHYSICIAN INTERACTION WITH INDIAN AND OTHER SOUTH ASIAN PAIN PATIENTS

This discussion has emphasized basic features of pain concepts and pain treatments in India and in diaspora populations. The major limitation in this presentation involves the dearth of first-hand data on pain-related clinical interactions between Indian and other South Asian patients and their physicians in Western countries. More medical anthropological and health-services research on these communities is necessary for the development of a more finely grained account of pain patients' experiences, therapeutic decisions, and attitudes towards their physicians. The recent call for a national health agenda for Asian Americans and Pacific Islanders[27] highlights the lack of close attention to Asian communities in the United States and urges support for research on health conditions and practices in these population groups.

Against this backdrop, the following suggestions, which are grounded in Indian culture and its health understandings and practices, offer some practical guidance for a clinically informed approach to pain among Indians and other South Asians.

Clinical Pearls
1. Cultural sensitivity should be displayed to family hierarchies, gender roles, and family decision-making processes as the norm in cases of chronic pain and disabling conditions.
2. Widespread pain is a common complaint among South Asians, and it has various possible interpretations. Patients may be reluctant to discuss issues of personal or family psychological strain, but physicians can practice sensitivity and rapport-building as a way to facilitate discussion.

3. It is culturally appropriate for physicians dealing with Indian and other South Asian pain patients to inquire about bodily processes such as digestion and elimination and patients' perceptions that particular food items pay contribute to pain.

4. A marked reticence about surgery may be noted when discussing treatment options for pain-related conditions.

5. Patients will often have marked concerns about the side effects of biomedical drugs.

6. Patients may use biomedical treatments along with traditional medicinal remedies and religious practices, but may not mention these remedies to biomedical practitioners.

7. It is culturally salient to recommend that patients incorporate the use of oils and massages in the management of pain conditions affecting the head, joints, muscles, bones, and skin.

8. Some pain patients may consider their body to be fragile or paralyzed, and hence they may avoid recommended exercise.[15]

9. The indication that Vitamin D deficiency may contribute to the widespread body pain often reported by South Asian patients offers an additional consideration in making a diagnosis. Note that cultural factors related to diet and clothing may be involved.

10. Overall, the expression of care and support is essential in building rapport and facilitating communication.[17,21]

REFERENCES

1. Helman C. *Culture, Health and Illness*. 5th ed. London: Hodder Arnold; 2007.
2. Norton JHK. *Global Studies: India and South Asia*. Boston, MA: McGraw Hill; 2010.
3. Pugh JF. The semantics of pain in Indian culture and medicine. *Cult Med Psychiatry*. 1991;15:19–43.
4. Pugh JF. Astrology and fate: the Hindu and Muslim experiences. In: Keyes CF, Daniel EV, eds. *Karma: An Anthropological Inquiry*. Berkeley: University of California Press; 1983:131–146.
5. Kakar S. *Shamans, Mystics, and Doctors: A Psychological Inquiry into India and its Healing Traditions*. New York: Knopf; 1982.
6. Bode M. *Taking Traditional Knowledge to the Market: The Modern Image of the Ayurvedic and Unani Industry, 1980–2000*. Hyderabad, India: Orient Longman; 2008.
7. Lad V. *Ayurveda: The Science of Self-Healing*. Sante Fe, NM: Lotus Press; 1984.
8. Pugh JF. Concepts of arthritis in India's medical traditions: Ayurvedic and Unani perspectives. *Soc Sci Med*. 2003;56:415–424.
9. Weiss MG, Desai A, Jadhav S. Humoral concepts of mental illness in India. *Soc Sci Med*. 1988;27:471–477.
10. Macfarlane GJ, Palmer B, Roy D, Afzal C, Silman AJ, O'Neill T. An excess of widespread pain among South Asians: Are low levels of vitamin D implicated? *Ann Rheum Dis*. 2005;64:1217–1219.
11. Jeffery R. *The Politics of Health in India*. Berkeley: University of California Press; 1988.
12. Madan TN. *Doctors and Society: Three Asian Case Studies*. New Delhi: Vikas; 1980.
13. Njobvu P, Hunt I, Pope D, Macfarlane G. Pain amongst ethnic minority groups of South Asian origin in the United Kingdom: a review. *Rheumatology*. 1999; 38:1184–1187.
14. Allison TR, Symmons DPM, Brammah T, Haynes P, Rogers A, Roxby M, et al. Musculoskeletal pain is more generalized among people from ethnic minorities than among white people in Greater Manchester. *Ann Rheum Dis*. 2002;61:151–156.
15. Rogers A, Allison T. What if my back breaks? Making sense of musculoskeletal pain among South Asian and African-Caribbean people in the North West of England. *J Psychosom Res*. 2004;57:79–87.

16. Palmer B, Macfarlane G, Afzal C, Esmail A, Silman A, Lunt M. Acculturation and the prevalence of pain amongst South Asian minority ethnic groups in the UK. *Rheumatology.* 2007;46:1009–1114.

17. Patel S, Peacock SM, McKinley RK, Carter D, Watson PJ. GPs' experience of managing chronic pain in a South Asian community—a qualitative study of the consultation process. *Fam Pract.* 2008;25(2):71–77.

18. Karasz A, Dempsey K, Fallek R. Cultural differences in the experience of everyday symptoms: a comparative study of South Asian and European American women. *Cult Med Psychiatry.* 2007;31:473–497.

19. Fenton S, Sadiq-Sangster A. Culture, relativism and the expression of mental distress: South Asian women in Britain. *Sociol Health Illn.* 1996;18(1):66–85.

20. Raguram R, Weiss MG, Keval H, Channabasavanna SM. Cultural dimensions of clinical depression in Bangalore, India. *Anthropol Med.* 2001;8(1):31–46.

21. Ahmed SM, Lemkau JP. Cultural issues in the primary care of South Asians. *J Immigr Health.* 2000;2(2):89–96.

22. Assanand S, Dias M, Richardson E, Waxler-Morrison N. The South Asians. In: Waxler-Morrison N, Anderson J, Richardson E, eds. *Cross-Cultural Caring: A Handbook for Health Professionals in Western Canada.* Vancouver, BC: University of British Columbia Press; 1990:141–180.

23. Ramakrishna J, Weiss MG. Health, illness, and immigration: East Indians in the United States. *West J Med.* 1992;57:265–270.

24. Lessinger J. *From the Ganges to the Hudson: Indian Immigrants in New York City.* Boston, MA: Allyn and Bacon; 1995.

25. Helliwell PS, Ibrahim G. Ethnic differences in responses to disease modifying drugs. *Rheumatology.* 2003;42:1197–1201.

26. Banerjee M. *Power, Knowledge, Medicine: Ayurvedic Pharmaceuticals at Home and in the World.* Hyderabad, India: Orient Blackswan; 2009.

27. Ghosh C. A national health agenda for Asian Americans and Pacific Islanders. *JAMA.* 2010;304(12):1381–1382.

/// 6 /// INSIGHTS ON THE PAIN EXPERIENCE IN MEXICAN AMERICANS

EVELYN RUIZ CALVILLO, RN, DNSC

Professor Emeritus of Nursing, School of Health & Human Services, California State University, Los Angeles, Los Angeles, California, USA

Key Points

- Much of the literature on pain among Mexican Americans includes the caveat that culture has a significant influence on the pain response.
- Pain assessment is of primary importance in managing pain and should take into account Mexican American traditional culture, traditional beliefs, values, and practices relevant to the pain experience.
- The extent to which traditional beliefs are held and adhered provides the healthcare provider information about the value of fatalism and suffering, stoicism, and self-control and how these are expressed during the pain experience.
- An assessment of actual responses to pain should include understanding the meaning of a particular pain-related behavior and/or vocalization.
- Pain management should consider and respect a patient's wish to use traditional interventions alone or in combination with standard medical treatment.
- The role of the family or social support network in providing any of these interventions should be assessed and accommodations should be made for family involvement.

INTRODUCTION

In 2002, there were 37.4 million Hispanics (Latinos) in the United States, representing 13.3% of the total population,[1] which increased by 58% nationally between 1990 and 2000. Among Hispanics, two-thirds (66.9%) were Mexican-American, referring to people of Mexican origin, both those born in Mexico and those born in the United States. Mexican Americans is a term for those of Mexican descent born in the United States but it will include Mexican immigrants as well in this chapter. Because Mexican Americans represent the largest Hispanic subgroup in the United States, understanding their pain experiences will advance the knowledge base needed to face a variety of challenges, such as treating pain effectively and developing skills to provide culturally competent care to this increasingly large and complex population.

The overall goal of this chapter is to provide insights into the pain experience of Mexican Americans. Health professionals in the United States often characterize various ethnocultural groups according to their reactions to pain and their ability to tolerate pain. Understanding includes recognizing the impact of acculturation and assimilation on the Mexican-American pain experience, becoming familiar with the evolution of traditional Mexican-American beliefs about the pain experience (including the influence of religion on the pain response), being familiar with cultural pain coping patterns, realizing how the traditional roles of the Mexican-American family affect the pain experience, and being aware of the use of traditional treatments for pain.

Much of the literature on pain in adults includes the caveat that culture has a significant influence on the pain response. Major studies or replications of cross-cultural pain research that include Mexican Americans are scarce or outdated; however, the findings of many outdated studies are consistent with more current research and will be included in the various sections of this chapter. More recent pain research that identifies Hispanics as the population of interest often do not distinguish subgroups within the population; that is, Mexican Americans, Puerto Ricans, Cubans, and so forth.[2] In addition, many studies that distinguish Mexican Americans are not focused on perceptions of pain but focus on ethnic differences in pain reports or disparities in medication treatment. [3,4] For example, racial differences are the focus in a study of women's prodromal and acute symptoms of myocardial infarction and serve to aid providers in their interpretation of women's symptoms.[5] Perceptions and meaning of the pain, which would have added more understanding were not measured in the study.

Studies of the pain response among Mexican Americans conducted since the 1980s contain inadequate and insufficient information on which to base sound recommendations. There is a clear shortage of current information about Mexicans' knowledge of preventive health practices, appropriate understanding of different illnesses, causes, and management related to the pain response. It is important to stress that the traditional values presented in this chapter represent broad generalizations that may or may not apply to any individual or in any given situation. Each person is unique and simultaneously formed by a variety of cultures and subcultures, not to mention personal choices and socioeconomic circumstances. Still, being aware of these values may help healthcare providers to understand a particular patient's behaviors and actions in the context of larger cultural inclinations.

ACCULTURATION, ASSIMILATION, AND LANGUAGE

In many studies, the length of time living in the United States serves as a proxy for in the extent of acculturation and assimilation, both of which affect pain perceptions.[2] In 2002, 37% (or 11.3 million) of the Mexican-origin people were foreign-born; 2.5 million of them were naturalized citizens.[1] Among the foreign-born Hispanic population in 2002, 52.1% entered the United States between 1990 and 2002, another 25.6% arrived in the 1980s, and the remainder (22.3%) entered before 1980.[1]

Mexican-American immigrants hold very strong bonds to their language, people, traditions, and homeland. For many, this closeness to their country of origin makes it harder to change, especially if there is still an attachment to family in Mexico. Some immigrants adapt quickly to survive in a new and often times stressful environment; others retain traditional cultural lifestyles to cope in a potentially hostile environment. Factors such as the level of assimilation into the dominant English-speaking culture of the United States are seen to affect behavior. Among all major immigrant groups in the United States, Mexican immigrants have long been known to maintain their native language tenaciously. Many Mexican Americans speak Spanish more fluently than English, or do not speak English at all, but there are also large numbers of Mexican Americans who cannot speak Spanish fluently. Factors that influence English language proficiency are multidimensional and can be attributed to immigration or nativity history, cohort effects, education level, and economic background, as well as residence and geographic area.

Investigating indigenous or traditional beliefs, while taking into account different acculturation levels, may help point to factors that can be useful in providing meaningful attention and care. Mexican Americans living in the United States experience the society in a variety of ways and for some, the culture changes rapidly, while others experience little change. Mexican Americans are a diverse group and the many intragroup differences among them could affect the pain response. Each person has different beliefs and traditions; however, unwarranted assumptions often are attached to a person because of his/her ethnicity, due to stereotypes about how Mexican Americans should respond to pain.[6] There are Mexican Americans who no longer believe or practice the folk medicine often associated with Mexican-American culture. Studies have shown that adherence to traditional ethnic health beliefs and practices is related to the degree of acculturation.[7,6] Nevertheless, a large percentage of Mexican Americans continue to hold traditional beliefs. Evidence suggests that a more intense adherence to the Mexican culture produces a more traditional health behavior.[8, 9, 6] The studies by Calvillo and Flaskerud,[8] and Castro, Furth, and Karlow,[9] which examined health-illness beliefs among Mexican, Mexican-American, and Anglo-American women, found that the acceptance of folk or traditional beliefs correlated with low acculturation scores.

Spanish, the language that represents Mexico, other Latin countries, and Spain, is the most prevalent of all foreign or non-English languages spoken in the United States. Language is unique to a cultural group and survival of the language is influenced by its continual usage. The widespread use of Spanish in the United States is due to a constant flow of Mexican immigrants, the proximity to Mexico, and the large size of this cultural group. Communication among Mexican-American people is not solely confined to verbal dialect, but also includes nonverbal communication. One element of this is the notion of *respeto*, or respect. Respect is the essence of acknowledging older individuals, by avoiding direct eye contact with those of higher status. There is an element of formality about this, especially when older persons are involved. In addition, Mexican-American people normally have shorter personal space standards than other North Americans; they routinely greet individuals with a hug, firm handshake, and a kiss on the cheek.

TRADITIONAL MEXICAN-AMERICAN BELIEFS ABOUT THE PAIN EXPERIENCE

Traditional beliefs provide culture-specific examples of values, attitudes, and experiences. Indigenous or traditional beliefs affect the perception of health and illness, which often includes expected behaviors in response to illness and pain. Beliefs are important constructs that lie at the core of "culture" and that are seen as antecedents of behavior.[9] For example, for many in Mexican-American culture the value of suffering and the concept of fatalism are accepted beliefs with religious undertones. Others believe that life has many difficulties, which must be accepted without complaint. One's fate is to suffer in this world and "submit with patience to one's allotted measure of suffering."[10] If a person is ill, that person bears the illness with dignity and courage.

Many newly arrived first-generation and many elderly Mexican Americans believe a healthy person is one who functions adequately, is well fleshed or robust, and is free of pain.[6,11] Functioning adequately means being able to do routine everyday tasks despite symptoms such as leg cramps or pain from a sore throat. Investigation of the ethno-medical beliefs and practices of Mexican Americans in a primary care setting in Texas discovered that usually two symptoms were considered in determining the severity of an illness: pain and the appearance of blood.[7] If those symptoms or signs subside, the person may stop treatment altogether, even when continuation of treatment is considered medically important. As with many cultures, frequently medical treatment is stopped because the symptoms subside or because an alternative treatment is sought.

INFLUENCE OF RELIGION ON THE PAIN RESPONSE

Themes of pain and suffering are deeply embedded in many facets of Mexican-American life, including religion.[12] Historical accounts of pain and suffering are important because they provide valuable insights into forces that have shaped the religious lives of many Mexican Americans today. With the colonization of Mesoamerica by the Catholic Spanish many indigenous cultures accepted the Catholic religion in order to survive and went "underground" with their indigenous beliefs. Because of the blending of Spanish Catholicism with the religious beliefs of indigenous cultures, some unique beliefs and rituals evolved, many of which are still in practice today.[13] While most Mexican Americans are influenced by the Catholic religion, some indigenous cultures still incorporate the spiritual beliefs of their ancestors, such as the Zapotec, Mayan, and Aztec. Others practice the principles of different Christian religions and do not necessarily share the same views.

It appears that some Mexican-American Catholics may be especially inclined to believe that pain and suffering are a necessary part of leading a religious life. If pain and suffering are a necessary part of living a religious life, then older Mexican Americans are likely to believe that bearing these difficulties serves some function.[14] For the most part many Mexican Americans value a religion that accepts the concepts of suffering and fatalism, believing that health and illness are due to "God's will" or fate, or both. Many are able to progress through an illness or through a recovery period with this attitude because "everything is in the hands of God."[9] Likewise, pain may be seen as punishment for immoral behavior. Suffering takes on a redemptive quality for some Mexican Americans; it is viewed as payment for their own misdeeds. In this religious context, many believe that cancer pain is just punishment and that suffering is part of life, to be endured in order to enter heaven.[15] Others believe that pain and suffering deepen one's faith, make people more sensitive to the plight of others, instill a sense of empowerment in late life, and provide payment or restitution for past sins.

Faith and prayer are necessary to maintaining and regaining health because illness and pain are divinely predetermined as God's will. Many older Mexican Americans have relied on their faith to help them deal with health and illness challenges, but there is still a great deal we do not know about the relationships among religion, pain, suffering, and health in Mexican-American culture. First, researchers need to know more about how religion shapes the belief structures that reinforce views on pain and suffering among older Mexican Americans. More specifically, greater insight is needed into what people think religion has to say about why pain and suffering exist, and researchers need to learn more about the social and psychological resources that are provided by religion to help Mexican Americans deal with these problems in their lives.

CULTURALLY DERIVED COPING PATTERNS OF MEXICAN AMERICANS

Health professionals in the United States often characterize various ethnocultural groups according to their reaction to pain and their ability to tolerate pain. Mexican Americans are often described as complainers who want immediate relief for their pain or have a low pain tolerance.[8] Yet studies of Mexican-American culture and cross-cultural studies of the pain experience and responses of Mexican Americans do not support this characterization.[16] Some Hispanics were less willing to admit loss of control and less likely to describe their pain as unbearable.[11] Their descriptions were consistent with the beliefs of a culture in which stoicism and self-control are highly valued. Many Mexican-American patients, especially women, moan when uncomfortable. Consequently, they are often identified as complainers who cannot tolerate pain. However, in the Mexican culture, crying out with pain is an acceptable expression and not synonymous with an inability to tolerate pain.[16] Wincing, groaning, and grimacing may be exhibited, and crying or moaning may function as a relief for pain, rather than communicate a request for help. Crying out with pain does not necessarily indicate either that the pain experience is severe or that the person is experiencing a loss of self-control. Neither does it mean that the person expects intervention. Some may react to mild pain by crying or moaning, but others may suppress overt behaviors in the presence of severe pain. This example points out clearly that any attempt to delineate cultural factors in the pain response should be made within the wider context of cultural attitudes and behaviors.

The concept of self-control and stoicism is a common value and an important element in the Mexican culture. One's ability to endure pain and cope by trying to work through the pain is highly valued.[16] Signs and symptoms of illness, such as pain, may not be acknowledged because lack of stamina and complaining are considered a sign of weakness. Mexican Americans endure illness and pain as a sign of strength and do not seek help until either becomes unbearable.[14] Self-control has been found to be a practice common to the Mexican American who is experiencing pain.[16,9] Self-control (*controlarse*) includes (1) the ability to withstand stress in times of adversity (*aguantarse*); (2) a passive resignation in which the person accepts his or her fate (*resignarse*); or (3) a more active cognitive coping characterized by working through a problem (*sobreponerse*).

EFFECT OF TRADITIONAL ROLES OF THE MEXICAN-AMERICAN FAMILY ON PAIN EXPERIENCE

A pervasive value in the Mexican culture is the family, including the extended family.[17] This concept of *la familia* or *familismo* influences and shape attitudes and beliefs and therefore can influence health-related knowledge and behaviors, including the pain experience. Pain is often seen as an accepted obligation of life; one's role within the family is to accept pain and suffering as something that one must bear, so as not to burden others.[14] On the other hand many older Mexican Americans indicate that it is important to reach out to family members and close friends when adversity arises. For some older Mexican Americans, suffering in silence is not a desirable way to deal with hard times because doing so forgoes the opportunity of benefitting from the help that significant others may provide. If a person has close ties with family members and friends, then suffering in silence may not be the coping response of choice. If an individual is embedded in a web of conflicted social ties, however, then suffering in silence may be a realistic response to a difficult interpersonal climate. This perspective also provides evidence that the decision to suffer in silence is shaped by more than religious principles alone. Instead, it is also influenced by social relationships outside the church.

A vast literature reveals that older people who make use of social support during stressful times tend to have better physical and mental health than older adults who remain isolated from others.[18] This is important because a well-developed literature suggests that being embedded in a tightly knit social network has health-enhancing effects. Family involvement often is critical in the health care of the patient and the family system should always be acknowledged as a source of support.

TRADITIONAL LATINO GENDER ROLES AND THE PAIN EXPERIENCE

Mexican-American men are socialized to think that they must endure pain to be considered a man and that expressing and admitting they have pain may show weakness and risks losing respect from others.[2] Men define illness and pain to include impairment that prevents a man from working and earning a living. Pain is seen as a major motivating factor for many men to seek health care. Care is sought not necessarily for the relief of pain but to continue doing what it takes to be a man. The ability to withstand pain is a sign of manhood and reliability.[2,19] *Machismo* is a concept familiar to most Mexican men. This idea of being *macho* has predominated and shaped Mexican society's idea of what one considers to be a man. Being tough, however, can lead to serious problems, especially if the person is in need of medical intervention. It is important that the patient be able to set aside this perception when health needs are a high priority. A challenge with being "big and tough," is the need to modify this thinking in order to facilitate appropriate healthcare interventions. To assist in dealing with *machismo*, one should let the patient know that despite their need for help, they are still considered to be strong. Although *machismo* prevails throughout Mexican society, it can be placed aside when facing severe, unrelenting pain.

The role for the woman is known as *marianismo*, referring to a woman who is self-sacrificing, religious, and responsible for running the household, raising the children, and caring for elderly relatives. Such women are likely to put the needs of all others ahead of their own needs. Although it is more socially acceptable for women to express pain, it is not uncommon for Mexican-American women to be as stoic as men. In the interest of not wanting her family members to worry about her a Hispanic woman who has been raised within a culture of *familism* may not report pain until it becomes very serious and intolerable.[20] Cultural traditions that emphasize women's obedience and obligation to sacrifice for their families can affect a woman's endurance of pain. The woman will endure the pain rather than allow the pain to keep her from fulfilling the multiple roles and responsibilities expected by her family. Because of *familism*, women may place their highest priority on family during the diagnosis and treatment process, including pain management. Being a woman may be a barrier to adequate pain management because being a mother in the Hispanic culture requires that women sacrifice for their children and place their own needs (including needs for pain management) second to those of other family members.

Traditional gender role behaviors of men and women may be different in public than at home. It is important to know that assimilation, acculturation, and the necessity for women to work in the United States have affected these gender roles. It is not unusual for roles to be reversed, or for power to be shared; however, in many instances gender roles still exist and are likely to be more pervasive in low-income families. In a study of marriages, Latino men and women shared decision-making within the family, but had different roles in their family life.[21] In families likely to have traditional roles, men were expected to provide the income for the family and the woman provide for the care of the children and the home.

Social norms dictate how and to what degree pain behavior may be expressed by men and women. It is more socially acceptable for women to complain. In Mexico, most men think they are strong and can stand pain, but it is all about machismo.[19] In contrast, women, as soon as they feel sick want to go to the doctor. Society forces one to act a certain way. When one cries as a small boy, one is likely to hear from a dad: "Don't cry. You're a big boy." Given these gender roles and expectations, it can be a challenge for the healthcare team to help keep patients comfortable.

USE OF ALTERNATIVE MEDICINE FOR TREATMENT OF PAIN

Although controversial, the use of traditional folk treatments and healers may still be a treatment option for many Mexican Americans. However, the effects of acculturation on the usage of folk remedies and belief in folk illnesses and *curanderos* have a direct inverse correlation.[13] Newly arrived immigrants, especially those from rural villages and towns are more likely to remain faithful to traditional Mexican values and health beliefs and practices than the US-born Mexican Americans who are influenced by a family that practices traditional care that integrates an individual's cultural values, beliefs, and customs.

Other cultural and social structure dimensions that may influence the use of folk medicine and folk healers are economics, education, immigration status, and mistrust of the professional health system. Numerous Mexican Americans do not trust modern day professional medical practitioners, whether it is due to lack of education, lack of communication, knowledge deficit, or inappropriate cultural care. There are Mexican Americans who sometimes choose to use ethno-medicine, sometimes choose to use conventional medical treatment, and sometimes choose to utilize both simultaneously. Although mothers use traditional Mexican teas, soups, or rubs, they also rely on over-the-counter medications and medical diagnosis to treat illness.

Cultural responses and expressions of pain, along with the hope that the pain will simply go away, may lead Mexican Americans to delay seeking medical treatment, often because of the lack of available treatment throughout Mexican-American communities and neighborhoods. People are able to purchase and find common herbs, tinctures, spices, etc. for customary home remedies in local shops referred to as *herbaria or yerberia (herb shops)*.[13] Herbalism dating from pre-Colombian times plays a key role in home remedies. Diagnoses are made and herbal prescriptions are brought home and made into broth or tea for the patient to drink. Families seek health information regarding over-the-counter medications for common ailments such as earaches, toothache, sore throat, and so on from neighborhood *boticas* (pharmacies) and botanicas, where oftentimes herbs and teas, potions, and spiritual icons are found for folk remedies and rituals. The proximity of the Mexican border enhances the availability and flexibility that allows Mexican Americans easy access to folk remedies that they cannot find in the United States.

Of particular importance in the Mexican-American population is the folk-healing practice *curanderismo,* which continues to be an important aspect of Mexican-American culture. Often integrating a religious component, *curanderismo* encompasses spiritual and emotional elements beyond the physiologic components of health. A review of ethnographic studies conducted across the lifespan[13] reveals how Mexican Americans consistently integrate cultural strategies, such as *curanderismo,* with conventional health methods and Western medicine in everyday life. This indicates that people do not view *curanderismo* and modern medicine as incompatible. Other studies find the use of cultural healers is minimal. Even when they grew up with a tradition of *curanderismo,* Mexican Americans do not rely solely on it to maintain family health, but also seek assistance from modern medicine when they experience more serious or chronic illness.

Many Mexican-American Catholics may turn to religious practices, such as praying, attending mass, anointment, communion, and blessing by the priest, to relieve or endure pain.[22] Traditional religious practices provide ways of prevention and "cures" through prayers to God, Christ, or saints. Some prayers are specific to certain conditions or illnesses and require a ritual with the prayer. Lighted candles, visits to churches or shrines, and wearing of religious and spiritual medals are popular practices.

CULTURALLY COMPETENT INTERVENTIONS

Clarifying or modifying treatment for pain to align with particular religious or cultural practices, as well as displaying a willingness to compromise about treatment goals when possible, are important during the negotiation process between providers and patients from unfamiliar cultures.[23,24] It is critical that providers be prepared to deliver culturally competent care for pain by increasing their own knowledge, adjusting their attitudes, and improving their skills.[14]

Culturally Sensitive Pain Assessment. A culturally sensitive pain assessment, as well as the use of a holistic approach to pain management, should be part of the plan of care. Most importantly, it is essential that providers remain sensitive to cultural influences on perceptions of and expressions of pain. Several guidelines have been developed to enhance the first step, which is assessment.[24] The first consideration when conducting an assessment is to avoid making stereotypical assumptions about cultural groups. Individual differences exist within Mexican-American culture; thus, the pain experience should be understood within the context of patients' beliefs, values, coping strategies, and life experiences. The meaning of pain should be explored because making sense of the pain experience is culturally bound and may be a powerful coping mechanism in dealing with it. Discussing with Mexican Americans a plan of care to manage pain enhances their sense of control and positively influences the quality of the provider-client relationship. When done in conjunction with cultural norms, cognitive-behavioral techniques such as self-monitoring and self-control have been found useful in guiding behavior change in patients with pain.

The plan for pain management should include sensitivity to Mexican cultural beliefs and approaches using traditional healing practices.[3] Healthcare providers are encouraged to elicit specific information about treatments used for symptoms of pain presented under common folk illnesses, types of folk medicines and healers used to treat illness, and whenever possible, to integrate folk medicine and biomedical therapies as part of treatment. In many cultures such as Mexican, it may be more appropriate to use nonpharmacological measures to reduce pain, or at least therapies that promote relaxation. Additionally, reliance on a higher power for many Mexican Americans may represent an effective coping mechanism that should be acknowledged and respected by determining religious beliefs. The fatalistic tone that is embedded in this view may convey a rather passive approach to dealing with difficult times. However, giving patients "permission" to use religious practices is comforting to them.

Establishing trust and sensitivity to nonverbal cues that may indicate pain and/or suffering is essential, as is encouraging honest expressions of the need for pain management. Mexican-American patients tend not to complain of pain[25] and therefore it is essential to assess pain by nonverbal cues. This is a concern because vast literature suggests that passive responses to stressors are often associated with undesirable health outcomes. Mexican

Americans value inner control and self-endurance. For example, in Mexican-American cancer patients, suffering often overshadowed the pain experience;[15] thus the level of suffering as well as pain should be assessed. Gender is another consideration that affects pain assessment. For some men, expressing pain shows weakness and possible loss of respect. Expression of pain socially is more acceptable in women; however, stoicism is also common.

Health Literacy. Inability to converse in English leads to miscommunication that can result in misperceptions, especially in healthcare settings. The Institute of Medicine (IOM) reports that nearly half of all American adults have difficulty understanding and acting upon health information.[26] For those whose native language is not English, health literacy issues are compounded by problems with basic communication and the specialized vocabulary needed to convey health information. This puts non-English speakers at risk for poorly informed health decisions that may negatively influence health outcomes. The US Census uses the term "linguistically isolated" to categorize those living in a household where no person aged 14 or above speaks English very well. According to the US Census almost 2 in 5 elderly Hispanic/Latinos who speak Spanish only are linguistically isolated.[27] Limited English proficiency has been reported as a barrier to accessing medical and social services for Mexican Americans. When in pain and anxiety, patients often use their primary language to express discomfort. If communication is not possible, Mexican Americans will not complain of pain, and therefore will suffer. Pain questionnaires and other educational materials in Spanish may help in communicating the quality of pain.[28]

Communication and the Therapeutic Relationship. Communication and the relationship between patient and healthcare provider are key to providing quality care [24]. Trust and interpersonal comfort are critical components of the relationship between the person who is ill and the healer. A curt healthcare provider may not learn of significant complaints or problems and may find the patient unlikely to return. It is uncommon for Hispanics to be aggressive or assertive in healthcare interactions or to use direct eye contact during them. Open disagreement with a provider is uncommon; the usual response to a decision with which the patient or family disagrees is silence and noncompliance.

The use of translators is often necessary and ideally they should be professional and of the same gender.[3] Family members or friends are sometimes used as translators, but this may result in avoidance of personal problems. The use of family or friends to interpret presents difficulty in communicating accurate instructions, such as pain medication regimens and side effects the patient must understand. Using children to translate puts the parent and child in a difficult position and misinterpretation can occur, especially if the child does not understand a medical term. In general, it is best to have Spanish-speaking staff, professional translators, or volunteers who have strong bilingual skills to translate. With staff whose primary function is translating, care should be taken that the translators confine themselves to the roles of translating and refrain from providing counsel, giving advice, or offering personal opinions, even if asked to do so. Translators need to be culturally competent by not including their own personal beliefs or opinions.

MANAGEMENT AND EVALUATION OF PAIN RESPONSE IN MEXICAN AMERICANS

Undermedication of Hispanic patients' pain might be a result of cultural differences between Hispanic patients and healthcare providers who have been trained in modern medicine based on Western culture.[20] Several factors could explain why pain management of Hispanic patients is inadequate[20, 15, 29]: (a) fewer resources and greater difficulty in accessing care and filling analgesic prescriptions, especially among patients of lower socioeconomic status; (b) stoicism, largely based in religious beliefs and fatalism among patients; (c) noncompliance with pharmacologic treatment because of the inability to understand instructions; (d) the tendency to perceive an illness such as cancer as destiny; and (e) having a sense of power-lessness or helplessness, therefore approaching pain with stoicism.

Another factor affecting the management of pain may be difficulty on the part of health-care providers in assessing pain because of differences in perception of pain, language fluency, and cultural background.[16] Differences in perception of pain occur even when the patient and provider share the same culture. There have been consistent differences between patients and healthcare staff in assessing the severity of Mexican-American and other Hispanic patients' pain.[16,4]

Studies of nurses have shown that the nurses' perceptions of pain did not coincide with those of the patients, which generally resulted in more suffering for the patient. Regardless of culture, nurses gave less medication for pain than ordered and less medication than patients needed to alleviate their pain. Other studies have shown that some doctors apparently arrive at the patient's bedside with preconceived notions about the patient's needs for pain medication that are tied to ethnicity and not to the illness per se.[30] A doctor who suggests that a patient is "making up" the pain for attention, sympathy, or pain medication can be very distressing and discouraging. The authors concluded that the physician's impression of the patient's pain, rather than the patient's expressions of pain were determinative factors in the extent to which pain was treated (or not treated) properly.

FUTURE MEXICAN AMERICAN PAIN RESEARCH

The research recommendations presented here are limited to Mexican Americans and suggest areas for study in both qualitative and quantitative approaches for the development of knowledge. Qualitative studies are needed to explore and describe the Mexican-American cultures' beliefs, values, and practices with respect to the pain experience; that is, the value of pain, the perception of pain, the response to pain, and the management of pain. These include: (1) descriptions of traditional health beliefs and practices related to pain, suffering, fatalism, and stoicism; (2) description of the meaning and function of behaviors and vocalizations associated with pain; (3) identification of traditional practices or self-control practices to alleviate pain used by individuals; and (4) identification of home and folk remedies used for pain. Quantitative studies needed include: (1) comparison of pain perception between cultural groups in clinical settings; (2) comparison of pain perception between health professionals and patients; (3) investigation of different interventions with patients from different cultural groups; and (4) comparison of requests for medication and the amount of medication provided to patients from different cultural groups for the same source of pain. Finally, research is needed which focuses on further development of pain assessment tools to use with Mexican Americans.

CONCLUSION

This chapter conveys a general knowledge of the concepts of culture and pain as specifically concerns the Mexican-American culture and its traditional beliefs, values, and practices as these relate to the pain experience. The most important concept presented may be the pain assessment, which should include the many aspects of the Mexican-American traditional culture. In conducting an assessment of a Mexican-American and his or her potential response to pain, the cultural beliefs, values, and practices of the client must be assessed with respect to suffering. The extent to which traditional beliefs are held and adhered to will give the healthcare provider information about the value of fatalism and suffering, stoicism, and self-control, and how these are expressed during the pain experience. An assessment of actual responses to pain should include gathering data on what a particular behavior and/or vocalization might mean in response to pain. For example, does it mean the pain is intolerable when a woman is crying and moaning? Is the function of these behaviors and vocalizations to relieve the pain? Or is the function to signal the nurse that pain intervention is being requested? The management of the patient's pain should include an assessment of the type of intervention the person desires. Does the patient wish traditional interventions, expressions of nurturance and compassion, psychological support, physical interventions, or a combination of traditional and medical treatment? The role of the family or social support network in providing any of these interventions should be assessed as well and accommodations made for family to become involved. These are a few of the most obvious implications for practice with Mexican-Americans who are experiencing pain.

REFERENCES

1. Ramirez RR, de la Cruz P. *The Hispanic Population in the United States: Current Population Reports.* Washington, DC: U.S. Census Bureau; June 2003.
2. Sobralske M, Katz J. Culturally competent care of patients with acute chest pain. *J Am Acad Nurse Pract.* 2005;17(9):342–349.
3. Hall-Lipsy EA, Chisholm-Burns MA. Pharmacotherapeutic disparities: Racial, ethnic, and sex variations in medication treatment. *American Journal of Health-System Pharmacology.* 2010;67:462–468.
4. Hernandez A, Sachs-Ericsson N. Ethnic differences in pain reports and the moderating role of depression in a community sample of Hispanic and Caucasian participants with serious health problems. *Psychosomatic Medicine.* 2006;68:121–128.
5. McSweeney JC, O'Sullivan P, Cleves MA, et al. Racial differences in women's prodromal and acute symptoms of myocardial infarction. *Am J Crit Care.* Jan 2010;19(1):63–73.
6. Harwood A. *Ethnicity and Medical Care.* Cambridge, MA: Harvard University; 1981.
7. Gonzalez-Swafford ML, Gutierrez MG. Ethno-medical beliefs and practices of Mexican Americans. *Nurse Pract.* 1983;8(10):29–34.
8. Calvillo E, Flaskerud J. Review of literature on culture and pain of adults with focus on Mexican Americans. *J Transcult Nurs,* 1993: 2:16–23.
9. Castro FG, Furth P, Karlow H. The health beliefs of Mexican, Mexican American, and Anglo American women. *Hispanic Journal of Behavioral Sciences.* 1984;6(4):365–368.
10. Calatrello RL. The Hispanic concept of illness: An obstacle to effective health care management? *Behavioral Medicine.* 1980;7(11):23–28.
11. Meinhart NT, McCaffery M. *Pain: A nursing approach to assessment and analysis.* Norwalk, Appleton-Century Crofts; 1983.
12. Krause N, Bastida E. Religion, suffering, and health among older Mexican Americans. *J Aging Stud.* 2009;23:114–123.
13. Clous VJ. *Mexican Home Remedies for Childhood Illnesses: A Handbook for Health Care Providers* [master's thesis]. Tucson: The University of Arizona; 2005:1–112.
14. Villarruel AM. Mexican American cultural meanings, expressions, self-care, and dependent-care actions associated with experiences of pain. *Res Nurs Health.* 1995;18(5):427–436.
15. Juarez G, Ferrell B, Borneman T. Cultural considerations in education for cancer pain management. *J Cancer Educ.* 1999;4:168–173.
16. Calvillo E, Flaskerud J. The evaluation of the pain response by Mexican American and Anglo American women and their nurses. *J Adv Nurs.* 1993;18:451–459.

17. Padilla YC, Villalobos G. Cultural responses to health among Mexican American women and their families. *Fam Community Health.* 2007;30(suppl 1):S24–S33.
18. Weaver GD, Kuo YF, Raji MA, Snih, SA, Ray L, Torres E, Ottenbacher KJ. Pain and disability in older Mexican-American adults. *Journal of the American Geriatric Society.* 2009;57:992–999.
19. Tran PD, Karina Garcia K. An international study of health knowledge, behaviors, and cultural perceptions of young Mexican adults. *Hisp Health Care Int.* 2009;7(1):5–10.
20. Im E, Guevara E, Chee W. The pain experience of Hispanic patients with cancer in the United States. *Oncol Nurs Forum.* 2007;34(4):861–868.
21. Skogrand L, Hatch D, Singh A. Understanding Latino families. Implications for family education. *Family Resources.* 2005; Utah State University, 1–3.
22. Davidhizar R, Giger JN. A review of the literature on care of clients in pain who are culturally diverse. *Int Nurs Rev.* 2004;51:47–55.
23. Betancourt J, Green A, Carrillo E. Hypertension in multicultural and minority populations: Linking communication to compliance. *Curr Hypertens Rep.* 1999;1:482–488.
24. U. S. Department of Health and Human Services Office of Minority Health. Physician Toolkit and Curriculum. Resources to Implement Cross-Cultural Clinical Practice Guidelines for Medicaid Practitioners. University of Massachusetts Medical School Office of Community Programs; March 2004.
25. Flores LY, Deal JZ. Work-related pain in Mexican American custodial workers. *Hisp J Behav Sci.* 2003;25(2):254–270.
26. Institute of Medicine. *IOM health literacy: A prescription to end confusion.* Institute of Medicine; 2004.
27. Lestina FA. *Analysis of the linguistically isolated population in Census 2000.* Final Report Planning, Research and Evaluation Division. U.S. Census Bureau; 2003.
28. Escalante A, Lichtenstein M.J, Rios, N, Hazuda HP. Measuring chronic rheumatic pain in Mexican Americans: Cross-cultural adaptation of the McGill Pain Questionnaire. *J Clin Epidemiol.* 1996;49(12):1389–1399.
29. Alvarado A J. *Cultural diversity: Pain beliefs and treatment among Mexican-Americans, African-Americans, Chinese-Americans and Japanese-Americans* [senior honors Thesis]. East Michigan University; 2008:1–47.
30. Anderson KO, Green CR, Payne R. Racial and ethnic disparities in pain: Causes and consequences of unequal care. *J Pain.* Dec 2009; 10(12):1187–204.

7

WE FEEL PAIN TOO

Asserting the Pain Experience of the Quichua People

MARIO INCAYAWAR, MD, MSC, DESS

Director, Runajambi–Institute for the Study of Quichua Culture and Health, Otavalo, Ecuador *and* Former Henry R. Luce Professor in Brain, Mind and Medicine, Cross-Cultural Perspectives, Claremont Colleges, Claremont, California, USA

SIOUI MALDONADO-BOUCHARD, MSC, PHD (CANDIDATE)

Research Assistant, Runajambi–Institute for the Study of Quichua Culture and Health, Otavalo, Ecuador *and* Doctoral Interdisciplinary Program in Neurosciences, Laboratory on Spinal Cord Injury Recovery, Texas A&M University, College Station, Texas, USA

Key Points

- There is a dearth of research on pain among Indigenous peoples and the pain experience of the Quichuas, the largest Indigenous nation in South America, is often misunderstood by non-Indigenous people in the region.
- The Quichuas have a multifactorial theory of pain causation, according to which emotions and comorbidity can worsen pain. Pain is more often attributed to psychosocial and supernatural causes than to physical conditions.
- The Quichuas believe both traditional healers and physicians can successfully treat pain, and that family and neighbors also play an important role.
- Quichua people consider talking about one's pain appropriate, but complaining about it undesirable (a sign of weakness). People express little pain to physicians.
- Better understanding the Quichuas' pain experience could promote pluralistic care, where biomedically trained physicians and traditional healers contribute to the treatment of patients' pain.
- Pain can kill a person, so it is of serious concern to the sufferer and his/her relatives; the majority prefers an effective treatment with immediate results.

INTRODUCTION

The variability of human pain experience has attracted the interest of many researchers for many decades. Zborowski's pioneering survey made at the Kingsbridge Hospital, Bronx, New York in the 1950s, showed intriguing differences in pain expression among Jewish, Italian, Irish, and "Old Americans."[1] The Jewish-American and the Italian-American were found to be more expressive as compared to the Irish-American and the protestant Anglo-American.[2] Zola found similar results in the early 1960s while conducting a study on the influence of culture on symptoms at the Massachusetts General Hospital and the Massachusetts Eye and Ear Infirmary in Boston.[3]

Since then, both experimental and clinical approaches have been adopted to study the responses to pain across ethnocultural groups worldwide. The experimental evidence has been scarce and mostly obtained from uncontrolled studies.[4,5] Nevertheless, these efforts have contributed toward developing the general view that the ability to perceive painful stimuli is culture-free.[6-9] It is worth noting, however, that these same experimental studies revealed cultural differences when they focused on pain tolerance (the point where the subject wants to stop receiving a painful stimulus).[10-14]

On the other hand, the abundant clinical, anthropological, and epidemiological evidence helped to determine that the expression of clinical pain varied according to cultural and other social factors.[15-17] Remarkable ethnocultural variability has been found in dental pain,[18] low back pain,[19] childbirth pain,[20] as well as in personality test performance among pain patients from different ethnic heritages,[21] pain experiences among hospitalized children,[22] and pain expression among specific ethnocultural groups such as the Bariba in Benin,[23] among others. Nevertheless, the above-mentioned cultural variability has been challenged by some researchers.[24-26]

The paucity of pain studies among the Indigenous Peoples of South America is striking. Its population is roughly equal to that of Canada—about 30 million people. Yet, to our knowledge, only three studies have been conducted in the region. A clinical study was published in 2004, exploring the frequency of signs and symptoms of temporomandibular disorders among 140 Tsachila and Quichua dental patients in Ecuador.[27] In 2006, an anthropological study examined the meanings attributed to headaches by women in Peru.[28] And in 2007, an anthropological survey of headache and migraine among the Tzeltal Maya (Mexico), Kamayur´a (Brazil), and Uru-Chipaya (Bolivia) also came out.[29] Evidently, much remains to be done;—we are only at the beginning. Comprehensive studies of the pain experience of different Indigenous Peoples of South America, for example, are much needed.

Given this lack of research, physicians continue to make clinical decisions based on their own popular beliefs and prejudice regarding Indigenous Peoples' pain experience. The generalized anecdotal view among the *mishu* (a Quichua name for Ecuadorian Latino), for example, is that Quichua people are stoical. This is reminiscent of the "savage" stereotype still present in the first half of the 20th century, which considered Amerindians incapable of feeling pain. According to it, only civilized people, usually from European origin, such as women, whites, and the rich were highly sensitive to pain. African Americans were even believed to have a disease called dysaesthesia aethiopis or an "obtuse sensibility of body" that rendered them "insensible to pain when subjected to punishment."[30,31] The American minister Samuel Stanhope Smith of Princeton University, who held honorary degrees from Yale and Harvard, and physicians of the American Enlightenment period believed that Amerindian people experienced little or no pain. Smith stated: "We know that among Indians the squaws do not suffer in childbirth. Among your red Indian and other uncivilized tribes, the parturient female does not suffer the same amount of pain during labour as the female of the white race."[32]

When Dr. Incayawar was completing his medical school training in Ecuador, he witnessed many cases of Quichua patients being undertreated for their pain. Their pain was easily ignored or dismissed. He observed that *mishu* physicians managed the Quichuas' (Inca) pain as though it were less severe than the mishus' pain. Physicians often assumed that the Quichua patients felt less pain than "usual," because they were stoical savages or third-class citizens; as a consequence, they decided the Quichua needed less pain medication.[33] Dr. Incayawar knew, from his personal experience, being himself a Quichua, that this was erroneous. Quichua patients obviously experienced pain as well; they merely expressed it differently. Indeed, we, the Indigenous Peoples of South America, have a rich and sophisticated system of beliefs and attitudes concerning the nature of pain and how to control it.[34] Unfortunately, it had until then never been studied systematically.

It is in part to start to fill this gap in cultural understanding that Dr. Incayawar conducted this first study discussed in the present chapter. He and his team surveyed the Quichua people of the Rumipamba area, southeast of the town of Ibarra, the capital of the Imbabura province in the northern highlands of Ecuador. Their goal was to explore the Quichuas' pain experiences—more precisely how they perceive, describe, and cope with pain. The Quichuas are demographically the most important Amerindian nation in South America. This unique exploratory description of pain experiences in the Andes should therefore be relevant for the culturally sensitive pain clinician.

THE QUICHUA PEOPLE OF THE ANDES

The Quichuas are an Amerindian nation with an estimated population of 28 million. They once made up a large proportion of the Tawantinsuyu, the Inca Confederation, which at its height included present-day Bolivia, Ecuador, and Peru, as well as parts of Argentina, Chile, and Colombia. In the 16th century, Spanish armies invaded and subjugated the Confederation and instigated a regime of domination and exploitation, which still persists today, despite the national independence from Spain gained by the aforementioned countries in the 19th century. Within Ecuador, for example, the ruling *mishu* (Latinos, people of mixed Spanish and Quichua ancestry who identify themselves as white westerners and repudiate their Amerindian roots) have replaced the Spaniards as perpetrators for the last 200 years. In present-day postcolonial Ecuador, there is a caste-like social stratification, along with a political structure that marginalizes indigenous peoples and supports institutionalized racism.[35] This long-lasting oppression and social exclusion has resulted in outrageously poor health status[33] and transformed the Amerindians into one of the most impoverished and dispossessed peoples in the world. For this reason, they are considered to live in the Fourth World.[36]

> *The pain would come and go, and would become most intense in the evenings, after having eaten. "Maybe it's the food that makes me feel such pain. It is almost unbearable." Mrs. X got up and walked to the kitchen to make some tea. "It is deep in the stomach that it hurts, and then the headache starts. It starts in the back of my head, and then it feels like someone is knocking in my head...." It was the same every evening lately. Her daughters and husband sympathized with her and understood that she was in pain, but they were running out of advice and ideas. Herbal tea did not help, warm blankets, or rest did not either. They had been to a traditional healer a few weeks earlier, and she had told him about the incessant pain. After his treatments, she had felt better for a week or two, but the*

pain had then re-emerged. They had tried to go to the doctor, but it was difficult for them to communicate her condition to him in Spanish, and he had most likely not grasped the extent of her suffering.

"What seems to be the problem Mrs. X?" the doctor had asked at the hospital. She had spoken softly. "I have trouble digesting certain foods." Those had been her only words to describe her situation. The doctor had applied pressure to her abdomen, to see if this hurt. She had only slightly shrugged. She just repeated, "It is when I eat ..." The doctor had told her it was nothing serious, that it would fade away by itself. He had prescribed her some medication for gastric acidity, and that was all. But the situation had persisted for Mrs. X. Several weeks later, she continued to experience a stomachache and headaches. Unfortunately, they could not afford to consult a doctor again.

THE SURVEY ON PAIN

The study was carried out using an exploratory qualitative/descriptive research design. Before starting the collection of data, informed consent was obtained from the participants following the Quichuas' requirements and customs. Any procedure that requires individuals to sign a document is regarded with extreme suspicion and is considered unacceptable for the Quichua. Therefore, family verbal consent was obtained instead of an individually signed consent document. The study was officially approved by the Community Council of Rumipamba. Community representatives closely monitored and participated in the study and considered it an important project for the region.

The questionnaire, called *Nanay Jahua Tapuicuna* [The Nature of Pain], was prepared in the Quichua language and explored the Quichuas' pain experience. It essentially followed the ethnographic approach developed by Zborowski.[2,37] The questionnaire sought to explore beliefs and behaviors in some depth and also roughly covered the notions of causation of pain, vulnerability to pain, responses to pain, aggravating factors, locations of pain, types of pain, duration, characteristics of pain, control of pain, pathways to care, and preventive measures concerning pain. The questionnaire contained 28 questions, of which most were multiple-choice or true/false questions, while some were open-ended questions.

The qualitative structured interview[38] on pain among the Quichuas was conducted using the *Nanay Jahua Tapuicuna* questionnaire. The study was a researcher-administered structured interview. The interviews were conducted in the Quichua language by a Quichua assistant native to the Rumipamba area. The questionnaire was administered verbally to all participants, including to those who had some years of schooling, for they unanimously preferred to respond to questions verbally.

The Quichuas who participated in our survey were 25 men and 15 women, aged 15 to 58 with a mean age of 32. They had completed very basic schooling; the average was 3.7 years (range 0 to 9). The main occupations of participants were: (a) merchants (mostly selling food); (b) weavers; and (c) farmers. Eighty-five percent of participants were married, 7.5% single, 5% widows, and 2.5 divorced. The vast majority were Catholics (95%).

THE QUICHUAS' PAIN EXPERIENCE

Contrary to common belief among the *mishu* in Ecuador, the Quichuas enjoy talking about pain and illness. They have an exquisite narrative and sophisticated theories on pain causation, predisposing factors, aggravating factors, clinical features, and diagnostic and treatment strategies. They not only hold elaborated concepts on pain prevention, but understand the value of social and community support, as well as the usefulness of good coping skills.

Origins of pain

Our survey revealed that the Quichuas hold a multifaceted notion of pain causation. For them, psychosocial factors, physical conditions (e.g., injury) and supernatural forces play important roles in the origin of pain.

Remarkably, psychosocial and supernatural causes were mentioned more frequently than physical conditions to explain the appearance of pain by our participants. Practically all respondents believed negative life events, losses, misfortunes, and *llaquicuna* can cause pain. *Llaqui* or the plural *Llaquicuna* is a complex Quichua concept referring to negative life events, sadness, and an illness category that resembles anxiety and depression.[39] Similarly, the great majority of respondents thought malign spirits (present in objects, animals, and humans) and sorcery can cause pain (see Table 7.1).

Although respondents did mention physical conditions such as wounds, trauma, and underlying diseases as causes of pain, 27% of them believed such physical injuries do not always cause pain. Interestingly, poor eating and personal hygiene, along with excessive work and fatigue, were also mentioned as potential causes of pain by a few participants. Local Quichua illnesses, including *mancharishca* (caused by sudden fright) and *wairashca* (caused by wind spirits), were also mentioned as potential causes of painful conditions.

Vulnerability to pain

According to our Quichua participants, some people are more susceptible than others to suffering from pain. The majority (84%) agreed that the elderly are the most vulnerable. An important proportion (65%) believed married people are prone to experiencing pain due to their economic and social responsibilities. In contrast, 91% believed single people do not suffer from pain due to their lack of familial and economic responsibilities; most of them are economically dependent on their parents. Third, among the most vulnerable are women, according to 57% of our respondents. Approximately half of the respondents believed newborns, young girls and boys, are very sensitive to pain. When questioned "Who else is vulnerable to pain?" our respondents mentioned the sick and the ones weakened by a disease. Some said that everybody is at risk of experiencing pain.

Responses to pain

The Quichua respondents appear to have an elaborated knowledge of the psychological and somatic effects of pain. Although their complex views on pain may suggest they are highly

TABLE 7.1 Origins of Pain

Attributed causes	N (40)	%
Negative life events, *llaquicuna*	39	97.5%
Malign spirits (objects, animals, humans)	38	95.0%
Sorcery	36	90.0%
Physical conditions (wounds, trauma)	29	72.5%
Underlying diseases	23	57.5%

Note: Respondents could answer more than one question and therefore the percentages do not total 100%. The sample includes males and females.

concerned with pain and its effects, they seem to favor a stoical attitude towards coping with pain.

It is remarkable that all interviewees agreed that a person with pain becomes depressed and profoundly tired or weak when in pain. The majority (two-thirds or more) thought people in pain become extremely irritable, anxious, fearful, and prone to crying/moaning easily. The consensus was equally strong concerning the somatic effects of pain as viewed in Table 7.2.

The majority believed that pain negatively impacts their appetite and sleep; it can prevent one from falling asleep and can affect one's sleep quality. Some of our respondents mentioned that pain limits the mobility of the sufferer and makes it difficult for him/her to walk and accomplish daily tasks. All our respondents believed that long-lasting or severe pain could be the cause of serious illness and even death. According to our respondents, pain can kill a person, so it is of serious concern to the sufferer and his/her relatives.

Now turning to their attitudes about coping with pain, 92% believed that remembering or thinking about a past pain experience could trigger pain. Moaning and complaining about pain was viewed as a sign of weakness by 78% of our interviewees. Although 55% believed that complaining does not help relieve pain, 29% believed it could help one endure pain. When asked whether they could endure any kind of pain, 33% responded positively, 54% believe they could endure pain to a certain extent, and 13% said they could not. For 31% of them, pain is not an important event or an experience with health implications. However, 92% preferred an effective treatment with immediate results when in pain. They did not express interest in knowing the cause of their pain before receiving an appropriate pain treatment. Effectively, our data suggests only a very few would be willing to wait to know further about the cause of their pain.

Aggravating factors

According to the Quichua, a wide range of factors including psychological disorders, physical diseases, and lifestyle can increase the severity of pain. The most frequently mentioned cluster of factors that can increase the severity of pain are the following: sadness, blues, worries, ruminating about problems, or suffering from *llaqui* (depression-anxiety illness category). This view was held by 97.5% of the interviewees.

TABLE 7.2 Responses to Pain

Effects of Pain	N (40)	%
Psychological		
Sadness and severe fatigue	40	100
Irritability, anxiety, fearf	39	97.5
Crying and moaning	32	80
Somatic		
Serious illness	40	100
Death	40	100
Lost of appetite	37	92.5
Sleep disturbances	36	90

Note: Respondents could answer more than one question and therefore the percentages do not total 100%. The sample includes males and females.

A quite unexpected finding was the view that exposure to cold or warm air drafts could also aggravate the severity of pain. Ninety percent believed cold drafts or sudden exposure to cold temperatures (locally, temperatures ranging between 10 to 18 degrees Celsius can be considered as cold) could increase pain. Only 10% believed cold is not related to an increase in pain. Interestingly, exposure to hot temperatures is also believed, by 74%, to increase pain severity.

A weaker agreement exists concerning the effect of comorbid conditions on pain. Sixty-two percent of respondents believed that the concomitant existence of other diseases can increase pain severity. For 38%, however, comorbidity is not related to an increase in pain severity.

Finally, respondents believed that lifestyle factors such as poor eating habits and lack of personal care and hygiene can aggravate pain.

Timeline and duration of pain

When asked whether pain appears preferentially in the morning, afternoon, night, or at midnight, most of our interviewees responded that it can appear essentially at any time. All respondents agreed that pain most frequently starts at night or midnight. Some people added that pain starts at a certain time of day depending on the underlying disease or illness.

Questioned on whether pain could persist for minutes, hours, or days, most respondents (95%) said that it could last for just minutes or persist for days. It is interesting to underline that for the Quichua, pain is usually present day and night. They also noted that pain could be episodic, with periods of intense pain and periods of relief.

Location of pain

According to the Quichua, the three most frequent locations of pain are the head, back, and abdomen. Other locations are listed in Table 7.3.

Types of pain

The best known and most frequently mentioned types of pain are headache, back pain, tooth pain, and abdominal pain (see Table 7.4). Four local Quichua illnesses are mentioned

TABLE 7.3 Locations of Pain

Location	N (40)	%
Head	37	93
Back	32	80
Abdomen	26	65
Heart	24	60
Hands	8	20

Mentioned by less than 16% of respondents: Legs, arms, foot, ears, eyes, tooth, and bone.

Note: Respondents could answer more than one question and therefore the percentages do not total 100%. The sample includes males and females.

TABLE 7.4 Types of Pain

Types	N (40)	%
Headache	30	75
Back pain	25	62.25
Tooth pain	19	47.5
Abdominal pain	11	27.5

Below are types of pain mentioned by very few respondents; therefore they are listed for information purposes only.

Pain related to *llaqui* subtypes: *Shuncu nanay* (seizure-like episodes) *Wairashca* pain, *Mancharishca* pain, *colerin* pain.

Pain located in anatomical regions and organs: lungs, bone, hernia, arms, chest, foot, muscle, eye, ear.

Pain related to diseases such as: cholera, parasitosis, tuberculosis, and calluses on hands and feet.

Note: Respondents could answer more than one question and therefore the percentages do not total 100%. The sample includes males and females.

by some interviewees as producing pain. The four categories listed here are subtypes of *llaqui* (depression-anxiety like syndrome),[39] a widespread Quichua illness experience: (1) *shuncu nanay* (seizure-like episodes); (2) *wairashca* (victims of malign spirits mobilized by the wind); (3) *mancharishca* (victim of malign spirits accruing after a sudden fright); and (4) *colerin* (experience of intense anger). These types of pain are distinctively unique to the Quichua culture.

Most severe pain reported

When the survey participants were asked to name a few of the most severe pains they knew, they mentioned a wide array of pains. Most agreed, however, that the following were the most severe types of pain: (1) pain caused by cholera-vibrio cholerae infection (73%); (2) pain caused by tuberculosis (56%); (3) certain types of headaches (32.5%); (4) abdominal pain (22.5%); and (5) tooth pain (30%). Other types of pain also considered to be severe included the following: pain caused by *llaqui* (depression-anxiety illness category), liver pain, chest pain, colic, muscle pain, pain caused by wounds, childbirth pain, ear pain, and pain caused by malaria. It is remarkable that only one person referred to cancer pain as the most severe pain known.

Quichua descriptors of pain

The Quichua in the Andes have a rich ensemble of descriptors for describing their pain experience. When invited to provide descriptors for their pain experience, the majority (80% or more) agreed that pain can have one or more of the following characteristics:

- Burning
- Blistering (something of lesser severity that burning)
- Itching

- Extremely debilitating (producing extreme weakness)
- Sickening
- Piercing (as a needle entering the flesh)
- Making breathing difficult or extremely difficult
- Inducing nausea and vomiting
- Pulsating
- Shooting
- Excruciating
- Unbearable (makes you want to die)
- Untreatable (so severe that no treatment could relieve pain)
- Like an electrical shock
- Like a living entity (behaves as a living being)
- Colic type
- Causing severe continuous cramps

Coping with pain

We explored this topic by asking some questions relating to who should treat pain and how pain should be treated. Nearly 85% of respondents believed pain does not disappear spontaneously and that therefore, seeking appropriate treatment is essential. Only 15 % admitted pain could remit spontaneously with time. Strikingly, 80% held the belief that distractions and efforts to ignore the pain are the best coping mechanisms.

It is remarkable that all our interviewees believed that both traditional healers and physicians can successfully treat pain. However, they admitted other individuals can also act as effective health agents. For example, 97% of them believed relatives and neighbors can help control pain. To our question of whether children can be helpful in controlling pain, all responded that children are unlikely to be of help. For their preferred ways to cope with pain, see Table 7.5.

Preventive measures

We found that participants attributed a preventive or protective role against pain to a disparate and interesting group of factors, especially when dealing with chronic pain. One unexpected factor was "not abusing our bodies and mind" with extreme acts or emotions.

TABLE 7.5 Pathways to Care

Agents of care	N (40)	%
Doctors	37	92.5
Healers	33	82.5
At home with herbs	15	37.5
Pharmaceuticals	7	17.5
Others: seeking help from relatives and neighbors, taking care themselves.		

Note: Respondents could answer more than one question and therefore the percentages do not total 100%. The sample includes males and females.

Extenuation from hard physical work, exposure to cold temperatures, worries about children, not earning enough money, exposure to frightening events, and extreme anger, among others, were mentioned as abuse of the body and mind. Therefore, balance and composure was recommended.

Interestingly, 90% of our respondents believed that education on matters related to pain, illness, and disease can prevent pain conditions. It was widely accepted (by 97%) as a good practice to take care of one's health, including visiting physicians, with the belief that it will favor early detection of pain-generating conditions. Personal hygiene and consumption of nutritious food were also mentioned as protective factors against pain.

DISCUSSION

Our survey on pain experience conducted among the Quichua in the northern highlands of Ecuador shows that they have a complex theory on the nature of pain, and strategies to cope with pain. Although we have chosen to explore and focus on the clinically relevant aspects of pain, it was also possible to note that the Quichua volunteers appeared to be familiar with all the dimensions of human pain, except, understandably, the neurobiological dimension of pain. Although they share commonalties with other societies studied, the pain experience of the Quichuas has quite distinct characteristics. As previously stated by pain researchers, culture is known to influence the way a person experiences and responds to pain.[2, 40, 41]

The Quichuas' multifactorial theory of pain causation comprises psychosocial and supernatural notions that are closely related to their theories of illness and worldview. Negative life events including the loss of loved ones, financial strains, and failure to maintain good relationships with neighbors, among others, seem to be important in originating illness, disease, and pain.[39,42] The Quichua emphasis on psychosocial causes of pain contrasts with the view of local Ecuadorian *mishu* medical practitioners who think the Quichua use a set of irrational or primitive beliefs to explain pain.[39] Nonetheless, supernatural explanations of pain remain important among the Quichua. This is in line with Murdock's observations when surveying the theories of illness from around the world, which revealed that supernatural explanations of illness and disease were among the most frequent.[43] It is now clear that the Quichua theory of pain causation includes both psychosocial and supernatural factors.

Turning to their beliefs about vulnerability to pain and its severity, the three groups most prone to suffer from pain are the elderly, married people, and women. Interestingly, this is concordant with published reports indicating that clinical pain is more prevalent among women and the elderly.[44–46] Interestingly, the Quichua consider married people as one of the groups most vulnerable to pain. This is consistent with the Quichua theory of emotional causation of illness and pain. According to the Quichua, married people are particularly concerned with raising a family and providing for it, educating their children, running a business, taking care of domestic animals, and cultivating their lands. Marriage clearly comes with several responsibilities and stressors. Everyday difficulties, life events, as well as social and interpersonal frictions can all potentially contribute, when severe, in originating illness, disease, and pain. The *llaquicuna* is a Quichua term that denotes suffering, fright, anger, worries, feelings of rejection, and sadness. It has been reported to be related with mental illness, especially depressive and anxiety disorders.[39,42] Because single people in the Andes usually live with their parents, they are viewed as people without serious responsibilities, and therefore protected from stressors and *llaquicuna*, and less susceptible to pain. Knowing some cultural details, and recognizing some striking parallels between the

Quichua belief system on pain and the scientific literature on predisposing factors, could facilitate patient-doctor communications, the sharing of views on susceptible groups, and the planning of pain-control strategies.

Strong emotional experiences hold an important place in the Quichuas' concept of the origin of psychological or physical illnesses, and are probably an ethos of the Quichuas of the Andes. Pain could be added to the list of factors that the Quichua view as potential causes of psychological suffering and diseases, including death. The Quichua interviewees demonstrated to possess a strong integrative biopsychosocial view of pain, considering pain as possibly leading to depression, anxiety, irritability, fearfulness, tiredness, sleep disturbances, poor appetite, and a range of serious diseases. That being said, some of their attitudes towards pain can be labeled as stoical. For example, moaning and complaining about pain was considered a sign of weakness by two-thirds of our interviewees, although they do not refrain from talking about pain. Thinking about or remembering pain is discouraged by the majority, which believes doing so will worsen or trigger the pain. This clearly is a cognitive strategy to deny or suppress pain. Overall, 87% responded they could endure any kind of pain. This stoical attitude is similar to what Zborowski noted among the Irish-Americans, who usually devalued the importance of their pain, and put the emphasis on learning to trivialize pain.[2] For the extremely impoverished Quichua people in the Andes,[47,48] where the poverty rate is 85% (living on $2 per day or less), complaining about pain with the aim of obtaining care is a useless strategy. It is better and more practical to learn how to endure pain, or ask the help of family members or traditional healers. Therefore, for the health practitioner, usually a *mishu* outsider, a Quichua patient may look defeated and passive in dealing with pain. It is remarkable that 80% of our interviewees favored ignoring pain as a coping strategy. This behavior is understandable considering that health care services are scarce for the majority of the millions of Quichua people and specialized services such as psychiatric care or pain control are nonexistent.[49]

With surprising similarity to biomedical and current psychological theories, the Quichua hold a firm view that emotions and comorbidity can aggravate pain. The central role of emotions in the origins and severity of illness, disease, and pain must be underscored. Some authors recognize that this emotional component is an important part of the widespread Latin American (Latino) theory of illness, which is rooted in Amerindian cultures.[50] The notion that exposure to relatively mild cold or hot temperatures could aggravate pain is another important feature of the Quichua belief system and those of other populations in Latin America.[51] Being aware that the Quichua patient could reject the use of warm or light clothing, reject the application of cold or warm pads to painful areas, or expect certain temperatures for their beverages and food, is useful for the pain clinician who could ask for a the patient's preferences and negotiate appropriate actions. The hot-cold theory is complex and present in many countries in Latin America.[51] It is not always related strictly to the actual temperature. It is widely accepted among the Quichua that food, plants, and medicines have intrinsic properties related to hot or cold, regardless of their temperature; for example white sugar is considered cold, while brown sugar is hot; the same goes for white bread and brown-color bread. Similarly, truly cold temperatures are viewed as a causal and aggravating factor for pain; therefore, Quichua patients can be reluctant to accept a pad of ice as treatment for acute pain caused by an injury.

The view that having specific dietary and hygiene habits can contribute to preventing pain, which some Quichuas hold, is unexpected and new in the region. It is probably the result of health education programs implemented in the last two decades by nongovernmental organizations and the Ecuadorian government. Those programs were intended to promote hygiene and eating good food in order to prevent malnutrition and infectious diseases (such as a severe epidemic of cholera, which affected the Imbabura region in 1996). Therefore, some Quichua people believe hygiene and good food can help control pain, decrease pain severity, or prevent pain. It is worth noting the salience of cholera when Quichuas try to determine the three most severe types of pain. The cholera epidemics that affected Ecuador during most of the 1990s clearly put this infectious disease in the forefront of the list of severely painful conditions.

The pathways to pain care that the Quichua people prefer are inclusive and pluralistic. The medical pluralism described in the Andes[52] resembles the new pluralism found among patients in the United States.[53] The Quichua of Imbabura, Ecuador, strongly embrace biomedicine and physicians, as well as Quichua traditional medicine and traditional healers, as sources of health care and pain control. Nonetheless, they have a preference for medicinal plants over pharmaceutical products. In addition, what differentiates them from patients in Western countries is the acceptance of family members and neighbors as valuable sources of care.

CLOSING REMARKS

The knowledge of some elements of the Quichuas' pain experience and their strategies to cope with it could help improve the clinical skills of pain practitioners who are working within a multicultural society or among patients from a cultural background different than their own. For instance, the knowledge that emotions, life events, comorbid conditions, and spirits, among other factors, play an important role in the origin of pain among the Quichuas could facilitate fruitful negotiations during the formulation of diagnoses. Becoming familiar with patients' preferences for inclusive and pluralistic care, including biomedical or traditional medicine methods, could facilitate the preparation of treatment plans, as well as patients' successful adherence to treatment recommendations.[54,55] Patient and family satisfaction could ensue from a culturally sensitive practice. Through a better understanding of patients' cultural preferences, pain professionals could, for instance, foster many patients' embrace for the support that family members and neighbors provide them. Effectively, they are often considered a valuable source of health care and pain control, as is the case among the Quichuas in the Andes. Consequently, what we have learned from the Quichuas' pain experience could contribute to gaining cultural competence in the cross-cultural clinical encounter. Finally, the knowledge of emic details of pain experience among the Quichuas of the Andes could be helpful for the health practitioner who is making efforts to provide high-quality medical care in rural and remote communities around the world.

ACKNOWLEDGMENT

This study was supported by a Doctoral Research Award granted by the Government of Quebec, Fonds FCAR, Canada. Many thanks to the Quichua people of Rumipamba in Imbabura, Ecuador for their support and participation. My deepest gratitude goes to the late Mr. Alberto Cacuango, a remarkable community leader and field research assistant, for his unconditional support in this study and for his friendship.

REFERENCES

1. Zborowski M. Cultural components in responses to pain. *J Soc Issues.* 1952;8(4):16–30.
2. Zborowski M. *People in Pain.* San Francisco: Jossey-Bass; 1969.

3. Zola IK. Culture and symptoms—an analysis of patients' presenting complaints. *Am Sociol Rev.* Oct 1966;31(5):615–630.

4. Wolff BB, Langley S. Cultural factors and the response to pain: a review. *Am Anthropol.* 1968;70:494–501.

5. Edwards CL, Fillingim RB, Keefe F. Race, ethnicity and pain. *Pain.* Nov 2001;94(2):133–137.

6. Zatzick DF, Dimsdale JE. Cultural variations in response to painful stimuli. *Psychosom Med.* Sep 1990;52(5):544–557.

7. Chapman CR, Sato T, Martin RW, et al. Comparative effects of acupuncture in Japan and the United States on dental pain perception. *Pain.* Apr 1982;12(4):319–328.

8. Campbell CM, Edwards RR, Fillingim RB. Ethnic differences in responses to multiple experimental pain stimuli. *Pain.* Jan 2005;113(1–2):20–26.

9. Young EE, Lariviere WR, Belfer I. Genetic basis of pain variability: recent advances. *J Med Genet.* Nov 2012;49(1):1–9.

10. Clark WC, Clark SB. Pain responses in Nepalese porters. *Science.* Jul 18 1980;209(4454):410–412.

11. Sternbach RA, Tursky B. Ethnic differences among housewives in psychophysical and skin potential responses to electric shock. *Psychophysiology.* 1965;1:241–246.

12. Woodrow KM, Friedman GD, Siegelaub AB, Collen MF. Pain tolerance: differences according to age, sex and race. *Psychosom Med.* Nov 1972;34(6):548–556.

13. Thomas VJ, Rose FD. Ethnic differences in the experience of pain. *Soc Sci Med.* 1991;32(9):1063–1066.

14. Edwards RR, Doleys DM, Fillingim RB, Lowery D. Ethnic differences in pain tolerance: clinical implications in a chronic pain population. *Psychosom Med.* Mar 2001;63(2):316–323.

15. Bates MS. *Biocultural dimensions of chronic pain—implications for treatment of multi-ethnic populations.* Albany: State University of New York Press; 1996.

16. Davitz LJ, Sameshima Y, Davitz J. Suffering as viewed in six different cultures. *Am J Nurs.* Aug 1976;76(8):1296–1297.

17. Good MJD. *Pain as Human Experience—An Anthropological Perspective.* Berkeley: University of California Press; 1994.

18. Moore R, Miller ML, Weinstein P, Dworkin SF, Liou HH. Cultural perceptions of pain and pain coping among patients and dentists. *Community Dent Oral Epidemiol.* Dec 1986;14(6):327–333.

19. Lau EM, Egger P, Coggon D, Cooper C, Valenti L, O'Connell D. Low back pain in Hong Kong: prevalence and characteristics compared with Britain. *J Epidemiol Community Health.* Oct 1995;49(5):492–494.

20. Weber SE. Cultural aspects of pain in childbearing women. *J Obstet Gynecol Neonatal Nurs.* Jan 1996;25(1):67–72.

21. Nelson DV, Novy DM, Averill PM, Berry LA. Ethnic comparability of the MMPI in pain patients. *J Clin Psychol.* Sep 1996;52(5):485–497.

22. Abu-Saad H. Cultural group indicators of pain in children. *Matern Child* Nurs J. 1984;13(3):187–196.

23. Sargent C. Between death and shame: dimensions of pain in Bariba culture. *Soc Sci Med.* 1984;19(12):1299–1304.

24. Pesce G. Measurement of reported pain of childbirth: a comparison between Australian and Italian subjects. *Pain.* Oct 1987;31(1):87–92.

25. Strassberg DS, Tilley D, Bristone S, Oei TPS. The MMPI and chronic pain: A cross-cultural view. *Psychol Assess.* 1992;4(4):493–497.

26. Lipton JA, Marbach JJ. Ethnicity and the pain experience. *Soc Sci Med.* 1984;19(12):1279–1298.

27. Jagger RG, Woolley SM, Savio L. Signs and symptoms of temporomandibular disorders in Ecuadorian Indians. *J Oral Rehabil.* Apr 2004;31(4):293–297.

28. Darghouth S, Pedersen D, Bibeau G, Rousseau C. Painful languages of the body: experiences of headache among women in two Peruvian communities. *Cult Med Psychiatry.* Sep 2006;30(3):271–297.

29. Carod-Artal FJ, Vazquez-Cabrera C. An anthropological study about headache and migraine in native cultures from Central and South America. *Headache.* Jun 2007;47(6):834–841.

30. Pernick MS. *A calculus of suffering—pain, professionalism, and anesthesia in nineteenth-century America.* New York: Columbia University Press; 1985.

31. Clark EB. "The sacred rights of the weak": pain, sympathy, and the culture of individual rights in antebellum America. *The Journal of American History.* 1995;82(2):463–493.

32. Pernick MS. "They don't feel it like we do": Social politics and the perception of pain. *A calculus of suffering—pain, professionalism, and anesthesia in nineteenth-century America.* New York: Columbia University Press; 1985:148–167.

33. Incayawar M, Maldonado-Bouchard S. The forsaken mental health of the Indigenous Peoples—a moral case of outrageous exclusion in Latin America. *BMC Int Health Hum Rights.* Oct 29 2009;9(1):27.

34. Incayawar M, Saucier JF. Pain in remote Andean communities—learning from Quichua (Inca) experience. *Rural Remote Health.* Apr 2010;10(3):1379.

35. Casagrande JB. Strategies for survival: the Indians of highland Ecuador. In: Whitten NE Jr, ed. *Cultural Transformations and Ethnicity in Modern Ecuador.* Urbana: University of Illinois Press; 1981:260–277.

36. Berger TR. *A long and terrible shadow—white values, native rights in the Americas, 1492–1992.* Vancouver: Douglas & McIntyre; 1991.

37. Moore R. Combining qualitative and quantitative research approaches in understanding pain. *J Dent Educ.* Aug 1996;60(8):709–715.

38. Gill P, Stewart K, Treasure E, Chadwick B. Methods of data collection in qualitative research: interviews and focus groups. *Br Dent J.* Mar 22 2008;204(6):291–295.

39. Maldonado MG. *Llaqui et dépression; une étude exploratoire chez les Quichuas (Équateur)*[thesis]. Montreal, QC: McGill University; 1992.

40. Fabrega H Jr, Tyma S. Language and cultural influences in the description of pain. *Br J Med Psycho.l* Dec 1976;49(4):349–371.

41. Bates MS. Ethnicity and pain: a biocultural model. *Soc Sci Med.* 1987;24(1):47–50.

42. Tousignant M, Maldonado M. Sadness, depression and social reciprocity in highland Ecuador. *Soc Sci Med.* 1989;28(9):899–904.

43. Murdock GP. *Theories of Illness: A World Survey.* Pittsburgh: University of Pittsburgh Press; 1980.

44. International Association for the Study of Pain, Task Force on Epidemiology, Crombie IK. *Epidemiology of pain—a report of the Task Force on Epidemiology of the International Association for the Study of Pain.* Seattle: IASP Press; 1999.

45. Elliott AM, Smith BH, Penny KI, Smith WC, Chambers WA. The epidemiology of chronic pain in the community. *Lancet.* Oct 9 1999;354(9186):1248–1252.

46. Wilson JF. The pain divide between men and women. *Ann Intern Med.* Mar 21 2006;144(6):461–464.

47. Van Nieuwkoop M, Uquillas JE. *Defining Ethnodevelopment in Operational Terms: Lessons from the Ecuador Indigenous and Afro-Ecuadoran Peoples Development Project.* Washington, DC: The World Bank; 2000.

48. Psacharopoulos G, Patrinos H. Indigenous People and poverty in Latin America. *Finance and Development.* Mar 1994:41–43.

49. Incayawar M. Indigenous peoples of South America—inequalities in mental health care. In: Bhui K, Bhugra D, eds. *Culture and Mental Health—a Comprehensive Textbook.* London, UK: Hodder Arnold; 2007:185–190.

50. Foster GM. Relationships between Spanish and Spanish-American folk medicine. *J Am Folklore.* 1953;66:201–217.

51. Currier RL. The hot-cold syndrome and symbolic balance in Mexican and Spanish-American folk medicine. *Ethnology.* 1966;5:251–263.

52. Koss-Chioino J, Leatherman TL, Greenway C. *Medical Pluralism in the Andes.* London: Routledge; 2003.

53. Kaptchuk TJ, Eisenberg DM. Varieties of healing. 1: medical pluralism in the United States. *Ann Intern Med.* Aug 7 2001;135(3):189–195.

54. Kleinman A. Culture, illness, and care: clinical lessons from anthropological and cross-cultural research. *Ann Intern Med.* 1978;88:251–258.

55. Gaw A. *Culture, Ethnicity, and Mental illness.* Washington, DC: American Psychiatric Press; 1993.

8

ALLYING WITH CHINESE PARENTS FOR ENHANCED CONTROL OF PEDIATRIC POSTOPERATIVE PAIN

HE HONG-GU, PHD, RN, MD
Assistant Professor, Alice Lee Centre for Nursing Studies, Yong Loo Lin School of Medicine, National University of Singapore, Singapore

KATRI VEHVILÄINEN-JULKUNEN, RN, PHD
Professor, Department of Nursing Science, Faculty of Health Sciences, University of Eastern Finland, Kuopio, Finland

Key Points
- Postoperative pain management for Chinese children is often suboptimal.
- Chinese culture may more readily expect and accept pain, as compared to some Western cultures.
- Understanding Chinese pain-related values and beliefs is important to interpreting a child's pain experience.
- Chinese parents experience a variety of negative emotions during their child's hospitalization for surgery.
- Clinicians should understand common postoperative pain-relief methods used by Chinese parents.
- Fear of addiction and side effects of analgesics are common among health professionals and patients.
- Excessive government regulation of opioid analgesic use in China serves as a barrier to optimal pain treatment.
- Parental feelings of usefulness and competency can be enhanced when they are involved in their child's care.

INTRODUCTION

China had a population of 1.3 billion in 2009, consisting of 56 ethnic groups.[1] Han is the largest of these ethnic groups, accounting for 92% of the population. Therefore, Han is considered the majority while other ethnic groups are termed minorities. These 55 minority ethnic groups are distributed widely throughout China. Many groups have been living in close proximity with Han people for centuries and their values and culture are very similar to those of Han people. Because of the multiple ethnicities in China, considerations of Chinese culture are complex. In most ethnic studies, "Chinese culture" and "Han culture" are viewed as indistinguishable. Researchers cautioned that classifying an individual as "Chinese" may gloss over large interethnic cultural differences in China.[2] Outside China itself, the Chinese are one of the most populous ethnicities worldwide.[3] Therefore, it is important to understand Chinese pain-related values and beliefs in order to provide culturally sensitive care to Chinese patients, whether in China or in other parts of the world.

The goal of this chapter is to provide insights into Chinese values and belief systems related to pain, by focusing on the attitudes, perceptions, and preferences of Chinese parents of hospitalized children in pain. Specifically, the following topics are included: Chinese values and beliefs related to pain experience, barriers to high-quality pain management in Chinese patients, Chinese parents' emotional feelings during their child's hospitalization for surgery, pain-relief methods used by Chinese parents for their children's postoperative pain, parents' perception of nursing support, parents' recommendations for health professionals in order to provide better postoperative pain care, and culturally competent care provided to children and their parents.

RATIONALE FOR FOCUSING ON CHINESE PARENTS' ATTITUDES, PERCEPTIONS AND PREFERENCES IN PEDIATRIC POSTOPERATIVE PAIN MANAGEMENT

Postoperative pain management for children has been deemed inadequate in many cultures.[4–7] Studies conducted in China report that most school-aged children experienced moderate and severe pain postoperatively, based on ratings by both children[6] and parents.[8]

Involving parents in pain care is beneficial both for child and parent[9–10] and may optimize pain management given that parents possess unique expertise in understanding and interpreting their child's behavior.[11–13] Generally, children readily convey their feelings of pain to a parent, but hesitate to inform a nurse. Parents are the best advocates for their children when pain is poorly managed and parents can also alert nurses to their child's concern.[12] Parents can define terms their children use to describe pain or predict how prior experience with pain might influence a child's outward behavior.[10] Caregivers must interpret the behaviors or reports generated by the patient in a socio-communication context where both the culture of the caregiver and the assumed culture of the patient have an impact.[2] Thus, the parental role is very important in terms of interpreting their children's pain behaviors and reports of postoperative pain. Previous research found that compared with nurses' ratings, parents' ratings of their children's pain are closer to the child's own ratings. [2,14–16]

Parental feelings of usefulness and competency can be enhanced when they are involved in their child's care.[17] Review papers related to parental roles in the care of a hospitalized child summarize that—with approval from nurses and with parents' increased confidence and competencies as caregivers—parents have strong desires and expectations to participate in their child's care during hospitalization, including performing many of their usual caregiving tasks.[18–19] However, parents often experience problems, such as lack of information and instruction in their child's postoperative pain management,[11,20–25] feelings of isolation or poor communication with nurses,[12,22,26]feelings of ignorance in relation to pain management, and being underutilized as a resource by health professionals.[27] All these obstacles might reduce the extent of parents' participation in their child's care. For example, some investigators[28–29] demonstrate that parents tend to underestimate pain intensity and under-medicate children for pain because (1) they have difficulty in estimating the children's pain intensity; (2) have not received instruction on pain assessment; and (3) lack knowledge of what appropriate actions to take.[9,12,20,22,23,25,26,30] Parents hold some misconceptions about pain treatment and they worry about analgesic side effects, tolerance, and even addiction, among their children.[31] Hence, they often use as little medication as possible or only as a last resort.[32]

In summary, many factors can affect parents playing an active role in their child's postoperative pain care. In mainland China, parents play a very important role in the care of their hospitalized children, especially if the child is their only child. China initiated a one-child policy in the 1980s and most couples have only one child. This only child is the center of the family. Therefore, one can assume that Chinese parents' role in taking care of a child who undergoes surgery may be even more maximized. It is of interest to know Chinese parents' attitudes, perceptions, and preferences when they are dealing with their hospitalized children in pain.

CHINESE CULTURE RELATED TO PAIN EXPERIENCE AND MANAGEMENT

Culture is often used as a proxy term for race or ethnicity.[2] Culture consists of many different concepts, such as religion, gender roles, language, and the view of older generations' role in society, all of which can create a barrier to adequate pain management.[33] The definition of pain is culturally influenced.[34] Six dimensions of pain have been identified by McGuire.[35] These include physiologic, sensory, affective, cognitive, behavioral, and social-cultural dimensions of pain. The author suggests that the socio-cultural dimensions of pain experience include demographic characteristics (e.g., age, sex, and race); ethnic background; and cultural, spiritual, religious, and social factors that influence an individual's perceptions of, and responses to, pain. Cultural background is an important aspect of the socio-cultural dimension of pain, because persons from different cultures perceive and respond to pain in different ways.

Culture plays an important role in beliefs and convictions of parents and health professionals regarding pediatric perioperative care.[36–37] Culture significantly affects pain assessment and management.[38] Our perceptions, meanings, attitudes, expressions, and care of pain are embedded in a cultural context. It is believed that the patients' culture does influence their pain behavior;[39]pain threshold and pain tolerance level;[40–42] pain perception or expression;[38–40,43] and pain coping,[43] as well as treatment preferences,[44] and consequently may influence individual pain experiences.[38,39,45] Many studies report significant differences in drug metabolism, dosing requirements, therapeutic response, and side effects among patients from different racial and ethnic groups.[46]

Historically, Chinese have treated pain as a disease entity, rather than a mere symptom.[31,47] Health professionals, children, and parents often regard postoperative pain as inevitable and to be tolerated to some extent [48] without resorting to analgesics.[49] Chinese culture may more readily expect and accept pain, as compared to some Western societies in which people expect pain, but do not expect to tolerate it as inevitable.[50] The philosophical and religious beliefs of Taoism, Buddhism, and Confucianism exert a major influence on Chinese perspectives on pain and pain-related behaviors.[47]

Confucianism heavily influences Chinese people's values and belief systems.
[51]Confucianism teaches that one should not do unto others what one does not want others to do unto oneself. If one suffers from pain, one should bear the burden alone, although one may derive some comfort from sympathetic relatives and friends.[47] Therefore, when a person suffers from pain, he or she would rather endure the pain and not report it to a clinician until the pain becomes unbearable.[49,52] Sometimes, patients will report pain only to close family members and ask the family members to report the pain to a member of the healthcare team.[53] This phenomenon is even more obvious in Chinese men. Chinese culture socializes men early in their childhood to be stoic and to hide pain when in public because it is a sign of weakness to do otherwise.[54,55] Men are not allowed to cry and express their emotions publicly.[56] Thus, Chinese men tend to be more passive in responding to pain and expressing their feelings than women. This is, in fact, similar to some Western cultures.[57]

Stoicism means repression of emotion, such as tolerance of pain, or indifference to pain as an adaptive coping strategy, and it is considered a positive trait for the Chinese. Stoicism in the sense of lack of expressiveness of pain is often associated with particular cultures, such as British in the American imagination.[57] However, a recent study does not support this prevalent view, [3] finding no difference in stoic attitudes between healthy Chinese and European or Canadian young adults experiencing acute pain. Explanations offered for the lack of stoicism include: Chinese attitudes of inhibition of emotions may not be generalized to acute pain situations, the endorsement of stoic attitudes with pain may be more pronounced in an older Chinese sample, and the influence of Confucianism may be declining in Chinese society as young Chinese people have more opportunities to explore and adapt to Western culture, especially those who have lived in other countries for a few years. Chinese participants tend to show more concern for their health and pursue good quality of life, and are more likely to request pain relief than ever, especially during the perioperative period.[31] Another important reason may be that all study subjects in the study by Hsieh et al were female.[3] Females in Chinese culture are allowed to show weakness and express their pain.[56] This gender difference between Chinese parents and their management of the postoperative pain of their boys or girls is reflected in a study conducted in China;[8] for example, fathers used positive reinforcement methods more frequently with their children than mothers, and both fathers and mothers used positive reinforcement more frequently with boys than girls.

In addition, fatalism (the belief that all events are predetermined and inevitable) and preference for specific complementary and alternative medicine approaches have important implications in symptom treatment among Chinese patients. Fatalism, a core construct in Chinese culture, also may affect pain expression and desire for treatment and the preference for treatment modalities.[58] Chinese patients tend to prefer specific complementary and alternative medicine approaches such as Traditional Chinese Medicine, acupuncture, and Chinese massage.

BARRIERS LEADING TO POOR MANAGEMENT OF PAIN IN CHINESE PATIENTS

Although it has improved over the last decade in China, pain management remains a critical patient care issue.[6,8,31] Aside from culture, other factors serve to limit pain management practices.[31] These factors include:

1. Excessive government regulation of pain medication use. Previously, opioids were strictly controlled by the government. The situation has been getting better since 1991 and the majority of health professionals consider the national policy of opioid

use restrictive, but adequate to satisfy clinical needs.[59] However, the morphine consumption per capita in China was very low (0.32mg), as compared to that of other Western countries (e.g., highest amount was 115.72 mg in Austria in 2004).[60]

2. Fear of addiction and side effects of pain medication by health professionals and patients themselves.[31]
3. Inadequate pain assessment and health professionals' lack of knowledge about pain management.[37]
4. Lack of access to more powerful analgesics[31] or poor-quality medicine.[61]
5. Economic reasons.[2,62] Some patients, especially those who need to use analgesics long-term, may choose not to use pain medication in order to reduce the costs of treatment.[31]
6. Chinese patients are reluctant to report pain and seek pain management.[31]
7. A shortage of nurses and whether professionals and administrators see pain prevention and treatment as a priority are also reasons for poor pain management.[2,37]

In mainland China, although patient-controlled analgesia is more popular for acute pain relief,[31] analgesics are still commonly administered through intramuscular injections on "as-needed" basis for postoperative pain, as has been reported in Taiwan.[58] In such cases, patients' unwillingness to report pain will impair postoperative pain control. Although "as needed" pain medication is often prescribed, proactive pain assessments are infrequent. Only when the patient asks for analgesics prescribed "as needed" will the nurse administer them.[63] However, Chinese patients may view requests to nurses for analgesics as distracting the nurse away from more important duties.[58,64] A client may view the nurse as an omniscient professional, who should know the client needs without being told, and, therefore, may wait passively for analgesics in the belief that if they are needed, they will be provided.[38] Some patients believe that pain medication can be given only at specified time intervals, and even if one is in pain, one cannot ask for medication until the interval is passed.[58] Other concerns about reporting pain and using analgesics among patients with postoperative pain include: fear of injections,[31,58] fear of inhibition of wound healing, desire to behave bravely,[31] desire to be a cooperative patient[31,58] and, therefore, remaining quiet and attempting to bear pain and wait for doctors and nurses.[49] For many reasons, postoperative pain has been poorly managed among Chinese patients.

CHINESE PARENTS' REACTION TO A CHILD'S HOSPITALIZATION

Parents struggle with complex emotional feelings while participating in their children's postoperative care. A descriptive questionnaire survey study conducted in China reported that Chinese parents experience a variety of emotions during their school-aged children's hospitalization for different types of surgery.[25] The feelings include worry, anxiety, fear, guilt, depression, helplessness, and anger.[20,22,23,26,65,66] Parents were asked to rate the level of these feelings using a five-point Likert scale ranging from "Totally agree" to "Totally disagree." The majority of parents experienced feelings of worry during their child's hospitalization, followed by anxiety. Other feelings, such as fear, guilt, depression, helplessness, and anger were less commonly experienced. An open-ended question inquired about the reasons for these feelings. A summary of responses revealed that parents' emotional feelings were mostly related to the surgical procedure their child had undergone,[67] such as risk of complications, risk of failure of the procedure and side effects of anesthesia. Other reasons included natural feelings related to parenthood,[68] such as parents' uncertainty about their child's condition and the prognosis of the procedure, lack of knowledge or capability to help their child, and seeing their child in pain.

The negative emotional feelings parents experience may lead to parental stress and decrease their ability to care for their child in pain.[22,23] The transmission of anxiety from parent to child has been recognized.[69] Children of highly anxious parents are often more frightened, anxious, or tend to be uncooperative following surgery. Previous studies have demonstrated that children, who have higher level of anxiety pre- or post-operatively, tend to experience higher levels of postoperative pain.[69–75] Therefore, greater attention is warranted in clinical practice to prevent and/or minimize the development of these feelings among parents. Parents need to be adequately provided with careful, relevant, and concurrent preoperative information from health professionals about the surgical procedure, anticipated sensory experiences, the recovery process, and pain-relieving methods. Such information could reduce their worries and anxiety [23,76] and could significantly contribute to their child's care in the postoperative period.[77]

CHINESE PARENTS' USE OF PAIN RELIEF METHODS

Previous studies show that parents use strategies familiar to them from everyday life when tending to their children's pain relief. These include emotional support such as comforting, holding, and remaining present, as well as help with daily activities.[13,78–80] Children prefer to have parents present and parents also prefer to accompany their hospitalized children.[81,82] Parents who choose to remain present may benefit from training in effective methods to help their child to cope.[78,83] Pain intervention studies[12,84] reveal that instructing parents to use nonpharmacological techniques could significantly reduce their children's pain during hospitalization and parents can use the knowledge they acquire to teach their child to use breathing techniques[85] and distraction[78,86] for pain relief.

He et al[8] conducted a questionnaire survey study in China, which examined what nonpharmacological methods Chinese parents used to relieve their children's postoperative pain and factors related to it. Results of the study revealed that Chinese parents use a variety of nonpharmacological methods, especially those convenient and familiar from everyday life, for children's pain relief. Consistent with other study findings,[24,79] He et al[8] found that methods commonly used by Chinese parents included emotional support and help with daily activities, as well as help with distraction and imagery. Other methods, such as physical methods and some cognitive-behavioral methods, including breathing technique, relaxation, and positive reinforcement were less frequently used. A survey study[87] examining parental guidance on the use of pain-relieving methods provided by Chinese nurses showed that more than half of the nurses guided parents to use methods of emotional support and help with daily activities; however, nurses themselves seldom used these methods.[37] This is consistent with the expectation that families are expected to provide direct postoperative care for their children.[36] The findings imply that optimal pain relief for children depends on providing sufficient instruction on pain-relief strategies to parents concerning their child's pain management.

Hospitalized children have been found to suffer from significant pain postoperatively in many different cultures.[6,79,88,89,90] In a study by He et al,[8] Chinese parents assessed their children's worst postoperative pain as moderate or severe. This finding offers evidence and a reason for Chinese health professionals to manage children's postoperative pain more aggressively, by using various pain relief methods, both pharmacological and nonpharmacological.

With regard to how child and parental background factors influence parents' use of pain-relief methods, He et al[8] revealed that fathers, and parents who were more educated, employed, and older were more active in using nonpharmacological methods with their children than mothers or parents without these characteristics. In addition, parents used some methods more frequently with boys, younger children, children admitted for selective operations, those with longer duration of hospitalization, and children with moderate or severe postoperative pain. More studies are needed to explore the reasons behind these findings.

CHINESE PARENTS' PERCEPTION OF SUPPORT RECEIVED FROM HEALTH PROFESSIONALS

Health professionals can provide various types of support to patients and their families, such as information giving, emotional support, and instrumental support. The support parents receive may influence the extent of their participation in their children's pain care. If parents receive sufficient and clear information and instruction about postoperative care, they may be more confident in their child's treatment[91] and may assume a greater role in caring for their children, with consequent improvements in their child's pain outcomes.[77,92,93] Well-prepared parents can transmit a sense of security to their child and may help reduce their child's pain.[9,78] However, parents often express the need for more information and support in pain management from nurses.[26,94] Parents need clear explanations of the surgical procedure (e.g., length and possible complications) and subsequent medical treatment (e.g., how to use pain medication) their child will undergo, expected roles, and time to validate their understanding.[9,12,20,21,22,23,26,30,95]

Parents provided inadequate preoperative preparation to their children, according to a survey study by He et al.[8] The reason might be that Chinese parents themselves lacked the related information, although nurses reported that they provided much cognitive information to parents.[87] Even so, nurses control the amount of parental participation through the information and support they provide and the way in which they communicate with parents.[18]

The survey study by He et al[25] reported that most Chinese parents received adequate information about the outcome of the procedure and the postoperative recovery process. However, information concerning pain and pain-relieving methods was insufficient. In addition, most parents reported having opportunities to consult nurses about pain management and subsequently receiving instructions on the use of pain relief methods. Nevertheless, only half of parents felt they had a clear idea about what they could do to help their child to relieve pain. These results might imply a gap between the information given by nurses and information understood and put into practice by parents. In fact, parents receiving more information than they could absorb might be still uncertain about their role.[96] Simons[97] also reported that nurses believed parents were well informed, whereas parents believed otherwise and were still anxious about pain-related issues. It is not enough to tell parents what to do, or simply to give them information.[96] Parents' understanding of information could be enhanced using a variety of methods, such as discussion between parents and health professionals, or using videotapes, written information, and picture books to convey information.[11,17,98] Information processing is affected by various factors, such as anxiety and cognitive ability of parents. Therefore, information given to parents should be individualized and adjusted according to their cultural and intellectual backgrounds, previous experience of their child's hospitalization, existing knowledge of pain management, and individual emotional needs.[98]

CHINESE PARENTS' RECOMMENDATIONS TO HEALTH PROFESSIONALS

Several studies have explored parents' recommendations to healthcare providers about their hospitalized children's pain care.[22,99–100] Most of the recommendations relate to the following areas: the continuity of care for their child, the use of pain medication, healthcare providers' willingness to listen to children and their parents, parents' defined roles in their child's care, information needs, as well as the need for greater involvement in their child's care and for adequate rest.

Chinese parents have offered several recommendations for improving their children's pain management.[25] The recommendations can be summarized into five themes: (1) applying nonpharmacological methods; (2) providing more information and instructions to the child and parents; (3) spending more time with their child; (4) showing friendly attitude toward their child; and (5) demonstrating concern toward their child. The majority of parents recommended that nurses apply nonpharmacological pain-relieving methods, such as comforting, positive reinforcement, and distraction to manage their child's pain, in addition to giving pain medication. In fact, these methods were most frequently introduced to parents by nurses and were used commonly by parents themselves to relieve their child's postoperative pain.[8,87] However, Chinese nurses themselves seldom used positive reinforcement as a pain-relieving method.[37] The parents' recommendations alerted nurses to the importance and necessity of using positive reinforcement while providing pain care to children, and through this, nurses also realized they could show friendly attitudes to children. Children are vulnerable, especially when they are hospitalized, so a friendly attitude and concern shown by nurses may make children feel more comfortable, thereby reducing their anxiety and fear of the hospital environment, and subsequently reducing their pain.[69,71,72]

PROVIDING CULTURALLY COMPETENT PAIN CARE TO CHINESE CHILDREN AND THEIR PARENTS

The sources of pain disparities among ethnic minorities are complex, involving patients (e.g., attitudes and the communication with healthcare providers), healthcare providers (e.g., decision making), and healthcare systems (e.g., access to pain medication) factors.[101] Cultural phenomena relative to the client, healthcare provider, and healthcare system must be considered when culturally sensitive strategies to alleviate pain are designed.[38] Davidhizar and Giger[38] proposed seven strategies for culturally appropriate assessment and management of pain that may be useful in providing culturally competent care to Chinese children and their parents (Table 8.1).

Healthcare providers must work closely with the client and family, in order to obtain accurate information about pain and then to provide culturally appropriate care.

Chinese people's perceptions of pain and their use of pain management strategies are influenced by different philosophies and religious beliefs, especially Confucianism.[47] These values and belief systems directly and indirectly influence children's pain experiences. For example, Chinese parents tend to tolerate and accept the pain caused by surgery, and thus may tend to encourage their children to tolerate pain. They may advise their children, especially boys, to be a 'brave child,'[8] and they may only report extreme postoperative pain when their child cannot bear it any longer. This hesitancy may be due to many reasons related to cultural values (e.g., stoicism and fatalism) and other reasons (e.g., fear of addiction and side effects, fear of bothering clinicians, or economic reasons).[47] Health professionals should understand this, and spend time with parents exploring and discussing parents' concerns and beliefs about their child's postoperative pain and pain management strategies.[47]

TABLE 8.1 Strategies for culturally appropriate pain assessment and management.

1. Utilize appropriate assessment tools;

2. Appreciate variations in affective response to pain across cultures;

3. Be sensitive to variations in communication styles across cultures;

4. Recognize that communication of pain may not be acceptable in a certain culture;

5. Appreciate that the meaning of pain varies between cultures;

6. Utilize knowledge of biological variations;

7. Promote personal awareness of values and beliefs, which may affect responses to pain.

Chinese parents experience negative feelings that impede their ability to provide postoperative care for their children. Parents desire more information and instruction about postoperative pain management, and health professionals should educate parents about various nonpharmacological pain alleviation methods available. In order to achieve optimal outcomes, they should also provide understandable information, instruction, emotional support, and additional time with the child and parents..

Healthcare providers are more likely to be responsive to communication concerning pain from an individual who shares the same culture.[38] Given that most of the previous studies examining the impact of culture on pain expression were conducted in North America,[50] what is needed is a comprehensive pain research agenda to address pain disparities among different cultures Such research is of potential importance to the more effective control of pain in all cultures.

FUTURE RESEARCH AND CLINICAL CHALLENGES

In order to improve children's postoperative pain management and care, future qualitative and quantitative studies are needed to focus on the following aspects: (1) the roles that parents have played in their child's postoperative pain management; (2) strategies to improve parental involvement, suggested by health professionals as well as parents and their children; (3) surveys of parents of Chinese origin who live in countries around the world about how their cultural values and belief systems influence their perception of pain and pain management among themselves and how this has influenced the pain management strategies they have used for their children postoperatively; (4) surveys of parents from different cultural backgrounds on their perception of their children's postoperative pain, and on maintaining their traditions and practices when dealing with children's suffering and pain.[62]

CONCLUSIONS

This chapter presents general knowledge of the concepts of culture, Chinese culture, values, and belief systems and their relationship to pain experiences and coping strategies to pain, and how these may influence Chinese parents' attitudes, perceptions, and preferences in dealing with their children in pain. Patients' pain has been poorly managed and apart from the cultural influences, other possible barriers are also discussed, which may arouse health professionals' interest as they try to improve the pain management practice for children. Chinese parents' feelings during their child's hospitalization for surgery, their commonly used nonpharmacological methods for their children's postoperative pain, the support and instructions they need from health professionals, as well as the recommendations they made for health professionals, were reported and discussed. Discrepancies were discovered during the research; for example, parents have various negative feelings that might impede their ability to take care of their hospitalized children, they tend to use the methods with which they are familiar from their daily life, and they need more information and instructions related to pain management. Attention to all of these factors may increase the culturally sensitive and competent care available to Chinese children and their parents. Future studies need to be conducted in order to get a better picture of the role parents play in their child's pain management, not only as it relates to cultural influences, but also to other influences, such as the provision of support, not only for postoperative pain, but also for other types of pain in children.

REFERENCES

1. National Bureau of Statistics of China. *National economy and social development statistics 2009 of China.* http://www.stats.gov.cn/tjgb/ndtjgb/qgndtjgb/t20100225_402622945.htm. Accessed March 15, 2011
2. Finley GA, Kristjánsdóttir Ó, Forgeron PA. Cultural influences on the assessment of children's pain. *Pain Res Manag.* 2009;14(1):33–37.
3. Hsieh AY, Tripp DA, Ji LJ, Sullivanz MJL. Comparisons of catastrophizing, pain attitudes, and cold-pressor pain experience between Chinese and European Canadian young adults. *J Pain.* 2010;11(11):1187–1194.
4. Helgadóttir HL. Pain management practices in children after surgery. *J Pediatr Nurs.* 2000;15(5):334–340.
5. Karling M, Renström M, Ljungman G. Acute and postoperative pain in children: A Swedish nationwide survey. *Acta Paediatr.* 2002;91(6):660–666.
6. He HG, Vehviläinen-Julkunen K, Pölkki T, Pietilä A-M. Children's perceptions on the implementation of methods for their postoperative pain alleviation: An interview study. *Int J Nurs Pract.* 2007;13(2):89–99.
7. Twycross A. Children's nurses' postoperative pain management practices: An observational study. *Int J Nurs Stud.* 2007;44(6):869–881.
8. He HG, Pölkki T, Pietilä A-M, Vehviläinen-Julkunen K. Chinese parents' use of nonpharmacological methods in children's postoperative pain relief. *Scand J Caring Sci.* 2006;20(1):2–9.
9. Kristensson-Hallström I. Strategies for feeling secure influence parents' participation in care. *J Clin Nurs.* 1999;8(5):586–592.
10. Rush SL, Harr J. Evidence-based paediatric nursing: does it have to hurt? *AACN Clin Issues.* 2001;12(4):597–605.
11. Simons J, Franck L, Roberson E. Parent involvement in children's pain care: Views of parents and nurses. *J Adv Nurs.* 2001;36(4):591–599.
12. Simons J, Roberson E. Poor communication and knowledge deficits: Obstacles to effective management of children's postoperative pain. *J Adv Nurs.* 2002;40(1):78–86.
13. Kankkunen P, Vehviläinen-Julkunen K, Pietilä A-M, Halonen P. Parents' use of non-pharmacological methods to alleviate children's postoperative pain at home. *J Adv Nurs.* 2003;41(4):367–375.
14. Jylli L, Olsson GL. Procedural pain in a paediatric surgical emergency unit. *Acta Paediatr.* 1995;84(12):1403–1408.
15. Craig KD, Lilley CM, Gilbert CA. Social barriers to optimal pain management in infants and children. *Clin J Pain.* 1996;12 (3):232–242.
16. Maciocia PM, Strachan EM, Akram AR, et al. Pain assessment in the paediatric Emergency Department: whose view counts? *Eur J Emerg Med.* 2003;10(4):264–267.
17. Greenberg RS, Billett C, Zahurak M, Yaster M. Videotape increases parental knowledge about paediatric pain management. *Anesth Analg.* 1999;89(4):899–903.

18. Corlett J, Twycross A. Negotiation of parental roles within family-centred care: A review of the research. *J Clin Nurs.* 2006;15(10):1308–1316.

19. Power N, Franck L. Parent participation in the care of hospitalized children: A systematic review. *J Adv Nur.* 2008;62(6):622–641.

20. Kristensson-Hallström I. Parental participation in pediatric surgical care. *AORN J.* 2000;71(5):1021–1024, 1026–1029.

21. Chapados C, Pineault R, Tourigny J, Vandal S. Perceptions of parents' participation in the care of their child undergoing day surgery: Pilot study. *Issues Compr Pediatr Nurs.* 2002;25(1):59–70.

22. Pölkki T, Pietilä A-M, Vehviläinen-Julkunen K, Laukkala H, Ryhänen P. Parental views on participation in their child's pain relief measures and recommendations to health care providers. *J Pediatr Nurs.* 2002;17(4):270–278.

23. Hug M, Tönz M, Kaiser G. Parental stress in paediatric day-case surgery. *Pediatr Surg Int.* 2005;21(2):94–99.

24. Tait AR, Voepel-Lewis T, Snyder RM, Malviya S. Parents' understanding of information regarding their child's postoperative pain management. *Clin J Pain.* 2008;24(7):572–577.

25. He HG, Vehviläinen-Julkunen K, Pölkki T, Pietilä AM. Chinese parents' perception of support received and recommendations regarding children's postoperative pain management. *Int J Nurs Pract.* 2010;16 (3):254–261.

26. Franck LS, Cox S, Allen A, Winter I. Parental concern and distress about infant pain. *Arch Dis Child Fetal Neonatal Ed.* 2004;89(1):F71–F75.

27. Carter B, McArthur E, Cunliffe M. Dealing with uncertainty: parental assessment of pain in their children with profound special needs. *J Adv Nurs.* 2002;38(5):449–457.

28. Zacharias M, Watts D. Pain relief in children: doing the simple things better. *BMJ.* 1998;316(7144):1552.

29. Lee Calvin R. Paediatric day surgery outcomes management: the role of preoperative anxiety and home pain management protocol. *AORN J.* 2000;71(3):695.

30. Kankkunen P, Vehviläinen-Julkunen K, Pietilä AM. Children's postoperative pain at home: family interview study. *Int J Nurs Pract.* 2002;8(1):32–41.

31. Liu W, Luo A, Liu HL. Overcoming the barriers in pain control: an update of pain management in China. *Eur J Pain.* 2007;1(1):10–13.

32. Nikanne E. *Ketoprofen for postoperative pain after day-case adenoidectomy in small children* [dissertation]. Kuopio, Finland: Kuopio University Printing Office; 1999.

33. D'Arcy Y. The effect of culture on pain. *Nursing Made Incredibly Easy.* 2009;7 (3):5–7. http://journals. lww.com/nursingmadeincrediblyeasy/Fulltext/2009/05000/The_effect_of_culture_on_pain.2.aspx. Accessed March 15, 2011.

34. Ludwig-Beymer P. Transcultural aspects of pain. In: Andrews MM, Boyle JS, eds. *Transcultural Concepts in Nursing Care*, 4th ed. Philadelphia: Lippincott Williams & Wilkins; 2003: 405–431.

35. McGuire DB. Comprehensive and multidimensional assessment and measurement of pain. *J Pain Symptom Manage.* 1992;7(5):312–319.

36. Alsop-Shields L. Perioperative care of children in a transcultural context. *AORN J.* 2000;71(5):1004–1006, 1008, 1011–1014, 1016, 1019–1020.

37. He HG, Pölkki T, Vehviläinen-Julkunen K, Pietilä AM. Chinese nurses' use of non-pharmacological methods in children's postoperative pain relief. *J Adv Nurs.* 2005;51(4):335–342.

38. Davidhizar R, Giger JN. A review of the literature on care of clients in pain who are culturally diverse. *Int Nurs Rev.* 2004;51(1):47–55.

39. MacLachlan M. *Culture and Health.* England: John Wiley & Sons Ltd; 1997: 160–167.

40. Beck SL. An ethnographic study of factors influencing cancer pain management in South Africa. *Cancer Nurs.* 2000;23(2):91–99.

41. Edwards RR, Doleys DM, Fillingim RB, Lowery D. Ethnic differences in pain tolerance: clinical implications in a chronic pain population. *Psychosom Med.* 2001;63(2):316–323.

42. Kim H, Neubert JK, San Miguel A, et al. Genetic influence on variability in human acute experimental pain sensitivity associated with gender, ethnicity and psychological temperament. *Pain.* 2004;109 (3):488–496.

43. Young KD. Pediatric Procedural Pain. *Ann Emerg Med.* 2005;45(2):160–171.

44. McCaffery M, Pasero C. *Pain: Clinical Manual.* St. Louis, MO: C.V. Mosby; 1999.

45. Craig KD. Pain in infants and children: Sociodevelopmental variations on the theme. In: Giamberardino MA, ed. *Pain 2002—An Updated Review. Refresher Course Syllabus.* 10th World Congress on Pain, San Diego, CA. Seattle: IASP Press; 2002: 305–314.

46. Salerno E. Race, culture, and medications. *J Emerg Nurs.* 1995;21(6):560–562.

47. Chen LM, Miaskowski C, Dodd M, Pantilat S. Concepts within the Chinese culture that influence the cancer pain experience. *Cancer Nurs.* 2008;31(2):103–108.

48. Xia P-Y. Actuality analysis and related strategies of postoperative pain management. *Chinese Journal of Current Clinical Medicine.* 2004;2(4B):563–564.

49. Wong EML, Chan SWC. The pain experience and beliefs of Chinese patients who have sustained a traumatic limb fracture. *Int Emerg Nurs.* 2008;16(2):80–87.

50. Hawthorn J, Redmond K. *Pain: causes and management.* UK: Blackwell Science Ltd; 1998: 70–85, 109–146.

51. Holroyd E. Developing a cultural model of caregiving obligations for elderly Chinese wives. *West J Nurs Res.* 2005;27(4):437–456.

52. Chung JY, Wong TK, Yang JS. The lens model-assessment of cancer pain in a Chinese context. *Cancer Nurs.* 2000;23(6):454–461.

53. Reel HG. *Confucius and the Chinese Way.* New York: Peter Smith Publisher; 2000.

54. Wills BS, Wootton YS. Concerns and misconceptions about pain among Hong Kong Chinese patients with cancer. *Cancer Nurs.* 1999;22 (6):408–413.

55. Tsai YF. Gender differences in pain and depressive tendency among Chinese elders with knee osteoarthritis. *Pain.* 2007;130 (1–2):188–194.

56. Higgins LT, Zheng M. An introduction to Chinese psychology—its historical roots until the present day. *J Psychol.* 2002;136(2):225–39.

57. Pain and Culture. *Pain research and western medicine, pain and knowledge, objectivity, and subjectivity.* http://www.answers.com/topic/pain-and-culture. Accessed 5 July, 2012.

58. Tzeng JI, Chou LF, Lin CC. Concerns about reporting pain and using analgesics among Taiwanese postoperative patients. *J Pain.* 2006;7(11):860–866.

59. Gu WP, Liu ZM. National surveys report on cancer pain in China. *Chin J Drug Depend.* 1999;8:4–5.

60. Pain and Policy Studies Group. *Availability of Morphine and Pethidine in the World, with a special focus on: Africa, Botswana, Ethiopia, Kenya, Malawi, Nigeria, Rwanda, Tanzania, and Zambia*]. Madison, WI: University of Wisconsin Pain & Policy Studies Group/WHO Collaborating Center for Policy and Communications in Cancer Care; 2006.

61. Brennan F, Carr DB, Cousins M. Pain management: a fundamental human right. *Anesth Analg.* 2007;105(1):205–221.

62. Kankkunen P, Vehviläinen-Julkunen K, Pietilä AM, Nikkonen M. Cultural factors influencing children's pain. *Int J Caring Sci.* 2009;2(3):126–134.

63. He H-G. *Non-pharmacological Methods in Children's Postoperative Pain Relief in China.* [dissertation]. Kuopio, Finland: University of Kuopio; 2006: 63.

64. Giger J, Davidhizar R. *Transcultural Nursing. Assessment and Intervention.* St. Louis, MO: C.V. Mosby Year Book; 1999.

65. Cimete G. Stress factors and coping strategies of parents with children treated by hemodialysis: a qualitative study. *J Pediatr Nurs.* 2002;17(4):297–306.

66. Thomlinson EH. The lived experience of families of children who are failing to thrive. *J Adv Nurs.* 2002;39(6):537–545.

67. Shirley PJ, Thompson N, Kenward M, Johnston G. Parental anxiety before elective surgery in children. A British perspective. *Anaesthesia.* 1998;53(10):956–959.

68. Coyne IT. Partnership in care: parents' views of participation in their hospitalized child's care. *J Clin Nurs.* 1995;4(2):71–79.

69. LaMontagne LL, Hepworth JT, Salisbury MH. Anxiety and postoperative pain in children who undergo major orthopedic surgery. *Appl Nurs Res.* 2001;14(3):119–124.

70. Palermo TM, Drotar D. Prediction of children's postoperative pain: the role of presurgical expectations and anticipatory emotions. *J Pediatr Psychol.* 1996;21(5):683–698.

71. Caumo W, Broenstrub JC, Fialho L, et al. Risk factors for postoperative anxiety in children. *Acta Anaesthesiol Scand.* 2000;44(7):782–789.

72. Ericsson E, Wadsby M, Hultcrantz E. Pre-surgical child behavior ratings and pain management after two different techniques of tonsil surgery. *Int J Pediatr Otorhinolaryngol.* 2006;70(10):1749–1758.

73. Kain ZN, Mayes LC, Caldwell-Andrews AA, Karas DE, McClain BC. Preoperative anxiety, postoperative pain, and behavioral recovery in young children undergoing surgery. *Pediatrics.* 2006;118(2):651–658.

74. Bringuier S, Dadure C, Raux O, Dubois A, Picot MC, Capdevila X. The perioperative validity of the visual analog anxiety scale in children: a discriminant and useful instrument in routine clinical practice to optimize postoperative pain management. *Anesth Analg.* 2009;109(3):737–744.

75. Crandall M, Lammers C, Senders C, Braun JV. Children's tonsillectomy experiences: influencing factors. *J Child Health Care.* 2009;13(4):308–321.

76. Dahl JB, Kehlet H. Postoperative pain and its management. In: McMahon SB, Koltzenburg M, eds. *Wall and Melzack's Textbook of Pain,* 5th ed. Philadelphia, PA: Elsevier/ Churchill Livingstone; 2006: 635–651.

77. Jonas DA. Parent's management of their child's pain in the home following day surgery. *J of Child Health Care.* 2003;7(3):150–162.

78. Kleiber C, Craft-Rosenberg M, Harper DC. Parents as distraction coaches during i.v. insertion: a randomized study. *J Pain Symptom Manage.* 2001;22(4):851–861.

79. Pölkki T, Vehviläinen-Julkunen K, Pietilä A-M. Parents' role in using non-pharmacological methods in their child's postoperative pain alleviation. *J Clin Nurs.* 2002;11(4):526–536.

80. Kankkunen P, Vehviläinen-Julkunen K, Pietilä A-M, Halonen P. Parents' perceptions of their 1-6-year-old children's pain. *Eur J Pain.* 2003;7(3):203–211.

81. Boie ET, Moore GP, Brummett C, Nelson DR. Do parents want to be present during invasive procedures performed on their children in the emergency department? A survey of 400 parents. *Ann Emerg Med.* 1999;34(1):70–74.

82. Boudreaux ED, Francis JL, Loyacano T. Family presence during invasive procedures and resuscitations in the emergency department: a critical review and suggestions for future. *Ann Emerg Med.* 2002; 40(2):193–205.

83. Broome ME. Helping parents support their child in pain. *Pediatr Nurs.* 2000;26(3):315–317.

84. Christensen J, Fatchett D. Promoting parental use of distraction and relaxation in pediatric oncology patients during invasive procedures. *J Pediatr Oncol Nurs.* 2002;19(4):127–132.

85. Powers KS, Rubenstein JS. Family presence during invasive procedures in the pediatric intensive care unit. *Arch Pediatr Adolesc Med* 1999;153(9):955–958.

86. McCarthy AM, Kleiber C. A conceptual model of factors influencing children's responses to a painful procedure when parents are distraction coaches. *J Pediatr Nurs.* 2006;21(2):88–98.

87. He HG, Pölkki T, Pietilä AM, Vehviläinen-Julkunen K. A survey of Chinese nurses' guidance to parents in children's postoperative pain relief. *J Clin Nurs.* 2005;14(9):1075–1082.

88. Paik HJ, Ahn YM. Measurement of acute pain after eye surgery in children. *Korean J Ophthalmol.* 2002;16(2):103–109.

89. Apfelbaum JL, Chen C, Mehta SS, Gan TJ. Postoperative pain experience: results from a national survey suggest postoperative pain continues to be undermanaged. *Anesth Analg.* 2003;97(2):534–540.

90. Pölkki T, Pietila A-M, Vehviläinen-Julkunen K. Hospitalized children's descriptions of their experiences with postsurgical pain relieving methods. *Int J Nurs Stud.* 2003;40(1):33–44.

91. McArthur E, Cunliffe M. Pain assessment and documentation—making a difference. *J Child Health Care.* 1998;2(4):164–169.

92. Kristensson-Hallström I, Elander G, Malmfors G. Increased parental participation in a paediatric surgical day-care unit. *J Clin Nurs* 1997;6(4):297–302.

93. Bishop-Kurylo D. Pediatric pain management in the emergency department. *Top Emerg Med.* 2002;24(1):19–30.

94. Kankkunen P, Pietilä A-M, Vehviläinen-Julkunen K. Families' and children's postoperative pain— Literature review. *J Pediatr Nurs.* 2004;19(2):133–139.

95. Tönz M, Herzig G, Kaiser G. Quality assurance in day surgery: do we do enough for the parents to prevent stress? *Eur J Pediatr.* 1999;158(12):984–988.

96. Hallström I, Runesson I, Elander G. Observed parental needs during their child's hospitalization. *J Pediatr Nurs.* 2002;17(2):140–148.

97. Simons J. Parents' support and satisfaction with their child's postoperative care. *Br J Nurs.* 2002;11(22):1442–1444, 1446–1449.

98. LeRoy S, Elixson EM, O'Brien P, Tong E, Turpin S, Uzark K. American Heart Association Pediatric Nursing Subcommittee of the Council on Cardiovascular Nursing; Council on Cardiovascular Disease of the Young. Recommendations for preparing children and adolescents for invasive cardiac procedures: A statement from the American Heart Association Pediatric Nursing Subcommittee of the Council on Cardiovascular Nursing in collaboration with the Council on Cardiovascular Diseases of the Young. *Circulation.* 2003;108(20):2550–2564.

99. Sclare I, Waring M. Routine venepuncture: improving services. *Paediatr Nurs.* 1995;7(4):23–27.

100. Lim SH, Mackey S, Liam LWJ, He HG. An exploration of Singaporean parental experiences in managing their school-aged children's postoperative pain: a descriptive qualitative approach. *J Clin Nurs.* 2012;21(5-6):860–869.

101. Green CR, Anderson KO, Baker TA, et al. The unequal burden of pain: confronting racial and ethnic disparities in pain. *Pain Med.* 2003;4(3):277–294.

9

UNDERSTANDING ANGLO-AMERICANS' CULTURE, PAIN, AND SUFFERING

SUSAN SHARP, MA, PSYD (STUDENT)
PGSP-Stanford PsyD Consortium, Palo Alto University, Stanford
Psychology and Biobehavioral Sciences Laboratory, Stanford
School of Medicine, Palo Alto, California, USA

CHERYL KOOPMAN, PHD
Associate Professor (Research), Department of Psychiatry
and Behavioral Sciences, Stanford University, Stanford,
California, USA

Key Points
- It is challenging to understand the evidence about pain experiences among Anglo-Americans due to the complexity and inconsistencies on how this group is self-identified and also how it is identified in the literature.
- Anglo-Americans tend to express less pain and have higher pain tolerance compared to persons of many other ethnic groups.
- Evidence suggests that Anglo-Americans differ from other ethnic groups in the expression of pain in the medical setting.
- Anglo-Americans, compared to other ethnic groups in the United States, are more likely to receive recognition of their pain and pain treatment with analgesics.
- As the dominant group in US culture, Anglo-Americans have heavily influenced medical thinking about pain and its treatment, not only within their subpopulation, but of patients more generally.
- In the United States, in assessing and treating patients' pain, healthcare providers need to be aware of the diversity of experiences and expressions of pain among Anglo-Americans as well as in other ethnic groups.

CHALLENGES OF UNDERSTANDING PAIN RESPONSES AND EXPRESSION AMONG ANGLO-AMERICANS

This chapter examines responses to pain among Anglo-Americans, the largest and culturally dominant group living in the United States. A major challenge in using the term

"Anglo-Americans" is that it has a variety of meanings, as do other ethnic constructs in the US context.[1] In this chapter, we will generally use the term broadly to refer to persons who identify as "white" and as "not Hispanic." In the 2010 US Census, a majority of Americans self-identified as "white" alone (223.6 million; 72.4%) or "white alone or in combination with one or more other races" (231 million; 74.5%).[2] In the 2010 census, "white" was identified as "a person having origins in any of the original peoples of Europe, the Middle East, or North Africa. It includes people who identify as "white" or reported entries such as Irish, German, Italian, Lebanese, Arab, Moroccan, or Caucasian."[2] Because people of European ancestry (e.g., English, German, Irish, or Italian) make up a majority of the white population in the United States, [3] the research on pain has been particularly focused on persons with European origins, and focused less on persons with origins in North Africa or the Middle East. This chapter will focus as much as the literature permits on pain specifically among Anglo-Americans who can trace their origins to northern European countries.

In the United States, people who identify as white rarely self-identify with the term "Anglo," even though pain researchers sometimes use it to refer to this population. The US Census 2010 found that slightly under two-thirds of the US population identified themselves to be non-Hispanic and "white."[2,3] Furthermore, matters are further complicated by participants sometimes being identified as "Caucasian"[1] or "of European origin." [1,4]

In most of the literature on responses to pain that can help to provide insight about Anglo-Americans, at least a sizable number of the participants or patients studied were identified simply as "white." Therefore, it is important to recognize such limitations in the existing literature for informing understanding of the Anglo-Americans' pain responses and expression.

This discussion of pain responses and pain management draws from a "multiculturalism" perspective that recognizes that pain-related experiences and reactions may be influenced by a person's culture, broadly defined. To understand these cultural influences, it is important to recognize not only differences in national origin, but also differences in gender, age, religious background, and social class, as has been emphasized in training psychologists[5] and physicians.[6-9] Culture encompasses beliefs, customs, and lifestyle choices.[10] Additionally, due to the historical processes of immigration and acculturation, people who originated from different countries may also exhibit important variations in their pain experiences. Because a variety of terms are used to address cultural groups in the United States, this chapter will generally use the group labels drawn directly from the literature, although our intended focus is on Anglo-Americans.

This chapter has three primary aims in reviewing the literature on responses to pain among Anglo-Americans. First, it discusses the literature on Anglo-Americans' responses to their own pain, particularly in their pain sensitivity, coping with their pain, and expression of their pain in the medical setting. Second, this chapter summarizes evidence suggesting that the dominance of Anglo-Americans among physicians and other health providers in the United States has unintended adverse consequences for pain management of ethnic minority patients. Finally, this review will conclude with recommendations for improvements in medical education and clinical practice as well as for future research. Throughout this discussion of pain experiences in the dominant American culture our intention is to suggest dimensions of cultural differences that should be considered in assessing pain and developing treatment strategies for managing and alleviating it. In discussing cultural differences, it must be emphasized that "there are differences within cultural groups that may be greater than the differences between the dominant culture and other cultures … Giving too much attention to the individual encourages neglect of the impact of the cultural group on the individual. Giving too much attention to the cultural group runs the risk of stereotyping the individual as a member of the cultural group and forgetting individual uniqueness." [11] Therefore, it is important to keep in mind that patients' cultural backgrounds may contribute to their clinical presentations of pain and suffering—while also considering each patient's individual characteristics.

BIOCULTURAL MODEL OF PAIN AND ETHNICITY

Pain is a highly complex psychobiological experience. [12] The experience of pain is understood to have physical, along with cognitive, emotional, and behavioral dimensions. [12–15] Pain experience is sometimes conceptualized as a distinctive dimension from the pain sensation, as there is evidence that the suffering can be lessened (e.g., when the sufferer is experiencing a hypnotic state), [16–17] and that the level of suffering depends upon the understanding of the meaning of one's pain (e.g., women's suffering experienced during labor is associated with cultural beliefs and contextual factors). [18]

In contrast to the purely medical model of pain-intervention solely via medical procedures, the biocultural model for pain as developed by Maryann S. Bates [19,20] is useful as a general approach for conceptualizing patients' experiences of pain and suffering. An important emphasis of the biocultural model is to acknowledge the relevance of factors beyond the biological aspects of medicine to also consider those that are psychological, social, and cultural. Furthermore, Bates' biocultural model [19,20] integrates theoretical and empirical advances in understanding pain; specifically, it integrates the gate-control theory developed by Melzack and Wall [21] that incorporates cognitive as well as neurophysiological aspects of pain with two theories drawn from the social sciences—social learning theory [22] and social comparison processes. [23] In the biocultural model, the pain response results from the interactions of the neurophysiological sources of pain with psychological variables that are influenced by social comparison and social learning processes that themselves are embedded within "ethnocultural group situations." [20,21] These social processes affect attitudes toward pain, prior pain experiences, and the attention given to pain and other cognitive processes, which in turn influence the sensory transmission of pain.

In the Western world, it is particularly important to understand the nature of chronic pain, given its high prevalence in most illnesses that people experience. [24] Bates drew considerable support for her biocultural model of chronic pain from her research comparing pain experiences of Anglo-Americans and persons from other ethnic groups recruited at a pain control center in New England, as well as comparing the New England Latinos and Anglo-Americans to a separate sample of native Puerto Ricans with back pain. [20] She found that persons from Anglo-American and Polish backgrounds were less demonstrative or emotional in expressing their pain compared to persons from Italian, New England Latino, or native Puerto Rican groups. Consistent with her biocultural model, she attributed much of this variation in the differences to " … home and family, where adults transmit to children the values and attitudes of their cultural or ethnic group. Attitudes, expectations, meanings for experiences, and appropriate emotional expressiveness are learned through observing the reactions and behaviors of others who are similar in identity to oneself." [20]

A multidisciplinary team approach for understanding and treating pain can significantly improve the quality of life of patients and their care providers. However, in the United States, cultural barriers can prevent an appropriate application of the biocultural model in assessing and managing pain. One type of cultural barrier is ignorance of how cultural differences can affect the experience and presentation of pain and suffering. Another type of cultural barrier is the high premium the dominant Anglo culture places on autonomy; this can interfere with treating pain adequately, especially in other cultural groups.

COMPARISONS OF PAIN SENSITIVITY OF ANGLO-AMERICANS WITH US MINORITY GROUPS

Several US studies suggest that Anglo-Americans demonstrate less pain sensitivity and greater pain tolerance than African Americans or Hispanics.[4,25–28] In regard to laboratory-induced pain, whites compared to African Americans have been found to show higher tolerances for cold-pressor pain,[29] ischemic pain, heat pain,[4,25] and thermal pain.[30] Similarly, in clinical settings, ethnic differences in pain severity have been found among people with various medical conditions, such as in chronic pain treated at an integrated pain management program[31] or following postoperative dental work.[32]

Chapman and Jones[33] studied cutaneous and visceral sensitivity to pain in 200 healthy participants. Their study compared two aspects of the pain experience—the pain threshold (at which individuals experience pain) to the tolerance threshold (at which they wince or withdraw from the pain stimulus). They found that participants of Northern European background demonstrated higher pain thresholds for experiencing pain compared with African Americans and persons of "Jewish and other Mediterranean" backgrounds. Furthermore, Northern European Americans exhibited pain tolerance that was considerably greater than their pain threshold, whereas African Americans and persons of Mediterranean backgrounds demonstrated levels of pain tolerance that were almost the same as their pain threshold.

These findings are particularly interesting because they suggest that Anglo-Americans may not only experience higher pain thresholds but also have greater pain tolerance compared to persons of other ethnic groups. This is consistent with the cultural notion among Anglo-Americans that it is desirable to react with a "stiff upper lip" to difficulties such as pain.

However, there are some mixed results in the literature comparing Anglo-Americans to persons of other ethnic backgrounds. Similarities in the experience of chronic pain have been found in comparing Anglo-American patients with African American patients and Hispanic patients, with no significant ethnic differences shown on measures of pain and pain-related disability.[34] Although a number of studies have found a significant relationship between reported pain severity and ethnicity, these findings should be interpreted with caution; variables such as age, sex, and psychosocial factors such as coping and working conditions may moderate the relationship between pain response and ethnicity.[1,35–36]

PAIN DIFFERENCES WITHIN ANGLO-AMERICAN CULTURE

Psychosocial factors appear to modulate pain and pain tolerance thresholds. For example, evidence with predominantly Anglo-American participants suggests that peoples' pain sensitivity decreases if they are educated in mindfulness techniques and know how to meditate.[37] Although a study of patients of European origin with early severe rheumatoid arthritis did not find socioeconomic status (SES) to be related to pain, SES was related to functional disability and depressive symptoms.[38] These findings suggest that having greater cognitive or social resources available may be beneficial for tolerating pain. This interpretation is also consistent with evidence that the pain threshold decreases with age among white persons;[26] it may be that older persons perceive pain at lower stimulus levels because of the depletion of cognitive and social resources associated with aging in the United States. However, alterations in affect may be a more potent influence on the capacity to tolerate pain: individuals' pain tolerances were lower after viewing negative pictures compared to viewing positive pictures.[39] Further research is needed to learn more about how individual experiences of emotion within the context of Anglo-American culture affect pain tolerance.

CULTURAL DIFFERENCES IN RESPONSES TO PAIN IN THE AMERICAN MEDICAL SETTING

Cultural differences in the expression of pain are important to consider because they may help to explain discrepancies in how pain is treated among different ethnic/racial groups.[40,41] In 1969, Zborowski reported that American patients of Jewish and Italian backgrounds expressed their pain more intensely than did "Old Americans" (of Northern European descent).[42] Also in the late 1960s, Zola reported among outpatients in Boston clinics, major differences in the expression of pain and other symptoms between patients who were of Italian and Irish backgrounds, in which the Italians expressed more symptoms, described more bodily areas in which they had physical complaints, and reported more types of bodily dysfunction.[43] He interpreted these differences as being due to their respective cultural differences with " … the Irish handling their troubles by denial and Italians theirs by dramatization."[43]

A subsequent study of Boston outpatients had similar findings to those encountered by Zola on ethnic differences in reporting pain. Koopman and colleagues[44] found that patients of an Anglo (Irish, English, or Scottish) background, compared to those of an Italian background, were significantly less likely to report pain. These differences were found in analyzing patients' responses to an open-ended question, "What troubles, problems, or difficulties do you feel you want help with today?" followed by a specific probe, "Have you been having any pain?" for those who did not mention aches or pains in response to the initial question. Interestingly, however, these ethnic differences were particularly pronounced among the older women in both ethnic groups, which the authors attributed to the likelihood that older women in particular in both ethnic groups had been socialized to carry on cultural traditions. However, because these studies of Anglo-Americans and other ethnic groups were conducted years ago, it is unclear as to what degree such differences are still present; these studies are therefore presented not so much as descriptions that are currently accurate but rather as examples of cultural forces at play in the expression of pain.

Anglo-Americans are more likely than are individuals from ethnic minority backgrounds to go to a medical care provider for treatment. For example, among those with mental health problems, Anglo-Americans are twice as likely to visit a mental health facility compared to Mexican Americans.[45] Also, when Anglo-Americans seek a medical care provider, they report less pain intensity and disability than do African Americans who have acute back pain[46] and vulvar pain,[47] and they also report less pain unpleasantness compared to African Americans.[48]

Most of the research on Anglo-Americans' responses to pain is focused on adults. In a southwestern US study of children with cancer undergoing a spinal tap or bone marrow aspiration,[49] Anglo children did not differ from Hispanic children in their perception and expression of pain and anxiety. However, Anglo parents of these children reported significantly lower levels of anxiety than did the Hispanic parents. In interpreting these results, the authors raise the question of whether the children's reactions were similar in these ethnic groups because they lacked sufficient exposure to attitudes, beliefs, and behaviors specific to their respective cultures. Perhaps with age, these children would embody their parents' cultural characteristics; although it is also possible that there is a cohort effect in which these cultural differences in responses to pain are vanishing among younger Americans.

MANAGEMENT OF PAIN IN THE UNITED STATES

The assessment and determination of a plan for alleviating pain is a very challenging and uncertain process due to the multiplicity of factors that must be considered, including those that are societal as well as those that are biological and intrapsychic. Furthermore, given the private nature of pain, particularly of chronic pain caused by factors that are not directly observable, the reactions of other people depend on "local moral worlds" in which a pain patient's reports of suffering are conceptualized as legitimate or illegitimate.[50–51] A patient's cultural background can then have an important effect on communications with medical providers and on subsequent pain management. Responses to the patient's report of suffering are influenced by other people's understanding of the meaning of this report within the cultural context.

An important disparity to understand is why Anglo-Americans reporting pain, when compared with individuals from US minority groups, are more likely to be treated with analgesics.[52–56] Providers' treatment decisions may be influenced by the ways in which they view their interactions with patients of other ethnic backgrounds. This is supported by evidence that for white pain patients, primary care physicians were more likely to prescribe a higher dosage or strength of opioid if the patient exhibited "non-challenging" behaviors. In contrast, for an African American patient, a decision to escalate pain medication was more likely if the patient used more challenging styles of communicating with the medical-care provider (e.g., anger or challenging the physician's authority).[57]

Despite such evidence for social and cultural differences, in the United States one can be oblivious that one's own views of and experiences with pain and suffering may not be representative of those of persons from other cultures. As will be discussed in the next section, the emphasis put on the value of autonomy in the dominant American culture may considerably influence the response to pain. This cultural preference for autonomy is in conflict with another aspect of Anglo-American culture that views pain as unacceptable, and therefore emphasizes the importance of responding compassionately to one's own as well as to others' pain.

AUTONOMY AND SYMPATHY IN PAIN AND SUFFERING

The stance of autonomy influences goals, ambitions, and aims in the American dominant culture, including views about how to evaluate and cope with pain appropriately.[58] From this perspective, human consciousness is autonomous from nature, which can be observed. Furthermore, this view emphasizes that, "The individual is a sovereign being, a distinct unit, prior to society and culture, and autonomous from them …."[58] According to Elaine Scarry, such thinking is embodied in Judeo-Christian scriptures in the form of narratives in which God reveals God's own existence through the alterations of the physical human body, such as its procreation, injury, and death.[59] She says that in this thinking, the individual person is objectified and has no voice of import, but gives rise to the opportunity for " … God's forceful shattering of the reluctant human surface and repossession of the interior."[59] In this view, little emphasis is placed on the social context of suffering, but rather people must individually redeem themselves in ways that are in accordance with God's will.

The view that individuals are autonomous and must bear their own suffering alone is highly prevalent among Anglo-Americans. White cancer patients express their concern with pain by doing their own research on pain management, controlling their pain, and anticipating the next step in the treatment process.[60] This pattern of response to pain contrasts with that of persons from other US ethnic groups such as African Americans who are more likely to turn to their families and other sources of social support for help in times of need.[31]

The Anglo-American emphasis on autonomy means that pain is something that the patient needs to control independently as the individualistic culture promotes self-reliance and autonomy; people are expected to take an active role in their recovery. Consistent with this notion, Anglo-American patients have reported having greater internal pain-coping strategies and higher perceived control over their chronic pain, compared with African American patients; they are also less likely to expect that others should focus on their pain.[31]

An adverse consequence of Anglo-Americans' emphasis on autonomy is that they do not have as many protective social factors that might serve as a buffer when they experience an external loss (e.g., illness) compared to persons from other cultural and ethnic groups. It has been suggested that the higher rate of suicides among Anglo-Americans compared to other ethnic groups may be attributed in part to their lack of close family ties.[61] Anglo-Americans are also less likely than are African Americans to turn to religion to help them cope with chronic pain. Because Anglo-Americans often rely on themselves to cope with their pain and suffering, it may be beneficial to help them recognize the limitations as well as the benefits of their emphasis upon self-sufficiency. A summary of this literature describing Anglo-Americans' responses to pain is presented in Table 9.1.

The value that Anglo-Americans place on individual autonomy in coping with pain is countered by the influence of humanitarian social movements promoting "a culture of sensibility" that emerged in England in the 1700s and spread to the United States.[62] According to Karen Halttunen, "Orthodox Christianity had traditionally viewed pain not only as God's punishment for sin (the English term is derived from the Latin *poena* or 'punishment') but also as a redemptive opportunity to transcend the world and the flesh by imitating the suffering Christ."[62]

TABLE 9.1 **Summary of the Literature about Anglo-Americans' Responses to Pain**

- Anglo-Americans tend to display less pain and greater pain tolerance than people from US minority groups, although not all studies find this ethnic difference.
- There may be a greater gap between perceiving and reacting to pain among Anglo-Americans compared to other ethnic groups.
- Compared to other ethnic groups, Anglo-Americans tend to be less expressive and emotional in reporting pain.
- Anglo-Americans are more likely to receive analgesics for their pain compared to individuals from US minority ethnic groups.
- As for other ethnic groups, pain responses among Anglo-Americans may differ by age, gender, socioeconomic status, national origin, and religious background, as well as by psychological (e.g., beliefs) and social factors (e.g., social norms).
- Because findings are based largely on convenience samples, focused on specific patient populations, and conducted at various points in time and geography, more research is needed on the effects of Anglo-Americans' responses to pain.

Halttunen asserts that the view of pain as necessary and deserved was dramatically challenged by the Anglo social movements that viewed pain as "loathsome and unacceptable."[62] The influence of these movements on Anglo culture led to thinking that when witnessing pain in others, it is virtuous to have a sympathetic response and to try to prevent or ameliorate the pain. She argues that this led to improvements in a wide range of social practices in Anglo-American culture, including revulsion at the use of flogging in the military, more humane treatment of prisoners and the mentally ill, concern for the treatment of animals, and efforts to stop the abuses of slavery and mistreatment of women and children. This movement is also credited with the rapid development and widespread use of anesthesia and pain medication. Thus there is ambivalence in Anglo-American culture about how to respond to pain, whether pain in oneself or in others; the cultural emphasis on the responsibility of the individual to cope with one's pain can conflict with the sense that pain is unacceptable and should be stopped.

An example of this ambivalence is exhibited by a 55-year-old Anglo-American female outpatient who complains to her physician about having chronic sinus congestion, labored breathing, headaches, difficulties in concentration, and irritated eyes, nose, and throat. She reports that she now realizes that she has had these symptoms for two months, but this is the first time she has sought medical attention. She attributes her symptoms to the presence of clouds of uncontrolled construction dust permeating her office building. Although her symptoms were virtually identical to those of other employees where she works, she has refrained for weeks from complaining about it to anyone else at the office. In fact, when others working in her office complained about their symptoms, she denied that she experienced similar symptoms, saying that she actually felt "just fine." She reports that while the other affected employees have now refused to continue working in the polluted office building, she has continued to work at her office, with her symptoms worsening. Now that she is finally taking the step of seeking help from her physician, she voices considerable regret that she did not react sooner to reduce her exposure.

WORKING WITH PATIENTS FROM OTHER CULTURES

There has been debate about whether practitioners consciously recognize that patients' cultural attributes affect their medical decisions or whether these influences on their decision-making operate unconsciously.[63] In the United States, Anglo-Americans, compared to other ethnic groups, are overrepresented among physicians.[64] Given that physicians can play a variety of roles with their patients,[65] this raises questions about whether identifying with the Anglo-American culture influences healthcare providers' encounters with pain patients, particularly with those from minority groups. Beliefs about other cultures can influence physician-patient interactions in important ways. For example, a survey of predominantly Anglo-American physicians' interactions with HIV seropositive patients revealed that healthcare providers viewed African American men as less likely than white men to adhere to their medication; this in turn affected the providers' treatment decisions about whether to prescribe highly active antiretroviral therapy.[66]

Evidence that Anglo-Americans' cultural beliefs affect medical decision making comes from a variety of studies. Anglo-American healthcare providers report that managing pain in persons of ethnic minority backgrounds is hindered by patients' opposition to reporting pain and taking opiates.[67] In a survey of 344 predominantly white cardiologists, only 33% agreed that there are disparities in how Hispanic or African Americans with cardiac disease or known risk factors are diagnosed or treated,[68] despite considerable evidence suggesting that such disparities exist;[69] the cardiologists surveyed were also more likely to attribute such disparities to patient characteristics or system level variables rather than to provider characteristics.[69]

Evidence suggests that physicians and nurses' underestimation of pain among minority patients plays a role in how much pain medication is provided. Among patients with metastatic or recurrent cancer, Anglo-American medical care providers were found to underestimate pain intensity for 74% of African American patients and 64% of Hispanic patients.[67] Another study found that although no differences were found in Anglo-American female patients' and Mexican American female patients' levels of cholecystectomy pain, their nurses rated the Anglo-American women's pain as significantly greater than they rated the Mexican American women's pain.[70]

Disparities in the providers' use of diagnostic and treatment procedures for patients of different ethnic backgrounds may be due in part to poor cross-cultural patient-physician communications. Johnson et al[71] found that physicians interacted differently with their African American patients than they did with their white patients; they were more verbally dominant and engaged in less patient-centered communication. They also found that the African American patients and their physicians, compared to the white patients and their physicians, demonstrated lower levels of positive affect. This suggests an emotional distance with African American patients that may interfere with communications and thereby result in less adequate treatment, including pain management. Of special interest in that study, about half of the participating physicians were white, but nearly all of the other physicians were either African American or Indian American. This raises the question about the extent to which physicians from US-ethnic-minority backgrounds adopt model styles of communicating with their ethnic minority patients that are similar to those used by physicians from the dominant Anglo culture.

In the United States, cultural differences between patients and medical care providers who identify with or are otherwise influenced by the dominant Anglo culture increases the risk of inadequate assessment and treatment of pain in minority patients.[72] A useful policy to aid in better assessment of pain in patients of diverse cultural backgrounds would be to standardize the tools used in these assessments.[72] Also, providers must pay careful attention to the social factors in pain management. Ethnic minority patients may receive inadequate pain medication because they lack material resources,[72] such as transportation to follow-up medical appointments.

An interesting implication of Bates' biocultural model of pain[19,20] for improving communication in medical settings in which Anglo-American perspectives dominate is to consider psychological as well as neurophysiological aspects of the patient's pain that are embedded within "ethnocultural group situations." Such considerations may be helpful in identifying sources of support, comfort, and meaning, such as patients' religion or spirituality that can play an important role in the management of disease[73] and the healing process.[74] Understanding patients' ethnocultural resources for coping with pain should inform plans for pain management by tailoring it accordingly. Although Anglo-American culture does not widely embrace Chinese medicine, many Chinese Americans diagnosed with cancer consider this approach to be an important part of their self-care.[75]

Although miscommunication is common in the United States when working with minority cultures, becoming aware of and understanding the patients' culture may facilitate correcting these misunderstandings. With regard to ethnic minority groups it is important to consider not only their host culture but also their culture of origin.[76] This can be facilitated by using open-ended questions and allowing patients to ask questions, which physicians do more frequently when communicating with Anglo-American patients compared to Hispanic patients.[77] Open-ended questions that might be helpful include: "What is your understanding of this pain?" and "What are you currently doing to manage this pain, and how is that working for you?" It can be helpful to communicate friendliness and build rapport, which physicians are less likely to do with ethnic minority patients than with their white patients.[77]

Among Chinese Americans, low acculturation may impede access to adequate pain management.[78] Because language barriers can impair the relationship between medical care providers and their patients,[77] it would be preferable for practitioners to have a professional interpreter present in situations where patients and their family members are not fluent in the language/s of the medical care provider.[72]

Research suggests that patients who have physicians from the same ethnicity as themselves rate their physicians as more participatory.[79] After a patient receives a diagnosis, it may be worthwhile to consider referring patients to outside providers and specialists who are knowledgeable about working with patients from a given cultural background. This might prove especially beneficial in situations where cultural differences between a patient and his or her health provider would otherwise become a barrier to an effective patient-provider relationship.

CONCLUSION

Considerable evidence suggests how Anglo-Americans as a group respond differently to pain compared to persons from other ethnic groups. Anglo-Americans have traditionally placed a great deal of emphasis on the expectation that people should demonstrate considerable autonomy in coping with their pain. Related to this, Anglo-Americans appear to be less expressive and emotional in communicating their pain compared to persons from other ethnic groups, yet Anglo-Americans are more likely to receive analgesic medication for their pain. As Anglo-Americans comprise the majority of physicians in the United States, their views have dominated the field of medicine. Therefore, as summarized in Table 9.2,

TABLE 9.2 Strategies to Improve Healthcare Providers' Competencies to Assess and Treat Pain in Anglo-Americans and Other Ethnic Groups

- Develop expertise in working with Anglo-American and other cultural groups to identify important aspects of patients' lives to consider in assessing and treating pain.
- Ensure that the development of expertise about Anglo-American and other US minority cultures' responses to pain also includes recognition that responses to pain may also differ by age, gender, socioeconomic status, national origin, religious background, and social and psychological factors.
- Improve multicultural training in all levels of medical education—including continuing medical education. Ideally, such training may require not only education about diverse cultures and how they may affect the patient, but also how cultural differences may affect patient-physician communications.
- Standardize the assessment of pain so that stereotypes and unconscious biases pertaining to patients of particular ethnic groups do not interfere with adequate pain assessment.
- Provide culturally and linguistically matched medical translation services as needed.
- Develop, evaluate, and disseminate evidence-based interventions that reduce ethnic disparities in the assessment and management of pain.

a good deal of emphasis needs to be placed on ensuring that Anglo-American providers gain understanding of their patients' cultures to enable better assessment and treatment of pain in patients from other cultural backgrounds.

More research is needed about how patient and provider characteristics and social interactions contribute to responses to pain among Anglo-Americans and others.[63] Also, considerable research is needed to inform our understanding about how organizational and societal level policies, such as alternative methods of reimbursement, court-based remedies, sanctions, and incentives might produce improvements in pain assessment and management.[63] We hope that a continued emphasis on considering the multifaceted dimensions of cultural differences will result in improved strategies for alleviating pain and suffering for people from all cultural backgrounds.

ACKNOWLEDGMENT

The authors acknowledge the contributions of Bethany Ketchen, Ph.D. and Susan Anderson, Ph.D. for their engagement, advice, and guidance.

REFERENCES

1. Edwards CL, Fillingim RB, Keefe F. Race, ethnicity and pain. *Pain,* 2001;94:133–137.
2. U.S. Census Bureau. Overview of race and Hispanic origin: 2010. March 2011. http://www.census.gov/prod/cen2010/briefs/c2010br-02.pdf. Accessed April 16, 2011.
3. Bureau USC. Selected social characteristics in the United States: 2008. http://factfinder.census.gov/servlet/ADPTable?_bm=y&-geo_id=01000US&-parsed=true&-ds_name=ACS_2008_1YR_G00_&-_lang=en&-_caller=geoselect&-format=. Accessed January 9, 2011.
4. Sheffield D, Biles PL, Orom H, Maixner W, Sheps DS. Race and sex differences in cutaneous pain perception. *Psychom Med,* 2000;62(5):517–523.
5. Speight S, Thomas A, Kennel R, Anderson M. Operationalizing multicultural training in doctoral programs an internships. *Professional Psychology: Research and Practice,* 1995;26(4):401–406.
6. Champaneria MC, Axtell S. Cultural competence training in US medical schools. *JAMA,* 2004;291(17):2142.
7. Godkin MA, Savageau JA. The effect of a global multiculturalism track on cultural competence of preclinical medical students. *Fam Med,* 2001;33(3):178–186.
8. Loudon RF, Anderson PM, Gill PS, Greenfield SM. Educating medical students for work in culturally diverse societies. *JAMA,* 1999;282(9):875–880.
9. Smith WR, Betancourt JR, Wynia MK, et al. Recommendations for teaching about racial and ethnic disparities in health and health care. *Ann Intern Med,* 2007;147(9):654–665.
10. Valle R. *Caregiving across cultures.* Washington, DC: Taylor & Francis; 1998.
11. Locke DC. *Increasing multicultural understanding: A comprehensive model.* Newbury Park: Sage; 1992.
12. Von Korff M, Jensen MP, Karoly P. Assessing global pain severity by self-report in clinical and health services research. *Spine,* 2000;25(24):3140–3151.
13. Labus JS, Keefe FJ, Jensen MP. Self-reports of pain intensity and direct observations of pain behavior: When are they correlated? *Pain,* 2003;102(1–2):109–124.
14. Price DD. Central neural mechanisms that interrelate sensory and affective dimensions of pain. *Mol Interv,* 2002;2(6):392–402.
15. Ducharme J. Acute pain and pain control: state of the art. *Ann Emerg Med,* 2000;35(6):592–603.
16. Chaves J, Barber, TX. *hypnotism and surgical pain. In M Weisenberg (ed), Pain: Clinical and experimental perspectives.* St. Louis: C.V. Mosby; 1975.
17. Kessler RC, Whalen T, eds. *Hypnotic preparation in anesthesia and surgery.* New York: Churchill Livingstone Inc.; 1999. Temes R, ed. Medical hypnosis: An introduction and clinical guide.

18. Lowe NK. The nature of labor pain. *Am J Obstet Gynecol,* 2002;186(5 Suppl Nature):S16–S24.

19. Bates MS. Ethnicity and pain: a biocultural model. *Soc Sci Med,* 1987;24(1):47–50.

20. Bates MS. *Biocultural dimensions of chronic pain: Implications for treatment of multi-ethnic populations.* Albany, NY: State University of New York; 1996.

21. Melzack R, Wall PD. *The challenge of pain.* New York: Basic Books; 1993.

22. Bandura A. *Social learning theory.* Englewood Cliffs, NJ; 1977.

23. Festinger L. A theory of social comparison processes. *Human Relat,* VII, 117–114, 1977 .

24. Encandela JA. Social science and the study of pain since Zborowski: A need for a new agenda. *Soc Sci Med,* 1993;36(6):783–791.

25. Campbell CM, Edwards RR, Fillingim RB. Ethnic differences in responses to multiple experimental pain stimuli. *Pain,* Jan 2005;113(1–2):20–26.

26. Woodrow KM, Friedman GD, Siegelaub AB, Collen MF. Pain tolerance: differences according to age, sex and race. *Psychosom Med,* 1972;34(6):548–556.

27. Rahim-Williams FB, Riley JL, 3rd, Herrera D, Campbell CM, Hastie BA, Fillingim RB. Ethnic identity predicts experimental pain sensitivity in African Americans and Hispanics. *Pain,* 2007;129(1–2):177–184.

28. McCracken LM, Matthews AK, Tang TS, Cuba SL. A comparison of blacks and whites seeking treatment for chronic pain. *Clin J Pain,* 2001;17:249–255.

29. Walsh NE, Schoenfeld L, Ramamurthy S, Hoffman J. Normative model for cold pressor test. *Am J Phys Med Rehabil,* 1989;68(1):6–11.

30. Edwards RR, Fillingim RB. Ethnic differences in thermal pain responses. *Psychosom Med,* 1999;61(3):346–354.

31. Tan G, Jensen MP, Thornby J, Anderson KO. Ethnicity, control appraisal, coping, and adjustment to chronic pain among black and white Americans. *Pain Med,* 2005;6(1):18–28.

32. Faucett J, Gordon N, Levine J. Differences in postoperative pain severity among four ethnic groups. *J Pain Symptom Manage,* 1994;9(6):383–389.

33. Chapman WP, Jones CM. Variations in cutaneous and visceral pain sensitivity in normal subjects. *J Clin Invest,* 1944;23(1):81–91.

34. Edwards RR, Moric M, Husfeldt B, Buvanendran A, Ivankovich O. Ethnic similarities and differences in the chronic pain experience: A comparison of African American, Hispanic, and white patients. *Am Acad Pain Med,* 2005;6(1):88–98.

35. Zatzick DF, Dimsdale JE. Cultural variations in response to painful stimuli. *Psychosom Med,* 1990;52(5):544–557.

36. Baker TA, Green CR. Intrarace differences among black and white Americans presenting for chronic pain management: The influence of age, physical health, and psychosocial factors. *Pain Med,* 6;(1):29–38.

37. Zeidan F, Gordon NS, Merchant J, Goolkasian P. The effects of brief mindfulness meditation training on experimentally induced pain. *J Pain,* 2010;11(3):199–209.

38. Berkanovic E, Oster P, Wong WK, et al. The relationship between socioeconomic status and recently diagnosed rheumatoid arthritis. *Arthritis Care Res,* 1996;9(6):257–262.

39. Rhudy JL, Dubbert PM, Parker JD, Burke RS, Williams AE. Affective modulation of pain in substance-dependent veterans. *Pain Med,* 2006;7(6):483–500.

40. Ortega RA, Youndelman BA, Havel RC. Ethnic variability in the treatment of pain. *Department of Surgery Faculty Papers and Presentations;* 1999, http://jdc.jefferson.edu/surgeryfp/11. Accessed April 18, 2011.

41. Zbowowski M. Cultural components in responses to pain. *J Soc Issues,* 1952;8:16–30.

42. Zborowski M. *People in pain.* San Francisco, CA: Joseey-Bass;1969.

43. Zola, IK. Culture and symtoms—an analysis of patients' presenteing complaints. *Am Sociol. Rev,* 1966:31(5):615–630.

44. Koopman C, Eisenthal S, Stoeckle JD. Ethnicity in the reported pain, emotional distress and requests of medical outpatients. *Soc Sci Med,* 1984;18(6):487–490.

45. Hough RL, Landsverk JA, Karno M, et al. Utilization of health and mental health services by Los Angeles Mexican Americans and non-Hispanic whites. *Arch Gen Psychiatry,* 1987;44(8):702–709.

46. Carey TS, Garrett JM. The relation of race to outcomes and the use of health care services for acute low back pain. *Spine,* 2003;28(4):390–394.

47. Harlow BL, Stewart EG. A population-based assessment of chronic unexplained vulvar pain: have we underestimated the prevalence of vulvodynia? *J Am Med Womens Assoc,* 2003;58(2):82–88.

48. Edwards RR, Doleys DM, Fillingim RB, Lowery D. Ethnic differences in pain tolerance: clinical implications in a chronic pain population. *Psychosom Med,* 2001;63(2):316–323.

49. Pfefferbaum B, Adams J, Aceves J. The influence of culture on pain in Anglo and Hispanic children with cancer. *J Am Acad Child Adolesc Psychiatry,* 1990;29:642–647.

50. Kleinman A. Pain and resistance: The delegitimation and relegitimation of local worlds. In Good MJD, Brodwin PE, Good BJ, Kleinman A. (eds), *Pain as human experience* (pp. 169–197), 1992, Berkeley: University of California Press,

51. Jackson JE. After a while no one believes you: Real and unreal pain. In Good MJD, Brodwin PE, Good BJ, Kleinman A. (eds), *Pain as human experience* (pp. 138–168), 1992, Berkeley: University of California Press,

52. Cintron A, Morrison RS. Pain and ethnicity in the United States: A systematic review. *J Palliat Med,* 2006;9(6):1454–1473.

53. Cleeland CS, Gonin R, Baez L, Loehrer P, Pandya KJ. Pain and treatment of pain in minority patients with cancer. The Eastern Cooperative Oncology Group Minority Outpatient Pain Study. *Ann Intern Med,* 1997;127(9):813–816.

54. Todd KH, Deaton C, D'Adamo AP, Goe L. Ethnicity and analgesic practice. *Ann Emerg Med,* 2000;35:11–16.

55. Todd KH, Samaroo N, Hoffman JR. Ethnicity as a risk factor for inadequate emergency department analgesia. *JAMA,* 1993;269:1537–1539.

56. Tamayo-Sarver JH, Hinze SW, Cydulka RK, Baker DW. Racial and ethnic dispairities in emergency department analgesic prescription. *Am J Public Health,* 2003;93:2067–2073.

57. Burgess DJ, Crowley-Matoka M, Phelan S, et al. Patient race and physicians' decisions to prescribe opioids for chronic low back pain. *Soc Sci Med,* 2008;67(11):1852–1860.

58. Kleinman A, Brodwin PE, Good BJ, Good MJD. Pain as human experience: An introduction. In Good MJD, Brodwin PE, Good BJ, Kleinman A. (eds), *Pain as human experience* (pp. 1–28), 1992, Berkeley: University of California Press,

59. Scarry E. *The body in pain: The making and unmaking of the world,* 1985. Oxford: Oxford University Press.

60. Im EO, Lee SH, Liu Y, Lim HJ, Guevara E, Chee W. A national online forum on ethnic differences in cancer pain experience. *Nurs Res,* 2009;58(2):86–94.

61. Oquendo MA, Ellis SP, Greenwald S, Malone KM, Weissman MM, Mann JJ. Ethnic and sex differences in suicide rates relative to major depression in the United States. *Am J Psychiatry,* 2001;158(10):1652–1658.

62. Halttunen K. Humanitarianism and the pornography of pain in Anglo-American culture. *American Historical Review,* 1995;100(2):303–334.

63. van Ryn M, Fu SS. Paved with good intentions: Do public health and human service providers contribute to racial/ethnic disparities in health? *Am J Public Health,* 2003;93(2):248–255.

64. U.S. Department of Health and Human Services, Health Resources and Services Administration, Bureau of Health Professions. Changing demographics: Implications for physicians, nurses, and other health workers. 2003. http://www.nachc.org/client/documents/clinical/Clinical_Workforce_Changing_Demographics.pdf. Accessed May 8, 2011.

65. Klabunde CN, Ambs A, Keating NL, et al. The role of primary care physicians in cancer care. *J Gen Intern Med,* 2009;24(9):1029–1036.

66. Bogart LM, Catz SL, Kelly JA, Benotsch EG. Factors influencing physicians' judgments of adherence and treatment decisions for patients with HIV disease. *Med Decis Making,* 2001;21(1):28–36.

67. Anderson KO, Mendoza TR, Valero V, et al. Minority cancer patients and their providers: pain management attitudes and practice. *Cancer,* 15 2000;88(8):1929–1938.

68. Lurie N, Fremont A, Jain AK, et al. Racial and ethnic disparities in care: The perspectives of cardiologists. *Circulation,* 2005;111(10):1264–1269.

69. Ford ES, Cooper RS. Racial/ethnic differences in health care utilization of cardiovascular procedures: a review of the evidence. *Health Serv Res,* 1995;30(1 Pt 2):237–252.

70. Calvillo ER, Flaskerud JH. Evaluation of the pain response by Mexican American and Anglo American women and their nurses. *J Adv Nurs,* 1993;18(3):451–459.

71. Johnson RL, Roter D, Powe NR, Cooper LA. Patient race/ethnicity and quality of patient-physician communication during medical visits. *Am J Public Health,* 2004;94(12):2084–2090.

72. Bonham VL. Race, ethnicity, and pain treatment: Striving to understand the causes and solutions to the disparities in pain treatment. *J Law Med Ethics,* 2001;29:52–68.

73. Polzer RL. African Americans and diabetes: spiritual role of the health care provider in self-management. *Res Nurs Health,* 2007;30(2):164–174.

74. Martin SS, Trask J, Peterson T, Martin BC, Baldwin J, Knapp M. Influence of culture and discrimination on care-seeking behavior of elderly African Americans: a qualitative study. *Soc Work Public Health,* 2010;25(3):311–326.

75. Chou FY, Dodd M, Abrams D, Padilla G. Symptoms, self-care, and quality of life of Chinese American patients with cancer. *Oncol Nurs Forum,* 2007;34(6):1162–1167.

76. American Psychiatric Association. *Diagnostic and statistical manual of mental health disorders,* 2000. Washington, D.C.: Author.

77. Schouten BC, Meeuwesen L. Cultural differences in medical communication: A review of the literature. *Patient Educ Couns,* 2006;64(1–3):21–34.

78. Edrington J, Sun A, Wong C, et al. Barriers to pain management in a community sample of Chinese American patients with cancer. *J Pain Symptom Manage,* 2009;37(4):665–675.

79. Cooper-Patrick L, Gallo JJ, Gonzales JJ, et al. Race, gender, and partnership in the patient-physician relationship. *JAMA,* 1999;282(6):583–589.

Culture and Pain Assessment

10

CROSS-CULTURAL USE AND VALIDITY OF PAIN SCALES AND QUESTIONNAIRES— NORWEGIAN CASE STUDY

HESOOK SUZIE KIM, PHD, RN
Professor Emerita, College of Nursing, University of Rhode Island, Kingston, Rhode Island, USA *and* Project Director for Research Programs, Institutt for helsefag, Buskerud University College, Drammen, Norway

DONNA SCHWARTZ-BARCOTT, PHD, RN
Professor, College of Nursing, University of Rhode Island, Kingston, Rhode Island, USA

INGER MARGRETHE HOLTER, PHD, RN
Project Coordinator, Norwegian Nurses Association, Norway

Key Points
- Pain is an internal, subjective phenomenon, and the gold standard of pain assessment is patient self-report.
- Pain assessment relies on scales and questionnaires, many of which measure intensity only, while others assess qualitative differences in pain and pain-related functional impairment.
- Pain assessment from the cross-cultural perspective utilizes both culture-specific and cross-culturally comparable instruments.
- The McGill Pain Questionnaire (MPQ) measures various characteristics of pain, and has been developed into different language versions.
- There are two types of non-English MPQs: those developed by the back-translation method and those developed applying the same instrument development technique used in the development of the original MPQ.
- The Norwegian case study in developing a version of the MPQ is presented to illustrate the utility and applicability of pain instruments from the cross-cultural perspective.

INTRODUCTION

Pain is one of the most universal human experiences, and has been explained by various combinations of neurophysiological, psychological, and cultural theories. Pain perception is fundamentally associated with injury or noxious stimuli, although the exact mechanisms and processes through which persons experience and express pain remain controversial. In addition to the specific noxious stimulus, the experience of pain is influenced by social circumstances and cultural background, as well as by the meanings of pain to the patient, and emotional states such as anxiety, fear, joy, and helplessness.[1] Pain is a subjective experience, therefore it fundamentally requires self-report.

Pain in the healthcare context remains challenging both in assessment and treatment. Research reveals that pain is underestimated and undermanaged in most countries, despite great advances in analgesics and nonanalgesic pain therapies, and efforts to improve pain assessment and treatment. Among these are the institutionalization of "pain clinics," pain specialization in healthcare fields, and the establishment of routine protocols for pain assessment in hospitals and nursing homes. Physicians and nurses are responsible for determining the intensity and quality of pain in their clients, in order to make decisions about pain management. Although health professionals often assess pain independently without relying on clients' expressions, there has been an increasing emphasis on obtaining clients' self-reports of pain to gain more valid information.

In clinical practice, there are two modalities for measuring pain: client self-report and independent assessment by professionals. Self-report of pain as the "gold standard" of pain assessment has been instituted in healthcare through the use of pain intensity scales and verbal reports or descriptions of pain. Healthcare professionals tend to use both pain intensity scales and, additionally, instruments such as behavioral observation scales for pain, especially when they are assessing pain in clients such as infants, children, or clients with dementia or confusion who are not able to express their pain optimally. Important discrepancies have been found between the self-reports by clients and the professionals' assessments.[2,3]

Although the principal objective of developing pain scales is their application in clinical practice, pain scales for research are also necessary. Measurement of pain for research purposes requires valid, objective instruments that can assess individual-to-individual differences and comparisons of pain responses. Various types of pain measurement tools have been developed and applied in studying pain experiences and pain responses. Reliable and valid detection of variations in pain across individuals, across different times in the same individual, and in different types of pain have been major issues in developing and applying pain scales for research. Cross-cultural use of pain scales is critical for developing knowledge about pain in different cultures and for understanding cross-cultural similarities and differences.[4,5] It is essential to develop knowledge about pain experiences across diverse cultures, in order to enhance our understanding of the nature of pain so that we can improve its management in the current multicultural scene.[6,7,8,9] Cross-cultural similarities and differences in pain response and experience are emerging in the literature and point to more in-depth investigations.[10,11,12,13,14] Cross-cultural knowledge on pain is enriched when researchers are able to compare research results from cross-culturally validated instruments and interpret findings from the cultural context. In this chapter, our discussion will focus on cross-cultural development and use of pain scales. We begin with a general discussion of existing pain assessment instruments.

TOOLS OF PAIN ASSESSMENT

Because pain is a felt-experience, the traditional convention of assessing pain is to ask the person with pain to describe the experience. Such personal descriptions provide critical and insightful information regarding how individuals experience pain, and are used by health-care professionals to gain in-depth understandings about pain experiences from their clients. Although this convention continues to be used by most professionals in their practice, there is increasing pressure to quantify and objectify pain experiences in order to standardize the language for pain assessment. In response to this movement, various measurement tools for assessing pain have been developed during the past 40 years, and used in both clinical practice and research. There are two types of pain measurement tools—self-report scales and professional assessment tools. Because pain is a subjective experience, it has been measured by the use of self-report instruments; at the same time, however, healthcare professionals responsible for managing pain have used observational instruments to measure pain in an objective fashion.

Self-report scales

Most self-report scales measure pain intensity using various graphic, numerical, or descriptive modes to represent differences. These include visual analog scales (VAS, the Sensation and Distress of Pain Visual Analogue Scale, and the Memorial Pain Assessment Card), the numerical pain scale (NMS or NRS-11), the Iowa Pain Thermometer, the pain faces scales (FPS & FPS-R, Wong-Baker Faces Pain Rating Scale, and Oucher pain scale for children), the verbal descriptor scale (VDS), and the verbal rating scale (VRS). Other pain scales measure not only the intensity but also the quality and characteristics of pain, such as the McGill Pain Questionnaire (MPQ & MPQ-SF),[4,15] Multidimensional Pain Inventory (MPI),[16] Brief Pain Inventory (BPI),[17] Pain Quality Assessment Scale (PQAS),[18] and the Multidimensional Affect and Pain Survey (101-MAPS).[19] Scales for pain in specific diseases or specific to pain-types also have been developed, such as back-pain scales (The Extended Aberdeen Spine Pain Scale[20]), the Neuropathic Pain Scale (NPS),[21] and various cancer-pain scales.

Observational pain scales

Clinicians use observational pain scales developed specifically for infants and children or for adults with cognitive difficulties, including behavioral rating scales and behavior checklists, such as CHEOPS,[22] the Colorado Behavioral Numerical Pain Scale,[23] Doloplus-2 Scale,[24] FLACC (Face, Legs, Arms, Cry, Consolability for children),[25] PACSLAC,[26] Pain Assessment in Advanced Dementia (PAINAD),[27] the Multidimensional Assessment of Pain Scale (MAPS),[28,29] CRIES Scale,[30] and the COMFORT scale.[31] Healthcare professionals also use various global pain intensity scales such as VAS and the numerical pain scale for assessing the intensity of pain based on observation. Table 10.1 gives a list of pain measurement tools commonly used in clinical practice and research. As shown in this table, numerous translated, non-English versions of pain scales are in use, suggesting cross-cultural sharing of pain instruments.

ASSESSING PAIN IN THE CROSS-CULTURAL CONTEXT

Assessing pain in different cultures requires using specific languages. With the movement toward standardized measures of pain instead of personal descriptions, there has been an active development of pain measurement tools for use in specific cultures and in different languages. Many pain measurement tools have been developed for use in specific cultures/languages for application in clinical practice and research. We found in the literature several pain scales developed independently in non-English languages in original forms, for example, the Brief, Descriptive Danish Pain Questionnaire (BDDPQ),[32] the

TABLE 10.1 List of Commonly Used Pain Measurement Tools

Type of Measurement	Name of Pain Scale	Description	Non-English Versions
Intensity Scales—For Self Report	Visual Analog Scale (VAS); Sensation & Distress of Pain VAS; The Memorial Pain Assessment Card	An intensity scale with 100 mm lines with two words that anchor two extreme pain spectra, such as "no pain" and "as bad as it can be." Pain intensity is combined for sensation and distress in the Sensation & Distress VAS. The Memorial Pain Assessment Card measures both pain intensity and mood.	
	The Numerical Pain Scale (NMS or NRS-11)	An intensity scale of rating in 0 to 10 or 0 to 100.	
	The Iowa Pain Thermometer	A picture of a thermometer with lines and an increasing shade of red specified by corresponding words for pain intensity from "No Pain" to "The Most Intense Pain Imaginable."	
	The Pain Faces Scales (FPS, FPS-R, Wong-Baker Faces Pain Rating Scale, The Oucher Pain Scale for Children)	A scale with 6 or 7 faces depicting the degree of hurt or pain. Used with children or adults with cognitive impairment or difficulty in communication.	
	The Verbal Descriptor Pain Scale (VDS); The Verbal Rating Scale (VRS)	A scale with 7 pain intensity descriptors from "no pain" to "the most intense pain imaginable."	
Quality of pain measurements—For Self Report	McGill Pain Questionnaire (MPQ)[7,15]	A pain questionnaire using 78 pain descriptor-adjectives in 21 categories characterizing pain and pain intensity.	Amharic, Arabic, Brazilian, Chinese, Czech, Danish, Dutch, Farsi (Iranian), Finnish, French, German, Greek, Hebrew, Hindi, Italian, Japanese, Korean, Norwegian, Polish, Slovak, Spanish, Swedish, Thai, Turkish, Urdu, Welsh

	Scale	Description	Languages
	The Multidimensional Pain Inventory (MPI)[16]	A measurement tool comprising of 61-items that include 5 scales for the perception of pain and pain reactions, 3 scales for others' responses to one's pain, and 4-scales for performance of everyday tasks.	Dutch, French, German, Italian, Swedish
	Brief Pain Inventory (BPI)[17]	A measurement for the intensity of pain and interference of pain with daily life (originally designed for cancer patients).	Chinese, French, German, Hebrew, Hindi, Italian, Japanese, Korean, Norwegian, Spanish, Thai, Turkish
	Pain Quality Assessment Scale (PQAS)[18]	A 20-item measure for pain quality, adopted from the Neuropathic Pain Scale to assess both neuropathic and non-neuropathic pain.	
	The Multidimensional Affect and Pain Survey (101-MAPS)[19]	A questionnaire containing 101 descriptors in sentences for three super-clusters of somatosensory pain, emotional pain, and well-being.	Japanese
Observational scales	The Colorado Behavioral Numerical Pain Scale[23]	An observational rating scale using behavioral descriptors developed for use with sedated patients.	
	Doloplus-2 Scale[24]	A rating scale originally developed in French with 10 items (5 somatic, 2 psychomotor, and 3 psychosocial items), each with four behavioral descriptors for ratings of 0–3. Developed for use with non-communicative patients (the elderly).	Chinese, Dutch, Japanese, Norwegian

(continued)

TABLE 10.1 (Continued)

Type of Measurement	Name of Pain Scale	Description	Non-English Versions
	PACSLAC[26]	A behavioral checklist with subscales for Facial Expressions, Activity/Body Movement, & Physiological Indicators/Eating/Sleeping Changes/Vocal Behaviors. Developed for use with cognitively impaired or non-communicative patients.	Dutch, French
	Pain Assessment in Advanced Dementia (PAINAD)[27]	A 5-item observational rating tool with a range of 0–10 for breathing, vocalization, facial expression, body language, and consolability. Developed for use with the cognitively impaired.	Chinese, Dutch, German, Italian
	The Behavioral Rating Scale (CHEOPS)[22]	A rating scale of the intensity, frequency, or duration of behaviors of pain obtained through observation, originally developed for pain assessment in children.	Japanese
	FLACC—Face, Legs, Arms, Cry Consolability For Children[25]	A 0–10 metric rating scale on 5 items scored 0–2 for pain in children measured through observation on face, legs, activity, cry, and consolability. Originally developed to be used with children, but has been applied with non-communicative patients.	Brazilian Portuguese, Hebrew, Korean
	Multidimensional Assessment of Pain Scale (MAPS)[28,29]	A 5-category, 10-point scale relying on observation for pain intensity and quality. Developed for use with pre-verbal children.	

	Scale	Description	Language
	CRIES Scale[30]	An observational scale for 5-categories (Crying, Requiring Oxygen, Increased Vital Signs, Facial Expression—Grimace, & Sleeplessness) rated 0–2 for intensity. Developed for use with infants.	Korean
	COMFORT Scale for Pain Assessment[31]	A 9-category rating scale for Alertness, Calmness, Respiratory Distress, Crying, Physical Movement, Muscle Tone, Facial Tension, Blood Pressure, and Heart Rate in the scale of 1–5. Developed to be used with children.	
	Behavioral Checklists (e.g., The Checklist of Nonverbal Pain Indicators)	Various versions of behavioral checklist indicative of pain.	
	Visual Analog Scale Observation (VASObs)	A visual analog scale rated by observation.	
	Global Behaviorally Anchored Rating Scale	A rating scale of 0–10 with behavioral anchors for "no pain" and "extreme pain"	
Specific pain scales	The Extended Aberdeen Spine Pain Scale[20]	A questionnaire to be used to elicit the nature of back pain	German
	The Neuropathic Pain Scale[21]	A rating scale with 2 items for the global dimension of pain intensity and pain unpleasantness, 8 items addressing specific qualities of neuropathic pain, and 1 item for temporal sequence of pain	

Dutch pain questionnaire,[33] the Finnish Pain Questionnaire,[34] the Questionnaire Douleur Saint-Antoine for French (QDSA),[35] the German (Berne) pain questionnaire,[36] the Italian Pain Questionnaire,[37] the Norwegian Pain Questionnaire,[38] the Korean Geriatric Pain Measure,[39] and the Chinese Cancer Pain Assessment Tool (CCPAT).[40] However, a great effort has been expended in developing pain measurement tools for cross-cultural stand-ardization especially during the past three decades.

Commonly used pain scales have been translated into many different languages. Pain measurement in the cross-cultural context is accomplished principally by (a) utilizing pain intensity rating scales such as VAS, FPS-R, and NMS, which require no translation except for instructions, and (b) translating and validating pain scales originally developed in English into specific languages for culture-specific applications.

As the McGill Pain Questionnaire (MPQ and MPQ-SF) has the longest history of development and use after its original proposal in 1975, the two versions of the MPQ have been translated into many languages. Costa et al[41] in their systematic review of cross-cultural adaptations of the McGill Pain Questionnaire list 29 long-form and 15 short-form non-English language versions of the MPQ, representing 26 different languages. However, some non-English versions of the MPQ were exact translations of the original scale retaining all of its descriptors and structure, while others were developed adopting only the methodology used to develop the original MPQ, resulting in language-specific descriptors and structures. Because the MPQ has pain descriptors as part of the scale to measure the quality of pain, the translation of the MPQ has involved validation of pain descriptors from the targeted language perspective. According to Costa et al[41] very few of these versions meet the "quality criteria for psychometric properties of health status questionnaires" suggested by Terwee et al.[42] Two issues in developing non-English versions of the MPQ were identified: (a) many did not follow rigorously and completely the process of cross-cultural adaptation of instruments including initial translation, synthesis, back translation, expert committee review, and pilot testing, with only four versions (the Brazilian-Portuguese, the Farsi, the Korean, and the Turkish) following all recommended guidelines; and (b) inadequate testing of measurement properties such as for internal consistency, construct validity, reproducibility, reliability, agreement, responsiveness, and floor and ceiling effects was evident in most of these instruments, with none of the versions meeting all of the criteria. (See Costa et al[41] for the detailed results of their analyses of the non-English MPQ versions regarding the quality criteria.)

Two other pain scales for assessing pain quality, originally developed in English, have been translated into various languages. The Brief Pain Inventory (BPI)[17] has been translated into Chinese,[43] French,[44] German,[45] Hebrew,[46] Hindi,[47] Italian,[48,49] Japanese,[50] Korean,[51] Norwegian,[52] Spanish,[53] Thai,[54] and Turkish.[55] The Multidimensional Pain Inventory (MPI)[16] has been translated into Dutch,[56] French,[57] German,[58] Italian,[59] and Swedish.[60] Several observational pain scales have also been translated into non-English languages as shown in Table 10.1. The need for clinically applicable pain scales has prompted the translation of disease-specific scales such as the Extended Aberdeen Back Pain Scale into German,[61] and of specialized scales such as DOLOPLUS-2 into Norwegian[62] and Japanese,[63] and PACSLAC into Dutch[64] and French.[65]

Our MEDLINE search of the literature from 1980 to 2010 revealed minimal use of these translated pain scales in published research reports. There are, in general, fewer than ten research publications for each language version of the MPQ, and even fewer applications of other translated pain scales in research. Furthermore, most pain research carried out in different countries tends to be limited to pain intensity measures, utilizing VAS, FPS, and the numerical rating scales. There also is a paucity of research on pain from the cross-cultural comparative perspective, possibly due to the lack of validated pain instruments for cross-cultural comparisons. While there is a need to develop pain scales for clinical applications in specific languages and to incorporate culture-specific expressions, there also is a need to develop pain scales for research, which can be used for cross-linguistic and cross-cultural comparisons in order to gain in-depth knowledge regarding similarities and differences.

The following case study illustrates how a Norwegian version of the MPQ was developed for cross-cultural research through direct translation of the original scale. Many of the earlier translated versions of the MPQ at the time were designed with an emphasis on cultural specificity and actually represent new versions rather than direct translations of the MPQ. The intent in this translation was to preserve the denotation and connotation embedded in the scale as well as the numerical scaling of the original MPQ so that the translated version could be applied to the study of universal and differential aspects of pain and its management from a cross-cultural comparative context.

A CASE STUDY—DEVELOPING A NORWEGIAN VERSION OF MCGILL PAIN QUESTIONNAIRE

This 1989 case study[66] was conducted in Norway. The original MPQ (also known as the long-form since the publication of the short-form) consists of a core component with a word list of 78 adjectives, clustered into 20 subclasses and reflecting three major dimensions of pain—sensory, affective, and evaluative. Each subclass contains two to five descriptors, each of which has an assigned value from 1 to 5 reflecting the level of intensity in that subclass. The instrument provides several measures. The most commonly reported scale, the pain-rating index total (PRIT), provides an estimate of overall pain intensity. This scale, obtained by summing all the descriptors selected from the 20 subclasses, has a possible range of 0 to 78. Similarly, separate scores for the three dimensions may be obtained by summing the values associated with the words selected from the subclasses that comprise a specific dimension. Scores for each of these dimensions vary in the range from 0 to 42 for the sensory dimension (PRIS), 0 to 14 for the affective dimension (PRIA), and 0 to 5 for the evaluative dimension (PRIE). In addition, the number of words chosen (NWC), which can range from 0 to 20, provides an indicator of how many of the subclasses were chosen by any one subject.

The process of Norwegian translation

The NMPQ was developed in three phases. The general aim throughout these phases was to create a translation that remained as faithful as possible to the underlying meaning, grouping, and intensity of the word descriptors in the original English version and that at the same time was acceptable to and easily understood by the average Norwegian. In the first phase, the MPQ was translated into Standard Norwegian by a well-known and highly experienced professional translator of English. A preliminary validation of this Norwegian translation was carried out by back-translation into English as the second phase. This is the standard method used for translating a psychometric research instrument from one language to another.[67,68,69] The translation of the initial version of the NMPQ back into English was performed by an American-born English teacher with fluency in Norwegian and over 15 years of teaching experience at the secondary and university levels in Norway. In the third phase, the English translation derived from the Norwegian translation was compared with the original English version of the MPQ and a consensus was reached on the final Norwegian version. This last phase was completed by a group of five bilingual Norwegian nurse educators.

This approach to the translation process, considered standard at the time, is somewhat different from that proposed by Beaton, Bombardier, Guillemin, and Ferraz,[70] whose model for translation of self-report measures contains four stages: Stage I—forward-translation by at least two translators, one translator being a naïve translator and the other with knowledge of the subject; Stage II—synthesis of the translations; Stage III—back-translation by at least two translators who are naïve translators; and Stage IV—consolidations of the translations for semantic, idiomatic, experiential, and conceptual equivalences. Although our method did not rigorously adhere to this four-stage process, the procedure followed met this process adequately.

All 78 descriptors from the original MPQ were translated into Norwegian. Single words (unlike the Italian version) were readily available in Norwegian and in most cases an appropriate word was relatively easily identified. When a choice between words was necessary, a word was selected that best (a) preserved the original qualities of each subclass (e.g., spatial, temporal); (b) expressed the same level of relative intensity in the ordering of the words; and (c) retained the same descriptive meaning. In only one case (tugging versus drawing), distinction could not be made between the two words in Norwegian, and the same Norwegian word (*trekkende*) was used twice, once for "tugging" under the sensory subclass of traction pressure, and another time for "drawing" under the second sensory miscellaneous subclass. (See Kim et al[66] for the list of Norwegian pain descriptors used in the NMPQ.)

Testing of the NMPQ for applicability and validity

The final version of the NMPQ was administered to a sample of 52 adult surgical patients two times during the postoperative period, initially on the second day after surgery and then subsequently on either the fourth or fifth postsurgical day. The sample was drawn from patients undergoing various sorts of surgery (such as soft-tissue, spinal, orthopedic, plastic, and Caesarian section) at one general hospital in Oslo, Norway, and consisted of patients ranging in age from 19 to 81 years with a mean of 45 years, and who were equally divided by gender, and ethnically homogeneous. The NMPQ was administered as a written self-report, with a question added at the end of the questionnaire for a description of pain in their own words.

No problem was encountered in administering the NMPQ with this sample. The respondents readily found words in the list to describe their pain and seemed to have little difficulty differentiating between words according to intensity. Descriptors from each of the 20 subclasses of the NMPQ were selected by the respondents at least once to describe their pain experience. The respondents used the same words that were in the NMPQ in describing pain, suggesting the accuracy, clarity, and cultural relevancy of the translated words. In response to the question to add other words that were not on the list to describe pain, only three new words were written in by one or two individuals. The research team reviewed these words and determined that there were words in the translated NMPQ having the same meanings as these new words.

The postoperative pain reported by these respondents on the NMPQ was rather circumscribed, mainly sensory and of moderate intensity, similar to that reported in the studies using the English version.[71,72,73] Eighty-four percent of the respondents selected 1 to 10 descriptors from the 20 possible subclasses, and all respondents selected at least one descriptor from a sensory subclass. The affective dimension was selected much less frequently to describe the postoperative pain. Over 75% of the sample at both time-points chose only one or none of the descriptors from the five subclasses reflecting the affective dimension. As expected for this sample, the intensity of pain was reported at the moderate range both on the second postoperative and the fourth or fifth postoperative days. In order to examine the sensitivity of the NMPQ, the respondents' two ratings were compared, with an expectation that patients would experience a decreasing amount of pain as the postoperative period extended. The NMPQ was sensitive in identifying the expected decrease in pain from the second to the fourth or fifth postoperative day, evident in the differences from the second postoperative day to the fourth or fifth postoperative day in PRIT, NWC, and PRIS.

Convergent validity was tested comparing the results of the NMPQ ratings with the results of the VAS (visual analogue scale) administered at the same time the NMPQ ratings were obtained. The correlations between the total and sensory pain scores of the NMPQ and the VAS scores were positive, moderately high, and statistically significant. These correlations are generally consistent with those reported in the literature,[7,73] although somewhat lower than those found by Taenzer.[71]

Divergent validity was examined by comparing the pain intensity scores from the NMPQ (PRIT, PRIS, and NWC) with the scores on the Spielberger State Anxiety Index (SSAI). The correlations between the NMPQ scale scores and the SSAI were statistically significant and at the moderate level for the first and second ratings for all sub-scales. These moderate levels of relationship between NMPQ and the anxiety scale suggest an adequate level of convergence and divergence between pain and anxiety.

These findings suggest that the NMPQ developed and tested in this work is culturally acceptable, relevant, and sensitive to fluctuations in pain and numerically consistent with the MPQ. This, along with the moderate level of validity attained with the scale, lends considerable assurance for its use for cross-cultural comparison. Thus, this translated version of the MPQ can be used for intracultural as well as for cross-cultural comparisons.

Direct versus language-specific translation

There are three versions of pain scales in Norwegian utilizing pain descriptors—the NMPQ developed in this work,[66] the adapted MPQ developed by Ljunggren,[74,75] and the Norwegian Pain Questionnaire (NPQ) developed by Strand & Wisnes.[63] While these three pain questionnaires share features of the MPQ, having adopted various parts of the MPQ development, they differ in the number of pain descriptors and the descriptors themselves, as well as in the methodological approaches used to develop them. Ljunggren[74,75] developed the adapted MPQ starting with the MPQ as the base for identifying the descriptors for low back pain, and finalized a questionnaire consisting of 47 somatosensory pain descriptors identified specifically for low back pain. Although based on the MPQ, its orientation to low back pain makes it of limited generalizability to other pain states.

To fashion a general pain questionnaire, Strand and Wisnes[58] developed the Norwegian Pain Questionnaire (NPQ) adopting methodology used to develop the original MPQ. Its final form consists of 106 words grouped into 18 categories obtained from the respondents' pain descriptions: twelve sensory, five affective, and one evaluative. The NPQ was developed with the specific perspective that there are culture-specific concepts and descriptions of pain, which are valid only within given target cultures.[76] Hence, the beginning of the NPQ development was a generation of pain descriptors by Norwegians, which were then filtered and arranged into groups. Strand and Ljunggren[77] noted that 39 descriptors of the adapted MPQ by Ljunggren were also found in the NPQ and five words in the adapted MPQ are not in the NPQ word lists. They also noted that only 46 descriptors of the NMPQ were also found in the NPQ. This means that 32 descriptors of the NMPQ's total 78 descriptors are not in the NPQ, while 60 descriptors among the NPQ's 106 words are not in the NMPQ. However, when the respondents were asked during the development of the NMPQ, all but two respondents felt no need for additional words to describe their pain. This raises a question regarding the method by which it should be possible to obtain both semantic and content validity when developing pain scales cross-culturally, for both the NMPQ and the NPQ.

The question regarding content and semantic validity when translating self-report scales into different languages is critical especially when viewed in terms of maintaining the applicability of scales in cross-cultural comparisons. The MPQ has been translated into 26 languages so far, and some of these are direct translations of the MPQ as is the NMPQ, while others are pain questionnaires developed with the same methodology used to develop the original MPQ, beginning with culture-specific collection of pain descriptors. Given that there are merits to both approaches, it may be useful to consider consolidating these two types of versions in order to develop a unified pain scale for a specific language, as suggested by Strand and Ljunggren.[77] However, this approach may not be as useful for cross-cultural comparisons as a direct back-translation approach, because a unified pain scale developed by consolidation would be different from the original MPQ and would not be appropriate for cross-cultural comparisons. Although we encountered no problem in finding corresponding descriptors in Norwegian for those in the English version of the MPQ, this may not be universal for all languages. Translating measurement tools such as the MPQ could be challenging when searching for corresponding descriptors in languages that are either richer or sparser in adjectives describing feelings than is English, especially non-European languages.

CONCLUSION

Even if the gold standard of self-report is universally accepted, measurement of pain is an elusive process, especially in terms of quantification and standardization. It is even more so in the cross-cultural context. One-dimensional, intensity-focused measurement tools are frequently used both for their simplicity of use and the difficulty in discriminating different dimensions of pain through measurement. Worldwide, the MPQ is one of the most widely used scales to measure pain through verbal expressions, rather than estimating pain intensity by approximate quantifications through various methods. As this tool has been converted into 26 different languages through translation and development, its application in cross-cultural comparisons and international communication is extensive. A rigorous translation of the MPQ based on back-translation methodology is the key approach for cross-cultural comparative studies of pain descriptions.[78] However, we must address the utility of developing various linguistic versions of the MPQ, as well as other pain measurement tools, applying different methodologies in light of linguistic and cultural variations in expression of pain. It is imperative to develop pain measurement tools in different languages specifically for intracultural application or for cross-cultural comparisons.

REFERENCES

1. Katz J, Melzack R. Assessment of pain. In: Aminoff MJ, Daroff RB, eds. *Encyclopedia of the Neurological Sciences*. Boston: Academic Press; 2003:716–722.
2. Sjöström B, Haljamäe H, Dahlgren LO, Lindström B. Assessment of postoperative pain: impact of clinical experience and professional role. *Acta Anaesthesiol Scand*. 1997;41(3):339–344.
3. Klopfenstein CE, Herrmann FR, Mamie C, Van Gessel E, Forster A. Pain intensity and pain relief after surgery. A comparison between patients' reported assessments and nurses' and physicians' observations. *Acta Anaesthesiol Scand*. 2000;44(1):58–62.
4. Thomas VJ, Rose FD. Ethnic differences in the experience of pain. *Soc Sci Med*. 1991;32(9):1063–1066.
5. Todd KH. Pain assessment and ethnicity. *Ann Emerg Med*. 1996;27(4):421–423.
6. Melzack R. *The Puzzle of Pain*. New York: The Basic Books; 1973.

7. Melzack R. The McGill Pain Questionnaire: major properties and scoring methods. *Pain*. 1975;1(3):277–299.

8. Morris DB. *The Culture of Pain*. Berkeley, CA: University of California Press; 1991.

9. Good MD, Brodwin PE, Good BJ, Kleinman A. *Pain As Human Experience: An Anthropological Perspective*. Berkeley, CA: University of California Press; 1992.

10. Edwards RR, Fillingim RB. Ethnic differences in thermal pain responses. *Psychosom Med*. 1999;61(3):346–354.

11. Cassisi JE, Umeda M, Deisinger JA, Sheffer C, Lofland KR, Jackson C. Patterns of pain descriptor usage in African Americans and European Americans with chronic pain. *Cultur Divers Ethnic Minor Psychol*. 2004;10(1):81–89.

12. Hobara M. Beliefs about appropriate pain behavior: cross-cultural and sex differences between Japanese and Euro-Americans. *Eur J Pain*. 2005;9(4):389–393.

13. Watson PJ, Latif RK, Rowbotham DJ. Ethnic differences in thermal pain responses: a comparison of South Asian and White British healthy males. *Pain*. 2005;118(1–2):194–200.

14. Koffman J, Morgan M, Edmonds P, Speck P, Higginson IJ. Cultural meanings of pain: a qualitative study of Black Caribbean and White British patients with advanced cancer. *Palliat Med*. 2008;22(4):350–359.

15. Dworkin RH, Turk DC, Revicki DA, et al. Development and initial validation of an expanded and revised version of the Short-form McGill Pain Questionnaire (SF-MPQ-2). *Pain*. 2009;144(1–2):35–42.

16. Kerns RD, Turk DC, Rudy TE. The West Haven-Yale Multidimensional Pain Inventory (WHYMPI). *Pain*. 1985;23(4):345–356.

17. Cleeland CS, Ryan KM. Pain assessment: global use of the Brief Pain Inventory. *Ann Acad Med Singapore*. 1994;23(2):129–138.

18. Jensen MP, Gammaitoni AR, Olaleye DO, Oleka N, Nalamachu SR, Galer BS. The pain quality assessment scale: assessment of pain quality in carpal tunnel syndrome. *J Pain*. 2006;7(11):823–832.

19. Knotkova H, Clark WC, Keohan ML, Kuhl JP, Winer RT, Wharton RN. Validation of the Multidimensional Affect and Pain Survey (MAPS). *J Pain*. 2006;7(3):161–169.

20. Williams NH, Wilkinson C, Russell I. Extending the Aberdeen Back Pain Scale to include the whole spine: a set of outcome measures to the neck, upper and lower back. *Pain*. 2001;94:261–274.

21. Galer BS, Jensen MP. Development and preliminary validation of a pain measure specific to neuropathic pain: the Neuropathic Pain Scale. *Neurology*. 1997;48(2):332–338.

22. McGrath PJ, Johnson G, Goodman JT, Schillinger J, Dunn J, Chapman J. CHEOPS: A behavioral scale for rating postoperative pain in children. In: Fileds HL, Dubner R, Cervero F, eds. *Adv Pain Res Ther*. Vol 9. New York: Raven Press; 1985:395–402.

23. Salmore R. Development of a new pain scale: Colorado Behavioral Numerical Pain Scale for sedated adult patients undergoing gastrointestinal procedures. *Gastroenterol Nurs*. 2002;25(6):257–262.

24. Lefebvre-Chapiro S; for The Doloplus-2 Group. The Dolopus-2 scale—Evaluating pain in the elderly. *European Journal of Palliative Care*. 2000;8:191–194.

25. Merkel S. Pain assessment in infants and young children: the Finger Span Scale. *Am J Nurs*. 2002;102(11):55–56.

26. Fuchs-Lacelle S, Hadjistavropoulos T. Development and preliminary validation of the pain assessment checklist for seniors with limited ability to communicate (PACSLAC). *Pain Manag Nurs*. 2004;5(1):37–49.

27. Warden V, Hurley AC, Volicer L. Development and psychometric evaluation of the Pain Assessment in Advanced Dementia (PAINAD) scale. *J Am Med Dir Assoc*. 2003;4(1):9–15.

28. Ramelet AS, Rees N, McDonald S, Bulsara M, Abu-Saad HH. Development and preliminary psychometric testing of the Multidimensional Assessment of Pain Scale: MAPS. *Paediatr Anaesth*. 2007a;17(4):333–340.

29. Ramelet AS, Rees NW, McDonald S, Bulsara MK, Huijer Abu-Saad H. Clinical validation of the Multidimensional Assessment of Pain Scale. *Paediatr Anaesth*. 2007b;17(12):1156–1165.

30. Krechel SW, Bildner J. CRIES: a new neonatal postoperative pain measurement score. Initial testing of validity and reliability. *Paediatr Anaesth*. 1995;5(1):53–61.

31. Ambuel B, Hamlett KW, Marx CM, Blumer JL. Assessing distress in pediatric care environments: the COMFORT scale. *J Pediatr Psycho.* 1992;17(1):95–109.

32. Perkins FM, Werner MU, Persson F, Holte K, Jensen TS, Kehlet H. Development and validation of a brief, descriptive Danish pain questionnaire (BDDPQ). *Acta Anaesthesiol Scand.* 2004;48(4):486–490.

33. Vanderiet K, Adriaensen H, Carton H, Vertommen H. The McGill Pain Questionnaire constructed for the Dutch language (MPQ-DV). Preliminary data concerning reliability and validity. *Pain.* 1987;30(3):395–408.

34. Ketovuori H, Pöntinen PJ. A pain vocabulary in Finnish—The Finnish pain questionnaire. *Pain.* 1981;11(2):247–253.

35. Boureau F, Luu M, Doubrère JF. Comparative study of the validity of four French McGill Pain Questionnaire (MPQ) versions. *Pain.* 1992;50(1):59–65.

36. Radvila A, Adler RH, Galeazzi RL, Vorkauf H. The development of a German language (Berne) pain questionnaire and its application in a situation causing acute pain. *Pain.* 1987;28(2):185–195.

37. De Benedittis G, Massei R, Nobili R, Pieri A. The Italian Pain Questionnaire. *Pain.* 1988;33(1):53–62.

38. Strand LI, Wisnes AR. The development of a Norwegian pain questionnaire. *Pain.* 1991;46(1):61–66.

39. Park J, Cho B, Paek Y, Kwon H, Yoo S. Development of a pain assessment tool for the older adults in Korea: the validity and reliability of a Korean version of the geriatric pain measure (GPM-K). *Arch Gerontol Geriatr.* 2009;49(2):199–203.

40. Chung JW, Wong TK, Yang JC. A preliminary report on the Chinese Cancer Pain Assessment Tool (CCPAT): reliability and validity. *Acta Anaesthesiol Sin.* 2001;39(1):33–40.

41. Costa LCM, Maher CG, McAuley JH, Costa LO. Systematic review of cross-cultural adaptations of McGill Pain Questionnaire reveals a paucity of clinimetric testing. *J Clin Epidemiol.* 2009;62(9):934–943.

42. Terwee CB, Bot SD, de Boer MR, et al. Quality criteria were proposed for measurement properties of health status questionnaires. *J Clin Epidemiol.* 2007;60(1):34–42.

43. Wang XS, Mendoza TR, Gao SZ, Cleeland CS. The Chinese version of the Brief Pain Inventory (BPI-C): its development and use in a study of cancer pain. *Pain.* 1996;67(2–3):407–416.

44. Poundja J, Fikretoglu D, Guay S, Brunet A. Validation of the French version of the brief pain inventory in Canadian veterans suffering from traumatic stress. *J Pain Symptom Manage.* 2007;33(6):720–726.

45. Radbruch L, Loick G, Kiencke P, et al. Validation of the German version of the Brief Pain Inventory. *J Pain Symptom Manage.* 1999;18(3):180–187.

46. Shvartzman P, Friger M, Shani A, Barak F, Yoram C, Singer Y. Pain control in ambulatory cancer patients—can we do better? *J Pain Symptom Manage.* 2003;26(2):716–722.

47. Saxena A, Mendoza T, Cleeland CS. The assessment of cancer pain in north India: the validation of the Hindi Brief Pain Inventory—BPI-H. *J Pain Symptom Manage.* 1999;17(1):27–41.

48. Caraceni A, Mendoza TR, Mencaglia E, et al. A validation study of an Italian version of the Brief Pain Inventory (Breve Questionario per la Valutazione del Dolore). *Pain.* 1996;65(1):87–92.

49. Bonezzi C, Nava A, Barbieri M, et al. Validazione della versione italiana del Brief Pain Inventory nei pazienti con dolore cronico. *Minerva Anestesiol.* 2002;68(7–8):607–611.

50. Uki J, Mendoza T, Cleeland CS, Nakamura Y, Takeda F. A brief cancer pain assessment tool in Japanese: the utility of the Japanese Brief Pain Inventory—BPI-J. *J Pain Symptom Manage.* 1998;16(6):364–373.

51. Yun YH, Mendoza TR, Heo DS, et al. Development of a cancer pain assessment tool in Korea: a validation study of a Korean version of the brief pain inventory. *Oncology.* 2004;66(6):439–444.

52. Klepstad P, Loge JH, Borchgrevink PC, Mendoza TR, Cleeland CS, Kaasa S. The Norwegian brief pain inventory questionnaire: translation and validation in cancer pain patients. *J Pain Symptom Manage.* 2002;24(5):517–525.

53. Badia X, Muriel C, Gracia A, et al. Validación española del cuestionario Brief Pain Inventory en pacientes con dolor de causa neoplásica. *Barc.* 2003;120(2):52–59.

54. Chaudakshetrin P. Validation of the Thai Version of Brief Pain Inventory (BPI-T) in cancer patients. *J Med Assoc Thai.* 2009;92(1):34–40.

55. Dicle A, Karayurt O, Dirimese E. Validation of the Turkish version of the Brief Pain Inventory in surgery patients. *Pain Manag Nurs.* 2009;10(2):107–113.e2.

56. Lousberg R, Van Breukelen GJ, Groenman NH, Schmidt AJ, Arntz A, Winter FA. Psychometric properties of the Multidimensional Pain Inventory, Dutch language version (MPI-DLV). *Behav Res Ther.* 1999;37(2):167–182.

57. Laliberté S, Lamoureux J, Sullivan MJ, Miller JM, Charron J, Bouthillier D. French translation of the Multidimensional Pain Inventory: L'inventaire multidimensionnel de la douleur. *Pain Res Manag.* 2008;13(6):497–505.

58. Kröner-Herwig B, Denecke H, Glier B, et al. Qualitätssicherung in der Therapie chronischen Schmerzes. Ergebnisse einer Arbeitsgruppe der Deutschen Gesellschaft zum Studium des Schmerzes (DGSS) zur psychologischen Diagnostik. IX. Multidimensionale Verfahren zur Erfassung schmerzrelevanter Aspekte und Empfehlungen zur Standarddiagnostik. *Schmerz.* 1996;10(1):47–52.

59. Ferrari R, Novara C, Sanavio E, Zerbini F. Internal structure and validity of the multidimensional pain inventory, Italian language version. *Pain Med.* 2000;1(2):123–130.

60. Bergström G, Jensen IB, Bodin L, Linton SJ, Nygren AL, Carlsson SG. Reliability and factor structure of the Multidimensional Pain Inventory—Swedish Language Version (MPI-S). *Pain.* 1998;75(1):101–110.

61. Osthus H, Cziske R, Jacobi E. A German version of the Extended Aberdeen Back Pain Scale: development and evaluation. *Spine (Phila Pa 1976).* 2006;31(5):571–577.

62. Hølen JC, Saltvedt I, Fayers PM, et al. The Norwegian Doloplus-2, a tool for behavioural pain assessment: translation and pilot-validation in nursing home patients with cognitive impairment. *Palliat Med.* 2005;19(5):411–417.

63. Ando C, Hishinuma M. Development of the Japanese DOLOPLUS-2: a pain assessment scale for the elderly with Alzheimer's disease. *Psychogeriatrics.* 2010;10(3):131–137.

64. Zwakhalen SM, Hamers JP, Berger MP. The psychometric quality and clinical usefulness of three pain assessment tools for elderly people with dementia. *Pain.* 2006;126(1–3):210–220.

65. Aubin M, Verreault R, Savoie M, et al. Validité et utilité clinique d'une grille d'observation (PACSLAC-F) pour évaluer la douleur chez des aînés atteints de démence vivant en milieu de soins de longue durée. *Can J Aging.* 2008;27(1):45–55.

66. Kim HS, Schwartz-Barcott D, Holter IM, Lorensen M. Developing a translation of the McGill pain questionnaire for cross-cultural comparison: an example from Norway. *J Adv Nurs.* 1995;21(3):421–426.

67. Berkanovic E. The effect of inadequate language translation on Hispanics' responses to health surveys. *Am J Public Health.* 1980;70(12):1273–1276.

68. Werner O, Schoepfle MG. *Systematic Fieldwork: Foundations of Ethnography and Interviewing.* Vol. 1. Beverly Hills, CA: Sage; 1987.

69. Bernard RH. *Research Methods in Cultural Anthropology.* Newbury Park, CA: Sage; 1988.

70. Beaton DE, Bombardier C, Guillemin F, Ferraz MB. Guidelines for the process of cross-cultural adaptation of self-report measures. *Spine (Phila Pa 1976).* 2000;25(24):3186–3191.

71. Taenzer, P. Postoperative pain: relationships among measures of pain, mood and narcotic requirements. In: Melzack R. ed. *Pain Management and Assessment.* New York: Raven; 1983:111–117.

72. Taenzer P, Melzack R, Jeans ME. Influence of psychological factors on postoperative pain, mood and analgesic requirements. *Pain.* 1986;24(3):331–342.

73. Fortin JD, Schwartz-Barcott D, Rossi S. The postoperative pain experience: a description based on the McGill Pain Questionnaire. *Clin Nurs Res.* 1992;1(3):292–304.

74. Ljunggren AE. Descriptions of pain and other sensory modalities in patients with lumbago-sciatica and herniated intervertebral discs. Interview administration of an adapted McGill Pain Questionnaire. *Pain.* 1983;16(3):265–276.

75. Ljunggren AE. Discriminant validity of pain modalities and other sensory phenomena in patients with lumbar herniated intervertebral discs versus lumbar spinal stenosis. *Neuro-Orthopedics.* 1999;11:91–99.

76. Sartorius N, Kuyken W. Translation of health status instruments. In: Orley J, Keyken W, eds. *Quality of Life Assessment: International Perspective.* Berlin: Springer-Verlag; 1994:3–18.

77. Strand LI, Ljunggren AE. Different approximations of the McGill Pain Questionnaire in the Norwegian language: a discussion of content validity. *J Adv Nurs.* 1997;26(4):772–779.

78. Hasegawa M, Mishima M, Matsumoto I, et al. Confirming the theoretical structure of the Japanese version of the McGill Pain Questionnaire in chronic pain. *Pain Med.* 2001;2(1):52–59.

11

THE CLINICAL ENCOUNTER

Implications for Pain Management Disparities

RAYMOND C. TAIT, PHD

Vice President, Research Professor, Department
of Neurology & Psychiatry Saint Louis University
Saint Louis, Missouri, USA

Key Points

- The assessment of chronic pain is a complex clinical undertaking that can be influenced by a range of social psychological factors that operate within the medical culture.
- Two types of cognitive processes inform judgments of patients with chronic pain: (1) speedy, largely intuitive processes that rely heavily on pre-existing cognitive schemes (mental shortcuts), and (2) rational, more laborious processes that are largely data-driven.
- Pre-existing cognitive schemes inform many clinical judgments of patients with chronic pain; such schemes are linked to factors related to the patient, the situation, and practitioner experience and characteristics.
- Negative cognitive schemes are likely to be activated when self-reported levels of pain are high; such schemes may lead practitioners to doubt the validity of reported symptoms.
- When questions arise about the validity of a pain report, the practitioner generally will treat a patient less aggressively than when the patient's report is considered valid.
- Negative cognitive schemas within the current medical culture are likely to contribute significantly to the widespread disparities that have been documented in the treatment of patients with chronic pain.

INTRODUCTION

For conditions such as chronic pain, where symptoms are subjective in nature and the likelihood of a cure often remote, the patient-provider encounter is of great importance. In that encounter, the clinician must evaluate the severity of the presenting pain complaint, its history, factors that contribute to its waxing and waning, and its multiple impacts. Based on this assessment, the clinician then makes a diagnosis (or diagnoses) and decides upon the treatment approach most likely to benefit. Subsequent encounters then guide changes in approach toward the goal of treatment that is optimally tailored to the patient's needs. In so doing, an enormous amount of information must be collected, considered, and weighed.

There is an extensive literature, however, that attests to systematic failures in meeting the latter goal. Not only does this literature identify frequent failures to optimize care, but it documents systematic disparities in treatment and in the outcomes of that treatment. Although disparities have been demonstrated across a number of medical conditions, those of interest in this chapter involve disparities associated with chronic pain. Indeed, because of the subjective nature of pain and the lack of objective medical evidence that often characterizes chronically painful conditions, chronic pain sufferers constitute a group that is particularly vulnerable to inadequate care.[1] While the literature is most extensive in regard to racial/ethnic disparities,[2,3] disparate care has been demonstrated across a range of other sociodemographic variables, including gender,[4] age,[5,6] and socioeconomic status (SES).[7]

In conjunction with the burgeoning recognition of disparities in pain care, there is increasing attention to the range of social psychological factors operating in the clinical encounter that may bias judgments and influence treatment decisions.[8,9] As shown in Figure 11.1, some of these factors are patient-related, such as the level of pain that is reported, the manner in which it is described, or the race/ethnicity of the reporter. Others are associated with features of the provider, such as their specialty training or their level of experience. Still others are associated with features of the situation in which the encounter occurs, such as the availability of medical evidence that supports the complaint or the stance of the insurance carrier providing financial coverage.

This chapter considers the social psychological factors referenced above as reflections of the medical culture relative to the practice of pain management. This view is clearly consistent with recent definitions of culture:[10] "...the values, beliefs, norms, and practices of a particular group that are learned and shared and that guide thinking, decisions, and

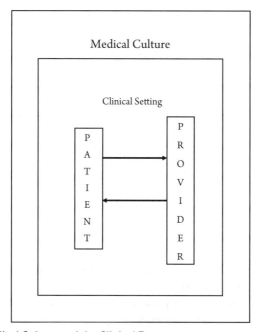

FIGURE 11.1 The Medical Culture and the Clinical Encounter

actions in a patterned way." Consequently, the chapter will examine the impact of these beliefs, norms, and practices on clinical judgments and decisions related to the care of patients with chronic pain. A close examination of these factors will identify practice patterns that contribute to disparities, particularly disparities that eventuate in systematic undertreatment. With a better understanding of these patterns, recommendations will emerge aimed at mitigating those disparities in healthcare delivery.

In choosing to focus on the medical encounter, we have chosen not to devote attention to other systemic, cultural factors that are associated with inequities in healthcare. In particular, we will not address larger societal contributors to these disparities, despite the ample evidence that a range of these factors contribute to the undertreatment of pain. This would include such factors as access to adequate analgesics (e.g., through neighborhood pharmacies) and adequate insurance coverage.[11,12] We have chosen to narrow our focus because we believe that cultural factors that inform the clinical encounter are often underappreciated, while these other societal factors have been better recognized. Hence, attention to social psychological aspects of the medical encounter is likely to highlight an underappreciated but important contributor to variability in the practice of pain medicine and disparities in pain treatment.

The chapter first provides a brief background on the psychology of social judgments, as these are central to decisions that flow from a clinical encounter. We pay particular attention to cognitive schemas commonly applied to patients with chronic pain, focusing on culturally derived stereotypes that can increase the "burden of proof" that must be adduced in order to establish the validity of a symptom (and to justify treatment). We then consider pain severity as an important mediating factor in whether these cognitive schemas are triggered, especially the levels of reported pain necessary to activate such schemas. The bulk of the chapter then involves an examination of the evidence related to patient, provider, and situational factors that systematically impact clinical judgments made about the care rendered to patients with chronic pain symptoms.

SOCIAL JUDGMENT AND CHRONIC PAIN

While pain generally is considered a medical problem, provider judgments of chronic pain conditions are influenced to a great degree by social psychological factors associated with the patient-provider interaction. Such social judgments are subject to processes that fall broadly under the umbrella of social cognition:[13] "the study of how people make sense of other people...." Indeed, because chronic pain conditions depend to such a degree on self-reports and because those self-reports may be discrepant from objective medical findings, clinical judgments of patients with chronic pain conditions are often characterized by relatively high levels of uncertainty, such that they may require considerable clinical judgment.

Recent research in social cognition has focused on processes that operate in conditions where judgments are uncertain.[14] Two distinguishable processes have been identified: one that relies on heuristics that are intuitive and relatively automatic, and another that uses processes that are deliberative and slow. The former process typically is driven by prior expectations and experiences, such that judgments can occur without reflection. This intuitive heuristic has the practical advantage of simplifying decision-making because it is almost reflexive and exacts little effort. By dint of their reflexive nature, intuitive processes are relatively immune to modification and often are maintained by the forces of habit and selective attention. By contrast, rational/deliberative processes are influenced not only by prior experience, but importantly by current circumstances. These processes are conscious, rule-governed, and sequential, making them slow and effortful. While more effortful, these processes also are much more amenable to learning and change than are intuitive processes.

Social cognition literature clearly shows that, when faced with uncertainty, we (humans) tend to operate as "cognitive misers" by defaulting to intuitive processes.[13] Moreover, the likelihood that this approach will be adopted is potentiated under certain conditions, such as when a high volume of material must be processed or when we are under time pressure, characteristics that describe the dynamics of much of modern clinical medicine. An extreme example might involve an Emergency Department (ED), where it is common for patients to be backlogged and for ED physicians to face considerable time pressure. Under these circumstances, social cognition predicts that physicians would be likely to rely on mental shortcuts (e.g., stereotypes, experiences with similar patients, "gut instincts") to facilitate rapid decision-making. Thus, the agitated patient complaining of severe headache and requesting a potent analgesic is unlikely to be seen as an ambiguous, complicated clinical picture with multiple psychosocial factors. Instead, that patient is likely to be seen as drug-seeking, so that the ED physician can default to a well-practiced alternative approach (e.g., prescribe a low potency analgesic and refer the patient to his/her primary care provider). While typical daily practice may lack some of the drama of this ED scenario, a busy clinical practitioner is likely to face demands of time urgency and the need for speedy decision-making, too.

Cognitive schemas

Cognitive schemas are "structures that represent knowledge about a concept or type of stimulus, including its attributes … that facilitate top-down or conceptually driven processing, as opposed to bottom-up or data-driven processing."[13] Typically, schemas operate at the earliest moments of perception and serve to facilitate decision-making processes (particularly intuitive processes like those described above) through the application of categories that organize and simplify those perceptions. Those categories typically are built around prototypes with particular attributes (e.g., visually prominent physical features, disease type). Once formed, the categories also impact memory for events; events that are consistent with a category (e.g., chronic pain → complaining, drug-seeking) are more readily encoded and remembered than are events that are inconsistent with a category. Hence, cognitive schemas tend to organize both our current and future experience of the social world.

Several schematic processes are of particular relevance to chronic pain. One such process involves the stereotype (i.e., the central prototype) constructed to represent the category of chronic pain patients. Another process of considerable importance has more to do with systematic biases that impact how a stereotype is applied, the fundamental attribution error. The fundamental attribution error references the ubiquitous tendency to attribute another's behavior to stable dispositional features (i.e., qualities specific to that person) rather than to situational factors.[13] The following sections speak to the implications of social stereotyping and attribution error for persons with chronic pain.

Chronic pain stereotypes

There is ample evidence that negative stereotypes of chronic pain pervade the medical culture. For example, a recent study of "illness prestige" asked physicians to rate disease categories by the level of prestige associated with those who provide treatment for that category.[15] Diseases that ranked at the top of the list (e.g., cardiovascular disease, cancer) were characterized by the availability of objective medical evidence and by their life-threatening nature. By contrast, diseases at the bottom of the list (depression, chronic pain) were more subjective in nature and less clearly life-threatening. While results of the study were framed in the context of career choice, it is impossible to miss the social stereotype implications: diseases characterized by largely subjective symptoms (such as pain) are devalued relative to other disease entities. Other studies also have shown that physicians harbor negative views of chronic pain patients.[16,17]

As noted above, stereotypes represent a shorthand way of characterizing a group of people who share a given attribute. The above paragraph describes a negative stereotype that can be ascribed to all patients with chronic pain conditions. Within that stereotype, of course, are other sociodemographic stereotypes, including those associated with racial/ethnic minority status, gender, and age, as well as nonsociodemographic stereotypes linked with constructs such as psychosomatic illness, compensation status, etc. While positive stereotypes predispose an observer to accept the validity of a self-report, negative stereotypes (such as those previously referenced) predispose to questioning the validity of a report and a tendency to discount it. Moreover, because it is easier for an observer to assimilate stereotype-consistent information than information inconsistent with a stereotype,[18] negatively stereotyped patients need higher levels of symptom-consistent information in order to counter the discounting effect referenced above (i.e., there is a higher "burden of proof").

For subjective complaints such as chronic pain, complaints that often lack confirmatory medical evidence or a recent inciting event, such "proof" can be difficult to find. Further, because negative stereotypes also affect the quality of social interactions, they also may interfere with communication, information gathering, and trust-building. Of course, the latter activities are required in chronic pain conditions in order to gather the very information that is necessary to meet the aforementioned burden of proof. Thus, a negative cycle can be engendered where negative stereotypes can contribute in several ways to inadequate clinical care.

The above dynamics are captured in a study that examined the impact of negative stereotypes on the assessment and treatment of non-specific chest pain.[19] In that study, videotapes were developed in which actresses portrayed a female patient with complaints of chest pain: one actress presented in a "business-like" manner (positive stereotype) and the other in a "histrionic" manner (negative stereotype). Internists viewed one of the videotapes and then indicated the likelihood that the patient had bona fide cardiac problems. They then were provided with test results and were asked again whether the patient had bona fide cardiac problems. Finally, they were asked whether they would be likely to provide subsequent follow-up. After watching the videotape, internists were significantly less likely to diagnose the histrionic patient with bona fide cardiac problems, a finding that reflected a negative bias toward the histrionic patient. When diagnostic evidence then was presented, diagnoses were revised so that there were no differences between the histrionic and the business-like patient. Despite the change in diagnosis, however, internists remained significantly less likely to pursue follow-up for the histrionic patient than for the business-like patient; the latter difference likely reflecting the negative dynamic that the internists anticipated.

The fundamental attribution error

As noted above, the fundamental attribution error involves the tendency to ascribe the cause of a behavior/problem to stable qualities of the person with the problem, rather than to situational features. Two sequelae of this attribution pattern are relevant to chronic pain. First, the latter attribution process is top-down (i.e., driven by pre-existing concepts), thereby narrowing the scope of information potentially relevant to judgments to be made (i.e., it limits consideration of data related to possible situational determinants). Second, attributions to stable personal qualities easily can translate into blame—the fundamental attribution error predisposes an observer to blame a problem on the person, rather than on situational factors.[20] Hence, the fundamental attribution error disadvantages people with chronic pain in two ways when they are seen by healthcare providers—it is likely to limit consideration of situational factors contributing to challenges faced by patients and predisposes providers to blame, rather than collaborative problem-solving.

In summary, conditions of uncertainty (common among chronic pain patients) can evoke cognitive schemas that engender negatively biased clinical judgments. Negative bias, in turn, can occasion questions regarding the validity of a patient's self-report, and can have prejudicial "downstream" effects on information gathering. The combination of negative stereotypes and the human tendency to blame people for problems that they encounter makes patients with chronic pain particularly vulnerable to clinical judgments that discount the severity of their symptoms and ultimately can occasion undertreatment.

The mediating influence of pain severity

While we will discuss pain severity as a factor in clinical judgment in greater detail later in the chapter, it is important to recognize that pain severity is likely to play a key role in whether or not cognitive schemas are activated. In particular, there is evidence that high pain reports are required in order to trigger cognitive schemas and symptom devaluation. When pain is reported to be low, there typically is little pressure in a clinical (or any other social) exchange for remedial or supportive action. Hence, the natural inclination is to accept the report as valid, irrespective of other social psychological (e.g., racial/ethnic stereotypes, fundamental attribution error) or medical factors (e.g., opiophobia). In a clinical setting, this is likely to translate into providing some minimal but adequate treatment.

On the other hand, high levels of reported pain intensity impact clinical judgment in several ways. First, there is evidence that a high level of reported pain, itself, occasions a consistent tendency among observers to discount pain estimates.[21] Second, high levels of pain appear to potentiate a range of factors contributing further to symptom discounting; data demonstrate an activating effect of high levels of pain severity for such factors as litigation status[22] and negative affect.[23] While the mechanisms of this effect are not clear, it is likely that high levels of pain "prime" psychological mechanisms such as negative stereotypes. This priming effect, then, further potentiates the skepticism that observers experience when facing people who report high levels of pain. Figure 11.2 illustrates this priming effect.

While the priming effect described above has empirical support, it falls short of an accepted construct in the field. Nonetheless, it has potential explanatory value in explaining some of the apparently discrepant findings reported in the literature. For example, a classic study examined Emergency Department (ED) records of patients who had been seen for treatment of long-bone fractures.[24] While pain levels were not described in the manuscript, it is reasonable to assume that patients were experiencing pain at moderate-to-high levels. In spite of the acute nature of the pain and the medical evidence supporting tissue damage, Hispanics received prescriptions for significantly less analgesia than non-Hispanic whites, a finding that was hypothesized to be mediated by discounted estimates of pain severity for the former group. A follow-up study of ED patients seen for sprain/strain diagnoses investigated that hypothesis by prospectively collecting pain severity assessments.[25] Results showed no ethnicity-related differences in pain estimates or in prescribed analgesics. The

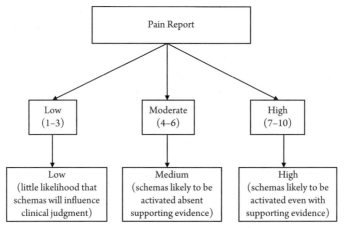

FIGURE 11.2 Pain Severity: Activation potential for cognitive schemas

estimates, however, showed low-to-moderate levels of pain (39/100), levels that may have been too low to activate symptom discounting. Although obviously speculative, the possibility that differing levels of pain severity mediated the apparently discrepant results is worthy of consideration.

THE CLINICAL ENCOUNTER

The following sections will review evidence for the systematic influence of patient, situational, and observer factors on judgments of symptoms in persons with chronic pain. The first section considers characteristics of the patient (the target about whom judgments are made). The next section considers characteristics of the observer (the health professional judging the patient's symptoms). The third section examines features of the situation, the context within which a clinical encounter occurs. The final section of the paper discusses implications for improving the quality of clinical decisions made when physicians face the uncertainties endemic to chronic pain and its management.

Patient characteristics

The impact of patient characteristics on pain assessment and treatment has received the most attention in the literature. This section will review that literature as it relates to the following patient characteristics: (1) the patient's symptom presentation, particularly the effects of differing levels of pain severity; (2) sociodemographic characteristics, including race, gender, and age; and (3) evidence of psychological distress.

Pain presentation
Pain intensity. It is well accepted that self-reports are the primary means by which to assess pain intensity and other pain-related characteristics (e.g., distribution, other sensory qualities). While the importance of patient self-reports is well accepted, there are data that attest to provider difficulties in accepting such self-reports when pain levels are described as high. Indeed, some of the most difficult clinical judgments must be made with patients whose pain is chronic, reported to be severe, and inconsistent with available objective medical evidence.

Obviously, providers are faced with their most difficult decisions when pain intensity is reported to be high. Under those conditions, providers typically are pressured to intervene. At the same time, research evidence indicates that observers are most likely to discount symptoms under conditions of high pain intensity.[23,26] For example, a study asked medical students to estimate "actual" pain for hypothetical patients reporting levels of pain ranging from low (3/10) to high (9/10).[21] Students inflated their pain estimates when reported intensity was low, accurately estimated pain of moderate intensity, and reduced estimates when pain was reported to be high. This pattern was moderated somewhat by the presence of supporting medical evidence; pain estimates were closer to patient reported levels of pain in the presence of such evidence, although still significantly lower than patient reports when pain was high (7/10, 9/10).

Such patterns, however, are not restricted to students. A strikingly similar pattern was found in a study of internists.[27] Evidence of this effect also has emerged from clinical studies.[28] The latter study examined levels of concordance between pain ratings provided by cancer inpatients (low, medium, high) and estimates made by the staff charged with their care (nurses, residents, and attending physicians). Concordance levels were high for patients reporting low levels of pain; they dropped substantially for patients reporting moderate pain; they were unfortunately poor for those patients who described high levels of pain. The latter finding, obviously, reflects observer estimates that were consistently lower than patient reports.

These and other studies suggest that observers, whether healthcare professionals or nonprofessionals, discount high levels of reported pain. Discounting appears to be allayed somewhat in the face of supporting medical evidence (apparently seen as "proof" of the validity of the self-report); even then, high levels of pain are subject to devaluation. While the mechanisms that underlie the tendency to devalue high intensity pain are unclear, the implications of this tendency certainly are clear: patients who describe pain at high levels, including those whose pain control needs are greatest, are most likely to have their symptom reports discounted.

Aside from the main effects of reported pain levels on provider pain discounting, previously referenced data speak to an apparent mediating effect of pain severity levels on other cognitive processes. In particular, those data suggest that high levels of reported pain are required in order to activate negative stereotypes. In turn, those stereotypes can occasion further pain discounting. Again, the mechanisms that underlie this mediating effect are unclear. That said, a possible explanation involves a social contract model.[29] According to this model, a patient who reports high levels of pain is placing implicit pressure on another for a response (e.g., an opioid prescription, an exemption from an obligation), pressure that is absent when pain levels are low. This model predicts that a pressured observer would be motivated to discount a pain report in order to reduce the social pressure to respond; by discounting the level of pain that the patient is judged to experience, the observer also reduces the response demand. While the latter explanation is intuitively appealing, it has received little direct study.

Chronicity. Because greater complexity attends patients with chronic pain relative to those with acute pain, there often is disagreement among healthcare providers as to how patients with chronic pain should be managed. Indeed, research has shown that the assessment and management of pain by primary care providers can be highly idiosyncratic.[30] The lack of an accepted management heuristic obviously enhances the vulnerability of chronic pain patients to undertreatment. This vulnerability is illustrated in a study from the nursing field.[31] In that study, floor nurses were asked to rate symptom severity for hypothetical patients with either acute or chronic pain who were depicted in vignettes. Compared to patients with acute pain, patients with chronic pain were estimated to have lower levels of pain severity, such that they also merited a lower intensity of treatment. While similar studies have not been conducted with other health professionals, there is little reason to believe that these views of chronic pain patients are idiosyncratic to the nursing field. Indeed, the previously referenced studies that document negative stereotypes for patients with chronic pain provide indirect evidence that such views are widely held.

Sociodemographic characteristics

Race/ethnicity. Racial/ethnic disparities have been a major focus of medical research over the past decade. Recent years have accrued considerable evidence specific to pain. Studies have demonstrated disparities in treatment across multiple patient groups, such as patients being treated for cancer pain[32] and patients undergoing treatment for back pain.[33] Not only are there disparities in treatment, but those disparities seem to engender disparate outcomes that also disadvantage minority patients.[34] Because several recent reviews have covered the extensive research on pain disparities, the interested reader is referred to those articles for a thorough treatment of that literature.[2,3]

While there is ample evidence of racial/ethnic disparities in pain care, research has yet to delineate the mechanisms that underlie those differences. In fact, multiple mechanisms are likely to be implicated, including socioeconomic factors and cultural factors, such as a well-documented distrust of the medical system among minorities.[35] Even though stereotypes have not been studied explicitly in this research, they are likely to be a significant contributing factor. Consider, for example, the classic ED study referenced earlier. Patients in that study presented with acute pain secondary to long-bone fractures, so the medical evidence was obvious and the need for healthcare was apparent. Moreover, the study controlled for differences in insurance status. Nevertheless, substantial disparities in analgesics prescribed for Hispanics were evident. Although the study did not ask why such differences occurred, it is hard to imagine that negative, race-based stereotypes (e.g., those related to drug use) did not play a role. Similarly, cross-cultural difficulties in communication, also well-documented in the medical literature, may have played a part.[36] Had the presenting pain complaint lacked credible medical evidence, the influence of psychological and/or other cultural factors would likely have been even greater.

Although this chapter focuses on the dynamics of the clinical encounter, a brief digression is warranted into the relative contributions of minority group membership and socioeconomic status (SES) on disparities in the provision of healthcare. As with race, there is substantial evidence that SES is associated with disparate treatment and with different outcomes of treatment, such that lower SES contributes to differences in care and in outcomes.[7,37] Because minority group membership is associated with lower SES, however, the effects of the two can be difficult to separate. For example, insurance coverage is highly correlated with SES; if minorities have poor insurance relative to non-minorities, both race/ethnicity and insurance coverage (SES) can occasion differences in care and outcomes.[7,12] Similarly, there is evidence that minorities tend to be concentrated in lower SES neighborhoods. Those neighborhoods are more likely to have pharmacies that lack common opioid analgesic medications, limiting the types of treatment available to those who use the pharmacy.[11] Again, it can be difficult to disentangle the relative effects of SES and minority status as both appear to play a part.

That said, there is recent research that reflects on the relative contributions of race and SES. These studies examined the intensity of treatment, as well as intermediate- (2-years post-settlement) and long-term (6-years post-settlement) outcomes in Workers' Compensation (WC) claimants with low back pain. Because the WC system guarantees treatment for workers who are injured on the job, the system controls for one of the factors (disparities in insurance coverage) that can confound disparities-related research. This research showed that both race and SES contributed to differences in the intensity of treatment rendered to WC claimants.[33,38] Race and SES also contributed to differences in intermediate-term outcomes.[34] In both cases, however, race contributed more substantially to those differences than SES. When long-term outcomes were examined, however, SES contributed more to differences in clinical and occupational adjustment.[39] The above pattern suggests that race-related factors played a greater role during and immediately following active treatment, while SES appeared to play a greater role in outcomes over time, possibly through SES-related differences in access to resources.

Gender. As with race/ethnicity, there is a body of research that has examined gender effects on pain assessment, much of it focusing on chest pain. That research, including a study cited earlier in this chapter, shows that men are more likely than women to receive a diagnosis of coronary heart disease when they present with chest pain.[19] Other painful presentations show a similar pattern; most research indicates that women have been underevaluated and undertreated for such conditions as postoperative pain, neck pain, and low back pain.[40,41,42] Similarly, studies have shown (although with some inconsistencies) that women are particularly vulnerable to misattribution of symptoms in the presence of co-existing stressors, suggesting a tendency among providers to attribute symptoms to psychological rather than physical causes.[43,44]

The data that show effects of patient gender on observer judgments of pain are consistent with "common sense" models of illness that evoke gender stereotypes. That stereotype conjures images of women as exaggerating their experience of pain and/or somatizing, particularly in the face of stress. Hence, the cultural stereotype of the female patient appears to place a greater burden of proof on them; without evidence consistent with their symptom reports, the validity of their symptoms is more likely to be questioned. Of course, in the case of chronic pain, such proof can be elusive.

Older age. The widespread belief that advancing age serves as an analgesic has received considerable attention in the neurologic and neuropsychiatric literature in recent years.[45] Some evidence suggests that older adults may have diminished sensitivity to pain; other evidence suggests that sensitivity to pain is unchanged or even enhanced. Absent consensus on the matter, standard care dictates that treatment be based on the assumption that age is not an analgesic.[46]

Nonetheless, pain in older adults often is undertreated.[45] A number of explanations have been advanced to account for this phenomenon. One involves the focus of care. If the primary focus of care is on other disease processes (e.g., treating a malignancy), pain control may be a secondary issue for the patient and the provider. If secondary to the patient, even the most sensitive provider will have little opportunity to intervene. A second possibility is related to provider knowledge; many providers lack an understanding of pharmacodynamics and pharmacokinetics of analgesics in older adults, making them hesitant to treat pain aggressively in this age group. Another pharmacological explanation involves the side effects and drug-drug interactions that can be severe in older adults, limiting pharmacologic treatment options. Several other explanations have been advanced that are directly relevant to medical culture: popular views of aging suggest that it often is accompanied by pain, making it a natural by-product of aging. If providers adopt that view, they are likely to downplay the importance that is ascribed to pain severity and give it little clinical attention. If patients adopt that view, they are likely to under-report it to providers (if they report it at all). Finally, a special (albeit common) case involves older adults with cognitive deficits that compromise communication. Because of the importance of self-report to effective pain assessment, the latter group is especially vulnerable to undertreatment. Whether because of these or other explanations, it is clear that current medical culture tolerates undertreatment of this population to a surprising degree.

Younger age. The literature on the treatment of pain in children parallels that for older adults, as pain in children also is frequently undertreated. In past years, the undertreatment was driven by the widespread misconception that the nervous system in children was insufficiently developed for them to experience pain as adults do.[47] Such misconceptions have been corrected, such that there is now evidence that early exposure to pain can sensitize infants to subsequent exposures (something already well-known to parents of children with an aversion to the pediatrician's office).[48]

While the latter misconception may have been dispelled, there is considerable evidence that pain remains undertreated in children of all ages and across a variety of settings, including the emergency department, the hospital, and at home.[49] Although a variety of explanations have been advanced for this persistent pattern, the single most persuasive explanation involves cultural elements: beliefs and communication. As noted above, the belief that children experience pain to a lesser degree than adults has been discredited. Other problematic beliefs remain, however, including parental beliefs that the aggressive treatment of pain in a postoperative child can lead to pernicious side effects; studies have shown that parents consistently undermedicate their children following painful medical procedures.[50] Relative to communication, there is now recognition that children can be anxious and deferential when approached by an authority figure (e.g., the white-coated physician). Under such circumstances, they may be loathe to complain of pain, making it difficult for even the most sensitive pediatrician to identify poorly controlled pain. Similarly, many of the rating scales that have been developed to facilitate pain assessment may be difficult for a young child to comprehend; considerable work has been done to develop scales that will be easily understood by children so as to facilitate pain-related communication with the treatment staff.[51]

Psychological presentation
Psychological distress. The attribution of symptoms to psychological, rather than medical causes, is a common mechanism by which symptom reports may be discounted. This tendency is evident in the research on Waddell's signs, the inappropriate signs and symptoms demonstrated by patients with low back pain that reflect the "clinical equivalent of psychological distress:"[52] superficial tenderness, nonanatomical tenderness, axial loading, simulated rotation, distracted straight leg raising, regional weakness, and over-reaction to examination. These signs are common in patients with low back pain. To the degree that they flag potential psychological distress, they indicate that psychological issues may complicate the clinical picture and, hence, require attention in their own right. They do not, however, preclude coexisting organic findings. Hence, it is recommended that these signs be viewed as evidence that a biopsychosocial perspective should be brought to the treatment.[53]

In practice, however, Waddell's signs often are viewed as discrediting the validity of a patient's complaints, reflecting a clinical predisposition to question painful symptoms when they are associated with psychological distress.[54] Given this predisposition, it is not surprising that some patients have developed ways of coping with this challenge.[55] For example, a study of patients with mixed chronic pain conditions showed that socially sophisticated patients reported high levels of pain and pain-related disability, but low levels of distress.[56] Less sophisticated patients, however, acknowledged higher levels of distress.

In short, the medical culture demonstrates a dynamic around patients with chronic pain conditions who experience comorbid psychological distress: the attribution of pain to psychological causes is associated with devaluation of physical contributions to chronic pain syndromes. In turn, the sophisticated patient may cope with this by magnifying physical aspects of his condition, while underplaying psychological aspects. This pas de deux is unfortunate on several levels. First, it greatly complicates the assessment of an already complicated problem. Second, by treating physical and psychological causation as mutually exclusive, the false dichotomy fails to recognize the frequency with which both elements contribute to clinical adjustment, such that each element deserves treatment.

Pain behavior. Attention to pain behaviors is integral to the assessment of chronic pain conditions. Not only do these behaviors convey information about how patients communicate their pain to others, but there is reasonable evidence that observers derive information about pain severity from assessments of both facial expressions and general motor activity.[57,58] In fact, both facial expressions and motor behaviors have been shown to correlate with patient reports of pain intensity. While observations of pain behavior can yield useful information, observer estimates of pain, whether based on facial expressions or motor behaviors, are consistently lower than patient reports.[59,60] As with other patient characteristics reviewed in this section, patients exhibiting high levels of pain behavior can be vulnerable to undertreatment.

The tendency to undertreat based on pain behaviors is exemplified in work examining pseudoaddiction, a condition characterized by agitation, anxiety, sleep disruption, and demands for increased analgesics. Typically, such patients have been viewed as addicts, so providers have resisted their analgesic requests. An alternative view has argued that pseudoaddictive behaviors reflect undertreatment of pain, such that withholding analgesics actually could exacerbate a pain problem.[61] A recent study investigated addiction likelihood and analgesic needs among patients with sickle cell pain who exhibited behaviors reflecting either genuine addiction or pseudoaddiction.[62] After reading vignettes that described these behavior patterns, hospital staff judged a patient's addiction likelihood and analgesic needs. Judgments of addiction likelihood showed sensitivity to pseudoaddiction issues; patients exhibiting pseudoaddictive behaviors were less likely to be viewed as addicted. On the other hand, this sensitivity did not translate into differences in treatment; analgesic recommendations were uniformly low, both for patients demonstrating actual and those exhibiting pseudoaddictive behaviors.

In summary, observer judgments of pain behaviors consistently underestimate pain relative to patient reports. Hence, judgments of behavior do not necessarily lead to corresponding judgments regarding treatment. The lack of linkage between symptom judgments and treatment decisions is clearly a matter of great clinical importance that deserves further attention.

Section summary

A broad range of patient characteristics had been studied, some directly and some indirectly related to clinical judgment. These characteristics can impact judgment in different ways. For some characteristics (e.g., pain severity, levels of psychological distress/pain behavior), the level of that characteristic (i.e., high vs. low) is a key determinant of its impact on judgment. For other characteristics (e.g., minority status, gender), its presence/absence is enough to occasion differences in judgment and/or clinical decision-making. Whether mediated by the magnitude or simply the presence of a characteristic, however, those characteristics systematically eventuate in underestimation of symptoms and accompanying undertreatment.

OBSERVER FEATURES

There is ample evidence that healthcare providers differ in their treatment of persons with pain.[63,64] Indeed, the evidence suggests that they demonstrate very little agreement in diagnostic and treatment decisions for patients, even in situations where they have access to identical information.[30] While there is documented variability across providers in their clinical judgments, there is surprisingly little information about provider factors that contribute to that variability. The following two sections review the relatively modest literature on the topic: (1) provider experience, and (2) other provider characteristics (affective valence, empathy).

Provider experience

Experience typically is thought to sharpen clinical judgments. In the realm of pain, sharpened judgments could reasonably be expected to increase levels of agreement between patient pain reports and provider estimates of pain that patients experience. Such expectations, however, are not supported by the literature. Indeed, most studies suggest that increased experience with pain predisposes providers to underestimation.

For example, an early study of patients receiving care on a burn unit showed significant differences in ratings that were associated with levels of nursing experience.[65] While nurses with more experience estimated patient pain at levels that were lower than patient reports, less experienced nurses estimated pain at levels higher than patient ratings. A similar phenomenon has been found among physicians. In a sample of emergency department physicians, more senior physicians have been shown to estimate pain at levels lower than those reported by patients, while the ratings of less experienced physicians were significantly higher than those of their more experienced colleagues.[66] Similar patterns have been reported for physical and occupational therapists. Videotapes of patients undergoing painful rehabilitation for shoulder injuries were viewed by either therapists or college students with no prior history of working with people in pain. Relative to the therapists, the college students consistently estimated the pain depicted in the videotapes to be higher.[67]

Among physicians with similar amounts of experience, there also is evidence that differences in types of experience mediate pain estimation. A recent study of hypothetical patients with low back pain compared estimates of pain severity and pain-related disability made by surgeons and internists.[68] The physician groups clearly differed in their types of experience, with neurosurgeons devoting more of their practice to hospital-based care and generally treating patients with higher pain acuity. Consistent with these differences in practice, neurosurgeon estimates of pain severity and disability were significantly lower than estimates made by internists, despite their exposure to identical descriptive information. While the results suggest that the physician cohorts may have used different standards against which to evaluate pain and disability, the research did not identify specific standards that may have mediated the different estimates.

Indeed, while there is substantial evidence that experience mediates provider judgments, the specific reason(s) for differences in judgments remain unclear.[69] The most accepted hypothesis is that frequent exposure to patients with severe pain may desensitize healthcare providers to pain complaints, possibly re-setting the anchor points that they use to judge pain.[67] According to this view, clinicians with extensive experience may, over time, have enough exposures to high levels of pain as to define the uppermost endpoint (e.g., "pain as bad as it can get") differently than those with less experience. Another hypothesis related to experience involves sensitivity to disconfirming information. Experienced clinicians may become progressively insensitive to information that could disconfirm their judgments, focusing selectively on information that supports the accuracy of their judgments.[70] A variation on the latter hypothesis focuses on attitudinal factors: providers with long exposure to patients with severe symptoms may develop negative attitudes that, in turn, may make them indifferent to pain that they confront on a regular basis.[71] A final hypothesis invokes the cognitive miser model: more experienced providers may default to well-established heuristics when assessing pain in others, rather than engage in more effortful processes that would require data-driven, patient-centered processes.

While there is no definitive study that would support one of these mechanisms over others (in fact, all of the mechanisms are likely to operate among providers), there is interesting evidence that suggests that the tendency to discount severe pain is largely found among health professionals. An interesting study examined a potential mediating factor that involves the nature of the relationship between the patient and the clinician (e.g., professional vs. nonprofessional). That study found that lay people who have been exposed to a fellow family member with a pain condition may be *more* sensitive to pain in others than are people who have not undergone such experience.[67] Hence, in a nonprofessional sample, experience may have a sensitizing effect, rather than a de-sensitizing one.

While the evidence suggests that health professionals are likely to underestimate pain intensity as they gain experience, there is some evidence that training may mitigate that effect. For example, physical and occupational therapists who are trained to recognize facial cues reflecting pain demonstrate increased sensitivity to patient discomfort.[72] Similarly, oncologists who have received specialized training in pain management seem to be more willing to prescribe opioids for cancer pain than those without such training.[73] Because neither of the latter studies examined corresponding changes related to judgment (e.g., attitudes), the mechanisms that account for training effectiveness are unclear. It may be that training recruits higher level cognitive processes (i.e., reasoning), mitigating the miserly approach that characterizes many cognitive processes. Whatever the mechanism, the changes described above certainly are consistent with judgments driven by clinical data.

Other provider characteristics

Affective valence. As noted previously, there is considerable evidence that the medical community holds negative views of patients with chronic pain. Negative affect associated with such views would be expected to bias inference processes negatively and trigger tendencies to blame patients for their symptoms.

Several studies (using vignettes depicting hypothetical patients) have investigated the effects of affective valence on observer judgments. Early studies manipulated the valence of the relationship between an undergraduate observer and a hypothetical person with chronic low back pain by depicting the latter in either a positive (calm and polite) or negative (upset and demanding) light.[23,26] When asked to rate the symptoms of the person who presented positively, observers in each study rated symptoms as significantly higher (i.e., more severe) than when the person presented negatively. Moreover, under positive affect conditions, persons without supporting medical evidence (i.e., those without "proof") were judged more charitably than when affective valence was negative. Thus, despite the lack of supporting evidence, their symptoms were judged more favorably, while those of the negatively valenced group were steeply discounted.

Efforts to conduct similar research with physicians, however, have proved problematic.[27] When internists were asked to rate symptom severity for hypothetical patients who presented in either a calm/polite or upset/demanding manner, they rated the symptoms of the latter group as more severe than those of the former, a pattern contrary to that of the under-graduates. The unexpected difference likely reflected a different appraisal of the patient behavior by physicians compared to undergraduates: while the undergraduates seemingly viewed the behavior relative to its interpersonal valence, the physicians apparently considered the behavior relative to the presenting problem. Hence, the upset demeanor apparently was viewed as reflecting pain-related distress, rather than a negatively toned relationship. Similarly, the calm demeanor was seen as reflecting no apparent distress, rather than a positive demeanor.

Empathy. Empathy, the ability to "put yourself into another person's shoes," is a characteristic that is recognized and valued in the medical field. It is seen as a critical component of patient-centered care that mediates good outcomes across a range of patient populations.[74,75] Moreover, it also has been shown to mitigate the risk of litigation.[76]

Interest in empathy related to pain research, however, has been primarily neuropsychological in nature. Pain researchers have studied empathy primarily because "empathic" neural circuits have been identified that are activated in response to pain behavior demonstrated by others.[77] The study of such circuitry has been enabled by technologic advances that permit examination of blood flow to various regions of the brain and by the recognition that the capacity to "intuitively experience the emotional distress of others" may be linked to a range of observer responses to pain behavior.[78]

Very little research, however, has examined relations between levels of empathy and clinical judgment. For example, one study showed that highly empathic nurses were likely to overestimate patient pain relative to both patient report and to less empathic nurses.[79] In another study focused more specifically on clinical judgment, surgeons were administered vignettes that described a patient with low back pain who first underwent (successful or failed) conservative treatment followed by a (successful or failed) surgery.[80] They then were asked to characterize the factors related to the surgical outcomes, including both physician attributes (generally reflecting skill) and patient attributes (generally reflecting psychological frailties). Interestingly, successful surgical outcomes were attributed primarily to physician skill, while unsuccessful outcomes were attributed to psychological frailties. Empathy, however, moderated the latter effect: surgeons with higher levels of empathy were less likely to blame patients for the surgical failures, while surgeons with lower levels of empathy were significantly more likely to do so.

Section summary

While obviously a crucial element in clinical judgments regarding pain (after all, they make those judgments), judges have been little studied. Research involving the effects of provider experience is more developed than that involving other characteristics, showing a tendency to discount patient pain reports as the level of experience increases. There also is suggestive evidence that the type of experience may mediate judgments. While less convincing evidence supports the role of other factors (e.g., affective valence, empathy) in provider judgments, the limited research on healthcare professionals and studies of nonprofessionals suggest that those characteristics are likely influences on clinical judgment.

SITUATIONAL FEATURES

Situational factors that impact clinical judgment fall into one of two general categories: (1) the availability of objective (supporting medical) evidence, and (2) patient litigation/

compensation status. Of course, other situational factors also could affect pain-related judgments. For example, time urgency and/or the likelihood of peer review also are situational candidates, but the impact of those features on judgments has not received much study. Therefore, the following sections only review the literature on the former two topics.

Medical evidence

The American Medical Association (AMA) guidelines for physicians evaluating impairment in patients with low back pain attach great importance to objective evidence of tissue damage in assessing impairment ratings.[81] The pain literature, however, shows that neither objective diagnostic results nor impairment ratings correlate with either reported pain intensity or pain-related disability.[82,83] Indeed, spinal pathology often exists among asymptomatic patients, sometimes at levels comparable to those in patients with low back pain.[84] Contrariwise, it is commonplace for patients to complain of severe pain without evidence of tissue damage. Despite the experimental evidence that demonstrates little association between objective medical evidence and the experience/impact of pain, evaluators still attach importance to confirming medical evidence when judging patients in pain.[85]

The importance of such evidence is readily apparent. For example, early studies of undergraduates used vignettes to describe hypothetical patients; each of these studies showed that students estimated pain to be higher when supporting medical evidence was present.[23,26] The second of those studies also examined the valence of the patient-observer relationship (positive vs. negative), finding that pain estimates were especially discounted when reported pain severity was high and relationship valence was negative. Thus, the absence of medical evidence undermined the apparent validity of the reported symptoms, and the presence of a negative relationship seemingly undermined it further.

Similar patterns have been found with medical students and with practicing healthcare providers. In a study with the former group, medical students estimated "actual" pain for hypothetical patients reporting one of four levels of pain severity (3/10, 5/10, 7/10, 9/10); supporting medical evidence was either present or absent at each level of pain.[21] Across all levels of pain severity, patients with medical evidence were credited with more severe pain than those without evidence. Studies of practicing professionals have shown that internists discount high levels of reported pain, especially when medical evidence is lacking.[27] Similarly, in the previously referenced study of "histrionic" and "business-like" patients presenting with complaints of chest pain, the symptoms of histrionic patients were less likely to be attributed to bona fide cardiac factors absent supporting medical evidence.[19]

Not surprisingly, clinical studies have yielded similar results. In a study of workers with occupational low back injuries, supporting medical evidence was strongly associated with disability ratings at the time of claim settlement, although only weakly associated with actual clinical adjustment.[86] A subsequent occupational medicine study showed that medical evidence strongly predicted impairment ratings when a claimant reached maximum medical improvement, as well as disability ratings at the time of claim settlement.[83]

Clearly, medical evidence weighs heavily when observers (lay or medical) are asked to judge the validity of pain-related symptoms, despite the fact that such evidence relates inconsistently (at best) to pain and pain-related disability. While a more rational approach would dictate that objective evidence not receive such weight (relative to its predictive validity), its intuitive appeal suggests that it will continue to weigh heavily as long as a medical (versus empirical) model guides clinical medicine.

Compensation status

There is a considerable literature regarding the effect of compensation status on symptom presentation and response to treatment in patients with chronic pain. The treatment literature shows that patients involved in litigation demonstrate poorer outcomes than nonlitigants.[87] The literature on symptom presentation is mixed: some shows evidence of apparent "symptom magnification," while some shows no such effects.[88,89] Despite the inconsistent empirical findings, the general attitude of the field attaches validity to the construct of "compensation neurosis" captured in the following quote from work that occurred over a half-century ago:[90] " ... a state of mind, borne of fear, kept alive by avarice, stimulated by lawyers, and cured by a verdict." Other pejorative terms have been linked to this construct over the intervening years, reflecting the widespread skepticism that providers hold toward patients involved in litigation proceedings: barristogenic illness, functional overlay, malingering, post-accident syndrome, psychogenic invalidism, railway spine, and secondary gain.[91]

Despite the widespread attitudes implicit in the terms cited above, there are few empirical data regarding the impact of compensation status on provider judgments. Not surprisingly, those data suggest that providers view litigating patients with skepticism. As with much of the judgment literature, those data are derived from vignette methodologies. One study found that lay observers did not discount the intensity of symptoms presented by compensation patients, but did question the legitimacy of those symptoms.[22] Another study, involving physical therapy trainees, examined the effects of instructional sets on judgments.[92] Some students were told to expect that some patients were faking pain, while others were given no such instruction. Despite the fact that all clinical information about the patient was held constant across both student groups, the former students rated pain intensity lower than did those who did not expect cheating.

In summary, litigation appears to trigger questions about the motivation of patients involved in compensation claims related to their pain conditions. In particular, litigation raises the specter of "secondary gain," where financial factors motivate symptom magnification. Whether or not that specter is justified, the negative cognitive set associated with litigation is intuitively appealing and likely to be relatively impervious to change.

DISCUSSION

This chapter has focused on cultural factors that operate at the medical encounter, particularly examining social psychological mechanisms that might influence judgments made in a patient-provider interaction. Mechanisms were identified that are associated with patient, provider, and situational features that can inform the interaction. An examination of those mechanisms clearly shows that beliefs and attitudes do influence how pain is judged and how pain management is practiced.

Factors implicated at the patient level derive from both sides of the patient-provider interaction. From the patient side, there is ample evidence of distrust of and dissatisfaction with medical care among racial/ethnic minorities. Leaving aside specific reasons why that distrust/dissatisfaction exists, a substrate of distrust/dissatisfaction can prejudicially affect the collaboration often required if pain management is to be effective. Further, there is evidence specific to treatments that are typically expected to mitigate pain (e.g., knee replacement surgery) that points to lowered expectations of benefit by minorities, dampening their willingness to undertake such interventions.[93]

Of course, this chapter focused primarily on factors operating on the provider side. Relative to patients, those factors center around negative sociodemographic stereotypes that can influence provider judgments, including stereotypes associated with minority status, female gender, and age (both old and young). Of these, there is particularly strong evidence that implicates negative racial/ethnic stereotypes as influencing the assessment of pain, as well as treatment decisions that flow from that assessment. Other patient factors, such as a patient's psychological presentation, also can influence provider judgments. In particular, manifestations of psychological distress may serve to offset/invalidate a patient's pain report, despite the wide recognition that psychological distress is a common comorbidity but a relatively infrequent cause of pain disorders.[94]

Situational factors also have a demonstrated impact on pain-related judgments. The presence or absence of medical evidence that supports a patient's pain report is of particular importance, despite the considerable documentation that shows little correlation between the presence of such evidence and the acuity of a pain complaint (and/or its functional impact). Nonetheless, the presence of such evidence greatly enhances the likelihood that pain will be validated in the eye of the beholder and that aggressive treatment will be pursued. In addition to medical evidence, another situational factor that can influence judgments involves compensation status. There is a long tradition in medical practice of doubting the complaints of patients who are involved in litigation secondary to financial gains that can accrue to magnified reports of pain and disability. While there is ample reason to consider litigation status as a potential complication in a chronic pain syndrome, the concept of secondary gain does not capture the nuances of that complication. In fact, many patients involved in litigation demonstrate no improvement once that litigation is resolved. Nonetheless, there is an evident tendency to view the presence of litigation as invalidating self-reports.

Given the focus of this chapter on factors that can influence provider judgments and occasion disparities in care, it is interesting that research specifically focusing on provider characteristics is the least developed of the three elements of the medical encounter. The topic that has been most examined involves the effects of provider experience. A preponderance of that evidence indicates that increasing experience attenuates provider estimates of pain: the more experienced providers tend to view pain as less severe than providers with less experience. Providers also may be influenced by the valence (positive/negative) of their relationship with a patient. Much of the latter research, however, is predicated on results derived from paper-and-pencil methodologies; more robust methodologies clearly are needed.

It is not surprising that a wide range of factors in the medical encounter can influence provider decisions. After all, we no longer operate under the illusion that providers function as automatons that make unbiased, probabilistic judgments. Nonetheless, as shown in Figure 11.3, it is somewhat daunting to realize that such factors not only can operate on behalf of positive outcomes, but that they also can operate to occasion disparities in clinical care.

Future directions

How should we proceed if we are to reduce such disparities? Several recommendations emerge from the foregoing discussion. First, we need to recognize that healthcare providers are subject to the same cultural factors that influence all of us. Indeed, providers may be subject to even more complex social psychological factors, given the relatively unusual

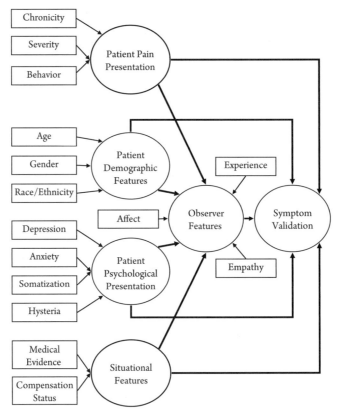

FIGURE 11.3 Social-psychological factors in clinical judgment. Adapted from Tait et al. *Pain Medicine*, 2009, 10, p.25.

nature of the patient-provider relationship and the vagaries of medical culture. Only if we recognize the potential impact of those factors can we move from intuition-driven to more rationally derived decision-making processes.

Second, there is evidence that education can be of some value in mitigating intuition-driven decision-making.[72,73] Of course, there also is evidence that the impact of educational initiatives is limited in the provider community.[95] While education is not a panacea, education that sensitizes providers to the pernicious effects of the biases described in this chapter is likely to constitute a necessary but not sufficient component of any fundamental change process.

Third, it is important to recognize that this chapter has focused on *individual* judgments, not judgments made by multidisciplinary teams. Multidisciplinary care, by dint of the team-based discussion that typically characterizes clinical decisions, has the potential to mitigate judgment bias through several mechanisms: (1) by structuring decision-making (i.e., through group discussion) in a manner that increases the likelihood of a thoughtful, albeit laborious, approach, and (2) by systematically introducing multiple perspectives into clinical decisions. Relative to the latter, selected members of the treatment team (e.g., nurses, social workers, psychologists) often are able to spend more time with patients, making them better able to speak to the social context in which the patient lives.

Finally, it is important to recognize that the cultural factors that can influence pain management judgments are well-established and not subject to easy change. In deference to that recognition, it also is important that considerable education/support be directed to the patients deemed most vulnerable to disparities in care, particularly those sociodemographic groups discussed above. To the degree that patients can advocate effectively for their own care, disparities are likely to be mitigated. Such training could be provided through a variety of channels, including patient advocates,[96] university- and/or clinic-based initiatives,[97] and community-based initiatives.[98] Indeed, given the obvious level of need documented in this chapter, each avenue should be pursued in an effort to touch all of the cultural elements that contribute to disparities in care.

REFERENCES

1. Tait RC, Miller L. Multidisciplinary treatment of chronic pain in vulnerable populations. In: Schatman ME, Campbell A, eds. *Chronic Pain Management: A Guidebook for Multidisciplinary Program Development.* New York: Informa Healthcare; 2008:129–150.
2. Green CR, Anderson KO, Baker TA, et al. The unequal burden of pain: confronting racial and ethnic disparities in pain. *Pain Med.* 2003;4:277–294.
3. Anderson KO, Green CR, Payne R. Racial and ethnic disparities in pain: causes and consequences of unequal care. *J Pain.* 2009;10:1187–1204.
4. McDonald DD. Gender and ethnic stereotyping and narcotic analgesic administration. *Res Nurs Health.* 1994;14:45–49.
5. Hamers JPH, Abu-Saad HH, van den Hout MA, Halfens RJG, Kester ADM. The influence of children's vocal expressions, age, medical diagnosis and information obtained from parents on nurses' pain assessments and decisions regarding interventions. *Pain.* 1996;65:53–61.
6. Fox PL, Raina P, Jadad AR. Prevalence and treatment of pain in older adults in nursing homes and other long-term care institutions: a systematic review. *Can Med Assoc J.* 1999;160:329–333.
7. Zuvekas SH, Taliaferro GS. Pathways to access: health insurance, the health care delivery system, and racial/ethnic disparities, 1996–1999. *Health Aff.* 2003;22:139–153.
8. Frantsve LME, Kerns RD. Patient-provider interactions in the management of chronic pain: current findings within the context of shared medical decision making. *Pain Med.*2007;8:25–35.
9. Tait RC, Chibnall JT, Kalauokalani D. Provider judgments of patients in pain: seeking symptom certainty. *Pain Med.* 2009;10:11–34.
10. Chang L, Toner BB, Fukudo S, Guthrie E, Locke GR, Norton NJ, Sperber AD. Gender, age, society, culture, and the patient's perspective in the functional gastrointestinal disorders. *Gastroenterology.* 2006;130:1435–1446.
11. Morrison RS, Wallenstein S, Natale DK, Senzel RS, Huang L-L. "We don't carry that"—failure of pharmacies in predominantly nonwhite neighborhoods to stock opioid analgesics. *N Engl J Med.* 2000;342:1023–1026.
12. Weinick RM, Zuvekas SH, Cohen JW. Racial and ethnic differences in access and use of health care services, 1977–1996. *Med Care Res Rev.* 2000;57(suppl 1):36–54.
13. Fiske ST, Taylor SE. *Social cognition.* 2nd ed. New York: McGraw-Hill; 1991.
14. Tversky A, Kahneman D. Availability: a heuristic for judging frequency and probability. *Cognit Psychol.* 1973;5:207–232.
15. Album D, Westin S. Do diseases have a prestige hierarchy? A survey among physicians and medical students. *Soc Science Med.* 2008;66:182–188.
16. Eccleston C, Williams A C de C, Rogers WS. Patients' and professionals' understandings of the causes of chronic pain: blame, responsibility and identity protection. *Soc Sci Med.* 1997;45:699–709.

17. Leclere H, Beaulieu MD, Bordage G, Sindon A, Couillard M. Why are clinical problems difficult? General practitioners' opinions concerning 24 clinical problems. *Can Med Assoc J.* 1990;143:1305–1315.

18. Bransford JD, Franks, JJ. The abstraction of linguistic ideas. *Cog Psychol.* 1971;2:331–350.

19. Birdwell BG, Herbers JE, Kroenke K. Evaluating chest pain: the patient's presentation style alters the physician's diagnostic approach. *Arch Intern Med.* 1993;153:1991–1995.

20. Heider F. *The Psychology of Interpersonal Relations.* New York: Wiley; 1958.

21. Chibnall JT, Tait RC, Ross L. The effects of medical evidence and pain intensity on medical student judgments of chronic pain patients. *J Behav Med.* 1997;20:257–271.

22. Chibnall JT, Tait RC. Social and medical influences on attributions and evaluations of chronic pain. *Psychol Health.* 1999;14:719–729.

23. Tait RC, Chibnall JT. Observer perceptions of chronic low back pain. *J Appl Soc Psychol.* 1994;24:415–431.

24. Todd KH, Samaroo N, Hoffman JR. Ethnicity as a risk factor for inadequate emergency department analgesia. *JAMA.* 1993;269:1537–1539.

25. Todd KH, Lee T, Hoffman JR. The effect of ethnicity on physician estimates of pain severity in patients with isolated extremity trauma. *JAMA.* 1994;271:925–928.

26. Chibnall JT, Tait RC. Observer perceptions of low back pain: effects of pain report and other contextual factors. *J Appl Soc Psychol.* 1995;25:418–439.

27. Tait RC, Chibnall JT. Physician judgments of patients with intractable low back pain. *Soc Sci Med.* 1997;45:1199–1205.

28. Grossman SA, Sheidler VR, Swedeen K, Mucenski J, Piantadosi S. Correlation of patient and caregiver ratings of cancer pain. *J Pain Symptom Manage.* 1991;6:53–57.

29. Kappesser J, C de C Williams A. Pain judgements of patients' relatives: examining the use of social contract theory as a theoretical framework. *J Behav Med.* 2008;31:309–317.

30. Chibnall JT, Dabney A, Tait RC. Internist judgments of chronic low back pain. *Pain Med.* 2000;1:231–237.

31. Taylor AG, Skelton JA, Butcher J. Duration of pain condition and physical pathology as determinants of nurses' assessments of patients in pain. *Nurs Res.* 1984;33:4–8.

32. Cleeland CS, Gonin R, Baez L, Loehrer P, Pandya KJ. Pain and treatment of pain in minority patients with cancer. *Ann Intern Med.* 1997;127:813–816.

33. Tait RC, Chibnall JT, Andresen EM, Hadler NM. Management of occupational back injuries: differences among African Americans and Caucasians. *Pain.* 2004;112:389–396.

34. Chibnall JT, Tait RC, Andresen EM, Hadler NM. Race and socioeconomic differences in post-settlement outcomes for African American and Caucasian workers' compensation claimants with low back injuries. *Pain.* 2005;114:462–472.

35. LaVeist TA, Nickerson KJ, Bowie JV. Attitudes about racism, medical mistrust, and satisfaction with care among African American and White cardiac patients. *Med Care Res Rev.* 2000;57(suppl 1):146–161.

36. Cooper-Patrick L, Gallo JJ, Gonzales JJ, Vu HT, Powe NR, Nelson C, et al. Race, gender, and partnership in the patient-physician relationship. *JAMA.* 1999;282:583–589.

37. Mayberry RM, Mili F, Ofili E. Racial and ethnic differences in access to medical care. *Med Care Res Rev.* 2000;57(suppl 1):108–145.

38. Chibnall JT, Tait RC, Andresen EM, Hadler NM. Race differences in diagnosis and surgery for occupational low back injuries. *Spine.* 2006;31:1272–1275.

39. Chibnall JT, Tait RC. Long-term adjustment to work-related low back pain: associations with socio-demographics, claim processes, and post-settlement adjustment. *Pain Med.* 2009;10:1378–1388.

40. Calderone KL. The influence of gender on the frequency of pain and sedative medication administered to postoperative patients. *Sex Roles.* 1990;23:713–725.

41. Hamberg K, Risberg G, Johansson EE, Westman G. Gender bias in physicians' management of neck pain: A study of the answers in a Swedish national examination. *J Womens Health Gend Based Med.* 2002;11:653–666.

42. Taylor BA, Casas-Ganem J, Vaccaro AR, et al. Differences in the work-up and treatment of conditions associated with low back pain by patient gender and ethnic background. *Spine*. 2005;30:359–364.

43. Martin R, Gordon EEI, Lounsbury P. Gender disparities in the attribution of cardiac-related symptoms: contribution of common sense models of illness. *Health Psychol*. 1998;17:346–357.

44. Martin R, Lemos K. From heart attacks to melanoma: do common sense models of somatization influence symptom interpretation for female victims? *Health Psychol*. 2002;21:25–32.

45. Hadjistavropoulos T, Herr K, Turk DC, Fine PG, Dworkin RH, Helme R, et al. An interdisciplinary expert consensus statement on assessment of pain in older persons. *Clin J Pain*. 2007;23(suppl):S1–S43.

46. Ferrell BA. Pain management in elderly people. *J Am Geriatr Soc*. 1991;39:64–73.

47. McGrath PJ, Unruh AM. *Pain in Children and Adolescents*. New York: Elsevier Science Publishers; 1987.

48. Taddio A, Shah V, Gilbert-MacLeod C, Katz J. Conditioning and hyperalgesia in newborns exposed to repeated heel lances. *JAMA*. 2002;288:857–861.

49. Howard RF. Current status of pain management in children. *JAMA*. 2003;290:2464–2469.

50. Swallow J, Briggs M. Semple P. Pain at home: children's experience of tonsillectomy. *J Child Home Health Care* 2000;4:93–98.

51. Stinson JN, Kavanagh T, Yamada J, Gill N, Stevens B. Systematic review of the psychometric properties, interpretability and feasibility of self-report pain intensity measures for use in clinical trials in children and adolescents. *Pain*. 2006;125:143–157.

52. Waddell G, McCulloch JA, Kummel E, Venner RM. Nonorganic physical signs in low-back pain. *Spine*. 1980;5:117–125.

53. Main CJ, Waddell G. Behavioral responses to examination: a reappraisal of the interpretation of "nonorganic signs." *Spine*. 1998;23:2367–2371.

54. Fishbain DA, Cole B, Cutler RB, Lewis J, Rosomoff HL, Rosomoff RS. A structured evidence-based review on the meaning of nonorganic physical signs: Waddell signs. *Pain Med*. 2003;4:141–181.

55. Marbach JJ, Lennon MC, Link BG, Dohrenwend BP. Losing face: sources of stigma as perceived by chronic facial pain patients. *J Behav Med*. 1990;13:583–604.

56. Deshields TL, Tait RC, Gfeller JD, Chibnall JT. The relationship between social desirability and self-report in chronic pain patients. *Clin J Pain*. 1995;11:189–193.

57. Craig KD, Hyde S, Patrick CJ. Genuine, suppressed, and faked facial behavior during exacerbation of chronic low back pain. *Pain*. 1991;46:161–172.

58. Keefe FJ, Block AR. Development of an observation method for assessing pain behavior in chronic low back pain patients. *Behav Ther*. 1982;13:363–375.

59. Prkachin KM, Berzins S, Mercer SR. Encoding and decoding of pain expressions: a judgment study. *Pain*. 1994;58:253–259.

60. Krause SJ, Wiener RL, Tait RC. Depression and pain behavior in patients with chronic pain. *Clin J Pain*. 1994;10:122–127.

61. Weissman DE, Haddox JD. Opioid pseudo-addiction: an iatrogenic syndrome. *Pain*. 1989;36:363–367.

62. Elander J, Marczewska M, Amos R, Thomas A, Tangayi S. Factors affecting hospital staff judgments about sickle cell disease. *J Behav Med*. 2006;29:203–214.

63. Green C, Wheeler J. Physician variability in the management of acute postoperative and cancer pain: a quantitative analysis of the Michigan experience. *Pain Med*. 2003;4:8–20.

64. Phelan SM, van Ryn M, Wall M, Burgess D. Understanding Primary Care Physicians' Treatment of Chronic Low Back Pain: The Role of Physician and Practice Factors. *Pain Med*. 2009;10:1270–1279.

65. Choiniere M, Melzack R, Girard N, Rondeau J, Paquin M-J. Comparisons between patients' and nurses' assessment of pain medication efficacy in severe burn injuries. *Pain*. 1990;40:143–152.

66. Marquie L, Raufaste E, Lauque D, Marine C, Ecoiffier M, Sorum P. Pain rating by patients and physicians: evidence of systematic pain miscalibration. *Pain*. 2003;102:289–296.

67. Prkachin KM, Solomon P, Hwang T, Mercer SR. Does experience influence judgments of pain behaviour? Evidence from relatives of pain patients and therapists. *Pain Res Manag*. 2001;6:105–112.

68. Tait RC, Chibnall JT, Miller L, Werner CA. Judging pain and disability: effects of pain severity and physician specialty. *J Behav Med.* 2011;34:218–224.

69. Solomon P. Congruence between health professionals' and patients' pain ratings: a review of the literature. *Scand J Caring Sci.* 2001;15:174–180.

70. Watts FN. Clinical judgment and clinical training. *Br J Med Psychol.* 1980;53:95–108.

71. Sharpe M, Mayou R, Seagroatt V, Surawy C, Warwick H, et al. Why do doctors find some patients difficult to help? *Quarterly J Med.* 1994;87:187–193.

72. Solomon PE, Prkachin KM, Farewell V. Enhancing sensitivity to facial expression of pain. *Pain.* 1997;71:249–284.

73. Cleeland CS, Cleeland LM, Dar R, Rinehardt LC. Factors influencing physician management of cancer pain. *Cancer.* 1986;58:796–800.

74. Banja JD. Empathy in the physician's pain practice: benefits, barriers, and recommendations. *Pain Med.* 2006;7:265–275.

75. Kaplan SH, Greenfield S, Ware JE. Assessing the effects of physician-patient interactions on the outcomes of chronic disease. *Med Care.* 1989;27:S110–S127.

76. Levinson W, Roter DL, Mullooly JP, Dull VT, Frankel RM. Physician-patient communication: the relationship with malpractice claims among primary care physicians and surgeons. *JAMA.* 1997;277:553–559.

77. Jackson PL, Brunet E, Meltzoff AN, Decety J. Empathy examined through the neural mechanisms involved in imagining how I feel versus how you feel pain. *Neuropsychologia.* 2006;44:752–761.

78. Goubert L, Craig KD, Vervoort T, Morley S, Sullivan MJL, Williams A C de C, et al. Facing others in pain: the effects of empathy. *Pain.* 2005;118:285–288.

79. Schupp CJ, Berbaum K, Berbaum M, Lang EV. Pain and anxiety during interventional radiologic procedures: effect of patients' state anxiety at baseline and modulation. *J Vasc Interv Radiol.* 2005;16:1585–1592.

80. Tait RC, Chibnall JT, Luebbert A, Sutter C. Effect of treatment success and empathy on surgeon attributions for back surgery outcomes. *J Behav Med.* 2005;28:301–312.

81. Cocchiarella L, Andersson GBJ, eds. *Guides to the Evaluation of Permanent Impairment.* 5th ed. Chicago: AMA Press; 2001.

82. Jensen CJ, Brant-Zawaszki MN, Obuchowski N, Modic MT, Malkasian D, Ross JS. Magnetic resonance imaging of the lumbar spine in people without back pain. *N Engl J Med.* 1994;331:69–73.

83. Tait RC, Chibnall JT, Andresen EA, Hadler NM. Disability determination: validity with occupational low back pain. *J Pain.* 2006;7:951–957.

84. Michel A, Kohlmann T, Raspe H. The association between clinical findings on physical examination and self-reported severity in back pain. *Spine.* 1997;22:296–304.

85. Carey TS, Hadler NM, Gillings D, Stinnett S, Wallsten T. Medical disability assessment of the back pain patient for the Social Security Administration: the weighting of presenting clinical features. *J Clin Epidemiol.* 1988;41:691–697.

86. Chibnall JT, Tait RC, Merys S. Disability management of low back injuries by employer-retained physicians: ratings and costs. *Am J Ind Med.* 2000;38:529–538.

87. Rohling ML, Binder LM, Langhinrichsen-Rohling J. Money matters: a meta-analytic review of the association between financial compensation and the experience and treatment of chronic pain. *Health Psychol.* 1995;14:537–547.

88. Mendelson G. 'Compensation neurosis' revisited: outcome studies of the effects of litigation. *J Psychosom Res.* 1995;39:695–706.

89. Rainville J, Sobel JB, Hartigan C, Wright A. The effect of compensation involvement on the reporting of pain and disability by patients referred for rehabilitation of chronic low back pain. *Spine.* 1997;22:2016–2024.

90. Kennedy F. The mind of the injured worker: its effect on disability periods. *Comp Med.* 1946;1:19–24.

91. Bellamy R. Compensation neurosis: financial reward for illness as nocebo. *Clin Orthopaed Rel Res.* 1997;336:94–106.

92. Kappesser J, Williams A, Prkachin KM. Testing two accounts of pain underestimation. *Pain.* 2006;124:109–116.

93. Ibrahim SA, Siominoff LA, Burant CJ, Kwoh CK. Differences in expectations of outcome mediate African American/white patient differences in "willingness" to consider joint replacement. *Arthrit Rheum.* 2002;46:2429–2435.

94. Gatchel RJ, Dersh J. Psychological disorders and chronic pain: are there cause-and-effect relationships? In: Turk DC, Gatchel RJ, eds. *Psychological Approaches to Pain Management: A Practitioner's Handbook.* 2nd ed. New York: Guilford Press; 2002:30–51.

95. Brown JB, Boles M, Mullooly JP, Levinson W. Effect of clinician communication skills training on patient satisfaction: a randomized, controlled trial. *Ann Intern Med.* 1999;131:822–829.

96. Kalauokalani D, Franks P, Oliver JW, Meyers FJ, Kravitz RL. Can patient coaching reduce racial/ethnic disparities in cancer pain control? Secondary analysis of a randomized controlled trial. *Pain Med.* 2007;8:17–24.

97. Shutty MS, DeGood DE, Tuttle DH. Chronic pain patients' beliefs about their pain and treatment outcomes. *Arch Phys Med Rehabil.* 1990;71:128–132.

98. Minkler M, Wallerstein N, eds. *Community Based Participatory Research for Health: From Process to Outcomes.* 2nd ed. San Francisco, CA: Jossey-Bass; 2008822–829.

12

SOCIAL CONTEXTS OF PAIN

Patients, Dentists, and Ethnicity

ROD MOORE, DDS, PHD, DR ODONT
Dental Anxiety Research and Treatment Center,
Royal Dental College, Faculty of Health Sciences,
Århus University, Århus, Denmark

Key Points

- Pain is a psychosocial contextual phenomenon, not just a physical sensation.
- Dentistry provides a useful model for exploring how social contexts affect pain perceptions, pain reactions, and preferences for alleviation or elimination of pain.
- Social expectations of pain, fear of painful treatment, and perceived remedies for pain vary from culture to culture.
- Dentists should be aware of cultural factors that influence their ability to manage pain and anxiety.
- Patient and dentist beliefs and expectations affect emotional meanings of dental pain in a mutually reinforcing manner.
- Patients and dentists should explore each other's pain-related expectations and beliefs in order to achieve superior outcomes.

DEFINING PAIN VS. DESCRIBING PAIN

Pain has been defined by the International Association for the Study of Pain (IASP) as: *An unpleasant sensory and emotional experience associated with actual or potential tissue damage, or described in terms of such damage. Note: Pain is always subjective. Each individual learns the application of the word through experiences related to injury in early life. Biologists recognize that those stimuli which cause pain are liable to damage tissue. Accordingly, pain is that experience which we associate with actual or potential tissue damage. It is unquestionably a sensation in a part or parts of the body, but it is also always unpleasant and therefore also an emotional experience.... There is no way to distinguish their experience from that due to tissue damage if we take the subjective report. If they regard their experience as pain caused by tissue damage, it should be accepted as pain. This definition avoids tying pain to the stimulus. Activity induced in the nociceptor and nociceptive pathways by a noxious stimulus is not pain, which is always a psychological state, even though we may well appreciate that pain most often has proximate physical cause....*[3]

Thus, pain is a psychosocial contextual phenomenon, not just a physical sensation. This means that there are perhaps also social ways to define pain more completely. Or perhaps a better word to use here is to "describe" pains, since defining implies limitation. Either way, the meaning of pain in its social context is the topic that is covered in this chapter. It is true that individuals in the course of their daily lives happen to experience painful sensations and learn conditioned responses to them (i.e., pain reactions). But these experiences are not devoid of social influences in the form of beliefs and learned expectations that a person has grown up with in the context of family and ethnic background that create an emotional meaning for the pain. That is, pain reactions must be seen in the social context within which they occur in order to fully understand them.[4]

EMOTIONAL MEANINGS OF PAIN—SOCIAL FRAMEWORKS FOR INDIVIDUAL PAIN EXPERIENCE

The influence of affect and meaning on the amount of pain reported has long been noted to weigh heavily on pain perception.[5-8] Thus, one hypothesis would be that certain emotional states may make pain more tolerable or may even extinguish it in certain situations, while other situations make pain worse. In everyday experiences we may note that a child running with joy or excitement does not notice a badly scuffed knee, yet will cry out with pain during a skin scratch test in the doctor's office. Sometimes children seek to have more control over parents, siblings, or other peers, by exaggerating or facilitating pains. Having a headache at an appropriate time can become a maneuver to avoid an unpleasant social situation. To gain advantages in football or soccer, where a penalty or free kick could determine the outcome of a heated game, players can also facilitate pain reactions. On the other hand, a football player may also not realize he had an injury during a close game, until after the final play. These types of phenomena were first documented by army physician Dr. Henry Beecher[5] whose observations of wounded soldiers after the battle at Anzio Beach in World War II indicated that pain expressions, reactions to injury, and use of pain medications were less than those of noncombatant surgical patients with similar injuries. The soldiers knew that they would be removed from battle and thus would survive, changing the meaning of their pain. Beecher[5] proposed to define pain not only as a sensory experience in response to injury, but also as an emotional experience where meaning is given to pain according to its social context.[5,6]

Of course, there are also emotional and social aspects of pain in dentistry. Pain or fear of pain is a phenomenon that must be dealt with almost on a daily basis in dentistry. Dental personnel may notice that some patients react in pain to drilling when the drilling has only been confined to superficial inorganic enamel surfaces of the teeth; that is, with little possibility for physiological dental pain stimulation. The personnel should register these events not just as troublesome or unrealistic, but rather as *messages* about a patient's psychosocial development. The message might be that the patient feels a need to communicate, perhaps only to ask for more anesthetic, or just to talk about the procedure and allay nervousness or fear that may be changing their pain perceptions and threshold. The pain is "real" to patients and they require some influence over it. In acute pain situations, regardless of whether fear of pain derives directly from painful past experiences or only on the expectation of pain, pharmacological agents can usually be employed successfully to control both physiological pain sensations and unpleasant psychological perceptions. However, the fear of pain must be recognized and addressed for lasting therapeutic impact using psychological or social means. The important distinction here is that anxiety or fear of pain may be persistent even after drug effects wear off after treatment in an acute or emergency episode. In other words, in the end it is better to help the patient to change underlying thoughts and beliefs that drive fear of pain or anxiety with the purpose of forming new healthcare attitudes and behavioral habits that maximize oral health and psychological coping.

If pain is expected, then it is reasonable to assume that this expectation has been learned, regardless of whether or not the pain is actually experienced. Expectations and beliefs are similar to suggestions in many ways.[9–11] According to Melzack[1] and Melzack and Wall,[12] some expectations and beliefs about pain are learned in larger culturally defined social contexts (e.g., familial, ethnic), while others are shaped by individual experience (e.g., trauma, emotional factors, degree of attention). From the discussion above about emotional meaning and social ways to define pains, it seems that the smallest "unit" of pain analysis is *"personal experiences within a framework of normative beliefs and social expectations about any particular pain phenomenon."* With the introduction of the Gate Control Theory[12] and Neuromatrix Theory (see Figure 12.1),[1] pain as a purely physical sensation no longer serves as the only pain research construct.

Several researchers took Beecher's findings a step further in search of pain context differences and how this might influence medical treatment. In 1952, Zborowski[13] reported that among a hospital sample of Italians, Jews, Irish, and Old Americans that the Irish were deniers and Americans belittlers of pain, but the Italians were non-optimistic expressers of pain, while the Jews were optimistic expressers. He concluded that behavioral response patterns to pain have different functions in various cultures and that pain coping modes adhere to these contexts.

Until 1986, most other empirical cross-cultural studies had largely confirmed Zborowski's,[14–16] pain reaction findings on Irish, Italians, and Anglo-Americans. One exception was a quasi-experimental study of dental pain and anxiety among African-American, Caucasian-American and Puerto Rican ethnic groups. Weisenberg et al[17] were first to explore possible contextual differences in dental anxiety and pain. They used an eight-item questionnaire developed by Zola[18] to measure attitudes toward pain by denial of pain or willingness to deal with pain. However, the Zola questionnaire had been developed for Italian, Irish, and Anglo-American samples and appeared not to have captured culturally significant pain beliefs of African Americans and Puerto Ricans fully. This distinction is

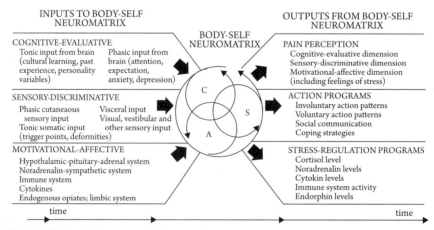

FIGURE 12.1 **Melzack's Neuromatrix**[1] Factors involved in a neuromatrix comprising sensory, affective, and cognitive aspects of perception that produce homeostatic and behavioral responses; a "body-self" perspective in which psychosocial aspects combine with brain physiology (courtesy of R Melzack[1]).

important because cultures have been shown to differ in typical linguistic reports and classifications of pain,[19,20] and these may have emotional significance or meaning in treatment contexts.[21]

Because it seemed plausible that cultural responses to pain, including description, self/care remedy, and local medical or dental practice modes, were linked to such perceptual sorting by emotional significance, a research strategy was devised[2,22,23] specifically intended to verify and describe the existence of ethnocultural contexts of pain, while testing a methodology for doing so. The ultimate goal of such cross-cultural research was to evaluate the power of expectations and beliefs in relation to social norms of pain perceptions, pain reactions, and remedy preferences, and how these can affect clinical practice. Common pains and remedies for them were described within different ethnocultural groups of first generation or immigrant mandarin Chinese, Danish, Swedish, and Anglo-American subjects from the greater Seattle area in the United States (54 patients and 31 dentists) in order to compare semantic categories of these pain/remedy perceptions.[2] All patient groups were demographically matched as closely as possible. Equal numbers of male and female patient subjects were chosen and matched by education, age, and socioeconomic status. In interviews, each was asked to answer the following questions in their native language: "What kinds of pain are there?" "What kinds of pain can one feel in the face and mouth?" "What kinds of pains can one feel at the dentist?" and "What kinds of ways are there to get rid of or ease these pains?" Based on patient responses, psychometric instruments of kinds of pains, pain descriptors, and pain coping remedies were developed and tested. Nearly all groups said they categorized the kinds of pains according to location, intensity, time, quality, curability, and cause dimensions. In addition to these, Western subjects named a mental/physical dimension differentiating emotional or "imagined" pain from physical or "real" pain.[2,24] Especially in interviews with dentists, this distinction was made clear and was often discussed as a negative perception about patient thinking. This raises the question of who determines when there is pain or not in clinical situations—patients or dentists? Answers to this complicated question were further explored in another study by Moore et al,[25] described further below.

The mind/body dichotomy of real vs. imagined pains was barely mentioned among Chinese subjects.[2] On the other hand, only Chinese subjects classified pains according to a *suan* or "sourish" dimension not previously described in the Western medical literature.[2] "*Suantong*" or sourish pain appeared to be most similar to quality and cause categories in Western concepts of pain, and varied according to body location, amount of area involved, and by depth. Tooth drilling suantong, for example, was described as dull, less intense, short-lasting pain that had a sourish, metallic characteristic. This was in contrast to Westerners who described dental pain to be sharp and intense and where Anglo-Americans specifically used "*excruciating*," an English word indicating great suffering as in death by *crucifixion*.[23]

Interview results showed that the frequencies with which certain pain concepts such as suantong and mental/physical pains were reported, clearly indicated qualitative differences among groups. Danish "*jagende*" (like intense shooting) and "*murrende*" (like nagging aching) were also considered to be ethno-specific terms with special sociolinguistic meanings. What may comfort patients was also often seen as culturally determined. Differences between patient and dentist perceptions of kinds of pain and descriptors were not as great as differences between pain coping remedies. In general, subjects categorized coping remedies as internally applied chemical agents, externally applied agents, changes of bodily function, psychosocial and healing-other dimensions, active pain tolerance, passive pain tolerance, ingestion of food or drink, and nontraditional medicine. Westerners named

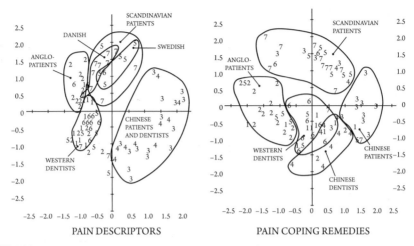

FIGURE 12.2 Multidimensional scaling representations of ethnic and dentist-patient pain and remedy beliefs[2]
(*Dentists*: 1 = American, 3 = Chinese, 6 = Scand.; *Patients*: 2 = American, 4 = Chinese, 5+7 = Scand.)

internally applied chemical agents most frequently, while Chinese patients most often named external agents such as salves and balms. Using multidimensional scaling of each subject's pain data profile, relationships of clusters of subject data points (see Figure 12.2) indicated that descriptions of pains were most influenced by ethnocultural groupings while all dentist groups had similar cognitive patterns concerning pain remedies and these contrasted with lay perceptions. Dentist perceptions did not differ from patient perceptions of pain description in any of these data. For example, Chinese dentists indicated closer ethnic affiliation with Chinese patients by perceptions of pain description than any other patient or dentist group. Ethnicity, therefore, appeared to have the major influence on pain description, whereas professional socialization had more influence on pain coping preferences in this population sample.

Besides providing rich ethnocultural data about perceptions and remedies for pain, the study described above also showed that this combination of interview and multidimensional scaling methods was a viable, valid, and reliable research program strategy.[26] These findings were followed up with a series of larger population studies, namely the US National Institutes of Health-funded *Pain in Context* studies that explored how sociocultural contexts provide a framework for individual pain and anxiety perceptions and reactions. One subsequent cross-cultural clinical epidemiological study focused on dental anxiety and related pain perceptions[27] among adults attending dental school clinics (N =951). Mandarin–speaking Chinese from Taipei, Taiwan (n=595) reported less use of dental anesthetics for same routine dental treatment and were less afraid of injections than Caucasian Americans from Iowa City, Iowa (n=395). Taiwanese and Americans with high dental anxiety (Dental Anxiety Scale > 12)[28] had similar occurrences of high fear of injections. Despite similar fears about dental drilling, however, high-anxiety Taiwanese reported using local anesthesia less frequently for routine treatments than did high-anxiety Americans. Only Americans reported negative dentist behaviors as significantly related to dental anxiety. Avoidance of appointment-making was high for all subjects afraid of injections and for Americans reporting negative dentist behaviors. Avoidance was highest in subjects with high dental anxiety regardless of ethnicity.

Thus, it was established that predominant characteristics or etiologies of dental anxiety could differ by ethnocultural background and dental healthcare system. These appear to be related to specific beliefs and/or expectations of patients within those systems. Within the normative patterns of these implicit, yet powerful psychosocial influences, each patient also brings along his/her own specific set of experiences and expectations[29] that have uniquely influenced their perceptions of dentists and/or dental procedures. For anxious individuals, these most often are negative beliefs and expectations.

In another *Pain in Context* study,[25] both dentists (n=129) and patients (n=396) were interviewed about the variance in use of local anesthetics for routine dental fillings among mandarin Chinese, Danes, Swedes and Anglo-Americans. Over half of Scandinavian patients (n=125) did not require local anesthetic for similar routine fillings (proximal), while 5% of mandarin-Chinese-speaking Taiwanese patients (n=159) and 95% of Anglo-American patients (n=112) required anesthetic.[25,30] Use of anesthetic was decided mainly by dentists in Taiwan and by patients in Western practices, but was readily available in all healthcare systems. Thus, perceptions of intensity and type of pain were dramatically different among the ethnic groups and indicated that psychosocial factors weigh heavily in perceived need for the use of local anesthetic. Most Western subjects who did not use anesthetic felt tooth drilling "did not hurt so much." But Danes had a special reason for not using local anesthesia. In spite of broad National Dental Health Insurance coverage in Denmark, patients are required to pay for "pain free" fillings. Danish national insurance does, however, officially only cover use of local anesthetic as included in the cost of extractions.[31] Non-use of anesthetic in Denmark was also reported by some dentists to be a "barometer of trust" in the dentist-patient relationship, directly linking trust of dentists with altered pain thresholds. This had its ultimate test in two reported cases where patients had extractions without use of local anesthetic.[25] Unless it was *suantong*, or "sourish pain," most Chinese dentists described tooth drilling as only "sourish," whereas dentists usually described injections to patients as outright "painful" (*tong*). There were few attempts by Chinese dentists to cognitively diminish the sensation of injections as Western dentists did when describing it only as a "pinch" or quick, short-lasting "discomfort." Thus, mandarin Chinese patients were frequently inhibited from using local anesthetic due to "fear of pain worse than drilling," even though it was readily available.

The conclusion drawn from these "Pain in Context" studies was that social expectations of pains, fear of painful treatment, and perceived remedies for pains varied from culture to culture and that these differences manifested themselves in beliefs and expectations of patient and dentist roles.

Earlier the question was raised: "Who determines when there is pain or not in clinical situations—patients or dentists?" The hypothetical question of decreasing patient suffering in the dentist-patient relationship, including elicitation of information about the patient's pain sensation, and subsequent meaningfulness of the response, is very important. Because the pain can have symbolic meaning and not just be a somatic sensation, the patient's perception of pain must not be taken lightly, or be based on false assumptions by healthcare professionals. In one *Pain in Context* study,[25] revealing discrepancies emerged among Chinese and Scandinavian dentists about use of local anesthetic for their own personal dental care compared with what they advised their patients. Chinese dentists in 90% of cases stated that they would have dental anesthetic for dental drilling of proximal fillings as did 93% of Scandinavian dentists.[25] This in comparison to 5% of mandarin-Chinese-speaking Taiwanese patients and about 50% of Scandinavian patients. One could ask if this is an indication of a double standard or merely a professional-lay difference in preference?

Or could there be other explanations, such as dentists' aversions to giving injections? At any rate, it points out the necessity for dentists to evaluate their own decision-making and communication processes, since attending to the meaning of a patient's pain is often highly related to satisfying therapeutic outcomes.[32–34] Although there have been no direct studies of discrepancies dentists may have with patients about pain control, there is some evidence that dentists or dental students perceive patients' pain responses more easily than they do anxiety or other emotional distress.[35] This is important since anxiety and other emotions, are mediators of pain behavior and can facilitate or exaggerate pain reactions. It is important that patients do not perceive the dentist as adversarial or judgmental about pain reactions, as this has been shown to increase the likelihood for continued reactions in similar treatments.[36]

ETHNOCULTURAL BELIEFS AND EXPECTATIONS IN DENTIST-PATIENT RELATIONS

Results from the studies above have explored many contextual meanings of pain and present an array of contrasting meaningful differences and expectations. But what are these expectations in operational terms as they exist in the dentist-patient relationship and how do they differ from beliefs? I suggest that beliefs are precursors to expectations. That is, beliefs "guide" or are the perceptual frameworks for our expectations and both can be limited by sociocultural context. I suggest that expectations are like "packages of motivation" that contain positive or negative energy and are exhibited and merchandised between patients and dentists in their interactions. Expectations are most often induced in the dental clinic through behavioral (nonverbal) cues (e.g., kindness or consideration vs. consternation; altruism vs. egoism). Historically, before the tremendous advent of technologically based biomedicine, the roles of healers in most ethnocultural groups recognized the importance of beliefs and expectations within the healing encounter. Doctors and "medicine men" took dominant roles in their societies and created complex rituals and ceremonies designed to elicit or foster positive expectations in participation from both the healer and the patient, and often times from the community as a whole.[37–40] This holistic approach to health care has been a fundamental component in the spiritual healing rituals of virtually all traditional native cultures,[37–39,41] similar to Balint's description of "The doctor is the drug."[42] With the coming of scientific research on neuropeptides and new cross-disciplinary branches such as "psychoneuroimmunology,"[43–46] there is new meaning to Balint's edict. An understanding of the importance of the healing process and healer roles by skilled dentists or therapists is required in order to facilitate and positively reinforce patient expectations.[47] Philosopher/psychologist Wilkins[48] wrote:

"In spite of the popular belief that psychotherapy outcome is strongly influenced by the expectancies a client holds about the benefits he may receive from therapy … a closer inspection of the studies conducted suggests that therapeutic improvements may be more appropriately attributed to the influence of the therapist rather than to clients' initial expectancies of improvement."

EXPECTANCY THEORY, THE ETHNOMEDICOGENESIS THESIS, AND EXPLANATORY MODELS

The thoughts in the previous citation were intended to provoke expectancy theorists. Expectancy theory as formulated by personality psychologists,[49–52] suggests that expectations are learned at the same time other learning events occur. For example, that a person who becomes anxious due to a previous experience of dental drilling also can expect to become anxious about drilling in subsequent attempts, given similar conditions. Studies have shown that both expectations of anxiety[49,50] and painful treatment[53,54] can create a kind of self-fulfilling prophecy[55] that makes it more likely for these events to be experienced. In the anxiety expectancy model, "fear of fear" makes people overly sensitive to anxiety and thus reinforces or exaggerates its negative affects.[49,52,56] In a broader ethnographic concept similar to psychological expectancy theory, medical anthropologists Hahn and colleagues[9,10,57,58] and others[59] have developed an *ethnomedicogenesis thesis*, which posits that beliefs and expectations of patients and healthcare workers influence or draw on positive or negative outcomes of treatments. Shapiro[60] called it *iatroplacebogenesis*. Extremes would include faith healing on the most positive side, and tribal Voodoo "death wish" rituals in Haiti on the negative side[9,10] (see Figure 12.3). These responses to nonspecific treatment effects have shown rates that vary between 7% and 60% in different settings.[59] There is some evidence to indicate that production of endogenous endorphins is linked to positive placebo responses.[61-64]

In researching such phenomena, it is important to consider both the perspective of providers and of patients and the social context from which they derive their expectations—their *explanatory models*, as psychiatrist-anthropologist Arthur Kleinman called them.[40,65] Explanatory models can also be used to explore possible iatrogenic or healing effects of dentist and patient interactions. This theory is graphically portrayed in Figure 12.3[9] as "positive" (hopeful) and "negative" (fearful) beliefs and expectations on the vertical axis, pathological and therapeutic outcomes on the horizontal, and a "property-space" of relations between expectations and outcomes, which also can be "side-effects" or paradoxical relationships. For example, it is unlikely in a western society that a belief such as "tooth extraction doesn't hurt" would be normative and thus does not require anesthetic. Yet there are individuals who, against dentist advice,[25] or due to allergy,[66] prefer sensations of tooth extraction to the use of local anesthetic.

Likewise, lack of patient faith in anesthetics may diminish their potency, and faith or skepticism about "pharmacologically inert" materials or practices (e.g., praying) may shift the results in positive directions by mere expectation. Thus, for any disease or treatment, one should consider at the same time the accompanying psychological process. There is a psychology of expectation, of hope, fear, and all variants in between in patient-care provider relating.[9-11,62,64] Giving patients hope and cognitive skills that improve their self-confidence, while also helping them to learn to appraise the dental environment and dentists less

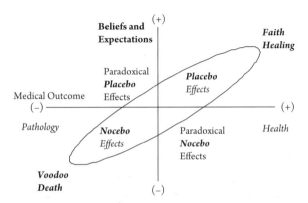

FIGURE 12.3 The Ethnomedicogenesis Thesis: Relationship between beliefs/expectations and health outcomes (courtesy of Robert Hahn[9]).

negatively, could be enough to improve their belief in their ability to reduce pain perceptions and reactions. This is not to say that it would be enough to eliminate anxiety completely, but perhaps enough to allay unnecessary suffering. Thus, the healing or iatrogenic
qualities of dentist behaviors are important to patient coping or enduring of extreme or
phobic dental anxiety or clinical pain.[2,22,25,27,67] Optimal communication skills and values
training would enhance a doctor or dentist's ability to understand their patients' feelings of
discomfort and thus facilitate decreased patient suffering.

CLOSING COMMENTS ABOUT EMOTIONAL SIGNIFICANCE OF PAIN PHENOMENA
AND ANXIETY WHEN PATIENTS MEET DENTISTS IN CULTURAL CONTEXTS

Patient and dentist beliefs and expectations affect emotional meanings of pain (and anxiety)
in dental clinics in a mutually reinforcing manner. This was found in all the clinical dental
settings of the *Pain in Context* study nations, such as the United States (Seattle, Columbus,
Ohio, and Iowa City, Iowa) Peoples Republic of China (Beijing and Guangdong), Republic
of China in Taiwan (Taipei), Denmark (Århus), and Sweden (Göteborg).

From the patient's perspective: As they signal harm or potential harm to physical or mental integrity of patients, pain and fear reactions can often be seen as crude forms of communication about suffering or expected suffering specific to emotional significance of the
clinical situation. In other words, these "messages" about feeling pain are directed toward
getting a dentist's attention and are unconscious or subconscious attempts to counteract
threatening negative outcomes in dentist-dominated relationships. Anxious patients need
to understand that they can attain power in the relationship through use of more effective
communication and social skills and state their fear of needles or drilling pain as positive
expectations. They also need to "re-learn" beliefs so that they can believe and expect that
the dentist is there to support them emotionally and to re-establish that patients, not dentists, are the *raison de être* of dental clinical activities. Finally, if patients can show the dental
staff that they appreciate their efforts, the staff will more likely respect them and become
engaged in allaying patient worries or concerns within the social context of those worries or
concerns. This requires a certain level of social or communication skills and self-confidence.
Depending on age or educational level, patients may or may not have these skills and therefore may require counseling. Normative beliefs or expectations about anxiety or pain with
dental treatment can undergo changes during a person's psychosocial development and as a
result of personal experiences over the years; that is, the belief building blocks are still there,
but actual painful or anxiety provoking experiences have modified or reinforced some of
them.

From the dentist's perspective: Infliction of pain and anxious patients are extremely stressful, if not the most stressful elements in everyday practice and probably are more so than
most dentists are willing to admit.[68,69] Stress reactions are cumulative, and dentists may often
be unaware or only subliminally aware of them.[69] Professional educational institutions need
to help dentists become more aware that there are choices of lifestyle and values that lead
to more mature decisions about dental practice and in relation to their lives as a whole, in
order to ensure psychological well-being for themselves and for their patients. Emotionally
mature dentists are less stressed, happier with practicing dentistry, and thus more naturally
involved with patients, which leads to less fear and fewer pain reactions for those patients.
A part of this understanding is inherent in a dentist's own ethnic context with patients.
They know what to say and do that helps. They can also ask patients, if uncertain. So, for
dental or other healthcare professionals, it is a matter of making choices that support their
patients and themselves in painful and anxious situations. As Rankin and Harris[70] so aptly

put it, "Dentistry is a two-way street. Whatever benefits the patient should in turn benefit the dentist as well."

ACKNOWLEDGMENT

Pain in Context studies were supported by Grant 5 R29 DE09945-04 NIH/NIDR, Bethesda, MD, USA.

REFERENCES

1. Melzack R. Pain and the neuromatrix in the brain. *J Dent Educ.* 2001;65:1378–1382.
2. Moore R, Miller ML, Weinstein P, Dworkin SF, Liou, HH. Cultural perceptions of pain and pain coping among patients and dentists. *Community Dent Oral Epidemiol.* 1986;14:327–333.
3. IASP Subcommittee on Taxonomy Pain terms: A list with definitions and notes on usage. *Pain.* 1979;6:249–252.
4. Moore R. *Psychosocial Aspects of Dental Anxiety and Clinical Pain Phenomena* [dissertation]. Aarhus, Denmark: Fællestrykkeriet for Sundhedsvidenskab, University of Aarhus; 2006.
5. Beecher HK. Relationship of significance of wound to pain experienced. *JAMA.* 1956;161:1609–1613.
6. Beecher HK. The measurement of pain. *Pharmacol Rev.* 1959;9:59–209.
7. Dworkin SF, Chen ACN. Pain in clinical and laboratory contexts. *J Dent Res.* 1982;61:772–774.
8. Dworkin SF, Chen AC, Schubert MM, Clark DW. Cognitive modification of pain: Information in combination with N2O. *Pain.* 1984;19:339–351.
9. Hahn RA, Kleinman A. Belief as pathogen, belief as medicine: "Voodoo death" and the "placebo phenomenon" in anthropological perspective. *Med Anthro Quarterly.* 1983;14:16–19.
10. Hahn RA. The nocebo phenomenon: Concept, evidence, and implications for public health. *Prev Med.* 1997;26:607–611.
11. Spiegel H. Nocebo: The power of suggestibility. *Prev Med.* 1997;26:616–621.
12. Melzack R, Wall PD. Pain mechanisms: A new theory. *Science.* 1965;150:971–979.
13. Zborowski M. *People in Pain.* San Francisco: Jossey-Bass; 1969.
14. Bates MS. Ethnicity and pain: a biocultural model. *Soc Sci Med.* 1987;24:47–50.
15. Koopman C, Eisenthal S, Stoeckle JD. Ethnicity in the reported pain, emotional distress and requests of medical outpatients. *Soc Sci Med.* 1984;18:487–490.
16. Lipton JA, Marbach JJ. Ethnicity and the pain experience. *Soc Sci Med.* 1984;19:1279–1298.
17. Weisenberg M, Kreindler M, Schachat R, Werboff J. Pain, anxiety and attitudes in black, white and Puerto Rican patients. *Psychosom Med.* 1975;37:123–135.
18. Zola IK. Culture and symptoms: An analysis of patients presenting complaints. *Am Sociol Rev.* 1966;31:615–630.
19. Fabrega H, Tyma S. Language and cultural influences in the description of pain. *Br J Med Psychol.* 1976;49:349–371.
20. Fabrega H, Tyma S. Culture, language and the shaping of illness: An illustration based on pain. *J Psychosom Res.* 1976;20:323–337.
21. Diller A. Cross-cultural pain semantics. *Pain.* 1980;9:9–26.
22. Moore R. Ethnographic assessment of pain coping responses. *Psychosom Med.* 1990;52:171–181.
23. Moore RA, Dworkin SF. Ethnographic methodologic assessment of pain perceptions by verbal description. *Pain.* 1988;34:195–204.
24. Jackson JE. "After a While No One Believes You": Real and Unreal Pain. In: Good M-JD, Brodwin PE, Good BJ, Kleinman A, eds. *Pain as Human Experience: An Anthropological Perspective.* Berkeley: University of California; 1992:138–168.
25. Moore R, Brødsgaard I, Mao T-K, Miller ML, Dworkin SF. Perceived need for local anesthesia in tooth drilling among Anglo-Americans, Chinese and Scandinavians. *Anesth Prog.* 1998;45:22–28.

26. Moore R, Brødsgaard I, Miller ML, Mao T-K, Dworkin SF. Consensus analysis: reliability, validity and informant accuracy in use of American and mandarin Chinese pain descriptors. *Ann Behav Med.* 1997;19:295–300.

27. Moore R, Brødsgaard I, Mao TK, Kwan HW, Shiau YY, Knudsen R. Fear of injections and report of negative dentist behavior among Caucasian American and Taiwanese adults from dental school clinics. *Community Dent Oral Epidemiol.* 1996;24:292–295.

28. Corah NL, Gale EN, Illing SJ. Assessment of a dental anxiety scale. *J Am Dent Assoc.* 1978;97:816–819.

29. Kent G. Cognitive processes in dental anxiety. *Br J Clin Psychol.* 1985;24:259–264.

30. Moore R, Brødsgaard I, Mao T-K, Miller ML, Dworkin SF. Acute pain and use of local anesthesia: tooth drilling and childbirth labor pain beliefs among Anglo-Americans, Chinese and Scandinavians. *Anesth Prog.* 1998;45:27–37.

31. Sygesikringens Forhandlingsudvalg, Dansk Tandlægeforening . [Agreement on Fees for National Dental Services] *Tandlægeoverenskomst—Landsoverenskomst om tandlægehjælp mellem Sygesikringens Forhandlingsudvalg (SFU), og Dansk Tandlægeforening.* 55.30.1 ed. Copenhagen: Ministry of the Interior; 2004:1–69.

32. Maggirias J, Locker D. Psychological factors and perceptions of pain associated with dental treatment. *Community Dent Oral Epidemiol.* 2002;30:151–159.

33. Corah NL, O'Shea RM, Bissell GD, Thines TJ, Mendola P. The dentist-patient relationship: Perceived dentist behaviors that reduce patient anxiety and increase satisfaction. *J Am Dent Assoc.* 1988;116:73–76.

34. Corah NL, O'Shea RM, Bissell GD. The dentist-patient relationship: Mutual perceptions and behaviors. *J Am Dent Assoc.* 1986;113:253–255.

35. Baron RS, Logan HL, Kao CF. Some variables affecting dentists' assessment of patients' distress. *Health Psychol.* 1990;9:143–153.

36. Eggly S, Tzelepis A. Relational control in difficult physician-patient encounters: negotiating treatment for pain. *J Health Commun.* 2001;6:323–333.

37. Kleinman A. On illness meanings and clinical interpretation: Not 'rational man,' but a rational approach to man the sufferer/man the healer. *Cult Med Psychiatry.* 1981;5:373–377.

38. Kleinman A. *The Illness Narratives: Suffering, Healing and the Human Condition.* New York: Basic Books, Inc.; 1988.

39. Kleinman A, Kleinman J. Suffering and its professional transformation: toward an ethnography of interpersonal experience. *Cult Med Psychiatry.* 1991;15:275–301.

40. Kleinman A. *Patients and Healers in the Context of Culture—An Exploration of the Borderland Between Anthropology, Medicine, and Psychiatry.* Berkeley: University of California Press; 1980.

41. Wirth DP. The significance of belief and expectancy within the spiritual healing encounter. *Soc Sci Med.* 1995;41:249–260.

42. Balint M. *The Doctor, His Patient and the Illness.* 2nd ed. London: Pitman Medical Publishing; 1964.

43. Zachariae B. *Den tænkende krop: essays om biologi, psykologi og sundhed* [The Thinking Body—Essays on Biology, Psychology and Health]. Copenhagen: Munksgaard-Rosinante; 2000.

44. Zachariae R. *Mind and Immunity: Psychological Modulation of Immunological and Inflammatory Parameters.* Copenhagen: Munksgaard-Rosinante; 1996.

45. Zachariae R, Hansen JB, Andersen M, Jinquan T, Petersen KS, Simonsen C, Zachariae C, Thestrup Pedersen K. Changes in cellular immune function after immune specific guided imagery and relaxation in high and low hypnotizable healthy subjects. *Psychother Psychosom.* 1994;61:74–92.

46. Zachariae R, Kristensen JS, Hokland P, Ellegaard J, Metze E, Hokland M. Effect of psychological intervention in the form of relaxation and guided imagery on cellular immune function in normal healthy subjects. An overview. *Psychother Psychosom.* 1990;54:32–39.

47. Rogers CR. *On Becoming a Person—A Therapist's View of Psychotherapy.* 4th ed. London: Constable; 1972.

48. Wilkins W. Client's expectancy of therapeutic gain: evidence for the active role of the therapist. *Psychiatry.* 1973;36:184–190.

49. Reiss S. Pavlovian conditioning and human fear: an expectancy model. *Behav Ther.* 1980;11:380–396.

50. Reiss S, Peterson RA, Gursky DM, McNally RJ. Anxiety sensitivity, anxiety frequency and prediction of fearfulness. *Behav Res Ther*. 1986;24:1–8.

51. Reiss S, Peterson RA, Gursky DM. Anxiety sensitivity, injury sensitivity, and individual differences in fearfulness. *Behav Res Ther*. 1988;26:341–345.

52. Reiss S, McNally RJ. The expectancy model of fear. In: Reiss S, Bootzin R, eds. *Theoretical Issues in Behavior Therapy*. New York: Academic Press; 1985:107–121.

53. Klages U, Ulusoy Ö, Kianifard S, Wehrbein H. Dental trait anxiety and pain sensitivity as predictors of expected and experienced pain in stressful dental procedures. *Eur J Oral Sci*. 2004;112:477–483.

54. Arntz A, Van Eck M, Heijmans M. Predictions of dental pain: The fear of any expected evil, is worse than the evil itself. *Behav Res Ther*. 1990;28:29–41.

55. Merton RK. The self-fulfilling prophecy. *Antioch Review*. 1948;8:193–210.

56. Taylor S. Anxiety sensitivity: theoretical perspectives and recent findings. *Behav Res Ther*. 1995;33:243–258.

57. Hahn RA. A sociocultural model of illness and healing. *Placebo: Clinical Phenomena and New Insights*. New York: Guilford Press; 1983.

58. Hahn RA, Kleinman A. Biomedical practice and anthropological theory: frameworks and directions. *Ann Rev Anthropol*. 1983;12:305–333.

59. Moerman DE. General medical effectiveness and human biology: placebo effects in the treatment of ulcer disease. *Med Anthro Quarterly*. 1983;14:3–15.

60. Shapiro AP, Morris LA. The placebo effect in medical and psychological therapies. In: Garfield SL, Bergin AE, eds. *Handbook of Psychotherapy and Behavior Change: An Empirical Analysis*. New York: John Wiley & Sons; 1978:269–410.

61. Amanzio M, Benedetti F. Neuropharmacological dissection of placebo analgesia: Expectation-activated opioid systems versus conditioning-activated specific subsystems. *J Neurosci*. 1999;19:484–494.

62. Brody H. The placebo response. Recent research and implications for family medicine. *J Fam Pract*. 2000;49:649–654.

63. Levine JD, Gordon NC, Smith R, Fields HL. Analgesic responses to morphine and placebo in individuals with postoperative pain. *Pain*. 1981;10:379–389.

64. Staats P, Hekmat H, Staats A. Suggestion/placebo effects on pain: negative as well as positive. *J Pain Symptom Manage*. 1998;15:235–243.

65. Kleinman A. The use of "explanatory models" as a conceptual frame for comparative cross-cultural research on illness experiences and the basic tasks of clinical care amongst Chinese and other populations. Chapter 36 In: Kleinman A, Kunstadter, P, Alexander, ER, Gale, JL eds. Medicine in Chines Cultures: Comparative Studies of Health Care in Chinese and Other Societies National Institutes of Health DHEW Publication No. (NIH) 75–653 Bethesda 1975;645–658.

66. Herod EL. Psychophysical pain control during tooth extraction. *Gen Dent*. 1995;43:267–269.

67. Kulich KR, Berggren U, Hallberg LR. Model of the dentist-patient consultation in a clinic specializing in the treatment of dental phobic patients: a qualitative study. *Acta Odontol Scand*. 2000;58:63–71.

68. Moore R. Danish dentists' career satisfaction in relation to perceived occupational stress and public image. *Tandlægebladet*. 2000;104:1020–1024.

69. Moore R, Brødsgaard I. Dentists' perceived stress and its relation to perceptions about anxious patients. *Community Dent Oral Epidemiol*. 2001;29:73–80.

70. Rankin JA, Harris MB. Patients' preferences for dentists' behaviors. *J Am Dent Assoc*. 1985;110:323–327.

Disparities and Inequities in Pain Management

13

IMPLICIT AND EXPLICIT ETHNIC BIAS AMONG PHYSICIANS

FATIMA RODRIGUEZ, MD, MPH
Brigham and Women's Hospital, Department of Medicine, Harvard Medical School, Boston, Massachusetts, USA

ALEXANDER R. GREEN, MD, MPH
Associate Director, The Disparities Solutions Center, Massachusetts General Hospital, Assistant Professor of Medicine, Harvard Medical School, Boston, Massachusetts, USA

Key Points
- A growing body of evidence documents disparities in medical care related to patient ethnicity, even when controlling for disease presentation, severity, and other potential confounding variables.
- Although most physicians endorse explicit egalitarian beliefs, recent evidence suggests that implicit bias may be an important contributor to disparities in health care generally, and in pain management specifically.
- Providers may unintentionally use nonmedical factors, including ethnicity and other sociodemographic characteristics, to guide clinical decision-making.
- Understanding the mechanisms by which providers may treat racial and ethnic minority patients differently than whites and how this can impact the doctor-patient relationship can be useful in addressing health disparities.
- Tools to measure bias include the Implicit Association Test (IAT) as well as novel techniques using neuroimaging modalities.
- Potential interventions to address bias include increasing physicians' awareness of their own potential biases, improving systems of care to mitigate the influence of bias, and increasing diversity in the healthcare workforce.

Clinical Vignette
Mr. Gonzalez is a 45-year-old immigrant from the Dominican Republic presenting to the emergency department after a work-related construction site injury. Mr. Gonzalez's English is limited but Dr. Jones, the attending physician, is able to exchange basic information with

him using her limited knowledge of medical Spanish and the patient's English skills. The Spanish medical interpreter is unavailable for the next hour and the telephone interpreter device is being used by another provider. A cursory review of the patient's electronic medical record describes a history of poorly controlled diabetes, hypertension, and previous alcohol abuse, as well as a distant history of an adverse reaction to morphine. A few notes mention that the patient has missed several appointments over the past three months due to "social issues."

Mr. Gonzalez appears uncomfortable but stoic. His vital signs are stable and he is cradling his right arm close to his body. Physical exam is notable only for diffuse tenderness along the right arm. A plain film demonstrates an isolated nondisplaced right humeral fracture. Given the language barrier, Mr. Gonzalez is not asked to quantify his pain using a formal pain scale. Dr. Jones instructs the nurse to give the patient 800 mg of ibuprofen and no reassessment is documented to determine analgesic effect and the patient is offered no stronger pain medication. Mr. Gonzalez remains in severe pain during his stay in the emergency department and for several days after his discharge.

As demonstrated in this clinical vignette, pain management decisions often rely on subjective factors that may be influenced by conscious or unconscious biases and stereotypes, communication barriers, and diagnostic uncertainty. Dr. Jones neglected to prescribe adequate pain medication to a patient with a documented long-bone fracture leaving him in severe pain for an extended period of time. Many factors could have contributed to this decision. Dr. Jones' prior experiences and socialization with Hispanic patients may have led to diminished empathy and attention to their suffering. In addition, she may have been influenced by certain conscious or unconscious assumptions. Such assumptions might include the following: (1) Stoic middle-aged male construction workers don't require or desire much pain medication; (2) patients with a history of substance abuse should not receive addictive medications such as opioids (despite the fact that he had abused alcohol rather than narcotics and this history was remote); (3) patients with a history of "noncompliance" are not trustworthy. Additionally, the recognized language barrier and the failure to employ tools to overcome it prevented the care team from obtaining a careful history and pain assessment that might have better informed Mr. Gonzalez's care. Instead, healthcare providers relied on historical data (such as the morphine reaction) and assumptions that provide a very limited and potentially erroneous clinical picture. Explicitly, Dr. Jones is unlikely to endorse racist beliefs about this patient. Her implicit attitudes about the patient, however, may have influenced her treatment decisions and thereby contributed to existing and well-documented disparities in pain management between minority patients (particularly black and Hispanic/Latino) and whites.

INTRODUCTION

A growing body of evidence documents disparities in medical care related to patient ethnicity, even when controlling for disease presentation, severity, and other potential confounding variables.[1,2] Research demonstrates that minority patients receive fewer cardiac procedures than whites with similar disease presentations,[3,4] less frequent referrals for renal transplantation,[5,6] lower quality of care for congestive heart failure and pneumonia,[7] and fewer preventive health services despite control for access-related factors.[8] Similarly, studies report that ethnic minority patients are less likely to receive appropriate analgesia for long-bone fractures in the emergency department[9,10] as well as for cancer and postoperative pain.[11,12] Although attention from national quality improvement initiatives has led to more aggressive use of analgesia in the emergency department, these well-documented disparities appear resistant to change.[13]

Many factors contribute to these observed disparities including those related to patients, providers, and the system itself. Physicians must often make decisions with incomplete information and may use unconscious cognitive shortcuts to help in the process. Drawing from cognitive psychology, explicit bias can be defined as conscious prejudgment of individuals that can lead to differential treatment and discrimination. On the other hand, implicit bias is derived from sociocultural learning over time and is primarily an unconscious process. In this chapter, we explore how biases, particularly implicit biases, shape clinical decision making and, in turn, may contribute to healthcare disparities.

MECHANISMS LINKING PHYSICIAN BIAS AND HEALTHCARE DISPARITIES

An influential report released by the Institute of Medicine, *Unequal Treatment*, identified three provider mechanisms that may contribute to healthcare disparities: (1) bias or prejudice; (2) clinical uncertainty; and (3) stereotypes held by the provider about minorities.[2]

Bias or prejudice

One potential factor that could contribute to medical treatment disparities is that healthcare providers hold minority patients in lower regard and provide them inferior treatment.[14] This may also be true for patients of lower socioeconomic status (or for other disadvantaged groups) and the contribution of these factors is difficult to distinguish from biases related to ethnicity. Prejudice is defined as an unjustified negative attitude based on a person's group membership.[2,15] Most healthcare providers are unlikely to endorse explicit prejudice or bias towards patients. In fact, research suggests that while providers generally rate themselves as just and fair on an explicit level, socially conditioned implicit bias may manifest in their nonverbal behaviors.[16,18] Green and colleagues observed that although physicians denied any explicit preference for white versus black patients, they demonstrated implicit biases favoring whites and viewed black patients as less cooperative.[19] More worrisome, in a case vignette study, this implicit pro-white bias was associated with a decreased likelihood of appropriately treating black patients for myocardial infarction.

Similarly, a well-publicized study by Schulman et al demonstrated that physicians were less likely to recommend cardiac catheterization procedures for women and African Americans presenting with identical complaints.[20] Other studies have documented that physicians' perceptions of their patients are influenced by nonmedical patient characteristics such as ethnicity, gender, and indicators of socioeconomic status.[21,22]

Studies have also revealed that physician bias is evident early in training. Rathore and colleagues studied medical students who viewed clinical vignettes of patients with identical symptoms of angina—either black females or white males.[23] Students were more likely to diagnose "definite" angina for white males and perceived black patients to have a lower quality of life with a worse health status. This difference was more pronounced among male medical students.

Clinical uncertainty

Healthcare providers frequently make decisions with incomplete information, oftentimes in busy and stressful environments. In the setting of uncertainty, clinical decision-making may be influenced by both conscious and unconscious assumptions related to a patient's ethnicity. Bogart et al surveyed a national sample of physicians about their decisions to prescribe antiretroviral therapy for HIV, a well-documented setting for disparities in care.[24] In the study, physicians reported that they would be less likely to prescribe antiretroviral therapy to patients they thought would not adhere to treatment regimens. The same physicians revealed later in the survey that they expected African Americans to be less compliant with antiretroviral therapy. Perceptions of lower rates of adherence among Blacks could be expected to impact the likelihood that a given African-American patient, absent any prior information about adherence, would receive antiretroviral therapy.[24] The extent of this uncertainty in a clinical encounter is often magnified when a patient is from a different ethnic background, due to cultural barriers, communication barriers, and potential mistrust. This then becomes a vicious circle whereby minority status leads to greater clinical uncertainty and uncertainty leads to reliance on subjective factors, such as biases based on ethnicity and other patient characteristics, further perpetuating disparities in care.[25]

Stereotypes

Numerous studies demonstrate that humans apply stereotypes in order to generalize and simplify multiple inputs from the environment.[26–28] Through informal socialization in the clinical and practice environment, providers may begin to link certain ethnic groups with specific health beliefs, behaviors, or other characteristics.[29] When healthcare providers assign a patient to a group, they may unconsciously assign these preconceived characteristics of the group to individual patients.

Similar to prejudice and bias, explicit stereotypes operate in a conscious or overt mode while more common implicit stereotypes are primarily unconscious. Stereotypes can adversely affect the patient-doctor relationship and result in mistrust, poor communication, and self-fulfilling prophecies whereby patients embody the negative characteristics projected by providers.[25] For example, African Americans have been shown to be more mistrustful of their clinical providers than whites.[29] This mistrust might in turn lead to lower adherence to medical recommendations, which would then confirm a provider's prior expectations that this group of patients is less likely to adhere to prescribed treatment regimens. In subsequent interactions with African-American patients, providers may incorrectly assume that they prefer less treatment or less aggressive treatment. Many other types of stereotypes may also operate that are more pertinent to pain management, including perceptions of minorities as more likely to seek opioid pain medication to abuse or sell, more likely to exaggerate their pain, or being generally less reliable.[11,12]

MEASURING IMPLICIT BIAS

The Implicit Association Test (IAT) is a computer-based test that includes cognitive tasks to identify implicit attitudes about ethnicity, skin color, gender, age, and sexual orientation, as well as other socialized characteristics.[30,31] The IAT measures the strength of associations between target categories (e.g., Black and White) and attributes (e.g., positive or negative words).[31] The stronger the mind makes the association, the faster the reaction time. The computer then calculates an aggregate score from the reaction time and can identify pro-white or pro-black preferences. More than 75% of white participants indicate an implicit preference for whites, even when this preference was denied in an explicit (self-reported) attitude and belief assessment.[32] Interestingly, almost 50% of blacks express some degree of pro-white implicit bias in the IAT, demonstrating that this preference is not fully accounted for by overt racism but instead part of a more subtle cognitive process shaped by socialization.[31] This is likely explained by the sociocultural advantages of whites in the United States that create pro-white preferences early in life.[33] Due to its high level of internal reliability and ease of administration, IAT measures have been used extensively in psychology and, more recently, health services research.[30,33-36] More information on this test can be found at www.implicit.harvard.edu.

Exploring the notion that ethnic or other prejudices and biases are largely experienced at an implicit level, recent studies have used neuroimaging and neurophysical testing to explore how individuals react empathically to the pain of another person. Avenanti and colleagues demonstrated that neural reactivity to others' pain is partially modulated by ethnic group membership and implicit ethnic bias.[37] The authors hypothesized that this may be largely explained by neural regions associated with the self that may underpin increased empathy for the pain of another member of one's own social group. Another study conducted by Xu et al used functional magnetic resonance imaging to identify regions in the brain that were activated by both ethnic in-group (same ethnicity) and out-group (different ethnicity) experiences of pain.[38] In this study, the authors demonstrated that both White and Chinese participants showed an empathetic bias toward in-group members during painful stimulations of concordant or discordant ethnicities. This growing evidence suggests that implicit bias may impair clinicians' assessment of and response to pain in patients from different ethnic backgrounds.

THE PATIENT-DOCTOR RELATIONSHIP

It is no surprise to learn that both explicit and implicit ethnic biases can lead to miscommunication and mistrust in the patient-doctor relationship. Whereas overt or explicit racism can shape intended action and lead directly to discrimination, implicit bias may shape care and decision-making both directly and indirectly.

Some more subtle effects of unconscious bias include changes in nonverbal behaviors such as eye-contact, blinking, and anxiety.[17] Trust, communication, and rapport are very subjective qualities and can be influenced as much by these nonverbal cues as by what the physician actually says. While nonverbal communication has not been directly correlated with disparities in clinical decisions, it is postulated that it may impact the patient-doctor relationship, leading to decreased trust and perhaps a lower likelihood of following clinical recommendations.

Interactions between ethnically or culturally discordant providers and patients may result in less empathetic responses from physicians, less exchange of information, and less shared decision-making.[39] In addition, minority patients, on average, have less trust in their providers than do white patients.[1] In one study conducted by Gordon and colleagues, Black patients viewed their ethnic discordant providers as less supportive and perceived that they received less information during their clinical encounters. Similarly, Latino patients report feeling less satisfied with their medical care, citing miscommunication as the primary concern.[41] These types of interactions can lead to cycles of mistrust by both patient and provider, thereby magnifying the underlying issue.

Treatment disparities caused by healthcare providers are particularly likely to occur when physicians must decide on "high-discretion procedures," particularly in situations fraught with clinical uncertainty.[2] High-discretion procedures are those in which the correct decision is not clear-cut and therefore is left to more subjective factors, such as the physician's experience and judgment, practice patterns, and characteristics of the patient that may make them seem more or less suitable for the procedure. Cardiac catheterization is a good example of this type of procedure, as is the use of analgesia, which is generally dependent on the patient's subjective description of the pain, the cause of the pain, and vital signs, along with the physician's judgment. In these situations, an unconscious (or conscious) bias can play a strong role in the physician's judgment of whether or not the patient should receive the procedure, as opposed to situations in which the decision is more clear-cut (e.g., whether to give antibiotics when a patient has a fever, cough, and obvious pneumonia on chest x-ray).

IMPLICATIONS FOR POLICY AND PRACTICE

As described in this chapter, a considerable body of evidence suggests that providers' explicit and implicit biases result in clinical decisions that may contribute to healthcare disparities. To best address these disparities, it is important to understand the sources of these biases and how they impact physicians' behaviors. This research will ideally lead to evidence-based interventions focused on both education and health systems change.

It is unrealistic to assume that providers are immune from bias, prejudice, or stereotyping. While explicit bias is unacceptable and less common in health care today, implicit biases exist in all of us but are difficult to recognize and address. Providers should be trained to understand their own implicit biases. Healthcare providers' awareness and acceptance of unconscious automatic processes would allow them to identify, inhibit, and overcome them before they have a detrimental impact on clinical decisions and care. Doctors should be trained to continually self-monitor and to be aware of the social cognitive shortcuts that they employ, particularly when dealing with unfamiliar situations.[29,36]

Cross-cultural education in health care should avoid teaching a unifying set of cultural norms or expectations for a given patient ethnic group. Instead, cross-cultural curricula should explore the patient-centered approach to care, where each patient's unique health beliefs, expectations, social and socioeconomic reality are carefully considered.[42,44] Academic programs in the health professions should target students' implicit attitudes about ethnicity with a goal of developing a "critical consciousness" about the self and others.[45,46] Similarly, students studying for the health professions should be taught to develop meaningful strategies, such as internal feedback and group reflection, to deal with implicit bias during patient encounters.[47]

Finally, systemic interventions should include developing and disseminating clinical guidelines that remove some of the subjectivity from clinical decisions, especially in areas that are demonstrably prone to bias and disparities, including pain management. Incorporating routine assessments of pain using standardized pain scales is an example of such an effort. In addition, more work is needed to increase workforce diversity in health care. By creating a diverse clinical and educational environment, positive personal experiences with colleagues across cultures are enhanced and these experiences may subsequently serve to reshape implicit and explicit biases.[48]

CONCLUSION

Bias in clinical decision-making among physicians and other healthcare providers is often implicit and subtle but can nevertheless have an important impact on patient care. In the setting of clinical uncertainty typical in most medical encounters, providers often employ cognitive shortcuts, such as stereotypes and pattern recognition, when working with patients from diverse, ethnic, cultural, and socioeconomic backgrounds. Even healthcare professionals who espouse egalitarian attitudes are susceptible to implicit biases, and these can contribute to ethnic disparities in care. Approaches to address these disparities include medical education using tools such as the Implicit Association Test to make providers aware of their unconscious biases; continual self-monitoring by providers to override the influence of unconscious bias on clinical practice; and evidence-based guidelines and other systems of care that limit the influence conscious and unconscious assumptions about particular groups can have on clinical decisions. More challenging still is changing our implicit biases. This will require recruiting more underrepresented minorities into the health professional workforce and providing students with positive experiences training among a diversity of both colleagues and patients. While our understanding of sociocultural biases among healthcare professionals is growing, our understanding of what to do about them is still in its infancy and will be an important field of study in the near future.

REFERENCES

1. La Veist TA. *Race, Ethnicity, and Health: A Public Health Reader.* San Francisco: Jossey-Bass; 2002.

2. Smedley BD, Stith AY, Nelson AR, eds. *Unequal Treatment: Confronting Racial and Ethnic Disparities in Healthcare.* Washington DC: National Academies Press; 2003.

3. Peterson ED, Shaw LK, DeLong ER, Pryor DB, Califf RM, Mark DB. Racial variation in the use of coronary-revascularization procedures. Are the differences real? Do they matter? *N Engl J Med.* 1997;336(7):480–486.

4. Einbinder LC, Schulman KA. The effect of race on the referral process for invasive cardiac procedures. *Med Care Res Rev.* 2000;57(suppl 1):162–180.

5. Ayanian JZ, Cleary PD, Weissman JS, Epstein AM. The effect of patients' preferences on racial differences in access to renal transplantation. *N Engl J Med.* 1999;341(22):1661–1669.

6. Epstein AM, Ayanian JZ, Keogh JH, et al. Racial disparities in access to renal transplantation—clinically appropriate or due to underuse or overuse? *N Engl J Med.* 2000;343(21):1537–1544.

7. Ayanian JZ, Weissman JS, Chasan-Taber S, Epstein AM. Quality of care by race and gender for congestive heart failure and pneumonia. *Med Care.* 1999;37(12):1260–1269.

8. Gornick ME, Eggers PW, Reilly TW, et al. Effects of race and income on mortality and use of services among Medicare beneficiaries. *N Engl J Med.* 1996;335(11):791–799.

9. Todd KH, Samaroo N, Hoffman JR. Ethnicity as a risk factor for inadequate emergency department analgesia. *JAMA.* 1993;269(12):1537–1539.

10. Todd KH, Deaton C, D'Adamo AP, Goe L. Ethnicity and analgesic practice. *Ann Emerg Med.* 2000;35(1):11–16.

11. Green CR, Anderson KO, Baker TA, et al. The unequal burden of pain: confronting racial and ethnic disparities in pain. *Pain Med.* 2003;4(3):277–294.

12. Ezenwa MO, Ameringer S, Ward SE, Serlin RC. Racial and ethnic disparities in pain management in the United States. *J Nurs Scholarsh.* 2006;38(3):225–233.

13. Pletcher MJ, Kertesz SG, Kohn MA, Gonzales R. Trends in opioid prescribing by race/ethnicity for patients seeking care in US emergency departments. *JAMA.* 2008;299(1):70–78.

14. Balsa AI, Seiler N, McGuire TG, Bloche MG. Clinical uncertainty and healthcare disparities. *Am J Law Med.* 2003;29(2–3):203–219.

15. Betancourt JR, Maina AW. The Institute of Medicine report "Unequal Treatment": implications for academic health centers. *Mt Sinai J Med.* 2004;71(5):314–321.

16. Dovidio JF, Gaertner SL, Validzic A. Intergroup bias: status, differentiation, and a common in-group identity. *J Pers Soc Psychol.* 1998;75(1):109–120.

17. Dovidio JF, Penner LA, Albrecht TL, Norton WE, Gaertner SL, Shelton JN. Disparities and distrust: the implications of psychological processes for understanding racial disparities in health and health care. *Soc Sci Med.* 2008;67(3):478–486.

18. Dovidio JF, Gaertner SL. Aversive racism and selection decisions: 1989 and 1999. *Psychol Sci.* 2000;11(4):315–319.

19. Green AR, Carney DR, Pallin DJ, et al. Implicit bias among physicians and its prediction of thrombolysis decisions for black and white patients. *J Gen Intern Med.* 2007;22(9):1231–1238.

20. Schulman KA, Berlin JA, Harless W, et al. The effect of race and sex on physicians' recommendations for cardiac catheterization. *N Engl J Med.* 1999;340(8):618–626.

21. van Ryn M, Burke J. The effect of patient race and socio-economic status on physicians' perceptions of patients. *Soc Sci Med.* 2000;50(6):813–828.

22. van Ryn M. Research on the provider contribution to race/ethnicity disparities in medical care. *Med Care.* 2002;40(suppl 1):I140–151.

23. Rathore SS, Lenert LA, Weinfurt KP, et al. The effects of patient sex and race on medical students' ratings of quality of life. *Am J Med.* 2000;108(7):561–566.

24. Bogart LM, Catz SL, Kelly JA, Benotsch EG. Factors influencing physicians' judgments of adherence and treatment decisions for patients with HIV disease. *Med Decis Making.* 2001;21(1):28–36.

25. Balsa AI, McGuire TG. Prejudice, clinical uncertainty and stereotyping as sources of health disparities. *J Health Econ.* 2003;22(1):89–116.

26. Kunda Z, Oleson KC. When exceptions prove the rule: how extremity of deviance determines the impact of deviant examples on stereotypes. *J Pers Soc Psychol.* 1997;72(5):965–979.

27. Kunda Z, Spencer SJ. When do stereotypes come to mind and when do they color judgment? A goal-based theoretical framework for stereotype activation and application. *Psychol Bull.* 2003;129(4):522–544.

28. van Ryn M, Fu SS. Paved with good intentions: Do public health and human service providers contribute to racial/ethnic disparities in health? *Am J Public Health.* 2003;93(2):248–255.

29. Betancourt JR. Not me! Doctors, decisions, and disparities in health care. *Cardiovasc Rev Rep.* 2004;25:105–109.

30. Greenwald AG, McGhee DE, Schwartz JL. Measuring individual differences in implicit cognition: the implicit association test. *J Pers Soc Psychol.* 1998;74(6):1464–1480.

31. Greenwald AG, Poehlman TA, Uhlmann EL, Banaji MR. Understanding and using the Implicit Association Test: III. Meta-analysis of predictive validity. *J Pers Soc Psychol.* 2009;97(1):17–41.

32. White-Means S, Zhiyong D, Hufstader M, Brown LT. Cultural competency, race, and skin tone bias among pharmacy, nursing, and medical students: implications for addressing health disparities. *Med Care Res Rev.* 2009;66(4):436–455.

33. Dunham Y, Baron AS, Banaji MR. The development of implicit intergroup cognition. *Trends Cogn Sci.* 2008;12(7):248–253.

34. Baron AS, Banaji MR. The development of implicit attitudes. Evidence of race evaluations from ages 6 and 10 and adulthood. *Psychol Sci.* 2006;17(1):53–58.

35. Krieger N, Carney D, Lancaster K, Waterman PD, Kosheleva A, Banaji M. Combining explicit and implicit measures of racial discrimination in health research. *Am J Public Health.* 2010;100(8):1485–1492.

36. Sabin J, Nosek BA, Greenwald A, Rivara FP. Physicians' implicit and explicit attitudes about race by MD race, ethnicity, and gender. *J Health Care Poor Underserved.* 2009;20(3):896–913.

37. Avenanti A, Sirigu A, Aglioti SM. Racial bias reduces empathic sensorimotor resonance with other-race pain. *Curr Biol.* 2010;20(11):1018–1022.

38. Xu X, Zuo X, Wang X, Han S. Do you feel my pain? Racial group membership modulates empathic neural responses. *J Neurosci.* 2009;29(26):8525–8529.

39. Ferguson WJ, Candib LM. Culture, language, and the doctor-patient relationship. *Fam Med.* 2002;34(5):353–361.

40. Gordon HS, Street RL Jr., Sharf BF, Kelly PA, Souchek J. Racial differences in trust and lung cancer patients' perceptions of physician communication. *J Clin Oncol.* 2006;24(6):904–909.

41. Morales LS, Cunningham WE, Brown JA, Liu H, Hays RD. Are Latinos less satisfied with communication by health care providers? *J Gen Intern Med.* 1999;14(7):409–417.

42. Carrillo JE, Green AR, Betancourt JR. Cross-cultural primary care: a patient-based approach. *Ann Intern Med.* 1999;130(10):829–834.

43. Beach MC, Rosner M, Cooper LA, Duggan PS, Shatzer J. Can patient-centered attitudes reduce racial and ethnic disparities in care? *Acad Med.* 2007;82(2):193–198.

44. Green AR, Betancourt JR, Carrillo JE. Integrating social factors into cross-cultural medical education. *Acad Med.* 2002;77(3):193–197.

45. Kumagai AK, Lypson ML. Beyond cultural competence: critical consciousness, social justice, and multicultural education. *Acad Med.* 2009;84(6):782–787.

46. Thompson BM, Teal CR, Scott SM, et al. Following the clues: teaching medical students to explore patients' contexts. *Patient Educ Couns.* 2010;80(3):345–350.

47. Teal CR, Shada RE, Gill AC, et al. When best intentions aren't enough: helping medical students develop strategies for managing bias about patients. *J Gen Intern Med.* 2010;25 (suppl 2):S115–S118.

48. Smedley BD, Butler AS, Bristow LR, eds. *In the Nation's Compelling Interest: Ensuring Diversity in the Health-Care Workforce.* Washington, DC: The National Academies Press, 2004.

14

ETHNIC DISPARITIES IN EMERGENCY DEPARTMENT PAIN MANAGEMENT

KNOX H. TODD, MD, MPH
Professor and Chair, Department of Emergency Medicine,
The University of Texas MD Anderson Cancer Center,
Houston, Texas, USA

MARK J. PLETCHER, MD, MPH
Associate Professor, In Residence, Departments of
Epidemiology & Biostatistics and Medicine, University of
California, San Francisco, San Francisco, California, USA

Key Points
- Pain is common and severe in the emergency department and emergency physicians may become desensitized to its presence.
- The emergency department is particularly prone to overreliance on heuristics and bias in pain management decision making due to transient relationships with patients and the time pressures of emergency medicine practice.
- Ethnic disparities in pain management are widespread and related to system, patient, and clinical factors.
- These disparities are not explained by comorbid medical conditions, socioeconomic status, or patient preference.
- Ethnic disparities in analgesic practice may be more readily predicted by provider characteristics than by patient factors
- Mechanisms that explain the provider contribution to ethnically biased pain practice deserve further study.

"Pain is a bio-psycho-social phenomenon. Nociception reflects anatomy and physiology, but culture and social factors (emphasis added) are the foundation for the expression and treatment of pain."[1]

Roselyne Rey, The History of Pain, 1995

THE EMERGENCY DEPARTMENT ENVIRONMENT

Emergency departments in the United States serve broad swaths of the population and are the single federally mandated source of universal health care access in the United States.[2] From 1997 to 2007, the number of emergency department visits increased from 95 to 117 million, while the number of departments actually decreased.[3] As a result, our emergency departments are commonly overcrowded and occasionally chaotic.[4,5] Emergency care providers treat a large scope of illnesses and injuries and do so under great time pressures. The lack of an established physician-patient relationship, limited continuity of care, frequency of diagnostic uncertainty, and time-sensitive nature of much emergent and urgent care renders the emergency department a prime setting for medical errors due to biased decision-making, stereotyping, and overreliance on misleading heuristics.[6]

PAIN IN THE EMERGENCY DEPARTMENT

Pain is the single most common reason patients seek care in the emergency department.[7] Despite its prevalence, pain is often seemingly invisible to emergency physicians. Multiple studies have documented that undertreatment of pain, or *oligoanalgesia*, is a frequent occurrence.[8] Oligoanalgesia is a cause of patient dissatisfaction with emergency care, hostility toward healthcare staff, potentially preventable returns to the emergency department or hospital readmissions, and delayed return to full health and function. As a result of failing to recognize and treat pain adequately, patients may experience anxiety, depression, sleep disturbances, and decreased ambulation with an attendant increase in the risk of venous thrombosis.

Emergency department oligoanalgesia was originally reported by Wilson and Pendleton in a pivotal 1989 paper published in the *American Journal of Emergency Medicine*.[9] The authors described 198 patients presenting to an emergency department in the midwestern United States with a wide variety of presumably painful conditions. Among their diagnoses were appendicitis, pancreatitis, ruptured ectopic pregnancy, kidney stones, gunshot wounds, fractures, and cardiac chest pain. Despite the painful nature of each of these diagnoses, a minority of patients (44%) received analgesics while in the emergency department, and of those receiving analgesics, 42% waited more than two hours before the initial dose. The authors attributed suboptimal emergency department pain management to a combination of tradition, hospital dogma, and physician misconceptions regarding the importance of acute pain treatment. In particular, they noted the priority emergency physicians placed on identification of the underlying cause of pain, and their concern that in treating pain, these diagnoses might be obscured.

RISK FACTORS FOR OLIGOANALGESIA

Risk factors for oligoanalgesia have been identified, including age and ethnicity. Selbst and Clark described analgesic use in the emergency department of Children's Hospital of Philadelphia and the Medical College of Pennsylvania in 1990.[10] They found that fully

60% of patients with painful conditions received no analgesics and that those younger than 19 and older than 65 were at greater risk for undertreatment. In 1994, researchers from Cincinnati Children's Hospital reported that only 62% of children with fractured bones received analgesics, while at Michigan State University, patients 20 to 50 years of age were more likely to be treated with analgesics than those above age 70.[11,12] Finally, a study of national emergency department data from 1997 through 2000 revealed that among all patients with fractured arms, legs, or clavicles, only 64% received some sort of analgesic and those at the extremes of age were less likely to be treated for pain.[13]

Ethnic disparities in health care have been documented in a wide variety of clinical settings, result in poor health outcomes, and are unacceptable.[14] Given the prevalence of oligoanalgesia and the nature of emergency medicine practice, it is perhaps not surprising that some of the earliest studies of ethnic disparities in pain management were conducted in the emergency department.

In 1993, we (KHT) published the first observations of disparities in physician pain management by patient ethnicity.[15] After anecdotal observations that among victims of major trauma, the pain treatment needs of Whites were more likely to be addressed than those of Latinos, we conducted the following retrospective cohort study. We examined emergency department pain management practices at the UCLA Medical Center for all Latino (generally of Mexican or Central American origin) and White patients between 15 and 55 years of age who were treated for an acutely fractured arm or leg. We excluded intoxicated patients and those injured more than six hours prior, while controlling for a variety of factors, including age, gender, insurance status, principal language spoken in the home, fracture severity, and mechanism of injury. We found that while 80 of 108 Whites (74%) received analgesics in the emergency department, only 14 of 31 Latinos (45%) received treatment for pain. After controlling for a number of potential confounders, we found that the relative risk of receiving no analgesic treatment was more than twice as great for Latinos than Whites. We could find no explanation for this disparity, including primary language of the patient. The latter finding was surprising, as we assumed that language barriers between patient and provider would provide at least a partial explanation for such a differential use of analgesics.

Although a small study, our findings were striking, and we considered a number of mechanisms by which ethnicity might influence pain management practice. The necessary elements preceding a decision to administer analgesics include perception of pain by the patient, communication of this pain experience to the clinician, and the ordering of an analgesic by the physician. Concerning pain perception, although experimental studies demonstrate ethnic differences in pain threshold and particularly for pain tolerance, these differences are of dubious clinical significance in the presence of a broken arm or leg.[16] We did not feel that the underuse of analgesics occurred because Latinos felt less pain than Whites. Of course, there are well described ethnic differences in the expression of pain and differential pain expression might explain our findings. Another explanation might be that physicians fail to appreciate pain in patients from ethnic groups unlike their own.

To narrow the list of causes for this disparity in analgesic practice, we conducted a second prospective study of cross-cultural pain assessment in the emergency department.[17] In this study, we questioned whether physicians assessed pain intensity among Whites and Latinos in similar fashions. We interviewed 207 White or Latino patients presenting to the emergency department with traumatic injury to an arm or leg and asked them to rate the intensity of their pain on a 100 mm visual analog pain scale. Treating physicians completed a questionnaire designed to imply that X-ray utilization was the focus of study. On this questionnaire, physicians rated their judgment of the patient's pain intensity.

As is true for most studies of similar design, patients tend to rate their pain intensity at a higher level than do physicians.[18] This is most likely due to the nature of the VAS pain scale, typically anchored at the lower bound by the statement, "no pain" and at higher bound, by "worst pain possible." Because emergency physicians tend to have a broader range of pain experience (by proxy), it is predictable that they ascribe less extreme values to painful events than patients. Although physician pain assessments differed from patient assessments, we were unable to find differences between Latino and White patient self-assessments of pain or in the assessment of their pain by physicians. Thus, the ethnic disparities in analgesic administration observed in our original study could not be explained by our physicians' lesser ability to assess the pain experience of Latinos.

Although physicians may grade pain in an "ethnic-blind" manner when prompted, it is possible that physicians in our original study were less likely to initiate a conscious pain assessment for Latino patients than for White patients. If this were true, incorporating routine pain assessments for all patients in the emergency department would hold great promise for changing disparate pain treatment practices. In fact, this effort was well under-way in the 1990s, with declaration of pain assessment as the "fifth vital sign" for medical encounters. However, if disparate analgesic prescribing by physicians occurs despite similar conscious pain assessments, effective interventions are much more difficult to envision.

To address the possibility of differing patient expectations for pain treatment between ethnic groups, Lee et al surveyed 58 Latino and 408 White patients presenting to the emergency department with a variety of painful conditions.[19] They questioned patients regarding their expectations for pain relief and how long it was reasonable to wait for administration of analgesics. Latino and Whites presented to the emergency department with similar levels of reported pain intensity, expectations regarding pain relief, and reasonable times to await analgesics.

In 2000, we published a third study from Emory University in Atlanta, Georgia to determine whether Blacks and Whites with broken arms or legs received disparate pain assessment or treatment.[20] Among 127 Black and 90 White patients, we found similar proportions of medical records noting the presence of pain (54% vs. 59%). While only 57% of Blacks received analgesics for pain, fully 74% of Whites were treated. Again, no obvious factor could explain this disparity.

A number of studies continue to explore the issue of ethnically-based analgesic disparities for various clinical conditions in the emergency department with disparate results. A retrospective study of 323 adults with long-bone fractures presenting to San Francisco General Hospital found no evidence of ethnic disparities in analgesic administration between Whites and non-Whites.[21] A study of emergency department patients at Royal London Hospital found no differences in the administration of analgesics between White and Bangladeshi patients with isolated long bone fractures.[22] In a large database study, investigators examined survey data for a nationally representative sample of US emergency departments collected from 1992 through 1998 and reported no difference in analgesic prescriptions for long-bone fractures between White children compared to African American and Latino children.[23] Among conditions other than fracture, Mills et al recently studied a retrospective cohort of 20,125 emergency department patients with back and abdominal pain. For both conditions, non-Whites were more likely to report severe pain and less likely to receive analgesics.[24]

GENDER AND OLIGOANALGESIA

Studies of patient gender from nonemergency department settings suggest that men tend to receive larger doses of higher potency analgesics.[25, 26, 27] However, in the emergency department, Raftery reported that women tend to present with higher pain levels and receive more analgesics.[28] Others have found little difference in pain intensity and analgesic treatment by patient gender.[29, 30, 31, 32]

OLIGOANALGESIA IN OTHER SETTINGS

Evidence for ethnic disparities in pain treatment extends beyond the emergency department setting. In 1994, Cleeland et al published a 54-site multicenter study of pain treatment for outpatients with metastatic cancer.[33] For 1308 patients treated within the Eastern Cooperative Oncology Group (ECOG), those treated in sites serving larger proportions of minority patients were three times as likely to receive inadequate treatment. In a 1997 follow-up study of ECOG sites, ethnic minority patients were less likely to receive adequate analgesic prescriptions than Whites (65% vs. 50%) with Latinos at particular risk for undertreatment.[34]

In 1996, Ng and Dimsdale published a retrospective review of pain management practices at the University of California San Diego Medical Center, including medical records of 454 patients prescribed patient-controlled analgesia (PCA) for postoperative pain over a six-month period in 1993.[35] PCA provides a useful model for studying disparities in analgesic prescribing because PCA allows patients to self-medicate by pressing a button, thus titrating administered analgesic to individual needs. While they found no difference in the amounts of analgesics self-administered by Whites, Blacks, Asians, and Latinos, the amount of analgesics prescribed by physicians differed by ethnic group, with higher amounts of opioids (narcotics) prescribed for Whites than for Latinos, and for Blacks than for Latinos and Asians.

Bernabei et al, in a 1998 analysis of the Systematic Assessment of Geriatric Drug Use via Epidemiology (SAGE) database, found that among 13,625 patients covered by Medicare for nursing home services, Blacks and Latinos were less likely to have pain assessments recorded, and members of ethnic minority groups were less likely to receive analgesics than Whites.[36] Blacks were 63% more likely to experience undertreated pain than Whites.

TRENDS IN ANALGESIC USE

By the end of the 1990s, self-reports of pain intensity were increasingly recorded as part of the routine emergency department intake process. A number of influential guidelines highlighted the importance of pain assessment as a means to improve analgesic practice. These included the Acute Pain Management Clinical Practice Guideline, published in 1992 by the Agency for Health Care Policy and Research (now the Agency for Healthcare Research and Quality), the 1994 Consensus Document on Emergency Pain Management from the Canadian Association of Emergency Physicians, and the American Pain Society Quality Improvement Guidelines for the Treatment of Acute Pain and Cancer.[37, 38, 39]

In 2008, we (MJP) published an analysis of the National Hospital Ambulatory Medical Care Survey (NHAMCS), a nationally representative survey of visits to US emergency departments (excluding federal, military, and Veterans Administration hospitals), with the goal of describing ethnic disparities in opioid prescribing for patients presenting to the ED with pain over time.[40] We analyzed survey years 1993–2005, and given campaigns by the Joint Commission on Accreditation of Healthcare Organizations and the Veterans Health Administration during the 1990s, our hypotheses were: (1) opioid prescribing would increase during this time period, and (2) ethnic disparities would shrink in magnitude. We focused on visits where the reason for visit was classified as "pain-related," analyzed results according to type and severity of pain, and described trends over time.

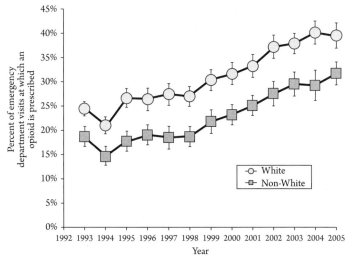

FIGURE 14.1 Trends in emergency department analgesic use.

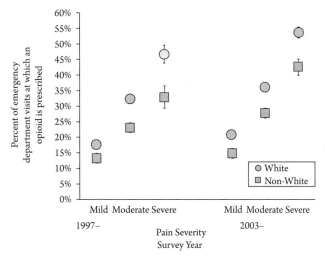

FIGURE 14.2 Ethnic disparities in emergency department analgesic use.

Among the 156,729 pain-related ED visits analyzed (42% of all ED visits), opioid prescribing increased from 23% in 1993 to 37% in 2005. This rising trend was more pronounced after 2000, coinciding with The Joint Commission's efforts. However, we found no narrowing in the gap between Whites and non-Whites (see Figure 14.1), with a gap of approximately 8% between Whites and non-Whites (40% and 32% respectively in 2005). Differential opioid prescribing was consistently present across different types of pain, across different levels of pain severity, for visits in which pain was the first or second/third reason for visit, and for two specific painful diagnoses, long-bone fracture and nephrolithiasis. Differences in prescribing between Whites and non-Whites were larger as pain severity increased (see Figure 14.2), and were particularly pronounced for patients with back pain, headache, and abdominal pain. Blacks were prescribed opioids at lower rates than any other ethnic group for almost every type of pain visit. Disparities were not explained by differences in types or severity of pain at presentation or other patient/visit characteristics, and were particularly pronounced among black and Hispanic children, blacks in government-owned (but nonfederal) hospitals those who self-paid, Asians/others with Medicare, and all non-Whites in hospitals located in the Northeast. Although the underlying reasons for differential prescribing by ethnicity could not be analyzed in this study, it is unlikely that it represents an appropriate pattern of care.

THE PROVIDER CONTRIBUTION

The influence of provider characteristics on differential treatment of pain has received little attention. Given that women constitute an increasing proportion of the medical workforce, differences in treatment decisions between male and female physicians are of increasing practical importance. Female physicians may be more nurturing, expressive, and have stronger interpersonal orientations than males.[41] In studies of physician-patient encounters, female physicians are reported to spend more time with patients, be more positive, make more partnership statements, ask more questions, and smile and nod more frequently.[42] Women may express higher levels of satisfaction when treated by female physicians, although satisfaction among male patients is unaffected by physician gender.[43] In general, female physicians tend to engage in more patient-oriented communication with a greater emphasis on patient psychosocial issues, emotions, and positive comments.[44]

In 2009, we (KHT) reported results from a prospective multicenter study of pain management at 19 emergency departments in the United States and Canada.[45] Of 842 patients, 56% were female. We found few differences in reported pain intensity or overall rates of analgesic administration between men and women, although the subset of females presenting with severe pain were less likely to receive analgesics than men (74% vs. 64%). Interestingly, female physicians were more likely to administer analgesics than males (66% vs. 57%). After controlling for multiple confounders of the relationship between gender and pain treatment, female physicians were more likely to administer any analgesics, and while female physicians were more likely to provide opioid analgesics to female patients, male physicians were more likely to provide them to males.

In a subsequent study, we (KHT) examined how provider ethnicity might influence pain outcomes in the emergency department.[46] We found that during an emergency department visit non-White (Latino, African-American and Asian-American) physicians were more likely to achieve clinically important reductions in pain intensity for their patients than White physicians. In this study, ethnic concordance between provider and patient did not predict a better pain outcome. This lack of impact is consistent with much of the literature on patient-provider ethnic concordance.[47] Interestingly, non-White physicians ordered analgesics at similar rates to White physicians (and opioids at lower rates), while achieving greater reductions in pain intensity. It seems likely that some unmeasured characteristic of the physician-patient interaction, separate from specific analgesic pharmacologic effects, influenced the observed reductions in pain. It is possible that non-White physicians were more successful in achieving a positive valence in the patient-physician interaction, thereby enhancing therapeutic effect, as has been proposed by Tait and Chibnall.[48]

THE EMERGENCY DEPARTMENT AS A HIGH COGNITIVE LOAD ENVIRONMENT

To the extent that provider characteristics determine ethnic disparities in pain treatment patterns and outcomes, a better understanding of mechanisms that determine such behaviors is deserving of scrutiny. In a 2002 review article, van Ryn et al describe a number of

Provider Contributions

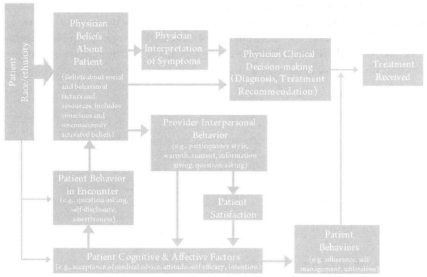

FIGURE 14.3 Hypothesized mechanisms of provider contributions to ethnic disparities in medical treatment.

complex mechanisms (see Figure 14.3) by which provider factors might result in ethnically disparate treatment patterns and outcomes.[49] Underlying these mechanisms are stereotypical beliefs about groups of patients (e.g., Latinos are illegal aliens, Asian Americans are high achievers, African Americans are lazy) that are automatically applied under the high stress conditions that exist in the emergency department. The emergency department typifies a "high cognitive load" environment, characterized by the need for providers to make multiple decisions in short periods of time, while enduring high rates of task interruption, and without the benefit of a long-term patient relationship.[50,51] Unfortunately, our emergency departments are increasingly crowded and high cognitive load conditions are more the norm than the exception.[52]

Burgess hypothesizes that in high cognitive load environments such as the emergency department, ethnic disparities in outcomes result from two mechanisms.[53] First, in such an environment, clinicians increasingly switch from conscious to automatic patterns of thought, relying on heuristics or "shortcuts" to arrive at decisions when constrained by time or other resources.[54] Although heuristics are essential to routine medical decision making, under ideal conditions clinicians should be able to employ more analytic processes when clinical conditions warrant, rather than being forced to overly rely on such shortcuts. High cognitive load conditions are expected to result in poorer care for all patients. Second, heuristics based on ethnic stereotypes are likely to be employed in these stressful environments and to the extent such stereotypes are both negative and clinically irrelevant, poorer outcomes for ethnic minorities are to be expected.

CONCLUSION

Ethnic disparities in pain treatment are well documented and although recognition of pain and the importance of pain treatment have increased over time, ethnic disparities in pain treatment are persistent. An increasing amount of research has been devoted to understanding the mechanisms underlying observed ethnic disparities in pain treatment and a better understanding of how these pathways work is important to fashioning interventions that promote equity in pain treatment. Apart from research efforts to understand its causes, routine monitoring of pain treatment patterns and disparate pain treatment should become a quality measure for the emergency department as well as other clinical settings. Clinicians and people with pain should advocate for such monitoring and for an increasing emphasis on continuing medical education to combat what are unacceptable inequities in pain practice.

REFERENCES

1. Rey, R. *The History of Pain*. Cambridge, MA: Harvard University Press; 1995.
2. Lee TM. An EMTALA primer: the impact of changes in the emergency medicine landscape on EMTALA compliance and enforcement. *Ann Health Law*. 2004;13:145–178.
3. Niska R, Bhuiya F, and Xu J. *National Hospital Ambulatory Medical Care Survey: 2007 Emergency Department Summary*. National health statistics reports; no 26. Hyattsville, MD: National Center for Health Statistics; 2010.
4. Richards, E. *The Knife and Gun Club: Scenes From an Emergency Room*. New York: Atlantic Monthly Press; 1989.
5. Pines JM, McCarthy ML. Executive summary: interventions to improve quality in the crowded emergency department. *Acad Emerg Med*. 2011;18:1229–1233.
6. Croskerry P, Sinclair D. Emergency medicine: a practice prone to error? *CJEM*. 2001;3(4):271–276.
7. Cordell WH, Keene KK, Giles BK, Jones JB, Jones JH, Brizendine EJ. The high prevalence of pain in emergency medical care. *Am J Emerg Med*. 2002;20:165–169.
8. Rupp T, Delaney KA. Inadequate analgesia in emergency medicine. *Ann Emerg Med*. 2004;43:494–503.
9. Wilson JE, Pendleton JM. Oligoanalgesia in the emergency department. *Am J Emerg Med*. 1989;7:620–623.
10. Selbst S, Clark M. Analgesic use in the emergency department. *Ann Emerg Med*. 1990;19:1010–1013.
11. Friedland LR, Kulick RM. Emergency department analgesic use in pediatric trauma victims with fractures. *Ann Emerg Med*. 1994;23:203–207.
12. Jones JS, Johnson K, McNinch M. Age as a risk factor for inadequate emergency department analgesia. *Am J Emerg Med*. 1996;14:157–160.
13. Brown J, Klein E, Lewis C, Johnston B, Cummings P. Emergency department analgesia for fracture pain. *Ann Emerg Med*. 2003;42:197–205.
14. Smedley BD, Stith AY, Nelson AR. *Unequal Treatment: Confronting Racial and Ethnic Disparities in Health Care*. Washington, DC: Institute of Medicine; 2002.
15. Todd KH, Samaroo N, et al. Ethnicity as a risk factor for inadequate emergency department analgesia. *JAMA*. 1993;269(12):1537–1539.
16. Rahim-Williams FB, Riley JL 3rd, Herrera D, Campbell CM, Hastie BA, Fillingim RB. Ethnic identity predicts experimental pain sensitivity in African Americans and Hispanics. *Pain*. 2007;129:177–184.
17. Todd KH, Lee T, Hoffman JR. The effect of ethnicity on physician estimates of pain severity in patients with isolated extremity trauma. *JAMA*. 1994;271:925–928.
18. Guru V, Dubinsky I. The patient vs. caregiver perception of acute pain in the emergency department. *J Emerg Med*. 2000;18:7–12.
19. Lee WW, Burelbach AE, Fosnocht D. Hispanic and non-Hispanic white patient pain management expectations. *Am J Emerg Med*. 2001;19:549–550.
20. Todd KH, Deaton C, D'Adamo AP, Goe L. Ethnicity and analgesic practice. *Ann Emerg Med*. 2000;35:11–16.
21. Fuentes EF, Kohn MA, Neighbor ML. Lack of association between patient ethnicity or race and fracture analgesia. *Acad Emerg Med*. 2002;9:910–915.
22. Choi DM, Yate P, Coats T, Kalinda P, Paul EA. Ethnicity and prescription of analgesia in an accident and emergency department: cross sectional study. *BMJ*. 2000;320:980–981.

23. Yen K, Kim M, Stremski ES, Gorelick MH. Effect of ethnicity and race on the use of pain medications in children with long bone fractures in the emergency department. *Ann Emerg Med.* 2003;42:41–47.

24. Mills AM, Shofer FS, Boulis AK, Holena DN, Abbuhl SB. Racial disparity in analgesic treatment for ED patients with abdominal or back pain. *Am J Emerg Med.* 2011;29:752–756.

25. Ochroch EA, Gottschalk A, Troxel AB, et al. Women suffer more short and long-term pain than men after major thoracotomy. *Clin J Pain.* 2006;22(5):491–498.

26. Peretti-Watel P, Bendiane MK, Obadia Y, et al. The prescription of opioid analgesics to terminal cancer patients: impact of physicians' general attitudes and contextual factors. *Palliat Support Care.* 2003;1(4):345–352.

27. Green CR, Wheeler JR, LaPorte F, et al. Clinical decision making in pain management: Contributions of physician and patient characteristics to variations in practice. *J Pain.* 2003;4(1):29–39.

28. Raftery KA, Smith-Coggins R, Chen AH. Gender associated differences in emergency department pain management. *Ann Emerg Med.* 1995;26(4):414–421.

29. Johnston CC, Gagnon AJ, Pepler CJ, et al. Pain in the emergency department with one-week follow-up of pain resolution. *Pain Res Manag.* 2005;10(2):67–70.

30. Heins JK, Heins A, Grammas M, et al. Disparities in analgesia and opioid prescribing practices for patients with musculoskeletal pain in the emergency department. *J Emerg Nurs.* 2006;32(3):219–224.

31. Kelly AM. Does the clinically significant difference in visual analog scale pain scores vary with gender, age, or cause of pain? *Acad Emerg Med.* 1998;5(11):1086–1090.

32. Lewis LM, Lasater LC, Brooks CB, et al. Are emergency physicians too stingy with analgesics? *South Med J.* 1994;87(1):7–9.

33. Cleeland CS, Gonin R, Hatfield AK, et al. Pain and its treatment in outpatients with metastatic cancer. *N Engl J Med.* 1994;330:592–596.

34. Cleeland CS, Gonin R, Baez L, Loehrer P, Pandya KJ. Pain and treatment of pain in minority patients with cancer. The Eastern Cooperative Oncology Group Minority Outpatient Pain Study. *Ann Intern Med.* 1997;127:813–816.

35. Ng B, Dimsdale JE, Rollnik JD, Shapiro H. The effect of ethnicity on prescriptions for patient-controlled analgesia for post-operative pain. *Pain.* 1996;66:9–12.

36. Bernabei R, Gambassi G, Lapane K, et al. Management of pain in elderly patients with cancer. SAGE Study Group. Systematic Assessment of Geriatric Drug Use via Epidemiology. *JAMA.* 1998;279:1877–1882.

37. US Department of Health and Human Services, Public Health Service, Agency for Health Care Policy and Research. Clinical Practice Guideline. *Acute Pain Management: Operative or Medical Procedures and Trauma* [AHCPR publication No. 92–0032]. Silver Spring, MD: Center for Research Dissemination and Liaison, AHCPR Clearinghouse; 1992.

38. Ducharme J. Emergency pain management: a Canadian Association of Emergency Physicians (CAEP) Consensus Document. *J Emerg Med.* 1994;12:855–866.

39. American Pain Society Quality of Care Committee. Quality improvement guidelines for the treatment of acute pain and cancer pain. *JAMA.* 1995;274:1874–1880.

40. Pletcher MJ, Kertesz SG, Kohn MA, Gonzales R. Trends in opioid prescribing by race/ethnicity for patients seeking care in US emergency departments. *JAMA.* 2008;299:70–78.

41. Weisman CS, Teitelbaum MA, Weisman CS, et al. Physician gender and the physician–patient relationship: Recent evidence and relevant questions. *Soc Sci Med.* 1985;20(11):1119–1127.

42. Hall JA, Irish JT, Roter DL, et al. Gender in medical encounters: An analysis of physician and patient communication in a primary care setting. *Health Psychol.* 1994;13(5):384–392.

43. Derose KP, Hays RD, McCaffrey DF, et al. Does physician gender affect satisfaction of men and women visiting the emergency department? *J Gen Intern Med.* 2001;16(4):218–226.

44. Roter DL, Hall JA, Aoki Y. Physician gender effects in medical communication: A meta-analytic review. *JAMA.* 2002;288:756–764.

45. Safdar B, Heins A, Homel P, et al. Impact of physician and patient gender on pain management in the emergency department—a multicenter study. *Pain Med.* 2009;10:364–372.

46. Heins A, Homel P, Safdar B, Todd K. Physician race/ethnicity predicts successful emergency depart-ment analgesia. *J Pain.* 2010;11:692–697.

47. Meghani SH, Brooks JM, et al. Patient-provider race-concordance: does it matter in improving minority patients' health outcomes? *Ethn Health.* 2009;14(1): 107–130.

48. Tait RC, Chibnall JT. Physician judgments of chronic pain patients. *Soc Sci Med.* 1997;45:1199–1205.

49. van Ryn M. Research on the provider contribution to race/ethnicity disparities in health care. *Med Care.* 2002;40:I-140–I-151.

50. Chisholm CD, Dornfeld AM, Nelson DR, Cordell WH. Work interrupted: a comparison of workplace interruptions in emergency departments and primary care offices. *Ann Emerg Med.* 2001;38:146–151.

51. Morrison JB, Rudolph JW. Learning from accident and error: avoiding the hazards of workload, stress, and routine interruptions in the emergency department. *Acad Emerg Med.* 2011;18:1246–1254.

52. Institute of Medicine. *Hospital-based Emergency Care: At the Breaking Point.* Washington, DC: National Academies Press; 2006.

53. Burgess DJ. Are providers more likely to contribute to healthcare disparities under high levels of cogni-tive load? How features of the healthcare setting may lead to biases in medical decision making. *Med Decis Making.* 2010;30:246–257.

54. Croskerry P. Achieving quality in clinical decision making: cognitive strategies and detection of bias. *Acad Emerg Med.* 2002;9:1184–1204.

15

PATIENT-PROVIDER ETHNIC CONCORDANCE IN PAIN CONTROL

Negotiating the Intangible Barrier

SALIMAH H. MEGHANI, PHD, MBE, CRNP
Assistant Professor, Biobehavioral and Health Sciences Division, University of Pennsylvania School of Nursing, Philadelphia, Pennsylvania, USA

OREN K. ISACOFF, BA, BSC, MD/MBA
Student, University of Pennsylvania, Philadelphia, Pennsylvania, USA

Key Points

- Social characteristics frequently play a role in providers' clinical decision-making resulting in unequal treatment for certain groups, including ethnic minorities.
- All healthcare interactions, including pain treatment, are embedded within a social context. The emergence of ethnic concordance literature is an attempt to approach ethnic disparities within this social framework.
- The hypothesis undergirding ethnic concordance research is that disparities in health may be ameliorated as a result of increased mutual respect, trust, communication, and satisfaction, which may exist more often in a ethnically concordant patient-provider relationship.
- Social identity research demonstrates that people tend to favor "in-group" members in the distribution of rewards (e.g., health care), even when the "out-groups" are arbitrary and pose no real threats.
- Although no reviews exist that synthesize evidence around ethnic concordance and pain outcomes, theoretical reasoning (subjective nature of pain and social construction of opioids) suggests a greater role of ethnic concordance in pain treatment than outcomes in objectively verifiable diseases.
- Despite theoretical appeal of the concept of ethnic concordance in pain treatment outcomes, most studies that have collected data on patient-provider characteristics have either not approached the specific question of concordance or have

failed to conclude with statistical significance the effect of ethnic concordance on pain assessment and treatment outcomes.

- The science of ethnic concordance is limited not only due to pragmatic and methodological considerations but also normative risks in espousing a concept that has the potential of creating a "separate but equal" ethnic divide within the healthcare sector.

INTRODUCTION

All healthcare interactions are embedded within a social context. General attitudes formed within and outside the healthcare system may influence patient-provider interactions, treatment decision-making, and health outcomes. Strong cumulative evidence suggests that social characteristics frequently play a role in providers' clinical decision-making resulting in unequal treatment for certain groups such as ethnic minorities. The emergence of ethnic concordance literature over the past two decades is an attempt to approach ethnic disparities within this social framework; the hypothesis undergirding ethnic concordance research is that disparities in health may be ameliorated as a result of increased mutual respect, trust, communication, and satisfaction, which may exist more often in a ethnically concordant patient-provider relationship.[1]

The general body of literature on ethnic concordance has failed to generate a consensus on the role of ethnic concordance and improvement in health outcomes for various ethnic groups. A qualitative review of 27 published studies on the topic found mixed evidence. Of the reviewed studies, patient-provider ethnic concordance was associated with positive health outcomes for minorities in only nine studies (33%), while eight studies (30%) found no association of ethnic concordance with the outcomes of interest and 10 (37%) presented mixed findings. Further analysis suggested that having a provider of same ethnicity did not improve "receipt of services" for minorities. However, no clear pattern of findings emerged in the domains of healthcare utilization, communication, preference, satisfaction, or perception of respect.[1]

No reviews exist that synthesize evidence around ethnic concordance, pain assessment, and pain treatment outcomes. In this chapter, we begin by presenting a theoretical discussion of why patient-provider ethnic concordance may matter in the specific context of pain outcomes and then review the extant literature to understand whether ethnic concordance finds support in the published literature as a predictor of pain treatment outcomes. We conclude with a discussion of methodological, pragmatic, as well as normative considerations in applying the concept of ethnic concordance in health care.

PATIENT-PROVIDER ETHNIC CONCORDANCE AND PAIN OUTCOMES

The primary thrust for understanding the relationship between patient-provider ethnic concordance and pain treatment outcomes stem from strong evidence of ethnic disparities in pain treatment.[2] When compared to Whites, ethnic minorities are less likely to receive analgesia in virtually all healthcare settings in the United States, including emergency departments;[3–7] inpatient and postoperative pain settings;[8–12] and outpatient, community, and nursing home settings.[13–16] They are also less likely than Whites to receive opioids[5,6,17–19] and NSAIDs with Cox-2 selectivity for arthritis pain.[20] Further, minorities are more likely to experience a step-down in analgesia at discharge from a hospital or emergency room[5,21,22] and to encounter longer wait times before receiving analgesics.[19,23]

While the concept of patient-provider ethnic concordance has been investigated widely in a number of healthcare settings and outcomes, it can be argued that the concept may have greater applicability for pain due both to the "nature of the condition" as well as the "nature of its treatment." Appropriate treatment of pain entails a covert interpretation of the complaint of pain and an overt negotiation between patients and providers.[24] The cycle of pain treatment can potentially break down at several levels during patient-provider interaction resulting in "disparity."[24] The Institute of Medicine report,[25] therefore, asserted that "given the role of cultural and linguistic factors in both patients' perception of pain and in physicians' ability to accurately assess patients' pain … it is reasonable to suspect that healthcare disparities might be greater in pain treatment … than in treatment of objectively verifiable disease."[25]

Unlike objectively verifiable conditions, appropriate treatment of pain depends, first and foremost, upon accurate assessment of pain. Despite significant advancement in the understanding of the complex biological mechanisms responsible for the genesis of pain, no clinical assay or objective test to date accurately measures the experience of pain. The clinical "gold standard" of pain assessment continues to be that defined by Margo McCaffrey more than two decades ago: pain is "whatever the experiencing person says it is."[26] This notion of "subjectivity" coupled with the notion of the "experiencing person" introduces room for bias in pain treatment decision-making.

Research on ethnic concordance relies mainly on the hypothesis of interaction between in-group and out-group memberships in the formation of bias. Relative to out-groups, providers may have favorable attitudes towards those they perceive as in-group members (e.g., members of similar ethnic groups and social classes) possibly because individuals view their fellow in-group members as conveyers of their own values potentially resulting in a scenario of *selective valuing*.[27] This theory stresses negative reciprocity between in-groups and out-groups especially in the face of a "conflict."[27]

The notion of "conflict" fits well with the paradigm of pain treatment. Treatment of pain is a "cognitively involved, higher level" mental task that presents many decisional risks, conflicts, and trade-offs for providers.[28] For instance: (1) Pain is a subjective condition and historical misconceptions about certain ethnic groups exist; (2) opioids are the cornerstone for the treatment of pain, but they also have a negative social construction as well as social risks; (3) many providers, especially those who see a preponderance of chronic pain patients, do not like to treat pain patients;[29,30] and (4) fear of legal actions is frequently on the minds of providers when prescribing opioids.[28] Feeding into these already complex mental trade-offs are the high volume/high pressure managed environments creating a conductive milieu for biased decision-making.[28]

Why ethnic concordance may matter? Some theoretical arguments

Theories of social cognition suggest that human beings are limited in their capacities to process complex information. When faced with circumstances that exceed cognitive reserves, individuals frequently rely upon automatic processes, e.g., mental shortcuts, a task in which one assigns new information to preconceived categories that are easy to process.[31] Automatic processes do not occur because of tardiness but rather out of necessity to maintain efficiency. Nonetheless, outcomes are usually suboptimal, misguided, and biased.[31] Taking this argument further, if biases leverage on "selective valuing," it may result in preferential treatment for in-group members and less than optimal treatment for members of the out-group.

Social identity research has consistently demonstrated that people tend to favor in-group members in the distribution of rewards (e.g., health care), even when the out-groups are arbitrary and pose no real threats, resulting in prejudice and bias.[32,33] Prejudice represents a negative attitude towards a person or a group due to perceived threat to one's supposed social identity.[33] Unfortunately, some types of biases may escape recognition because they are "implicit" and dissociated from conscious processes. In one study (albeit in a non-pain setting), physicians stated no "explicit" preference for treating white or black patients, but the *Implicit Association Test* revealed an implicit preference for favoring white patients and an implicit stereotype for disfavoring black patients.[34] Authors demonstrated a direct relationship between physicians' pro-White implicit bias and their likelihood of offering more treatment to Whites and less treatment to Blacks (P = .009).[34]

Other distinct psycho-cognitive mechanisms, such as stereotypes and clinical uncertainty, also intervene in shaping patient-provider clinical interactions. Stereotypes are processes "by which people use social categories (e.g., ethnicity, gender) in acquiring, processing, and recalling information about others."[35] Burgess et al elucidated two distinct processes ("automatic" stereotyping and "goal-modified" stereotyping) responsible for bias in clinical decision making.[35] Automatic stereotyping occurs via "diffuse, associative process" and is most likely to occur when limited cognitive resources are available to attend to and incorporate individual patient information. Contrarily, goal-modified stereotyping leverages on providers' specific comprehension needs for a clinical encounter (e.g., consideration of the relative prescription drug abuse rates between Blacks or Whites in the setting of chronic pain treatment). When compared to automatic stereotyping, goal-modified stereotyping may draw more heavily on aspects of ethnic stereotypes and is especially prominent when less objective data are available to physicians.[35,36] Thus, the subjective paradigm of pain treatment may serve as a conducive medium for channeling, through distinct psycho-cognitive mechanisms, preconceived social beliefs about certain individuals or groups, ultimately resulting in discordance and disparities.

PATIENT-PROVIDER ETHNIC CONCORDANCE AND PAIN OUTCOMES

Below we discuss evidence from published literature to examine if patient-provider ethnic concordance results in improved pain assessment and treatment outcomes.

Todd et al published one of the first studies of pain undertreatment among ethnic minorities.[3] Researchers found that the risk of receiving no analgesia in emergency departments (ED) for long-bone fractures was more than twice as much for Hispanic patients as for Whites (Hispanics, n= 31; Whites, n=108). Although a specific analysis of patient-provider ethnic concordance was not presented, authors reported that various stratified analyses controlling for specific covariates including physician ethnicity did not change ethnic disparity in ED analgesia. Further, the findings persisted after controlling for the primary language used by the patient, suggesting that differential use of analgesia could not be attributed to acculturation or ability to communicate with providers. In a subsequent study,[37] authors investigated whether disparate prescription of analgesics observed in the previous study could be attributed to disparities in assessment of pain between Hispanics and Whites (n= 209). Although physicians rated pain in Whites as slightly more severe than in Hispanics (33.6 mm v. 29.7 mm), this finding was not statistically significant despite 80% statistical power to detect a difference of 10 mm or more on a visual analogue scale. Again, the specific question of ethnic concordance was not investigated, and only eight Hispanics (of 69) were ethnically concordant with their physicians. Nevertheless, in adjusted analysis, none of physician characteristics, including ethnicity or gender, predicted disparity in patient-physician pain assessment. Authors concluded that disparities in analgesic treatment for Hispanics could not be explained by differential assessment of pain by providers.

In yet another study, Todd et al found that the risk of receiving no analgesia in the ED was 66% greater for black patients than for white patients (RR, 1.66, 95% CI, 1.11–2.50), an effect that persisted in an adjusted analysis.[4] Authors did not find an association between physician ethnicity and analgesic prescribing patterns in the ED. However, authors acknowledged that the small number of minority physicians in the study precluded an analysis of patient-physician concordance and pain treatment outcomes.[4] Based on insights gained from several studies,[3,4,37] authors concluded that the primary culprit contributing to undertreatment of pain among ethnic minorities "is not the failure of physicians to assess pain, but the failure to administer analgesics."[4]

However, the role of patient-provider agreement on pain assessment in the genesis of disparities remains unsettled and may very well be setting-dependent. Studies conducted in cancer and noncancer pain settings report significant discordance in patient-provider assessment of pain. In a survey of healthcare professionals treating minority cancer patients with recurrent or metastatic cancer, Anderson et al found that physicians underestimated the severity of pain in 74% of African Americans and 64% of Hispanic patients. Inadequate pain assessment was cited by majority of providers (71%) as a major barrier to optimal pain treatment.[16]

Two studies specifically examined pain assessment disparities in the cancer setting.[14,15] Cleeland et al examined how sufficiently the cancer-associated pain in minority patients was treated in the outpatient setting. The Eastern Cooperative Oncology Group (ECOG) randomly selected minority patients and their physicians (N = 281) to grade pain severity, pain-related functional impairment, and success of analgesia-induced pain relief. Patients treated in minority communities or academic centers were more likely to receive inadequate analgesia than those treated in nonminority community treatment settings (77% compared with 52%; P = 0.003). Furthermore, greater numbers of minority patients had pain severity underestimated by physicians (P < 0.04), desired more potent analgesia (P < 0.001), and felt that their physicians had underprescribed to achieve adequate pain control (P < 0.001). Like many other studies, ethnic concordance was not directly assessed in this study and treatment location was used as a proxy for patients' ethnicity.[14]

Bernabei et al.[15] investigated cancer-pain assessment and treatment in minority and elderly patients treated in the nursing home setting (N = 13,625). The study found that patients aged 85 years and older were less likely to receive analgesia than those aged 65 to 74 years (13% vs. 38%, respectively). The study did not examine ethnic concordance, but rather demonstrated that ethnic minorities, especially African Americans, were less likely to have their pain recorded by providers than were white patients. Also, minority background served as an independent predictor for receiving "no analgesia."

Two studies published as part of a larger project of Patient Physician Perception of Pain[38,39] also documented significant disparities in physician-patient assessment in the chronic nonmalignant pain setting. The study investigated patient-provider agreement on pain across 12 primary care centers in the United States (n = 455). Findings demonstrated discordance in patient-provider estimates of pain in 54% of encounters.[38] Patient-provider discordance in pain assessment (defined as two or more points of difference on an 11-point numeric rating scale) was significantly associated with poor physical functioning, as well as worse bodily pain, in this sample.[38] A subsequent study in this series showed that physicians were twice as likely to underestimate pain in black patients compared to all other ethnicities combined.[39] Interestingly, in further analysis with the subset of patients who had their pain overestimated by their physicians, physicians were more likely to overestimate pain in non-black patients. The authors acknowledged that the small sample (6%) of black physicians in this sample did not allow an explicit analysis of the effect of ethnic concordance on pain treatment outcomes for black patients.[39]

In a recently reported study, Heins et al.[18] investigated the association between patient-provider ethnic concordance and effectiveness of pain treatment among patients presenting to 20 EDs across the United States and Canada (n =776). The primary outcome variable of effectiveness of pain treatment was defined as a 2-point or greater reduction in pain intensity score on an 11-point rating scale. The outcome of significant reduction in pain intensity was predicted by arrival pain scores, receipt of any ED analgesia, and being treated by a nonwhite physician. In effect, being treated by a nonwhite physician was the strongest predictor of reduction in pain intensity scores in the multivariable analysis, no matter the ethnicity of the patient. Interestingly, nonwhite physicians achieved better pain control while prescribing opioids at lower rates than white providers. Authors speculated that characteristics of the clinical encounter and the physician-patient interaction rather than specific pharmacological treatments provided may have influenced the outcome of clinically significant reductions in pain intensity. However, the authors did not find an association between ethnic concordance and the primary outcome of reduction in pain intensity scores. It is important to note that investigators dichotomized patient and physician ethnicity as Whites/non-Whites due to small numbers of individuals within each ethnic category. For instance, only 2% (n =18) of the providers were African Americans, 4% (n =28) were Hispanics, and 5% (n =42) were Asians, potentially precluding meaningful ethnic concordance analysis.

To circumvent the ubiquitous problem of a small sample of minority providers in clinical studies, some authors have employed clinical vignettes to understand the role of patient-physician characteristics in pain treatment decision-making;[40–43] however, no clear pattern of findings has emerged. Burgess et al.[40] investigated the impact of ethnicity (white or black) and verbal and nonverbal behavior (challenging or nonchallenging; and confident, dejected, or angry) in achieving adequate pain treatment by administering written clinical vignettes to randomly selected primary care physicians (N= 382). The analysis found significant interaction between patients' ethnicity and verbal behavior that influenced physician decision to prescribe opioids. Physicians were significantly more likely to prescribe higher doses of opioids to challenging patients versus nonchallenging patients who were African Americans. The opposite was true when prescribing to Whites. In another vignette study, Nampiaparampil et al.[41] explored whether an interaction between patients' ethnicity and insurance status (African Americans with Medicaid versus Caucasians with Blue Cross insurance) might affect physicians' decisions for managing chronic pain. Physicians were more likely to prescribe opioids to Caucasians although this finding did not reach statistical significance. Also, rates of referral for nerve block were significantly higher for Caucasian patients.

Tamayo-Sarver et al.[42] surveyed whether physicians were predisposed to varied treatment decisions dependent upon patient ethnicity, and if those predispositions were altered when physicians received additional information about patient socioeconomic status. Emergency physicians (N= 5,750) received one of three clinic vignettes that provided patient ethnicity along with varying details about patient socioeconomic demographics. The study found that patient ethnicity (white, African American, or Hispanic) had no observed influence on the opioid prescription and that the knowledge of socioeconomic factors only modestly increased opioid prescription rates. Similarly, Weisse et al.[43] also did not find evidence of ethnic disparities in their vignette study investigating the influence of ethnicity and gender on pain treatment decisions for back pain or renal colic. However, they found an interesting interaction between gender and ethnicity; female physicians prescribed lower doses of opioids to male patients. In the setting of renal colic, lower doses were prescribed to black versus white patients when the patient was female, whereas the reverse was true when patients were male. Thus, ethnic concordance did not appear to play a role in the provision of pain treatment in this study. These vignette studies have been of limited value in characterizing the association between ethnic concordance and pain outcome because they used scenario analysis to extrapolate conclusions about actual patient care. In doing so, they have been unable to provide a consistent picture of how physicians may think and behave in actual care delivery settings.

METHODOLOGICAL LIMITATIONS

Despite theoretical appeal of the concept of ethnic concordance in pain treatment outcomes, most studies that have collected data on patient-provider characteristics have either not approached the specific question of concordance or have failed to conclude with statistical significance the effect of ethnic concordance on pain assessment and treatment outcomes. Understanding the relationship among ethnic concordance and various health outcomes is methodologically challenging and complex. Some studies that collected data on provider characteristics were unable to present an analysis of ethnic concordance due to small samples of minority patients, providers, or both.[3,4,39,44] This methodological reality also meant that even those studies that have presented an explicit analysis of patient-provider ethnic concordance on pain outcomes have investigated main effects without accounting for complex interactions among theoretically important variables. The small sample of providers was a problem across studies, mirroring the fact that most research on disparities originates from academic medical centers, and ethnic minorities comprise a small proportion of faculty staff at these institutions.[39] Studies that are unable to exert statistical rigor are unlikely to provide clinically or socially meaningful conclusions. Studies of clinical scenarios, while adequately powered and theoretically useful, have a limited quantifiably justified relationship to actual clinical behavior. Furthermore, most of the ethnic concordance studies have been conducted in the United States and contribute little knowledge to non-African American and non-Hispanic minority groups who are either not included or grouped together as part of so-called "other" minority groups.

Thus, based on this review, we conclude that many gaps remain in our understanding of the role of ethnic concordance in influencing pain assessment and treatment outcomes. There appears to be a setting level effect with lack of discordance in patient-provider pain assessment in acute care settings (ED) versus chronic pain settings. However, studies have not consistently approached the question from the perspective of patient-provider ethnic concordance, limiting any definitive conclusions. Similarly, while an overwhelming body of literature exists on ethnic disparities in pain treatment, a critical mass of literature is absent, specifically investigating the contribution of patient-provider ethnic concordance to these outcomes. Adequate sampling of minority patients and providers is necessary for any attempt to broach this topic.

CONCLUSIONS AND IMPLICATIONS

Treatment of pain is a subjective and value-laden process that lends itself to a greater possibility of implicit (unconscious) bias. In theory, the outcome of unequal pain treatment resulting from implicit bias may be intercepted, at least in part, by the availability of a concordant patient-provider relationship. This hypothesis has been the subject of many investigations and policy recommendations. An idea calling for a policy change must meet pragmatic and normative criteria.

Pragmatic considerations in approaching ethnic concordance

It has been demonstrated that, if given a choice, patients from some ethnic groups (e.g., African Americans, Hispanics, and Asians) are more likely to chose providers of the same ethnicity.[45] However, the ability to choose requires the availability of sufficient numbers of ethnically concordant providers.[45] The reason that most studies failed to achieve an adequate sample of minority providers is reflective of the macro-level problem of the disproportionate composition of the minority healthcare workforce. Despite African Americans and Hispanics being the fastest growing segments of the US population, they are also the groups that are most severely under-represented in healthcare. For instance, in the United States, only 16.8% of the total registered-nurse workforce is of minority ethnicity.[46] Of these, only 5.8% are Blacks and only 3.6% are Hispanics. Among physicians, only 3.5% are Blacks and only 5% are Hispanics.[46] Diversity within the workforce is an indispensible goal that ensures that the health system is representative of a nation's demographics and is responsive to the healthcare needs of diverse populations. However, the issue of diversity should be considered separately from the issue of ethnic concordance. For instance, international medical graduates (IMGs) who graduate from medical school outside of the United States comprise 25% of actively practicing physicians in the country.[47] These graduates are also more likely than Whites to serve minorities and work in primary care shortage areas where they are more likely to encounter patients with pain.[48] The majority of these providers come from South Asian countries and are not white, black, or Hispanic. Discussion about this large body of physician workforce in the context of concordance is largely absent from the literature.[48] Further, in the 2010 Census, 9 million people identified themselves as multiracial or belonging to more than one race[49] (up from 6.8 million in 2000).[50] This trend is expected to increase in coming years. Further, the idea of ethnic concordance undermines vast heterogeneity that exists within racial and ethnic categories.[1] For instance, Asians represent one of the six National Institutes of Health racial categories, but in essence Asians range from Japanese to Pakistani. These two "Asian" groups are as removed from each other as any other group outside of this racial category. These pragmatic realities call for a paradigm shift in approaching the question of patient-provider ethnicity and health outcomes.

Normative considerations

Regardless of theoretical advantages, the science of ethnic concordance is limited not only due to pragmatic considerations but also normative risks in espousing a concept that has the potential to create a racial divide in the healthcare sector. As a society, we have strived to move away from the "separate but equal" social paradigm. This paradigm contends that "equality" cannot be fully achieved in the face of a racial divide.[51] Thus the concept of ethnic concordance has some potential to create a racially segregated healthcare system.[1] Further, it imparts a sense of exoneration among providers that only certain types of patient-provider relations are expected to produce optimal outcomes. Thus, the concept of ethnic concordance may inadvertently serve as a "red herring"[52] in advancing the goal of equity in health outcomes. Rather, emphasis should be placed on learning what may be unique about ethnic-concordant relationships and transferring this knowledge to any patient-provider relationship. This includes developing respect for diversity and difference, cultural sensitivity, mutual trust, and language access and communication, as well as taking part in sensitization training to overcome implicit and explicit biases that frequently seep into pain treatment decision-making. Heins and colleagues[18] recently demonstrated that therapeutic alliance between patients and providers may not necessarily depend upon ethnic concordance but rather upon experiences and attitudes that providers may bring to the pain treatment setting. In the specific context of pain treatment, focus should also be placed on targetable professional characteristics that have been found to be significant, e.g., type and duration of training and experience,[5,18,39] in impacting pain treatment outcomes.

REFERENCES

1. Meghani SH, Brooks JM, Gipson-Jones T, Waite R, Whitfield-Harris L, Deatrick JA. Patient-provider race-concordance: does it matter in improving minority patients' health outcomes? *Ethn Health.* 2009;14(1):107–130.

2. Meghani SH, Byun E, Gallagher RM. Time to Take Stock: A Meta-Analysis and Systematic Review of Pain Treatment Disparities in the United States. *Pain Med.* 2012;13(2):150–174.

3. Todd KH, Samaroo N, Hoffman JR. Ethnicity as a risk factor for inadequate emergency department analgesia. *JAMA.* 1993;269(12):1537–1539.

4. Todd KH, Deaton C, D'Adamo AP, Goe L. Ethnicity and analgesic practice. *Ann Emerg Med.* 2000;35(1):11–16.

5. Heins JK, Heins A, Grammas M, Costello M, Huang K, Mishra S. Disparities in analgesia and opioid prescribing practices for patients with musculoskeletal pain in the emergency department. *J Emerg Nurs.* 2006;32(3):219–224.

6. Quazi S, Eberhart M, Jacoby J, Heller M. Are racial disparities in ED analgesia improving? Evidence from a national database. *Am J Emerg Med.* 2008;26(4):462–464.

7. Singer AJ, Thode HC Jr. National analgesia prescribing patterns in emergency department patients with burns. *J Burn Care Rehabil.* 2002;23(6):361–365.

8. Atherton MJ, Feeg VD, el-Adham AF. Race, ethnicity, and insurance as determinants of epidural use: analysis of a national sample survey. *Nurs Econ.* 2004;22(1):6–13, 3.

9. Ng B, Dimsdale JE, Rollnik JD, Shapiro H. The effect of ethnicity on prescriptions for patient-controlled analgesia for post-operative pain. *Pain.* 1996;66(1):9–12.

10. Glance LG, Wissler R, Glantz C, Osler TM, Mukamel DB, Dick AW. Racial differences in the use of epidural analgesia for labor. *Anesthesiology.* 2007;106(1):19.

11. Ng B, Dimsdale JE, Shragg GP, Deutsch R. Ethnic differences in analgesic consumption for postoperative pain. *Psychosom Med.* 1996;58(2):125.

12. Rust G, Nembhard WN, Nichols M, et al. Racial and ethnic disparities in the provision of epidural analgesia to Georgia Medicaid beneficiaries during labor and delivery. *Am J Obstet Gynecol.* 2004;191(2):456.

13. McNeill JA, Sherwood GD, Starck PL. The hidden error of mismanaged pain: a systems approach. *J Pain Symptom Manage.* 2004;28(1):47.

14. Cleeland CS, Gonin R, Baez L, Loehrer P, Pandya KJ. Pain and treatment of pain in minority patients with cancer. The Eastern Cooperative Oncology Group Minority Outpatient Pain Study. *Ann Intern Med.* 1997;127(9):813–816.

15. Bernabei R, Gambassi G, Lapane K, et al. Management of pain in elderly patients with cancer. SAGE Study Group. Systematic Assessment of Geriatric Drug Use via Epidemiology. *JAMA.* 1998;279(23):1877–1882.

16. Anderson KO, Mendoza TR, Valero V, et al. Minority cancer patients and their providers: pain management attitudes and practice. *Cancer.* 2000;88(8):1929–1938.

17. Pletcher MJ, Kertesz SG, Kohn MA, Gonzales R. Trends in opioid prescribing by race/ethnicity for patients seeking care in US emergency departments. *JAMA.* 2008;299(1):70.

18. Heins A, Homel P, Safdar B, Todd K. Physician race/ethnicity predicts successful Emergency Department analgesia. *J Pain.* 2010;11(7):692–697.

19. Epps CD, Ware LJ, Packard A. Ethnic Wait Time Differences in Analgesic Administration in the Emergency Department. *Pain Manag Nurs.* 2008;9(1):26.

20. Dominick KL, Bosworth HB, Hsieh JB, Moser BK. Racial differences in analgesic/anti-inflammatory medication use and perceptions of efficacy. *J Natl Med Assoc.* 2004;96(7):928.

21. Moore C, Siu A, Maroney C, et al. Factors associated with reductions in patients' analgesia at hospital discharge. *J Palliat Med..* 2006;9(1):41.

22. Heins A, Grammas M, Heins JK, Costello MW, Huang K, Mishra S. Determinants of variation in analgesic and opioid prescribing practice in an emergency department. *J Opioid Manag.* 2006;2(6):335–340.

23. Wheeler E, Hardie T, Klemm P, et al. Level of pain and waiting time in the emergency department. *Pain Manag Nurs.* 2010;11(2):108–114.

24. Meghani SH. *Factors affecting the negotiation of treatment for cancer pain among African Americans [dissertation].* Philadelphia: University of Pennsylvania; 2005. *Available from ProQuest.* http://repository.upenn.edu/dissertations/AAI3179777

25. Smedley BD, Stith AY, Nelson AR. Institute of Medicine Committee on Understanding and Eliminating Racial and Ethnic Disparities in Health Care: *Unequal treatment: confronting racial and ethnic disparities in health care.* Washington, DC: National Academies Press; 2003.

26. McCaffery M. Pain: *Clinical Manual for Nursing Practice.* 2nd ed. St. Louis: Mosby; 1989.

27. McCallion MJ. In-groups and out-groups. In: Ritzer G, ed. *Blackwell Encyclopedia of Sociology Online.* http://www.sociologyencyclopedia.com/public/. Accessed: June 27, 2012.

28. Meghani SH. Corporatization of pain medicine: implications for widening pain care disparities. *Pain Med.* 2011;12(4):634–644.

29. Mitchinson AR, Kerr EA, Krein SL. Management of chronic noncancer pain by VA primary care providers: when is pain control a priority? *Am J Manag Care.* 2008;14(2):77–84.

30. Dobscha SK, Corson K, Flores JA, Tansill EC, Gerrity MS. Veterans affairs primary care clinicians' attitudes toward chronic pain and correlates of opioid prescribing rates. *Pain Med.* 2008;9(5):564–571.

31. Fiske ST, Taylor SE. *Social Cognition.* 2nd ed. New York: McGraw-Hill, Inc.; 1991.

32. Balsa AI, McGuire TG. Prejudice, clinical uncertainty and stereotyping as sources of health disparities. *J Health Econ.* 2003;22(1):89–116.

33. Pettigrew TF, Meertens RW. Subtle and blatant prejudice in Western Europe. *Eur J Soc Psycholy.* 1995;25:57–75.

34. Green AR, Carney DR, Pallin DJ, et al. Implicit bias among physicians and its prediction of thrombolysis decisions for black and white patients. *J Gen Intern Med.* 2007;22(9):1231–1238.

35. Burgess DJ, van Ryn M, Crowley-Matoka M, Malat J. Understanding the provider contribution to race/ethnicity disparities in pain treatment: insights from dual process models of stereotyping. *Pain Med.* 2006;7(2):119–134.

36. Tait RC, Chibnall JT. Physician judgments of chronic pain patients. *Soc Sci Med.* 1997;45(8):1199–1205.

37. Todd KH, Lee T, Hoffman JR. The effect of ethnicity on physician estimates of pain severity in patients with isolated extremity trauma. *JAMA.* 1994;271(12):925–928.

38. Panda M, Staton LJ, Chen I, et al. The influence of discordance in pain assessment on the functional status of patients with chronic nonmalignant pain. *Am J Med Sci.* 2006;332(1):18–23.

39. Staton LJ, Panda M, Chen I, et al. When race matters: disagreement in pain perception between patients and their physicians in primary care. *J Natl Med Assoc.* 2007;99(5):532–538.

40. Burgess DJ, Crowley-Matoka M, Phelan S, et al. Patient race and physicians' decisions to prescribe opioids for chronic low back pain. *Soc Sci Med.* 2008;67(11):1852–1860.

41. Nampiaparampil DE, Nampiaparampil JX, Harden RN. Pain and prejudice. *Pain Med.* 2009;10(4):716–721.

42. Tamayo-Sarver JH, Dawson NV, Hinze SW, et al. The effect of race/ethnicity and desirable social characteristics on physicians' decisions to prescribe opioid analgesics. *Acad Emerg Med.* 2003;10(11):1239–1248.

43. Weisse CS, Sorum PC, Dominguez RE. The influence of gender and race on physicians' pain management decisions. *J Pain*. 2003;4(9):505–510.

44. Karpman RR, Del Mar N, Bay C. Analgesia for emergency centers' orthopaedic patients: does an ethnic bias exist? *Clin Orthop Relat Res*. 1997;334:270–275.

45. Traylor, AH, Schmittdiel, JA, Uratsu, CS, Mangione, CM, & Subramanian, U. The Predictors of Patient–Physician Race and Ethnic Concordance: A Medical Facility Fixed-Effects Approach. *Health Serv Res*. 2010;45(3):792–805.

46. Health Resources and Services Administration. *The Registered Nurse Population: Findings from the 2008 National Sample Survey of Registered Nurses*. http://bhpr.hrsa.gov/healthworkforce/rnsurvey2008.html Accessed June 27, 2012.

47. Association of American Medical Colleges. 2009 *State Physician Workforce Data Book*. Washington, DC: Association of American Medical Colleges. 2009.

48. Meghani SH, Rajput V. Perspective: the need for practice socialization of international medical graduates—an exemplar from pain medicine. *Acad Med*. 2011;86(5):571–574.

49. U.S. Census Bureau. 2010 *Census Shows America's Diversity*. U.S. Census Bureau. http://2010.census.gov/news/releases/operations/cb11-cn125.html. Accessed June 27, 2012.

50. Economics and Statistics Administration. US Census Bureau. *Census 2000 Brief: Overview of Race and Hispanic Origin*. Washington, DC: US Department of Commerce; 2001. http://www.census.gov/prod/2001pubs/c2kbr01-1.pdf. Accessed April 10, 2011.

51. Washington HA, Baker RB, Olakanmi O, et al. Segregation, civil rights, and health disparities: the legacy of African American physicians and organized medicine, 1910–1968. *J Natl Med Assoc*. 2009;101(6):513–527.

52. Khorana AA. Concordance: how does a physician who is neither black nor white decide when race is a factor? *Health Aff*. (Millwood) 2005; 24(2):511–515.

THE EFFECT OF ETHNICITY ON PRESCRIPTIONS FOR PATIENT-CONTROLLED ANALGESIA FOR POST-OPERATIVE PAIN

BERNARDO NG, MD, DFAPA
Clinical Assistant Professor, Department of Psychiatry, University of California, San Diego, La Jolla, California, USA *and* Medical Director, Sun Valley Behavioral Medical Center, Imperial, California, USA

"Pain is an interpersonal signal" Beecher, 1956[1]

Key Points

- Ethnic disparities in pain management may result from cultural and psychosocial factors that influence pain expression and assessment.
- Patient-controlled analgesia (PCA) may minimize communication problems associated with pain control in the inpatient setting.
- Ethnic disparities in PCA dosing have been documented by a number of researchers.
- Specific psychosocial indicators may predict those for whom PCA would be most beneficial.
- Although PCA use can improve pain outcomes, it should not become a barrier to clinician-patient communication.
- Genetic and pharmacogenomic factors may be incorporated in future more personalized PCA prescribing.

INTRODUCTION

Psychiatrists frequently are asked to evaluate the "appropriateness" of patients' pain behaviors. Consultees sometimes wonder about the disparity between patients' illnesses and their complaints of pain. This disparity may lead to patients being described as "stoical," "histrionic," or "drug seeking."[2] In a seminal study by Marks and Sachar, consultation liaison psychiatrists from Montefiore Hospital found that "in virtually every case" in which inpatients displayed marked emotional responses to pain; treatment was inadequate.[3]

The psychiatrist's task in such settings is greatly complicated when either the patient or staff members are from different cultural backgrounds. The complications arise because cultural and psychosocial factors play such a powerful role in the way humans understand and respond to pain.[4] In other words, the provision of good analgesia is influenced by ethnic differences in how pain is expressed, the attitudes of patients and health professionals towards pain management, and pharmacological differences in the responses to opioids.[5]

The use of patient-controlled analgesia (PCA) can minimize some of the problems that may occur because of poor communication between the patient and healthcare staff. Nevertheless, in multicultural societies, health professionals should be conscious of the many factors that influence the effects of prescribed treatment to manage pain in different ethnic groups.[6]

PATIENT CONTROLLED ANALGESIA

PCA has been used since 1970 for postoperative pain management, potentially reducing the interaction between patient and staff, and increasing patient's control in the treatment of his/her own pain. PCA hardware includes a pump that delivers intravenous analgesics at the patient's command. The main variables of a standard PCA prescription are drug of choice (i.e., morphine versus fentanyl), bolus dose, and lockout interval. The bolus dose is the amount of drug administered with successful activation of the pump, and the lockout interval is the period after successful activation of the device during which no additional analgesic can be administered. The initial set up of the device is done by a pain specialist who relies on his or her clinical impression of the patient (i.e., age, gender, weight, type of surgery, tissues involved, duration of surgery, and opioid consumption in the recovery room), and his/her own clinical knowledge and experience. PCA parameters can be adjusted later according to patient's analgesic response.[7,8]

PCA AND ETHNICITY

We first studied ethnicity and postoperative pain after publication of a study of emergency department pain management for long-bone fractures, in which Hispanics were found less likely to receive analgesics than non-Hispanic Whites.[9] We initially reviewed 250 consecutive admissions to the University of California, San Diego (UCSD) Medical Center for open reduction and internal fixation of a limb fracture, and found that the average consumption of daily morphine equivalents varied according to ethnic group. Caucasians received 21.7 mg/day, African Americans 16 mg/day, and Hispanics 12.8 mg/day (P<.002), while the use of non-steroidal anti-inflammatory drugs was no different. In this study, postoperative analgesics were generally prescribed on an as-required (PRN) basis, such that the actual administration of medication depended both on the patient's demand and on the nurse's perception of the patient's pain.[2]

Staff attitudes toward patient's pain complaints can vary according to the staff member's own ethnic and educational background, as well as their familiarity with individual patients. On the other hand, the differences in the patient's demand for pain control may be related to the manner in which patients understand their illness, as well as their expectations for pain control and demand for medical services. Additionally, we recognized the possibility that pharmacokinetic differences across the ethnic groups could contribute to our findings.

In order to reduce the bias introduced by the patient-nurse interaction in our study, we decided to study postoperative patients treated with PCA immediately after surgery.[8] We abstracted medical records of 454 postoperative patients from four ethnic groups; a summary of our findings is presented in Table 16.1.

TABLE 16.1 Summary of findings.

	African American	Asian American	Caucasian	Latino	
N	30	37	314	73	Sum=454
Prescribed opioid (mg/h)	12.13	10.21	11.03	9.53	P<0.5
Age (years)	41.17	46.19	46.85	37.82	P<.001
Private insurance (%)	40	46	52.9	13	P<.001
Intraoperative opioids (%)	60.7	51.3	65.02	74.29	NS
Former opioid use (%)	13.3	8.1	10.5	6.85	NS
Gender (% male)	73.3	51.3	64.65	53.42	NS

Adapted from Ng et al 1996.

The variables that differed among ethnic groups were private insurance, age, and analgesic prescribed. The latter was based on the initial prescription made by the pain specialist once the patient was admitted to the surgical floor. A higher amount of opioid was prescribed for Caucasians than Latinos, and for African Americans than Latinos and Asians (P<.05). We also examined the amount of opioids prescribed, as a function of: age, gender, preoperative use of opioids, insurance status, and pain site. Age correlated negatively with self-administered opioid ($r = -.154$, P<.01) and men were prescribed more analgesics than women (11.32 mg/hr vs. 10.27 mg/hr, P<.03). Opioid prescriptions were unrelated to health insurance status. Patients with a prior history of opioid use self-administered more opioids (59.61 mg/hr vs. 28.37 mg/hr, p <.001). Patients with more than one pain site had more opioids prescribed (14.21 mg/hr vs. 10.49 mg/hr, P<.02). In order to determine whether variables such as pain site were accounting for the differences in PCA prescriptions across the ethnic groups, we performed an ANOVA with covariates (age, gender, preoperative use of opioids, health insurance, and number of pain sites), using the amount of prescribed opioids as the dependent variable. Ethnicity persisted as an independent predictor of the amount of opioid prescribed even after controlling for these covariates, and in spite of the fact that previous use of opioids and the use of intraoperative opioids were not significantly different among the ethnic groups.

Other investigations into this area were identified in searches of the medical literature. A PubMed search of the keyword "PCA" resulted in 6,461 publications, yet if the keyword "ethnicity" is added, the number of retrieved citations falls to 21 publications, of which five (including ours) studied two ethnic groups or more, and two reported on one ethnic group.

The most recent study is from Tan et al, who studied 1,034 Indian and Chinese women in Singapore undergoing elective cesarean sections. Indian women had more pain complaints and higher morphine consumption regardless of age, body mass index, or duration of surgery (P<.001).[10] Another publication by Adams et al, reported a retrospective study of 30 Hispanic and 30 Caucasian patients who were prescribed PCA for postoperative pain control. No differences in the amount of prescribed morphine were found between Hispanics and Whites (11.2 +/– 3.2 mg/hr vs. 11.1 +/– 4.3 mg/hr respectively, p = 0.85) or self-administered

TABLE 16.2 Summary of Inter-ethnic and PCA studies

Author	Country	N	Ethnic groups	
Tan et al (2008)	Singapore	1,034	Indian > Chinese	P<.001
Adam et al (2004)	United States	60	Latino = Caucasian	NS difference
Ng et al (1996)	United States	454	African American > Caucasian > Asian > Latino	P<.05
Perry et al (1994)	United States	99	African American = Latino = Caucasian	NS difference
Houghton et al (1992)	Hong Kong	22	European > Asian	P<.05

morphine ($2.6 +/- 2.0$ mg/hr vs. $3.3 +/- 3.0$ mg/hr, p = 0.27) were seen.[11] Perry et al found that anxiety traits and age rather than ethnic factors influenced the amount of analgesic consumption and pain complaints. Their sample was multiethnic (N = 99) and included 70% Caucasian, 28% African American, and 2% Hispanic women who underwent simple hysterectomy with no known cancer. They also reported that non-Caucasians reported less of a need to be "in control" of their pain medications; however, they felt this association was of minor clinical significance.[12] Finally, Houghton et al, in a very small study (eight European and 14 Asian adult postoperative patients), reported lower analgesic PCA demands among Asians (P<.05).[13]

Published investigations within single ethnic groups include one by Chia et al, in Taiwan, who found that among 2,298 postoperative patients, analgesic consumption was predicted by gender (males > females) and intensity of incident pain (that occurring with movement).[14] Li et al, from Guangzhou, China, studied 180 elder Chinese postoperative patients to establish the optimal pain assessment instrument . They compared the Faces Pain Scale Revised (FPS-R), the Numeric Rating Scale (NRS), and the Iowa Pain Thermometer (IPT), finding that all scales correlated well with the PCA opioid consumption. The scale most preferred was the IPT (54.7%), followed by the FPS-R (28.5%), and the NRS (15.6%). No significant differences were noted in participant preference by age and cognitive status, but preference for the IPT and the FPS-R were significantly related to gender and education level.[15]

PCA for postoperative pain control has recently been used as a setting in which to address genetic determinants of opioid consumption. Zhang et al, in Zhengzhou China, studied patients undergoing gynecological surgery (N = 74) during the postoperative period and assessed pain sensitivity, opioid consumption, and the presence of the A118G polymorphism of the mu opioid receptor gene (OPRM1). Homozygotes for A118G consumed more opioid than the heterozygote or homozygotes for A118A carriers.[16]

DISCUSSION

PCA is a useful and practical, yet understudied and underutilized, research and clinical tool. It is clinically useful by removing barriers in the delivery of analgesia. By giving patients the ability to self-dose, it decreases the need to interact with healthcare staff, and allows precise tracking of drug consumption. It is difficult to generalize results of existing evidence involving PCA use so that they are applicable to any ethnic group as a whole. One wonders whether the number of publications in this area are limited because it has become a non-issue, or because it is such a complicated one that researchers prefer to focus in other areas. Regardless, PCA remains a very useful clinical tool that deserves wider use.

Nevertheless, PCA does not eliminate the need for clinician-patient communication, where ethnicity plays such an important role. In fact, if clinically used in an attempt to "avoid" interacting with the patient, PCA can lead to negative consequences in the doctor-patient-nurse interaction. A vignette of an actual case illustrates this very issue below:

Case Vignette

Mr. L was a 59-year-old separated Caucasian male referred for depression and uncontrolled pain. He had a history of a previous surgery and "recurrent and persistent" abdominal pain, as described by his own words. He was in his third day of PCA and unhappy with it. After working on developing rapport—he was initially offended that a psychiatrist was there to see him—he explained his problem. He claimed he needed to have available an opioid for "breakthrough pain" because the drug obtained through the PCA device took 30–45 minutes after the first morning dose for him to experience any relief. He was reminded that the PCA machine allowed him to self-dose more often than that. He then explained that while asleep through the night, he did not recall to wake up and dose himself, such that after sleeping five to six hours he would wake up with "literally no pain medication left [in his body]."

When asked about his personal life, he first stated "everything is fine in my life." He was visiting his parents in town and actually lived about 300 miles away. He reported that he had been "asked" by his parents to spend a few weeks "for my health, but everything is OK with my health." He reported that he was a retired disabled veteran who "owned" two businesses. He had sold one to his former business partner, and the other one was being run by his wife from whom he was actually in the process of separation. He refused to give any more details regarding his business and marital situation, as he claimed it had nothing to do with his current condition.

He insisted that he needed more medication, and that it was probably not clear to staff because the anesthesiologist did not speak English well. ("He's Chinese or something."). Mr. L also did not feel understood by most nurses, who were either Latino or Asian. He was then told that his insistence on having more pain medication might lead staff to believe that he wanted opioid medication for reasons other than pain, when, in fact, they were confident that the PCA device was sufficient. This information added to his perceived "language [cultural]" barrier. He was also reminded that as a patient with chronic pain, he was probably experienced with the fact that pain relief many times did not mean complete elimination of pain. If he was not waking up during the night to self-dose, it was probably because the pain was not severe enough. After much reluctance, he agreed to give PCA a chance for at least one more day, but remained unwilling to discuss further any ongoing stressors in his life that could be leading to depressive symptoms.

In this particular case, the patient felt staff did not understand him, and had opted to give him a "machine" and "ignore" him afterwards. When made aware of the advantages of self-dosing, and of the possible interpretation of his behavior, he seemed willing to give PCA another chance. Cases like this illustrate how a better understanding of the PCA-ethnicity interface is so necessary. It is so unfortunate that such an important research tool has not been studied further for this purpose.

On one hand the PCA machine remains a unique device, as it acts as a silent witness that due to its nature can keep reliable track of opioid consumption as a consequence of a human interaction. It records every dose prescribed by the one programming it and every dose dispensed by the patient. On the other hand, it adds another layer of interaction, patient-staff versus patient-PCA machine-staff, calling for the need for multiple disciplines to improve research models and better understand the implications of existing literature including our findings and those of others. Thus, PCA has positive and negative effects. It simplifies the relationship between patient and caregivers to some extent, but also introduces a new "player" into the interaction. As to the negative effects, programming a PCA device is not free of errors; for some patients it might be better to deal with a person than with a machine and, of course, the use of a PCA does not prevent patients from experiencing the side effects of opioids. It is also known that culture and ethnicity play a major role in the manifestation of side effects and the reaction to complications.

A study by Tsui et al of 1,233 Chinese patients in Hong Kong concluded that the majority of PCA users welcomed the device, as 76% of them reported the experience as "good." All patients were started with the same parameters as were given Caucasian patients in the same hospital (Caucasians were not included in the study), allowing variation in consumption that ranged from 18 to 30 mg/day; suggesting that the device may be well received in the majority of cases.[17] As to the staff's reaction, reports are available about efforts made with nursing staff to minimize PCA programming errors, which occur with some frequency.[18] In the end, no matter how useful the pump is, it does not completely replace the necessary communication required to make an appropriate assessment of the patient's needs, not only for the initial prescription, but also for maintenance dosing and assessment of ongoing side effects and level of effectiveness. Let us not forget that staff members (i.e., doctors, nurses, pharmacists) also have their own educational and ethnic background. As to the available evidence, the study by Li et al, using the IPT, is quite encouraging in demonstrating that communication can be improved with instruments designed in the United States and used in other locales.[16]

It is difficult to compare the results of studies involving two or more ethnic groups, due to sample and methodological differences.[8,11] Nevertheless, it is remarkable that the two studies with the largest samples found definite differences in the amount of opioid prescription. On the other hand, it is interesting to point out that the study by Adam et al,[12] done in Arizona with similar ethnic groups as ours, happened to find equivalent amounts of analgesic prescribed postoperatively to all ethnic groups, and at the end of the study, found that consumption was not different across the groups. This underscores the importance of clinical assessment over predictions based on patient's ethnicity, as well as research in much larger and diverse populations, where other factors such as socioeconomic status, education, health disparities and health outcomes can be included among the variables studied.

As to the clinical assessment, our research group has come up anecdotally with what we call "psychosocial indications" for PCA. In other words, we consider this pump very useful and beyond the patients' ethnicity and surgical features, some psychosocial features can be considered to be "indications" for PCA treatment.

First, these indications carry the following goals:

1. Provide proper pain management.
2. Prevent deterioration of the patient-nurse relationship.
3. Prevent burnout of the nursing staff that can result in patient neglect.
4. Keep accurate record of analgesic consumption.
5. Promote a faster postoperative recovery.

The indications would be the following:

1. Personality style, in general would be those individuals who under stress are "required" to be in "control" of their environment, or have a hard time communicating their needs.
   a. Obsessive Compulsive
   b. Avoidant
   c. Narcissistic
   d. Antisocial
2. Psychiatric diagnoses would include those who have a low pain threshold and those fearful of receiving high dosages of opioid at one time, and would rather not ask for medication.
   a. Active substance abuse, especially opioids (i.e., heroin or opioid analgesic), and not stabilized on methadone or buprenorphine.
   b. No diagnosis of substance abuse, but history of high tolerance to opioids.
   c. History of alcohol dependence or other kind of dependence.
   d. Generalized Anxiety disorder.

CONCLUSIONS

At this point, the available literature demonstrates the feasibility of PCA research in different ethnic groups and in different countries. This research explores the complexity of theoretical models that attempt to explain PCA-ethnicity interactions and supports the use of PCA in patients with specific psychiatric profiles. The literature also suggests the importance of factors other than ethnicity in the postoperative-pain PCA prescribing decision. Clearly, there is no reason to prescribe any more or less analgesic based on the patient's ethnicity alone. In the future, it is very likely that genetic and/or pharmacogenomic features will enter the equation that determines our prescribing practices.

ACKNOWLEDGMENTS

The author thanks Dr. Joel E. Dimsdale for his invaluable help and support in this project.

REFERENCES

1. Beecher HK. Measurement of subjective responses. *Quantitative Effects of Drugs*. New York: Oxford University Press; 1959
2. Ng B, Dimsdale JE, Shragg P, Deutsch R. Ethnic differences in analgesic consumption for postoperative pain. *Psychosom Med*. 1996;58:125–129.
3. Marks RM, Sachar EJ. Undertreatment of medical inpatients with narcotic analgesics. *Ann Intern Med*. 1973;78(2):173–181.
4. Bates MS. Ethnicity and pain: A biocultural model. *Soc Sci Med*. 1987;24:47–50.
5. Lee A, Gin T, Oh TE. Opioid requirements and responses in Asians. *Anaesth Intensive Care*. 1997;25(6):665–670.
6. Green CR, Anderson KO, Baker TA, et al.. The unequal burden of pain: confronting racial and ethnic disparities in pain. *Pain Med*. 2003;4(3):277–294.
7. Smythe, M (1992) Patient-controlled analgesia. A review. *Pharmacotherapy*. 1992;12(2);132–143.
8. Ng B, Dimsdale JE, Rollnik JD, Shapiro H. The effect of ethnicity on prescriptions for patient-controlled analgesia for post-operative pain. *Pain*. 1996;66(1):9–12.

9. Todd K. Samaroo N, Hoffman J. Ethnicity as a risk factor for inadequate emergency department analgesia. *JAMA*. 1993;269:1537–1539.

10. Tan EC, Lim Y, Teo YY, Goh R, Law HY, Sia AT. Ethnic differences in pain perception and patient-controlled analgesia usage for postoperative pain. *J Pain*. 2008;9(9):849–855.

11. Adams RJ, Armstrong EP, Erstad BL. Prescribing and self-administration of morphine in Hispanic and non-Hispanic Caucasian patients treated with patient-controlled analgesia. *J Pain Palliat Care Pharmacother*. 2004;18(2):29–38.

12. Perry F, Parker RK, White PF, Clifford PA. Role of psychological factors in postoperative pain control and recovery with patient-controlled analgesia. *Clin J Pain*. 1994;10(1):57–63.

13. Houghton IT, Aun CS, Gin T, Lau JT. Inter-ethnic differences in postoperative pethidine requirements. *Anaesth Intensive Care*. 1992;20(1):52–55.

14. Chia YY, Chow LH, Hung CC, Liu K, Ger LP, Wang PN. (2002). Gender and pain upon movement are associated with the requirements for postoperative patient-controlled iv analgesia: a prospective survey of 2,298 Chinese patients. *Can J Anaesth*. 2002;49(3):249–255.

15. Li L, Herr K, Chen P. Postoperative pain assessment with three intensity scales in Chinese elders. *J Nurs Scholarsh*. 2009;41(3):241–249.

16. Zhang W, Chang YZ, Kan QC, et al. Association of human micro-opioid receptor gene polymorphism A118G with fentanyl analgesia consumption in Chinese gynaecological patients. *Anaesthesia*. 2010;65(2):130–135.

17. Tsui SL, Tong WN, Irwin M, et al. The efficacy, applicability and side-effects of postoperative intravenous patient-controlled morphine analgesia: an audit of 1233 Chinese patients. *Anaesth Intensive Care*. 1996;24(6):658–664.

18. Ferguson R, Williams ML, Beard B. Combining quality improvement and staff development efforts to decrease patient-controlled analgesia pump errors. *J Nurses Staff Dev*. 2010;26(5):E1–E4.

17

DISPARITIES IN HEALTH CARE AND PAIN MANAGEMENT FOR AMERICANS WITH SICKLE CELL DISEASE

JOSEPH TELFAIR, DRPH, MSW, MPH

Professor, Public Health Research and Practice *and* Director, UNCG Center for Social, Community and Health Research and Evaluation, University of North Carolina at Greensboro, Greensboro, North Carolina, USA

LORI E. CROSBY, PSYD

Associate Professor of Clinical Pediatrics, University of Cincinnati College of Medicine, Division of Behavioral Medicine and Clinical Psychology, Cincinnati Children's Hospital Medical Center, Cincinnati, Ohio, USA

Key Points

- Recurrent pain is the hallmark of sickle cell disease and the chief reason those with the disease seek medical care.
- No randomized, controlled clinical trials exist to inform the management of chronic pain among adults with sickle cell disease.
- Sickle cell disease disproportionately affects immigrants, ethnic minorities, and other socio-economically disadvantaged families and groups.
- Individualized treatment plans are optimal for management of pain.
- Sociocultural background has a major influence on how persons with sickle cell disease perceive and react to acute and chronic pain.
- Healthcare utilization among those with sickle cell disease is not simply a function of physiological disease severity or psychological/psychiatric comorbidity but, rather, a complex interaction of biological, psychological, and sociocultural variables.

INTRODUCTION

Sickle cell disease (SCD) is an autosomal, recessively inherited disorder of the red blood cells that affects a significant number of Americans, particularly those of African, Mediterranean, Middle Eastern, and Asian Indian descent.[1] Data from the US National Newborn Screening Information System (NNSIS) indicate that approximately 1700 babies are born each year with some form of the disease and in excess of 75 000 are identified as carriers of related abnormal hemoglobinopathies.[2] While the true prevalence of SCD in the United States is unknown, it is estimated to be between 72 000 and 98 000.[3] African Americans carry most of the burden of sickle cell disease in the United States, where the disease occurs in about one out of every 365 births.[3] It is estimated that 10% of individuals with SCD are of Hispanic ethnicity.[4] Sickle cell disease is a lifelong blood disorder, but the first three years of life are especially critical; without preventive measures those years see the highest mortality due mainly to infection.[5-7]

Sickle cell disease is characterized by intermittent vaso-occlusive events and chronic hemolytic anemia. Patients with SCD may experience several complications such as vaso-occlusive pain crisis, stroke, and pulmonary hypertension, all of which can contribute to a loss of 20–30 years of life. Vaso-occlusive events result in tissue ischemia leading to acute and chronic pain, as well as organ damage that can affect any organ in the body including the bones, lungs, liver, kidneys, brain, eyes, and joints. Like individuals with similar chronic conditions, these variations are reported to have a profound impact on the biological, psychological, and social development of individuals with SCD, as well as implications for their overall disease management.[8] Understanding the impact that sickle cell disease has on the lives of those with the condition, and the areas where disparities exist, must begin with a basic understanding of the condition itself. This chapter provides a brief overview of issues specific to pain management and health care of persons with SCD.

PAIN MANAGEMENT OF SICKLE CELL DISEASE

Because sickle cell disease (SCD) pain can be acute or chronic, it is often difficult to manage. For patients who experience only acute SCD pain episodes, the potential for positive outcomes is high, provided the pain can be managed adequately.[9] For patients with more frequent acute pain episodes, or chronic pain, the outlook may not be as promising. Unlike other pain conditions where research has revealed effective strategies for pain management, there have only been approximately ten published randomized clinical trials examining acute pain in SCD. Further, the authors were unable to find any randomized clinical trials examining chronic pain in adults with SCD. As a result, the rationale for current treatment regimens have been derived from clinical observation, consensus opinion, and literature relating to other pain conditions.[10] Despite the relative paucity of the literature, the American Pain Society (APS) established Guidelines for pain assessment and management in SCD in 2000.[9] In addition, a review by Cochrane et al (2006) identified some empirically supported treatments for SCD pain including nonsteroidal anti-inflammatory medicines (NSAIDs), opioids, and steroids which tend to be utilized the most.[11]

The majority of sickle cell pain is managed at home with a combination of fluids, acetaminophen, acetaminophen with hydrocodone, NSAIDS such as ibuprofen, or opioid analgesics.[12,13] Consistent with APS Guidelines, most patients initially manage pain with acetaminophen and NSAIDs.[9] Some patients may also combine oral opioids with ibuprofen, which appears to have some empirical support.[14] Despite the empirical support for these treatments, home management of pain using these medications may not be effective because patients often fail to take medications as frequently as recommended.[12]

In addition to taking medications for pain management, patients also use a variety of nonpharmacological methods. Some of the most commonly used techniques include rest, distracting activities (e.g., watching TV, reading, conversation), prayer (or attending worship),[14-18] massage, and heat.[17,19,20] Although alternative pain management strategies including guided imagery and cognitive-behavioral strategies have received some empirical support, they are utilized less often. This lack of use may be due to limited patient access or reluctance to receive treatment from behavioral health providers trained in these types of strategies.[21] Furthermore, APS Guidelines indicate that these types of interventions should be used in combination with more traditional treatments, such as opioids.[9]

Longer and more severe pain episodes are typically treated in the emergency department. While the goal of treating these episodes is to make the pain tolerable, managing pain in hospital settings remains a challenge.[9] First, patients are often frustrated by the lack of success of home management. Second, patients may be fearful because the type of pain or pain site is different or novel and may imply a worsening of their disease. In addition, the lack of biological markers to guide SCD pain management, and the necessity to tailor opioid regimens to individual patients, may lead to frustration among the emergency department staff.[9,12] Given the aforementioned negative events associated with emergency department visits, patients may delay seeking treatment, thereby increasing their risk of infection or medical complications and subsequently negatively impacting quality of life.

In an effort to address these issues and enhance the management of SCD pain, many healthcare systems have developed day hospital programs where patients with SCD can be treated by a consistent set of providers familiar with the disease.[22] Not surprisingly, day hospital programs have been found to improve SCD pain management, patient satisfaction, and patient functioning, as well as to decrease overall healthcare costs.[22]

The most severe pain episodes require hospitalization. In these instances, the APS recommends that pain be managed aggressively the first two to three days of hospitalization via bolus doses of opioids intravenously and intermittent administration using a fixed schedule or patient-controlled analgesia (PCA) pump.[23] "As needed" administrations should be avoided as they may inadvertently reinforce inappropriate pain management strategies by patients, such as clock watching. Dosing schedules and the types of analgesics used will vary based on opioid tolerance, pain severity, and individual pharmacokinetics (i.e., rates of absorption, metabolism, etc.). Transdermal fentanyl and continuous epidural infusions of fentanyl have shown promise in reducing pain for patients unresponsive to intravenous analgesic therapy.[24,25] Once pain has lessened, patients can be switched to oral medications.

Despite the effectiveness of opioids to decrease pain, their long-term use also has several negative consequences. First, for some patients, long-term opioid use can lead to heightened sensitivity to pain, termed hyperalgesia.[22] In addition, patients may develop anxiety regarding addiction to opioids. Third, repeated use of opioids leads to high levels of tolerance and physical dependence (not to be confused with psychological dependence).[26-28] To avoid the negative consequences of long-term opioid use, some providers have utilized sedatives or anxiolytics; however, such medications should not be used alone to treat SCD pain, as they mask behavioral pain symptoms without providing pain relief.[9]

To achieve optimal pain management, the healthcare team should partner with the patient to create an individualized treatment plan outlining medications and strategies to be utilized for mild, moderate, and severe pain. Treatment decisions should be guided by data on patient response to medication type, order of medications, and route of administration. While individualized treatment plans are currently the most effective strategy for pain management, additional research is needed to discover more effective treatments for the clinical management of pain in SCD.

DISPARITIES IN THE DELIVERY OF HEALTH CARE TO PERSONS WITH SICKLE CELL DISEASE: OVERVIEW

Sickle cell disease (SCD) disproportionately affects immigrants, ethnic/racial minorities, and other socio-economically disadvantaged families and groups; populations already challenged with accessing and navigating the system of care, and with understanding and managing the symptoms of the disease.[29] As a result of their diagnosis, persons with SCD and their families must learn to navigate a complex healthcare system including case managers, primary and specialty care providers, and emergency department providers. In addition to the demands of managing SCD, many individuals with SCD and their families face barriers to access and delivery of healthcare services. Despite major advances in the treatment of SCD in the last 30 years, disparities remain in the delivery of healthcare services. While there are significant health implications of these disparities, health and human services outcomes (i.e., access, utilization, and cost-of-care) have received little attention in published literature.[8,30]

In the current atmosphere of medical and healthcare reform in the United States, this lack of research presents a serious problem for those in the SCD community (i.e., clients, families, providers, and researchers). Specifically, comprehensive care centers at the tertiary and community-levels serving persons with SCD, are finding themselves ill-prepared to address the many new demands of a rapidly changing system.[31,32] While the health-reform literature indicates that information regarding client characteristics and patterns of care utilization is key to planning, developing, and implementing healthcare financing, quality guidelines, and access (how and for whom) decisions,[33] there is a lack of literature documenting these characteristics in individuals with SCD.[31,34]

To reduce disparities in the delivery of healthcare services, it is also important to understand the relationship between sociocultural diversity and the effective treatment of pain. Sociocultural background has long been recognized as a major influence in how persons with SCD perceive and react to their acute and chronic pain experiences. For example, Kleinman[35] and Narayan[36] point out that pain has both personal and cultural meanings. Because culture significantly affects both the assessment and management of people in pain, these cultural meanings influence decisions about healthcare delivery and analgesic use by both the person with SCD and those caring for them.[8,37]

PERSONAL AND CULTURAL NARRATIVE OF PAIN

Researchers recognize that healthcare utilization by this population is not simply a function of physiological disease severity or psychological/psychiatric comorbidity but, rather, a complex interaction of biological, psychological, and sociocultural variables.[37] Recurrent pain is the hallmark of sickle cell disease and the chief reason people seek medical care. Although pain episodes are implicated in the majority of hospital and emergency department visits,[38–42] their etiology is poorly understood. While clients may experience similar treatment conditions, pain responses may differ dramatically.[36] When treating persons with SCD, the client's concern for alleviation of symptoms must be addressed with as much concern as the physical symptoms themselves. The cultural reality is that persons with SCD (like those in the general public) attribute meaning to their pain; they attempt to order the experience of their pain, and understand what pain means to them and those close to them, through collective and personal narratives of their illness.[35,43] Both personal and cultural meanings are important in the experience and treatment of pain. An appreciation of the influence of culture on communication about pain, affective response to pain, conditioning for pain, meaning of pain, and biological differences of pain is important if patients are to be treated effectively.[36]

Multidisciplinary providers of care for persons with SCD are more sensitive to pain and recognize that unrelieved pain has significant physiological and psychological effects on patients.[38] Research shows that undertreated and unrelieved pain can slow the process of recovery from an acute pain episode, create burdens for patients and their families, and increase the cost of care.[13] Therefore, research that generates a full understanding of sickle cell–related pain treatment and management, as well as pain-related health care utilization may significantly contribute to the development of targeted programs and services that minimize costs to patients and other taxpayers while optimizing comprehensive patient care.[44]

CONCLUSION

Sickle cell disease is a varied and complicated disorder. Insights into treatment of pain and health care management of persons with the disease serve to highlight this complexity. Because of the unique ethnic, religious, and racial makeup of persons with sickle cell disease, it is critical that the influence of cultural issues on health service delivery be central to any treatment plan or culturally competent system of care. Individuals with SCD, as part of a diverse group, share a myriad of historical experiences, which commonly bind them together as a unique group within our society. Many, however, experience varying degrees of complex health disadvantages, which are exacerbated by a combination of economic disadvantages, racial bias, ignorance, and a history of challenges to the attainment (access) of adequate, quality medical and health services. It is notable that individuals experience such problems from different economic, class, and interpersonal perspectives that may affect the individual's (or their family's) relationship with providers and their adherence to treatment regimens. Because family and other caregivers are critical for the successful treatment of a child with sickle cell disease, parent and caregiver education is essential for successful navigation of the system of care.[45] Furthermore, it is critical when addressing the pain experience of persons with sickle cell disease that the complexity of the healthcare environment itself, in which treatment is provided, is considered as an influencing factor on the treatment and management of pain for persons with sickle cell disease.

ACKNOWLEDGMENTS

The authors would like to express gratitude to those persons with sickle-cell disease and their families, as well providers and others in the SCD community who unselfishly shared their insights and work to make this chapter possible. The authors are grateful to Ms. Amanda Story and Ms. Meghan McGrady for their editorial assistance in the refinement of this chapter.

REFERENCES

1. National Heart, Lung and Blood Institute. Who is at risk for Sickle Cell Disease? http://www.nhlbi.nih. gov/health/dci/Diseases/Sca/SCA_WhoIsAtRisk.html. Accessed November 8, 2010.
2. National Newborn Screening and Genetics Resource Center. *National Newborn Screening Information System—Hemoglobinopathies.* 2009.http://genes-r-us.uthscsa.edu/Accessed November 30, 2010.
3. Hassell KL. Population estimates of sickle cell disease in the U.S. *Am J Prev Med.* Apr 2010;38(suppl 4):S512–S521.
4. Brousseau DC, Panepinto JA, Nimmer M, Hoffmann RG. The number of people with sickle-cell disease in the United States: national and state estimates. *Am J Hematol.* Jan 2010;85(1):77–78.

5. Ebrahim SH, Khoja TA, Elachola H, Atrash HK, Memish Z, Johnson A. Children who come and go: the state of sickle cell disease in resource-poor countries. *Am J Prev Med.* Apr 2010;38(suppl 4):S568–S570.

6. Quinn CT, Rogers ZR, McCavit TL, Buchanan GR. Improved survival of children and adolescents with sickle cell disease. *Blood.* Apr 29 2010;115(17):3447–3452.

7. Gaston MH, Verter JI, Woods G, et al. Prophylaxis with oral penicillin in children with sickle cell anemia. A randomized trial. *N Engl J Med.* Jun 19 1986;314(25):1593–1599.

8. Telfair J. Sickle Cell Disease: Biosocial Aspects. In: Livingston L, ed. *The Praeger Handbook of Black American Health: Policies and Issues Behind Disparities in Health.* 2nd ed. Westport, CT:The Greenwood Publishing Group; 2004:129–146.

9. Preboth M. Management of pain in sickle cell disease. *Am Fam Physician.* Mar 1 2000;61(5):1544, 1549–1550.

10. Taylor LE, Stotts NA, Humphreys J, Treadwell MJ, Miaskowski C. A review of the literature on the multiple dimensions of chronic pain in adults with sickle cell disease. *J Pain Symptom Manage.* Sep 2010;40(3):416–435.

11. Dunlop RJ, Bennett KC. Pain management for sickle cell disease. *Cochrane Database Syst Rev.* 2006(2):CD003350.

12. Dampier C. Pain in Sickle Cell Disease. In Gary A. Walco and Kenneth R. Goldschneider (eds) *Pain in Children: A Practical Guide for Primary Care* . Totwa, NJ: SpringerLink; 2008:201–207.

13. Smith WR, Bovbjerg VE, Penberthy LT, et al. Understanding pain and improving management of sickle cell disease: the PiSCES study. *J Natl Med Assoc.* Feb 2005;97(2):183–193.

14. Dampier C, Ely E, Brodecki D, O'Neal P. Home management of pain in sickle cell disease: a daily diary study in children and adolescents. *J Pediatr Hematol Oncol.* Nov 2002;24(8):643–647.

15. Anie KA, Steptoe A, Bevan DH. Sickle cell disease: Pain, coping and quality of life in a study of adults in the UK. *Br J Health Psychol.* Sep 2002;7(Part 3):331–344.

16. Cotton S, Grossoehme D, Rosenthal SL, et al. Religious/Spiritual coping in adolescents with sickle cell disease: a pilot study. *J Pediatr Hematol Oncol.* May 2009;31(5):313–318.

17. Dampier C, Ely E, Eggleston B, Brodecki D, O'Neal P. Physical and cognitive-behavioral activities used in the home management of sickle pain: a daily diary study in children and adolescents. *Pediatr Blood Cancer.* Nov 2004;43(6):674–678.

18. Harrison MO, Edwards CL, Koenig HG, Bosworth HB, DeCastro L, Wood M. Religiosity/ Spirituality and Pain in Patients With Sickle Cell Disease. *J Nerv Ment Dis.* 2005;193(4):250–257.

19. Bodhise PB, Dejoie M, Brandon Z, Simpkins S, Ballas SK. Non-pharmacologic management of sickle cell pain. *Hematology.* Jun 2004;9(3):235–237.

20. Yoon SL, Black S. Comprehensive, integrative management of pain for patients with sickle-cell disease. *J Altern Complement Med.* Dec 2006;12(10):995–1001.

21. Chen E, Cole SW, Kato PM. A review of empirically supported psychosocial interventions for pain and adherence outcomes in sickle cell disease. *J Pediatr Psychol.* Apr-May 2004;29(3):197–209.

22. Benjamin L DC, Jacox A, Odesina V, et al. *Guideline for the management of acute and chronic pain in sickle-cell disease.* Glenview, IL: American Pain Society.: 2007.

23. Jacob E, Miaskowski C, Savedra M, Beyer JE, Treadwell M, Styles L. Quantification of analgesic use in children with sickle cell disease. *Clin J Pain.* Jan 2007;23(1):8–14.

24. Christensen ML, Wang WC, Harris S, Eades SK, Wilimas JA. Transdermal fentanyl administration in children and adolescents with sickle cell pain crisis. *J Pediatr Hematol Oncol.* Nov 1996;18(4):372–376.

25. Yaster M, Tobin JR, Billett C, Casella JF, Dover G. Epidural analgesia in the management of severe vaso-occlusive sickle cell crisis. *Pediatrics.* Feb 1994;93(2):310–315.

26. American Psychiatric Association. *Diagnostic criteria for substance abuse and substance dependence.* 4th ed. Washington, DC: American Psychiatric Association; 2000.

27. Goldstein RZ, Alia-Klein N, Tomasi D, et al. Is decreased prefrontal cortical sensitivity to monetary reward associated with impaired motivation and self-control in cocaine addiction? *Am J Psychiatry.* Jan 2007;164(1):43–51.

28. Kirsh KL, Whitcomb LA, Donaghy K, Passik SD. Abuse and addiction issues in medically ill patients with pain: attempts at clarification of terms and empirical study. *Clin J Pain.* Jul-Aug 2002;18(suppl 4):S52–S60.

29. Flores G, Abreu M, Tomany-Korman SC. Limited English proficiency, primary language at home, and disparities in children's health care: how language barriers are measured matters. *Public Health Rep.* Jul-Aug 2005;120(4):418–430.

30. Haque A, Telfair J. Socioeconomic distress and health status: the urban-rural dichotomy of services utilization for people with sickle cell disorder in North Carolina. *J Rural Health.* Winter 2000;16(1):43–55.

31. Blumenthal D, Meyer GS. Academic health centers in a changing environment. *Health Aff (Millwood).* Summer 1996;15(2):200–215.

32. Lottenberg R, Hassell KL. An evidence-based approach to the treatment of adults with sickle cell disease. *Hematology Am Soc Hematol Educ Program.* 2005:58–65.

33. Smith LA, Oyeku SO, Homer C, Zuckerman B. Sickle cell disease: a question of equity and quality. *Pediatrics.* May 2006;117(5):1763–1770.

34. Midence KE, *Sickle Cell Disease: A Psychosocial Approach.* New York: Radcliffe Medical Press; 1994.

35. Kleinman A. *Patients and Healers in the Context of Culture: An Exploration of the Borderland between Anthropology, Medicine, and Psychiatry.* Berkeley: University of California Press; 1980.

36. Narayan MC. Culture's effects on pain assessment and management. *Am J Nurs.* Apr 2010;110(4): 38–47; quiz 48–39.

37. Bediako S, Lavender A, Yasin Z. Racial centrality and health care utilization among African American adults with sickle cell disease. *J Black Psychol.* 2007;33(4):422–438.

38. Ballas SK. Complications of sickle cell anemia in adults: guidelines for effective management. *Cleve Clin J Med.* Jan 1999;66(1):48–58.

39. Grant MM, Gil KM, Floyd MY, Abrams M. Depression and functioning in relation to health care use in sickle cell disease. *Ann Behav Med.* Spring 2000;22(2):149–157.

40. Platt OS, Thorington BD, Brambilla DJ, et al. Pain in sickle cell disease. Rates and risk factors. *N Engl J Med.* Jul 4 1991;325(1):11–16.

41. Schwartz LA, Radcliffe J, Barakat LP. The Development of a Culturally Sensitive Pediatric Pain Management Intervention for African American Adolescents With Sickle Cell Disease. *Child Health Care.* Aug 1 2007;36(3):267–283.

42. Sutton M, Atweh GF, Cashman TD, Davis WT. Resolving conflicts: misconceptions and myths in the care of the patient with sickle cell disease. *Mt Sinai J Med.* Sep 1999;66(4):282–285.

43. Mousa SA, Al Momen A, Al Sayegh F, et al. Management of painful vaso-occlusive crisis of sickle-cell anemia: consensus opinion. *Clin Appl Thromb Hemost.* Aug 2010;16(4):365–376.

44. Woods K, Karrison T, Koshy M, Patel A, Friedmann P, Cassel C. Hospital utilization patterns and costs for adult sickle cell patients in Illinois. *Public Health Rep.* Jan-Feb 1997;112(1):44–51.

45. Wilson RE, Krishnamurti L, Kamat D. Management of sickle cell disease in primary care. *Clin Pediatr (Phila).* Nov-Dec 2003;42(9):753–761.

18

UNAVAILABILITY OF PAIN MEDICINES IN MINORITY NEIGHBORHOODS AND DEVELOPING COUNTRIES

LAURA P. GELFMAN, MD
Fellow in Palliative Medicine, Brookdale Department of Geriatrics and Palliative Medicine, Mount Sinai School of Medicine, New York, New York, USA

R. SEAN MORRISON, MD
Professor, Geriatrics and Medicine, Department of Geriatrics and Palliative Medicine, Mount Sinai School of Medicine, New York, New York, USA

Key Points
- Pain is a treatable symptom of illness.
- With enhanced education, drug policy, and access to opioids, the barriers to adequate pain control can be targeted.
- Minority groups are particularly vulnerable to lack of access to opioids.
- Several studies have demonstrated the barriers to filling opioid prescriptions for individuals living in minority neighborhoods.
- In addition, lack of opioid availability in developing countries illustrates how the tight regulatory policies for opioid distribution impede access to pain relief.
- The small number of original research studies conducted to evaluate opioid availability in these populations limits the scope of the chapter.

INTRODUCTION

Pain is a common and dreaded symptom of illness. Multiple studies of diverse populations have demonstrated that pain is not being appropriately managed, particularly in minority

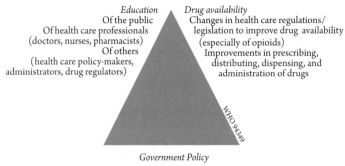

FIGURE 18.1 The WHO foundation measures for implementing cancer pain relief programs World Health Organization (1996) Cancer pain relief with a guide to opioids availability. Handbook. Second Edition. WHO, Geneva. Page 43.

groups.[1,2,3] There are many barriers to adequate pain control, including education and training of prescribers, fear of dependence and drug abuse, legal restrictions on use of opioids, and unavailability of pain medications.[4] The World Health Organization (WHO) mapped the foundation measures for implementing cancer pain relief with a three-pronged approach including education, government policy, and drug availability (Figure 18.1).[5] This approach emphasizes solutions to the primary barriers to pain relief.

In this chapter, we will examine the focus point of drug availability, specifically in minority neighborhoods in the United States as well as developing countries. Several studies have demonstrated the barriers to filling opioid prescriptions for individuals living in minority neighborhoods. Similarly, examining opioid availability in developing countries illustrates how the tight regulatory policies for opioid distribution and dispensing hinder access to pain relief. Therefore, availability to opioid analgesics for ambulatory patients living in minority neighborhoods in the United States and patients in developing countries must remain a priority.

BARRIERS TO FILLING OPIOID PRESCRIPTIONS IN MINORITY NEIGHBORHOODS

Several studies have shown that socioeconomic factors influence availability of opioids in outpatient pharmacies.[6] More specifically, studies have been conducted to determine the availability of commonly prescribed opioids in a number of cities and states, including New York City, Michigan, and Washington State.

The first study conducted by Kanner et al in 1986 was designed to determine the availability of opioid analgesics for ambulatory cancer patients with pain in the Bronx, New York.[7] The study comprised an initial telephone survey of pharmacists at 42 randomly selected pharmacies in the Bronx, New York evaluating whether they routinely stocked various classes of opioids, followed by a survey of 112 pharmacies around New York City. In the city-wide pharmacy survey, 94 pharmacies responded to the survey. Of these, 29% carried no Class II (medications designated as having highest abuse liabilities) opioids, 25% carried only oxycodone/aspirin or acetaminophen combinations, 20% stocked levorphanol, 15% carried hydromorphone, 3% carried oral morphine, and 2% stocked methadone. In the telephone surveys of the pharmacists, the most common reason for not stocking opioids was fear of robbery, followed by lack of prescription demand. Based on the results of this 1986 study, the authors cited three main priority areas to be addressed to improve opioid availability: (1) physician education regarding prescription practices, (2) pharmacy inducements to stock appropriate medications, and (3) protection of pharmacists once medications are stocked.[7]

In 1998, Morrison et al observed that many black and Hispanic patients who received palliative care at a major urban teaching hospital were unable to obtain prescribed opioids from their neighborhood pharmacy upon hospital discharge. Based on this observation, Morrison et al conducted a study to determine the availability of commonly prescribed opioids in New York City pharmacies.[8] The study surveyed a random sample of 30% of New York City pharmacies to obtain information about their opioid stock, and correlated the pharmacy locations with US Census information about racial and ethnic composition of the neighborhoods as well as the proportion of residents who were 65 years or older.

In this study, opioids were divided into four categories on the basis of the Agency for Health Care Policy and Research (AHCPR) guidelines: (1) combination products for the treatment of moderate pain, (2) short-acting opioid tablets for dose-finding in patients with severe pain and for the treatment of breakthrough pain, (3) short-acting opioids in liquid form for the treatment of severe pain in patients with swallowing difficulties or in those in whom precise dose adjustments are required, and (4) long-acting opioids for the extended treatment of severe pain. The stock of each pharmacy was categorized as (1) complete (if the pharmacy had in stock an agent in each of the four medication categories), (2) nearly complete (if the pharmacy had in stock sufficient medication to treat a patient in moderate or severe pain, (3) incomplete (if the pharmacy did not have either a long-acting or a short-acting opioid preparation in stock), or (4) absent (if the pharmacy did not carry any opioids but did stock other prescription medications). Finally, the pharmacists representing pharmacies with inadequate supplies, including classifications of both incomplete or absent, were interviewed with open-ended questions about why opioids were not fully stocked in their pharmacy. In addition, using US Census data, the investigators determined the racial and ethnic composition of the neighborhood around each pharmacy surveyed, defined as the area within 0.4 km radius of the pharmacy. The neighborhoods around each sampled pharmacy were classified based on percentage of white, black, Hispanic or Asian residents in the designated area. The adequacy of opioid supplies was analyzed according to the categories of racial and ethnic composition.

Across the five boroughs of New York City, 503 pharmacies were identified (160 in Manhattan, 130 in Brooklyn, 114 in Queens, 72 in the Bronx and 27 on Staten Island), of which 431 pharmacies met the inclusion criterion and 347 agreed to participate. Of the 347 pharmacies, 176 (51 percent) did not have opioid supplies that were sufficient to provide adequate treatment for a patient with severe pain. Although 116 of the 122 pharmacies with incomplete supplies (95 percent) had a combination product in stock that could be used for the treatment of moderate pain, only 55 (45 percent) carried a strong opioid preparation that could be used for the treatment of severe pain.

Twenty-five percent of pharmacies in predominantly nonwhite neighborhoods (those in which less than 40 percent of residents were white) had adequate opioid supplies, as compared with 72 percent of pharmacies in predominantly white neighborhoods (those in which at least 80 percent of residents were white) (odds ratio for adequate supplies in predominantly nonwhite neighborhoods, 0.13; 95 percent confidence interval, 0.07 to 0.26). Sixty-six percent of pharmacies that had no opioids in stock were in predominantly nonwhite neighborhoods.

Adjusting for age and rates of burglary, robbery, and drug-related arrests, the authors demonstrated that pharmacies in predominantly nonwhite neighborhoods were significantly less likely to supply opioids than were pharmacies in predominantly white neighborhoods. Two-thirds of the pharmacies that did not carry any opioids were in neighborhoods where the majority of the residents were nonwhites. This finding, together with reports that nonwhite patients are significantly less likely than white patients to receive prescriptions for analgesic agents recommended by the AHCPR, suggests that minority patients are at increased risk for inadequate pain control.[10]

Pharmacists cited (1) low demand for these medications, (2) regulations with regard to disposal, (3) fear of fraud and illicit drug use, and (4) fear of theft as the primary reasons for not carrying an adequate supply of opioids. In open-ended interviews, pharmacists named the close oversight of regulatory agencies as an additional barrier for not stocking opioids. More specifically, they cited the regulatory oversight and monitoring of these medications, the additional paperwork of state and federal drug-enforcement agencies, and fear of penalties imposed by state and federal agencies. In predominantly nonwhite neighborhoods, pharmacists were more likely to report a low demand for opioids or expressed concern about their disposal.

Morrison's study demonstrates that many New York City pharmacies do not stock sufficient medication to treat patients with severe pain. Given the limitations imposed on availability of opioids, pharmacists would benefit from an education program about safe and appropriate use of opioid analgesics. In addition, the potential harm resulting from inadequate pain relief calls for re-evaluation of regulations that hinder pharmacists from stocking these controlled substances. These results suggest that nonwhite patients may be at even greater risk for the undertreatment of pain than previously reported.

FILLING OPIOID PRESCRIPTIONS IN MICHIGAN

Spurred by similar reports from minority patients regarding barriers to filling opioid prescriptions at their local pharmacies after the publication of the New York study, Green et al conducted a similar study comparing opioid availability in predominantly minority areas with availability in predominantly white areas across Michigan. While the study by Morrison et al was conducted only in the urban area of New York City, the study by Green examined the entire state of Michigan, including urban and rural settings. In addition, this study investigated opioid availability based on pharmacy type (corporate and noncorporate) to gain an understanding of how income affects availability.[10]

In a fashion similar to Morrison, Green et al categorized pharmacies based on the ethnic composition of the zip code in which the pharmacy was located: (1) zip codes with more than 70% minority residents were designated as minority zip codes and (2) zip codes with more than 70% white residents were classified as white zip codes. Next, pharmacies were randomly sampled in both white and minority zip codes for an adequate representation of both groups.

Pharmacy managers were interviewed about the availability of the following 15 opioid analgesics: long-acting (i.e., controlled release oxycodone, controlled release morphine, fentanyl, levorphanol, and methadone); short-acting (i.e., immediate release oxycodone, immediate release morphine, hydromorphone, butorphanol, and meperidine); or combination products (i.e., propoxyphene, acetaminophen and hydrocodone, acetaminophen and codeine, aspirin and oxycodone, acetaminophen and oxycodone, and oxycodone terephthalate). Opioid availability was classified as (1) available, if at least one of the medications in each opioid category was available; if not, it was coded as not available, (2) sufficient supply, if a pharmacy had all three categories of opioids; if not, it was coded as insufficient.

Using a phone survey, Green et al collected data about reasons for insufficient supplies of opioids and barriers to opioid availability among Michigan pharmacies. Pharmacy managers' responses were categorized as (1) low demand, (2) worries about illicit use, (3) excessive paperwork, (4) fear of robbery, (5) drug disposal regulations, and (6) other concerns. In addition, data about socioeconomic status, the proportion of residents who were 65 years or older, as well as information about hospital proximity (if there was a hospital within walking distance, designated up to 0.5 mile radius, from the pharmacy) was collected.

Based on a sample of 95 white and 93 minority pharmacies, analyses of interviews of these pharmacy managers between June 2003 and April 2004 found that (84.1%) met criteria to be designated as having sufficient opioid supply (Table 18.1). However, pharmacies located in white zip codes more frequently had sufficient opioid supplies as compared with pharmacies located in minority zip codes (86.9% versus 54.2%; $p < 0.01$). Corporate pharmacies were less likely to have sufficient opioid stock when compared with noncorporate pharmacies (58.8% versus 91%; $p < 0.01$).

In a multivariate model, the most commonly cited barrier for lack of opioid supply by the pharmacy managers was low demand (93.1%), followed by fear of opioid usage for illicit purposes; this barrier was associated with pharmacies with insufficient supplies when compared with pharmacies with sufficient supplies (30.3% versus 4.3%; $p < 0.01$). The pharmacies in the white zip codes were more likely to have sufficient opioid supplies than pharmacies in minority zip codes (Table 18.2). When comparing the subgroup of zip codes with a median income greater than or equal to the mean income for

TABLE 18.1 Sociodemographic Characteristics and Sufficiency of Opioid Analgesic Supplies

Sociodemographic Characteristics	N	Pharmacies In Minority Zip Codes (N = 93)	Pharmacies In White Zip Codes (N= 95)	P Value*
Median zip code age (mean yrs±SE)	188	32.3±0.9	36.5±0.9	<.01
Median zip code household income (mean $±SE)	188	$32,034±$2,076	$49,434±$2,160	<.01
Proportion of residents ≥65 years within each zip code (mean proportion ± SE)	188	.109±.008	.129±.005	<.05
Rural zip code (%yes)†	132	0.0	13.2	.28
Pharmacy type (% corporate)	188	64.3	59.9	.61
Hospital in the zip code (% yes)	188	31.7	43.2	.42

Abbreviations: N, sum of normalized sampling weights; SE, design based standard error for the estimated mean, taking clustering by zip code into account.

*Reported P values are for tests (for age, median income, and proportion ≥65 years) and design-based Rao–scott χ^2 tests.

†Zip codes located across rural and urban areas were not included in this analysis

Green CR, Ndao-Brumblay SK, West B, et al. Differences in prescription opioid analgesic availability: comparing minority and white pharmacies across Michigan. *J Pain.* October 2005;6 (10):694.

TABLE 18.2 Results from the Multivariate Models for Sufficient Supply

| Predictor | Income Group* | | | |
| | ≥ Mean Zip Code Income | | < Mean Zip Code Income | |
	Odds Ratio	95% CI	Odds Ratio	95% CI
White	13.36	(1.09–164.17)	54.42	(6.27–472.02)
Noncorporate	24.92	(3.03–205.18)	3.61	(1.11–11.77)
Median age	.77	(.60–1.00)	1.06	(.99–1.14)
Hospital in the zip code	.63	(.12–3.44)	2.01	(.62–6.52)

Abbreviation: CI, confidence interval

*Pharmacies are divided into 2 income groups: those in zip codes with a median income that is greater than or equal to the average median zip code income and those with a median income that is less than the average median zip code income.

Green CR, Ndao-Brumblay SK, West B, et al. Differences in prescription opioid analgesic availability: comparing minority and white pharmacies across Michigan. *J Pain.* October 2005;6 (10):695.

all zip codes, pharmacies in white zip codes were more than 13 times more likely than pharmacies in minority zip codes to have sufficient opioid stock (odds ratio (OR) 13.36; 95% confidence interval (CI) 1.06–164.17). In addition, noncorporate pharmacies were more likely to have sufficient opioid supplies than corporate pharmacies (OR 24.92; 95% CI, 3.03–205.18) and pharmacies in zip codes with a higher median age were less likely to have sufficient opioid supply (OR, 0.77; 95% CI, 0.60–1.00). In contrast, when looking at the zip codes with median income less than the mean income for all zip codes, pharmacies in white zip codes were approximately 54 times more likely than pharmacies in minority zip codes to have sufficient opioid analgesic supply (OR, 54.42; 95% CI, 6.27–472.02). The highly significant association between minority zip code and having insufficient opioid supply is much larger in low-income zip codes than in high-income zip codes.

This study by Green et al further demonstrates that Michigan pharmacies with sufficient opioid supplies were less likely to be found in predominantly minority zip codes than predominantly white zip codes. These findings confirm the results of Morrison et al and broadened these findings by providing evidence that pharmacies in low-income areas are more likely to have insufficient opioid stock than pharmacies in high-income areas, regardless of race. Overall, they found that if an opioid is prescribed to patients living in either minority zip codes or low-income zip codes, they are less likely to be able to fill that prescription. These findings further validate that both populations who fill opioid prescriptions at pharmacies near minority and low-income populations are at increased risk of that prescription not being filled, and therefore at risk for inadequate pain relief. Interestingly, they found that income also affects opioid availability in white communities, but had little impact in minority zip codes, presenting the likelihood that poor whites also face obstacles in accessing prescriptions for opioids in their communities.

These differences in access to opioids in Michigan have significant implications for access to quality pain care. Individuals living in minority zip codes throughout Michigan are less likely to have access to sufficient opioid supplies than those living in white zip codes, regardless of income, yet income did impact opioid supplies in high-income white areas. However, individuals in minority and low-income zip codes have less access to opioids than individuals in high-income white zip codes. This study further demonstrates how opioid availability is a fundamental barrier to quality pain care for vulnerable populations.

THE CASE OF WASHINGTON STATE

Because prior population-based studies were conducted only in New York City and Michigan, an additional study was conducted to clarify whether rural-urban or socioeconomic differences impact the availability of commonly prescribed opioids in pharmacies throughout Washington State.[11] Similar to the prior described studies, pharmacies were matched to zip codes and the pharmacies surveyed about availability of different classes of opioids. Pharmacy zip code data were linked to socioeconomic and demographic data from the 2000 Census. Again, opioids were classified by groups: (1) short-acting opioids and combination products (immediate-release morphine, oxycodone, oxycodone with acetaminophen, hydrocodone with acetaminophen, codeine, codeine with acetaminophen, tramadol, meperidine, and hydromorphone) and (2) the long-acting opioids (sustained-release oxycodone, sustained-release morphine, transdermal fentanyl, and methadone). Pharmacies that did not stock two or more of the opioids in either of the two classes were categorized as deficient.

Most pharmacies surveyed carried most opioids and only 14 pharmacies were deficient in access to short-acting opioids and 16 pharmacies deficient in access to long-acting opioids. The pharmacies designated as deficient were more likely to be located in zip codes with more residents living below poverty [OR 1.06; 95% confidence interval (CI) 1.01–1.12 for short-acting opioids; OR 1.07; 95% CI 1.01–1.12 for long-acting opioids], and a higher percentage of nonwhite residents (OR 1.06; 95% CI 1.02–1.08 for short-acting opioids; OR 1.06; 95% CI 1.04–1.08 for long-acting opioids). In multivariate logistic regression, Mayer et al found that pharmacies in nonwhite zip codes were more likely to be deficient in access to both short- and long-acting opioids, when controlling for the percentage of residents living in poverty (OR 1.05; 95% CI 1.02–1.08 for short-acting; OR 1.05; 95% CI 1.03–1.08 for long-acting).

The findings in Washington State differ from those from New York City and Michigan State, in that most of the Washington State responding pharmacies carried both long- and short-acting opioids. These authors give multiple potential explanations for these differences in opioid availability in Washington State including less racial diversity and socioeconomic variation, more rural and isolated areas, lower burglary rate, greater outreach efforts to educate patients and providers on pain management, as well as different sampling methods and sample size than prior studies. This study raises the possibility of geographic variation in opioid availability, but differences in the categorization of classes of opioids stocked make comparison difficult.

These multiple studies confirm the concerns of clinicians and researchers by demonstrating that individuals living in minority neighborhoods and low-income neighborhoods are limited in ability to access opioids for pain relief. Although these barriers have significant implications for disparities in quality of care, they also present opportunities for change and improvement. With an emphasis on education of pharmacists and review of oversight regulations of opioids, access to opioids for minorities could be drastically improved.

ACCESS TO OPIOIDS IN DEVELOPING COUNTRIES

Looking beyond the scope of the ambulatory patients in minority neighborhoods in the United States, in 1996, the World Health Organization (WHO) published a report about opioid availability, with a focus on patients with cancer, on a more global scale.[5]

In this report, the WHO cites many barriers to relief of cancer pain, including the following: (1) absence of national policies on cancer pain and palliative care; (2) lack of awareness of health care workers, administrators, policy makers, and the public that cancer pain can be relieved; (3) shortage of financial resources and limitations of healthcare delivery systems and personnel; (4) concern that opioids will produce psychological dependence and drug abuse; and (5) legal restrictions on the use and the availability of opioids.[12] The WHO created a strategy to combat these barriers including three primary development goals: (1) national or state policies that support cancer pain relief through government endorsement of education or drug availability; (2) educational programs for the public, healthcare personnel, regulators, and others; and (3) modification of laws and regulations to improve the availability of drugs, especially opioid analgesics.[5]

In an effort to evaluate improvements in pain management, the WHO monitors morphine consumption for each individual country. Since the WHO began to emphasize the importance of opioids in cancer pain management in 1984, morphine consumption has tripled globally from 1984 to 1992.[13] Nevertheless, obtaining opioids presents challenges for many countries due to inadequate funding of health services, lack of funding of health infrastructure, and inadequate facilities for the storage and distribution of medications.

The WHO has aimed to address these barriers through the Action Program on Essential Drugs, which strives to establish both a national policy on essential drugs that should exist in every country, as well as an action plan to guarantee availability at a reasonable cost for a limited number of drugs of significant therapeutic value. As of the publication of this report, more than 100 countries had adopted this list of essential drugs.[14] Nevertheless, morphine and other opioids are not available in many countries because of national laws targeting drug abuse.

Different international organizations have created treaties and committees to regulate opioids globally. One such treaty by the United Nations is the Single Convention on Narcotic Drugs, initially written in 1961, and amended in 1972, with the overarching purpose to both (1) prevent the abuse of narcotics or opioids and (2) guarantee the availability of opioids for medical usage. As such, the treaty explains the steps on how to make morphine and other opioids available for pain management and eliminate barriers to their availability. Critical to understanding these barriers is an understanding of how drugs are distributed—starting with the importation or manufacturing of opioids, to the distribution to hospitals and pharmacies, and finally, to the dispersal to patients by healthcare providers. The treaty mandates that all individuals or enterprises in the distribution system must be licensed or authorized, and that opioids may only be transferred between authorized parties.

In addition, the International Narcotics Control Board (INCB), an independent and quasi-judicial control organization for the implementation of the United Nations drug conventions, acknowledged that opioids are underutilized in cancer pain treatment and requested that countries re-evaluate their individual needs.[15] Each year, national drug regulatory authorities estimate these countries' opiate needs for the following year and the Single Convention mandates that the amount of opioids either imported or manufactured in a country must not exceed that estimate provided to the INCB. Therefore, it is the responsibility of the national government to determine the amount of opioid needed to meet the medical needs of its country. Because the supply of opioids in a given country is determined by regulatory authorities, it is critical that healthcare personnel communicate with their government about the importance of pain relief, and similarly, that healthcare personnel understand the opioid distribution system and regulatory measures to prevent abuse and diversion.[5]

The import and export of opioids in the distribution system is closely monitored and regulated under the Single Convention with a step-by-step process dictated under the treaty to ensure that the amount of opioid stays within the approved estimate of need by the importing country. INCB receives quarterly reports on all of the imports and exports of opioids by national drug regulatory authorities. These authorities must create an annual inventory and report the total amount of opioid manufactured, consumed, and in stock. The INCB then uses these data to monitor production and consumption of opioids.[16]

In spite of these efforts, the INCB reports that the medical need for opioids is not yet being fully met, especially with respect to cancer pain; as a result, they made the following suggestions to government, medical providers, and the WHO to: (1) improve methods of assessing medical needs; (2) develop a supervisory system to demonstrate whether medical needs for opioids are being met and to indicate corrective actions required; (3) identify obstacles to the appropriate use of opioids and facilitate their availability in cases of severe pain; (4) establish national policies and guidelines on the appropriate medical use of opioids; (5) ensure that healthcare providers are adequately trained in opioid use and informed about drug dependence; and (6) urge medical instructors and professional medical associations to promote the rational use of opioids for medical purposes while taking measures to ensure that they are not abused.[13]

The INCB recognizes the withholding of opioids from medical use does not necessarily guarantee prevention of the abuse of illicitly procured opioids. The Drug Control and Access to Medicines (DCAM) Consortium provides information about consumption of opioids in 2008 on a global scale (Figure 18.2). The consumption statistics are displayed in milligrams of morphine per capita, which is calculated by dividing the total amount of opioid consumed in kilograms by the population of the country for that particular year, based on United Nations population data. This provides a population-based statistic that allows for comparisons between countries.

For example, based on data from 2008, the United States consumed 66.6 mg of morphine per capita. In comparison, India consumed 0.16 mg of morphine per capita and China consumed 0.68 mg of morphine per capita. The interactive map demonstrates the disparity in consumption of opioids.[18] The restrictions imposed by government agencies may cause unnecessary suffering of a population in need of pain relief.

SUMMARY

Returning to the foundation measures of education, government policy, and drug availability mapped by the WHO, it is clear that many opportunities exist to improve pain relief for individuals living in minority neighborhoods and those in developing countries. By focusing on the education of clinicians, pharmacists, government regulators, and patients, as well as reviewing the government regulations to ensure restrictions do not present barriers to pain relief, the availability of opioids for the millions of patients suffering from pain from multiple disorders can be better ensured.

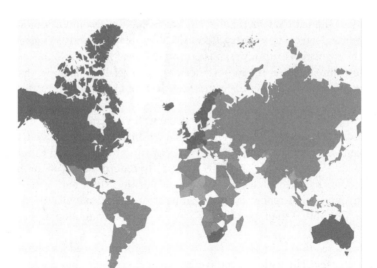

• mg/Capita

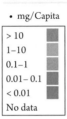

> 10	
1–10	
0.1–1	
0.01– 0.1	
< 0.01	
No data	

FIGURE 18.2 Morphine Consumption Map. Copyright © 2009–2011 The Board of Regents of the University of Wisconsin System.
Sources: International Narcotics Control Board; United Nations population data

REFERENCES

1. Cleeland CS, Gonin R, Baez L, Loehrer P, Pandya KJ. Pain and treatment of pain in minority patients with cancer. The Eastern Cooperative Oncology Group Minority Outpatient Pain Study. *Ann Intern Med.* Nov 1 1997;127(9):813–816.

2. Todd KH, Samaroo N, Hoffman JR. Ethnicity as a risk factor for inadequate emergency department analgesia. *JAMA.* Mar 24–31 1993;269(12):1537–1539.

3. McDonald DD. Gender and ethnic stereotyping and narcotic analgesic administration. *Res Nurs Health.* Feb 1994;17(1):45–49.

4. Joranson DE. Availability of opioids for cancer pain: recent trends, assessment of system barriers, New World Health Organization guidelines, and the risk of diversion. *J Pain Symptom Manage.* Aug 1993;8(6):353–360.

5. World Health Organization. *Cancer Pain Relief with a Guide to Opioid Availability. Handbook.* 2nd ed. Geneva: WHO; 1996:1–70.

6. Cleeland CS, Gonin R, Baez L, Loehrer P, Pandya KJ. Pain and treatment of pain in minority patients with cancer. The Eastern Cooperative Oncology Group Minority Outpatient Pain Study. *Ann Intern Med.* Nov 1 1997;127(9):813–816.

7. Kanner RM, Portenoy RK. Unavailability of narcotic analgesics for ambulatory cancer patients in New York City. *J Pain Symptom Manage.* Spring 1986;1(2):87–89.

8. Morrison RS, Wallenstein S, Natale DK, Senzel RS, Huang LL. "We don't carry that"—failure of pharmacies in predominantly nonwhite neighborhoods to stock opioid analgesics. *N Engl J Med.* Apr 6 2000;342(14):1023–1026.

9. Jacox A, Carr DB, Payne R, et al. *Management of Cancer Pain. Clinical Practice Guideline No. 9.* Rockville, MD: Agency for Health Care Policy and Research, US Department of Health and Human Services, Public Health Services; March 1994. AHCPR publication no. 94–0592.

10. Green CR, Ndao-Brumblay SK, West B, et al. Differences in prescription opioid analgesic availability: comparing minority and white pharmacies across Michigan. *J Pain.* Oct 2005;6(10):689–699.

11. Mayer JD, Kirlin B, Rehm CD, Loeser JD. Opioid availability in outpatient pharmacies in Washington State. *Clin J Pain.* Feb 2008;24(2):120–123.

12. Foley KM. Management of cancer pain. In: DeVita VT Jr, Hellman S, Rosenberg SA, eds. *Cancer: Principles & Practice of Oncology.* 5th ed. Philadelphia: Lippincott-Raven; 1997:2820–2823.

13. International Narcotics Control Board. *Narcotic Drugs: Estimated World Requirements for 1992.* New York: United Nations; 1991.

14. World Health Organization. *The Use of Essential Drugs: Sixth Report of the WHO Expert Committee.* Geneva: World Health Organization, 1995. WHO Technical Report Series, No. 850.

15. International Narcotics Control Board. *Demand For and Supply of Opiates for Medical and Scientific Needs.* New York: United Nations, 1989.

16. International Narcotics Control Board. *Report of the International Narcotics Control Boards for 1990.* New York: United Nations; 1990.

17. Opioid Consumption Map. Available at: http://www.dcamconsortium.net. Accessed January 18, 2010.

Cross-Cultural Management of Pain

19

DISPARITIES IN TREATMENT OF CANCER PAIN IN ETHNIC MINORITY PATIENTS

KAREN O. ANDERSON, PHD, MPH

Associate Professor, Department of Symptom Research,
The University of Texas MD Anderson Cancer Center,
Houston, Texas, USA

Key Points

- Ethnic minority patients are at risk for inadequate treatment of pain associated with cancer, cancer treatment, and cancer survivorship.
- Multiple barriers related to patients, healthcare providers, and the healthcare system lead to less-than-optimal cancer pain treatment for ethnic minority patients.
- Patients who experience cancer-related pain often report attitudes, beliefs, and coping strategies that can influence their pain treatment.
- Healthcare provider–related barriers to optimal pain management may include limited knowledge and training related to cancer pain, inadequate assessment of pain, poor communication skills, and preconceptions regarding minority patients.
- Healthcare system–related barriers to optimal pain treatment may include lack of insurance or underinsurance, limited access to pain specialists, and limited availability of resources needed for high-quality pain treatment.
- Multi-component interventions are needed to reduce disparities in cancer pain and cancer pain treatment in ethnic minority patients.

INTRODUCTION

Ethnic disparities in health care and health outcomes are a major public health problem in the United States. Particularly, disparities related to cancer incidence, treatment, and outcomes have been well documented. The Institute of Medicine published a report in 1999, *The Unequal Burden of Cancer: An Assessment of NIH Research and Programs for Ethnic Minorities and the Medically Underserved,*[1] which acknowledged the unequal burden of cancer in minority patients. For example, minority patients have higher incidence rates of lung, colorectal, prostate, and cervical cancer, as compared to nonminority patients.[2] Ethnic minority patients with cancer are also more likely than nonminority patients to experience disparities in cancer treatment and outcomes. In general, minority patients with cancer are more apt than nonminority patients to experience delays in diagnosis, follow-up after positive screening tests, and the initiation of evidence-based treatment plans.[3-7] Minority patients also have disproportionately high rates of morbidity and mortality from certain types of cancer.[1,8]

Several studies have documented disparities in disease characteristics, treatment, and outcomes between African-American and white patients with cancer. For example, African-American women with breast cancer are more likely to be younger, to be diagnosed at a more advanced disease stage, and to experience higher mortality rates than white women with breast cancer.[9,10] Disparities in breast cancer treatment have also been demonstrated: African-American women are more likely than white women to undergo mastectomies and less likely to receive adjuvant treatments.[11] Among patients with colorectal cancer, African Americans have lower 5-year survival rates than whites.[2] Incidence rates for lung cancer are significantly higher for African-American men than for white men.[2] African-American men are also at risk for poorer outcomes associated with prostate cancer, as evidenced by more advanced disease stage at diagnosis, poorer performance status, younger age, and higher mortality rates than white men.[12]

DISPARITIES IN CANCER PAIN AND ITS TREATMENT

Inadequate treatment of cancer-related pain in minority patients has been reported in multiple studies over the past 15 years. Most of the research has been cross-sectional investigations of two or more ethnic groups that showed that minority patients with cancer were at risk for more severe pain than white patients.

In one of the earliest studies, over 1300 white and ethnic minority outpatients with metastatic or recurrent cancer were surveyed, and the results showed that 42% of the patients with pain were prescribed analgesics that were less potent than those recommended by the World Health Organization guidelines for cancer pain treatment.[13] Patients seen at centers treating primarily minorities were three times more likely than nonminority patients to be undertreated for pain. In a subsequent study, pain treatment was examined in 281 minority outpatients with recurrent or metastatic cancer.[14] The majority of Hispanic (74%) and African-American (59%) patients with pain did not receive sufficiently potent analgesics, given the intensity of their pain. In addition, minority patients reported less pain relief than white patients, and their pain was less likely to be adequately assessed. A later study that focused on economically disadvantaged Hispanic and African-American patients with cancer-related pain found that 65% of the patients reported severe pain (>7 on a 0–10 scale).[15] Although most patients received appropriate types of analgesics, the high levels of pain may have been associated with inadequate dosages and/or patient nonadherence to analgesic regimens. The majority of the Hispanic and African-American patients reported taking their analgesics less often than prescribed by their oncologists. In addition, the physicians underestimated the pain severity of over half the patients.

A descriptive study of 116 low-income women who had undergone breast cancer surgery found that African-American and Hispanic women were more likely to report pain and lymphedema than white women.[16] A higher number of symptoms was associated with having a lower income, being Hispanic, having undergone a mastectomy, and having received chemotherapy. Telephone interviews of older African-American and white breast cancer survivors revealed that both groups reported frequent pain, joint stiffness, and fatigue

5–9 years after diagnosis.[17] The symptoms experienced by both ethnic groups were similar, and symptom management was often inadequate.

A study of 87 multiethnic (African American, white, and Latina) women with breast cancer-related pain who were receiving care at urban outpatient oncology clinics in New York found that average pain severity was higher in Latinas with Spanish language preference and those with lower incomes.[18] Spanish language preferring Latinas also reported greater distress and perceived barriers to pain management relative to whites.

Ethnic differences in pain and symptom reports were found in a survey of 480 multiethnic cancer patients.[19] Asian Americans had the lowest pain scores on multiple types of scales, and Hispanic patients had the highest scores on visual analog, pictorial, and numerical pain scales. In contrast to previous research findings, the visual analog and verbal descriptor pain scores of the African Americans were significantly lower than those of the white and Hispanic participants. The samples, however, may not have been representative of larger population groups. All of the participants were recruited from community sites and Internet support groups. A survey study of 281 outpatients with solid tumors and cancer-related pain found African-American patients reported higher pain intensity ratings than white patients.[20]

Most of the studies of disparities in cancer-related pain have been cross-sectional. Only a few longitudinal investigations have evaluated pain in diverse samples of patients with cancer.[21–25] A clinical trial of over 1000 women with metastatic breast cancer and at least one bone metastasis included regular pain assessments for one year.[21] The results indicated that pain severity increased more rapidly in nonwhite women than in whites.

Patients with cancer-related pain often experience breakthrough pain, a transitory flare-up of moderate to severe pain in the context of well-controlled baseline pain.[26] Breakthrough pain is usually treated with rescue doses of analgesics. A recent longitudinal study that examined breakthrough pain in a sample of 68 white and 28 nonwhite patients with advanced cancer found that nonwhite patients reported significantly greater severity of breakthrough pain at its greatest and lowest intensity and at the initial assessment. Consistent with findings reported in previous research, nonwhite patients also reported greater severity of general or background pain.[24,25]

The literature on disparities in cancer pain management has generally focused on African-American and Hispanic patients. The results of a few studies indicate that other minority groups are also at risk for undertreatment of cancer-related pain. For example, focus group studies of Native Americans suggest individuals in this minority group are at risk for poor assessment and undertreatment of cancer-related pain.[27,28] Prospective longitudinal studies are needed to evaluate cancer pain management in all potentially vulnerable and underserved minority populations.

Disparities in pain management in the palliative and end-of-life care setting

Minority patients with cancer who receive palliative care in a nursing home are especially at risk for inadequate treatment of cancer-related pain. A chart review of over 13,000 Medicare recipients in nursing homes found that minority patients with cancer were less likely than nonminority patients to have a pain score recorded in their charts.[29] In addition, they were less likely to receive pain medication, even when a pain score was documented. African-American patients were 63% more likely not to receive pain treatment than white patients. A recent retrospective chart review in 12 nursing homes revealed no ethnic disparities in pain treatment.[30] White residents, however, were more likely than minority residents to have living wills, do-not-resuscitate orders, and healthcare proxies. The authors concluded that minority patients' end-of-life care, including pain management, might have been adversely affected by limited advance care planning.

A small amount of research has indicated that significant ethnic disparities exist in palliative and end-of-life care for patients with cancer. A review of the literature on palliative care for women with breast cancer concluded that differences in pain management and the use of hospice care exist between African-American and white women.[31] The findings suggest that these differences adversely affect pain-related outcomes and quality of life for African-American women with breast cancer.

Minority patients with cancer are less likely than nonminority cancer patients to enroll in hospice care. For example, fewer than 9% of patients who receive hospice care in the United States are African American, and fewer than 6% are Hispanic.[1,32] Similarly, most patients who receive Medicare hospice benefits are white.[33] Economic barriers to palliative and end-of-life care for minority patients include the lack of health insurance or inadequate insurance.[34] Limited knowledge of hospice procedures and goals among minority patients and their physicians may also contribute to limited hospice enrollment. Cultural values and beliefs regarding end-of-life care also affect hospice enrollment.[35,36] Given that optimal pain management is an important goal of hospice care, the limited utilization of hospice programs by minority patients with cancer may contribute to increased pain and disparities in pain treatment at the end of life.

A study of 90 patients with advanced cancer, congestive heart failure, or chronic obstructive pulmonary disease who were receiving palliative care in a general medicine clinic found no significant differences among minority groups with regard to their self-reports of pain.[37] The African-American, Hispanic, and Asian-American patients, however, reported more severe pain than white patients. Pain treatment was generally inadequate for all patients, as indicated by the limited number of opioid prescriptions. A cross-sectional study of patients with cancer who were receiving pain medications from home health or hospice agencies found that Hispanic patients reported more severe "worst" pain ratings than non-Hispanic white and African-American patients.[38] African-American patients, however, reported the most severe "average" pain ratings.

Cancer pain and health-related quality of life disparities

Given the disparities in cancer pain that have been noted in ethnic minority patients, it is not surprising that differences in health-related quality of life have also been found. Cancer-related pain has been associated with impaired quality of life in diverse samples of patients with cancer.[39] Several studies of men with prostate cancer have found that minority men reported lower quality of life and physical well-being than nonminority men.[40–43] A longitudinal study of men age 65 or older with newly diagnosed prostate cancer found that African-American men reported a lower quality of life at baseline than white men.[22] In addition, African-American men reported more severe pain and urinary symptoms at the end of one year. Rao et al studied a large sample of patients with diverse types of cancer.[44] Compared to white patients, African-American patients reported greater malaise (i.e., "feeling ill") and a lower ability to work but less severe fatigue and treatment side effects. Overall, African-American patients reported poorer social and physical well-being and physical functioning but better emotional well-being than white patients. A recent survey of cancer survivors in Michigan found that almost 20% of the survivors reported current pain.[45] The African-American survey respondents reported greater pain severity since diagnosis and more pain-related interference and disability than white respondents.

Factors associated with disparities in cancer pain and cancer pain treatment

Multiple barriers to optimal pain treatment for ethnic minority patients are related to patients, healthcare providers, and the healthcare system. Barriers related to patients may include differences in pain sensitivity, thresholds, and tolerance among ethnic groups, as discussed in Chapter 21. Genetic factors also may play a role in cancer pain disparities . In addition, the patients' attitudes and beliefs about pain often impact their pain treatment and outcomes. Provider-related barriers often include a lack of knowledge and training related to cancer pain, inadequate assessment and treatment of pain, ineffective communication skills, and preconceptions regarding minority patients. Minority patients also face barriers in the healthcare system that can prevent optimal pain treatment, including the lack of insurance or underinsurance, limited access to care, and limited availability of the resources needed for optimal pain management.

Patient-related variables

Patients who experience cancer-related pain often report beliefs and coping strategies that can influence their pain treatment and outcomes.[46-49] For example, patients with cancer are often most concerned about treating their underlying disease and do not want to distract their physicians from focusing on cancer therapies such as chemotherapy, radiotherapy, or immunotherapy. Patients also may have fears related to their pain, such as concerns that the pain cannot be controlled or that pain indicates disease progression. Several studies have found that minority patients with cancer report some concerns about pain more frequently than nonminority patients.[15,47,49-51] For example, many Hispanic and African-American patients endorse stoicism and the belief that cancer pain is inevitable.[38,50-52] They are often concerned about taking opioids because they fear that they will become addicted, develop tolerance, or experience severe side effects.[14,15,50] Many minority patients rely on alternative and complementary pain treatments and prefer to take analgesics only when pain is very severe.[38,50,53,54] They are also more likely to believe that gender and ethnicity influence access to pain care and to feel they should have been referred to a pain specialist sooner.[55]

In addition to these beliefs, strategies for coping with cancer pain may vary among ethnic groups.[54,56] Several studies have found ethnic differences in coping with non-cancer-related pain. For example, African-American and Hispanic patients with chronic non-cancer-related pain are more likely than non-Hispanic whites to use prayer and other religious coping strategies.[57-61] Tan and colleagues found that African-American patients with chronic non-cancer-related pain were more apt than white patients to use external coping strategies that were associated with increased emotional distress and disability.[62] Future research should evaluate possible ethnic variability in coping with cancer-related pain and the relationship between coping and pain outcomes.

Patients' self-efficacy or confidence in their ability to cope with cancer and cancer-related pain also may influence pain outcomes. A survey of outpatients with cancer-related pain found that perceptions of their control over pain helped to explain ethnic differences in pain-related distress and function.[20] Only disparities in pain intensity between African-American and white patients remained when perceptions of control over pain were held constant. A recent study of a diverse sample of breast cancer patients with pain found that self-efficacy for seeking and understanding medical information was associated with fewer reported barriers to pain management.[18]

Healthcare provider-related variables

Relatively little research has examined provider-related variables that contribute to ethnic disparities in cancer pain and its treatment. Accurate and regular pain assessment is needed for physicians to provide quality pain treatment. Ethnicity can affect pain assessment, especially if a language or other cultural barrier exists. Research results have documented that physicians often underestimate the severity of cancer-related pain in minority patients.[14,15]

Physicians and nurses treating low-income minority patients with cancer were asked to rank a list of potential barriers to optimal cancer-pain management in their clinical settings.[15] Inadequate pain assessment and insufficient staff knowledge regarding cancer pain treatment were reported as the most significant barriers by more than half the healthcare providers. A lack of staff time to attend to patients' pain was also described as a significant barrier. Physicians, nurses, and other healthcare providers often receive limited education on pain assessment and treatment during their training. Multiple studies have found that many clinicians lack expertise in pain treatment and the ability to provide culturally competent care for ethnic minority patients.[15,63–65]

The ethnicity and language skills of the provider may influence outcomes. Research findings have suggested that patients can relate to and interact more with providers who share their values and cultural background.[66] A study of African-American and white patients with lung cancer who were receiving treatment at a Veterans Affairs medical center found that ethnic discordance between patients and physicians did not predict physicians' information-giving. However, analysis of information-giving that was prompted by the patient showed that patients in a ethnically concordant consultation received more information-giving statements from their physicians.[67] A recent review of patient-provider ethnic concordance, however, did not conclusively support the hypothesis that patient-provider ethnic concordance is associated with positive health outcomes for minority patients.[68]

Recent research suggests that other provider characteristics may influence pain treatment and outcomes.[69] In a study of Medicare recipients, Bach and colleagues found that African-American patients were more likely than white patients to have primary care physicians who were not board certified and who reported difficulty achieving high-quality care for their patients and obtaining access to high-quality subspecialists' services.[70] The empathy of the healthcare provider also may influence the adequacy of pain treatment. In three recent laboratory experiments, undergraduate students and nurses enrolled in graduate school watched videos of African-American and white patients' facial expressions of pain and provided pain treatment recommendations.[71] The subjects demonstrated significant pain treatment biases in favor of white patients. An empathy-inducing, perspective-taking intervention required the subjects to imagine how the patients' pain affected their lives. The subjects who participated in the intervention exhibited a 55% reduction in pain treatment bias compared to a control group who did not participate in the intervention.

Overall, currently available research indicates that patients' ethnicity influences the quality of pain management delivered by healthcare providers. Variability in the assessment and treatment of pain in minority patients has been well documented. Additional research is needed to investigate how provider-related variables contribute to disparities in pain assessment and treatment. Further evaluation of provider interventions is also needed to promote optimal pain treatment for all patients.

Healthcare System-related Variables

Minorities and individuals with limited incomes are more likely to be uninsured or underinsured than nonminorities and people with higher incomes.[72] The lack of adequate health insurance limits access to the evaluation and treatment of all types of pain, including cancer-related pain. Although federal and state health insurance programs such as Medicare and Medicaid are designed to help the elderly, persons with disabilities, and children from low-income families, these programs provide less-than-optimal coverage for pain management. The availability and cost of analgesic medications are additional barriers to pain treatment. The results of a recent survey indicated that African-American individuals were more likely than whites to report an inability to afford health care and difficulty paying for health care despite having insurance. Moreover, chronic pain was described by the African-American respondents as a major problem, even when they had access to pain specialists.[55] The minority respondents also believed that ethnicity, ethnocultural groups, and gender influenced access to health care and pain treatment.

In addition to individual income and socioeconomic status, the socioeconomic level of patients' neighborhoods also can influence access to healthcare services such as pain treatment programs.[73] When patients do receive pain treatment, substandard living conditions and other structural barriers in neighborhoods may adversely affect pain treatment outcomes.[74] For example, limited availability of opioids in pharmacies located in minority neighborhoods has been documented.[75,76] Research has demonstrated that minority patients remain at risk for disparities in pain treatment even when neighborhood socioeconomic status is held constant.[77]

STRATEGIES FOR REDUCING DISPARITIES IN CANCER PAIN TREATMENT

Interventions for reducing disparities in cancer pain treatment have focused on the patient, the healthcare provider, or the healthcare system.

Previous research suggested that patients could benefit from education in pain management that addresses patient-related barriers. Several randomized clinical trials with largely nonminority samples of patients with cancer found that education on pain management produced significant reductions in pain intensity ratings.[78–82] Our randomized clinical trial of underserved African-American and Hispanic patients with cancer, however, found that education alone did not improve the long-term pain experience of the minority patients.[83] The results suggested that patients might benefit more from individualized education that targets specific patient-related barriers.

A recent randomized trial evaluated an individualized pain education and communication intervention in female patients with breast cancer. Patients with pain in the intervention group received 30 minutes of individualized education on barriers to pain treatment and also received training in communicating with their physician about their pain.[84] The intervention group patients reported a significant decrease in barriers to pain management (e.g., concerns about analgesic addiction) but not in pain severity. The patients who reported fewer barriers demonstrated less distress and better emotional well-being. The patients who scored higher in active communication (e.g., asking questions, giving information) reported fewer barriers and better pain relief. The women who viewed their physicians as being more receptive reported better pain management.

Provider-based interventions that focus on implementing recommended pain treatment protocols (e.g., National Comprehensive Cancer Network pain treatment guidelines) for all patients are needed.[85,86] Research that evaluates pain treatment guidelines should include an analysis of the efficacy of pain treatment for minority patients. Training healthcare providers in empathy, communication skills, the appropriate use of interpreters, and cultural competence are other promising interventions that need further development.

One recent laboratory study found that perceptual training to differentiate other-race faces led to reduced ethnic bias.[87] A model of shared decision-making between the patient and healthcare provider may also encourage patients to be partners in their pain treatment.

Many patients with cancer, especially those with metastatic disease, require opioid medications for cancer-related pain. One healthcare system barrier to optimal pain management for minority patients has been the decreased availability of opioid medications in minority neighborhood pharmacies. Research that evaluates strategies to ensure access to opioids and other pain medications in minority neighborhoods is needed. Given the multiple patient, provider, and healthcare system variables related to cancer pain treatment disparities, multi-component interventions are needed to reduce disparities in pain and pain treatment among ethnic minority patients.

CONCLUSIONS

Ethnic disparities in cancer pain have been well documented in the literature. Most of the research to date has focused on African-American and Hispanic patients with cancer-related pain. Multiple studies across adult age ranges and treatment settings have found that cancer pain in these populations is often inadequately assessed and treated. Very few studies have included other ethnic groups, such as Asian American, Arab American, native Hawaiian, Pacific Islander, Native American, or Alaskan native. Heterogeneity within the ethnic groups that have been studied has also not been addressed. For example, subgroups within the non-Hispanic white population have ethnic identities that can influence pain treatment.[88,89] In addition, very little research has evaluated possible disparities in the treatment of cancer-related pain in pediatric patients.[90] The literature on pediatric pain suggests that children with cancer are vulnerable to poor assessment and undertreatment of pain.[91] Studies of possible disparities in pediatric cancer pain related to minority status and developmental stage are needed.

A patient's country of origin, immigration status, and years in the United States are additional variables that may influence cancer pain and treatment outcomes. Acculturation is a related variable that may affect individuals' experiences of cancer pain as well as their interactions with healthcare providers and the healthcare system. Acculturation is defined as a process in which individuals in one cultural group adopt the beliefs and behaviors of another (typically dominant) group in a society.[92] Future research on pain-related disparities should address the issues of acculturation and ethnic group heterogeneity and how they may affect pain treatment and outcomes.

Although a few promising interventions to reduce cancer pain disparities have been developed, more research is needed to develop multi-component and multi-level interventions that target healthcare providers, patients, and the healthcare system. In an age of healthcare reform, reducing disparities in cancer pain and cancer pain treatment should be an important public health issue and priority.

ACKNOWLEDGMENTS

Supported by American Cancer Society grant #RSGT-05–219–01-CPPB.

REFERENCES

1. Haynes MA, Smedley BD, Institute of Medicine, Committee on Cancer Research among Minorities and the Medically Underserved. *The Unequal Burden of Cancer—an Assessment of NIH Research and Programs for Ethnic Minorities and the Medically Underserved.* Washington, DC: National Academies Press; 1999.

2. Jemal A, Siegel R, Xu J, Ward E. Cancer statistics, 2010. *CA Cancer J Clin.* 2010;60(5):277–300.

3. Elmore JG, Nakano CY, Linden HM, Reisch LM, Ayanian JZ, Larson EB. Racial inequities in the timing of breast cancer detection, diagnosis, and initiation of treatment. *Med Care.* 2005;43(2):141–148.

4. Kerner JF, Yedidia M, Padgett D, et al. Realizing the promise of breast cancer screening: clinical follow-up after abnormal screening among Black women. *Prev Med.* 2003;37(2):92–101.

5. Shavers VL, Brown ML. Racial and ethnic disparities in the receipt of cancer treatment. *J Natl Cancer Inst.* 2002;94(5):334–357.

6. Shavers VL, Harlan LC, Winn D, Davis WW. Racial/ethnic patterns of care for cancers of the oral cavity, pharynx, larynx, sinuses, and salivary glands. *Cancer Metastasis Rev.* 2003;22(1):25–38.

7. Shavers VL, Harlan LC, Stevens JL. Racial/ethnic variation in clinical presentation, treatment, and survival among breast cancer patients under age 35. *Cancer.* 2003;97(1):134–147.

8. Newman LA, Griffith KA, Jatoi I, Simon MS, Crowe JP, Colditz GA. Meta-analysis of survival in African American and white American patients with breast cancer: ethnicity compared with socioeconomic status. *J Clin Oncol.* 2006;24(9):1342–1349.

9. Newman LA, Carolin K, Simon M, et al. Impact of breast carcinoma on African-American women: the Detroit experience. *Cancer.* 2001;91(9):1834–1843.

10. Shinagawa SM. The excess burden of breast carcinoma in minority and medically underserved communities: application, research, and redressing institutional racism. *Cancer.* 2000;88(suppl 5):1217–1223.

11. Tammemagi CM. Racial/ethnic disparities in breast and gynecologic cancer treatment and outcomes. *Curr Opin Obstet Gynecol.* 2007;19(1):31–36.

12. Mettlin CJ, Murphy GP, Cunningham MP, Menck HR. The National Cancer Data Base report on race, age, and region variations in prostate cancer treatment. *Cancer.* 1997;80(7):1261–1266.

13. Cleeland CS, Gonin R, Hatfield AK, et al. Pain and its treatment in outpatients with metastatic cancer. *N Engl J Med.* 1994;330(9):592–596.

14. Cleeland CS, Gonin R, Baez L, Loehrer P, Pandya KJ. Pain and treatment of pain in minority patients with cancer. The Eastern Cooperative Oncology Group Minority Outpatient Pain Study. *Ann Intern Med.* 1997;127(9):813–816.

15. Anderson KO, Mendoza TR, Valero V, et al. Minority cancer patients and their providers: pain management attitudes and practice. *Cancer.* 2000;88(8):1929–1938.

16. Eversley R, Estrin D, Dibble S, Wardlaw L, Pedrosa M, Favila-Penney W. Post-treatment symptoms among ethnic minority breast cancer survivors. *Oncol Nurs Forum.* 2005;32(2):250–256.

17. Gill KM, Mishel M, Belyea M, et al. Triggers of uncertainty about recurrence and long-term treatment side effects in older African American and Caucasian breast cancer survivors. *Oncol Nurs Forum.* 2004;31(3):633–639.

18. Mosher CE, Duhamel KN, Egert J, Smith MY. Self-efficacy for coping with cancer in a multiethnic sample of breast cancer patients: associations with barriers to pain management and distress. *Clin J Pain.* 2010;26(3):227–234.

19. Im EO, Chee W, Guevara E, et al. Gender and ethnic differences in cancer pain experience: a multiethnic survey in the United States. *Nurs Res.* 2007;56(5):296–306.

20. Vallerand AH, Hasenau S, Templin T, Collins-Bohler D. Disparities between black and white patients with cancer pain: the effect of perception of control over pain. *Pain Med.* 2005;6(3):242–250.

21. Castel LD, Saville BR, Depuy V, Godley PA, Hartmann KE, Abernethy AP. Racial differences in pain during 1 year among women with metastatic breast cancer: a hazards analysis of interval-censored data. *Cancer.* 2008;112(1):162–170.

22. Jayadevappa R, Johnson JC, Chhatre S, Wein AJ, Malkowicz SB. Ethnic variation in return to baseline values of patient-reported outcomes in older prostate cancer patients. *Cancer.* 2007;109(11):2229–2238.

23. Bonham VL. Race, ethnicity, and pain treatment: striving to understand the causes and solutions to the disparities in pain treatment. *J Law Med Ethics.* 2001;29(1):52–68.

24. Green CR, Montague L, Hart-Johnson TA. Consistent and breakthrough pain in diverse advanced cancer patients: a longitudinal examination. *J Pain Symptom Manage.* 2009;37(5):831–847.

25. Montague L, Green CR. Cancer and breakthrough pain's impact on a diverse population. *Pain Med.* 2009;10(3):549–561.

26. Portenoy RK, Hagen NA. Breakthrough pain: definition, prevalence and characteristics. *Pain.* 1990;41(3):273–281.

27. Hutson SP, Dorgan KA, Phillips AN, Behringer B. The mountains hold things in: the use of community research review work groups to address cancer disparities in Appalachia. *Oncol Nurs Forum.* 2007;34(6):1133–1139.

28. Elliott BA, Johnson KM, Elliott TE, Day JJ. Enhancing Cancer Pain Control among American Indians (ECPCAI): a study of the Ojibwe of Minnesota. *J Cancer Educ.* 1999;14(1):28–33.

29. Bernabei R, Gambassi G, Lapane K, et al. Management of pain in elderly patients with cancer. SAGE Study Group. Systematic Assessment of Geriatric Drug Use via Epidemiology. *JAMA.* 1998;279(23):1877–1882.

.30. Reynolds KS, Hanson LC, Henderson M, Steinhauser KE. End-of-life care in nursing home settings: do race or age matter? *Palliat Support Care.* 2008;6:21–27.

31. Payne R, Medina E, Hampton JW. Quality of life concerns in patients with breast cancer: evidence for disparity of outcomes and experiences in pain management and palliative care among African-American women. *Cancer.* 2003;97(suppl 1):311–317.

32. NHPCO Facts and Figures: Hospice Care in America. Alexandria, VA: National Hospice and Palliative Care Organization, January 2012.

33. Christakis NA, Escarce JJ. Survival of Medicare patients after enrollment in hospice programs. *N Engl J Med.* 1996;335(3):172–178.

34. Francoeur RB, Payne R, Raveis VH, Shim H. Palliative care in the inner city. Patient religious affiliation, underinsurance, and symptom attitude. *Cancer.* 2007;109(suppl 2):425–434.

35. Crawley L, Payne R, Bolden J, Payne T, Washington P, Williams S. Palliative and end-of-life care in the African American community. *JAMA.* 2000;284(19):2518–2521.

36. Reese DJ, Ahern RE, Nair S, O'Faire JD, Warren C. Hospice access and use by African Americans: addressing cultural and institutional barriers through participatory action research. *Soc Work.* 1999;44(6):549–559.

37. Rabow MW, Dibble SL. Ethnic differences in pain among outpatients with terminal and end-stage chronic illness. *Pain Med.* 2005;6(3):235–241.

38. Juarez G, Ferrell B, Borneman T. Cultural considerations in education for cancer pain management. *J Cancer Educ.* 1999;14(3):168–173.

39. Wang XS, Cleeland CS, Mendoza TR, et al. The effects of pain severity on health-related quality of life: a study of Chinese cancer patients. *Cancer.* 1999;86(9):1848–1855.

40. Eton DT, Lepore SJ, Helgeson VS. Early quality of life in patients with localized prostate carcinoma: an examination of treatment-related, demographic, and psychosocial factors. *Cancer.* 2001;92(6):1451–1459.

41. Krupski TL, Sonn G, Kwan L, Maliski S, Fink A, Litwin MS. Ethnic variation in health-related quality of life among low-income men with prostate cancer. *Ethn Dis.* 2005;15(3):461–468.

42. Lubeck DP, Kim H, Grossfeld G, et al. Health related quality of life differences between black and white men with prostate cancer: data from the cancer of the prostate strategic urologic research endeavor. *J Urol.* 2001;166(6):2281–2285.

43. Penedo FJ, Dahn JR, Shen BJ, Schneiderman N, Antoni MH. Ethnicity and determinants of quality of life after prostate cancer treatment. *Urology.* 2006;67(5):1022–1027.

44. Rao D, Debb S, Blitz D, Choi SW, Cella D. Racial/Ethnic differences in the health-related quality of life of cancer patients. *J Pain Symptom Manage.* 2008;36(5):488–496.

45. Green CR, Hart-Johnson T, Loeffler DR. Cancer-related chronic pain: Examining quality of life in diverse cancer survivors. *Cancer.* 2011;117(9):1994–2003.

46. Cleeland C. Research in cancer pain. What we know and what we need to know. *Cancer.* 1991;67(suppl 3): 823–827.

47. Meghani SH, Keane A. Preference for analgesic treatment for cancer pain among African Americans. *J Pain Symptom Manage.* 2007;34(2):136–147.

48. Ward SE, Goldberg N, Miller-McCauley V, et al. Patient-related barriers to management of cancer pain. *Pain.* 1993;52(3):319–324.

49. Ward SE, Hernandez L. Patient-related barriers to management of cancer pain in Puerto Rico. *Pain.* 1994;58(2):233–238.

50. Anderson KO, Richman SP, Hurley J, et al. Cancer pain management among underserved minority outpatients: perceived needs and barriers to optimal control. *Cancer.* 2002;94(8):2295–2304.

51. Meghani SH, Houldin AD. The meanings of and attitudes about cancer pain among African Americans. *Oncol Nurs Forum.* 2007;34(6):1179–1186.

52. Im EO, Lim HJ, Clark M, Chee W. African American cancer patients' pain experience. *Cancer Nurs.* 2008;31(1):38–46.

53. Juarez G, Ferrell B, Borneman T. Influence of culture on cancer pain management in Hispanic patients. *Cancer Pract.* 1998;6(5):262–269.

54. Campbell LC, Andrews N, Scipio C, Flores B, Feliu MH, Keefe FJ. Pain coping in Latino populations. *J Pain.* 2009;10(10):1012–1019.

55. Green CR, Baker TA, Ndao-Brumblay SK. Patient attitudes regarding healthcare utilization and referral: a descriptive comparison in African- and Caucasian Americans with chronic pain. *J Natl Med Assoc.* 2004;96(1):31–42.

56. Green CR, Anderson KO, Baker TA, et al. The unequal burden of pain: confronting racial and ethnic disparities in pain. *Pain Med.* 2003;4(3):277–294.

57. braido-Lanza AF, Vasquez E, Echeverria SE. En las manos de Dios [in God's hands]: Religious and other forms of coping among Latinos with arthritis. *J Consult Clin Psychol.* 2004;72(1):91–102.

58. Cano A, Mayo A, Ventimiglia M. Coping, pain severity, interference, and disability: the potential mediating and moderating roles of race and education. *J Pain.* 2006;7(7):459–468.

59. Edwards RR, Moric M, Husfeldt B, Buvanendran A, Ivankovich O. Ethnic similarities and differences in the chronic pain experience: a comparison of African American, Hispanic, and white patients. *Pain Med.* 2005;6(1):88–98.

60. Griswold GA, Evans S, Spielman L, Fishman B. Coping strategies of HIV patients with peripheral neuropathy. *AIDS Care.* 2005;17(6):711–720.

61. Jordan MS, Lumley MA, Leisen JC. The relationships of cognitive coping and pain control beliefs to pain and adjustment among African-American and Caucasian women with rheumatoid arthritis. *Arthritis Care Res.* 1998;11(2):80–88.

62. Tan G, Jensen MP, Thornby J, Anderson KO. Ethnicity, control appraisal, coping, and adjustment to chronic pain among black and white Americans. *Pain Med.* 2005;6(1):18–28.

63. Green CR, Wheeler JR, LaPorte F. Clinical decision making in pain management: Contributions of physician and patient characteristics to variations in practice. *J Pain.* 2003;4(1):29–39.

64. van Ryn M. Research on the provider contribution to race/ethnicity disparities in medical care. *Med Care.* 2002;40(suppl 1):I140-I151.

65. Von Roenn JH, Cleeland CS, Gonin R, Hatfield AK, Pandya KJ. Physician attitudes and practice in cancer pain management. A survey from the Eastern Cooperative Oncology Group. *Ann Intern Med.* 1993;119(2):121–126.

66. Bissell P, May CR, Noyce PR. From compliance to concordance: barriers to accomplishing a re-framed model of health care interactions. *Soc Sci Med.* 2004;58(4):851–862.

67. Gordon HS, Street RL, Jr., Sharf BF, Souchek J. Racial differences in doctors' information-giving and patients' participation. *Cancer.* 2006;107(6):1313–1320.

68. Meghani SH, Brooks JM, Gipson-Jones T, Waite R, Whitfield-Harris L, Deatrick JA. Patient-provider race-concordance: does it matter in improving minority patients' health outcomes? *Ethn Health.* 2009;14(1):107–130.

69. Payne R. Racially based disparities in pain management: something old, something new, but what to do? *Pain Med.* 2009;10(3):432–434.

70. Bach PB, Pham HH, Schrag D, Tate RC, Hargraves JL. Primary care physicians who treat blacks and whites. *N Engl J Med.* 2004;351(6):575–584.

71. Drwecki BB, Moore CF, Ward SE, Prkachin KM. Reducing racial disparities in pain treatment: The role of empathy and perspective-taking. *Pain.* 2011;152(5):1001–1006.

72. Garson A Jr. The uninsured: problems, solutions, and the role of academic medicine. *Acad Med.* 2006;81(9):798–801.

73. Fiscella K, Franks P, Gold MR, Clancy CM. Inequalities in racial access to health care. *JAMA.* 2000;284(16):2053.

74. Ward E, Jemal A, Cokkinides V, et al. Cancer disparities by race/ethnicity and socioeconomic status. *CA Cancer J Clin.* 2004;54(2):78–93.

75. Green CR, Ndao-Brumblay SK, West B, Washington T. Differences in prescription opioid analgesic availability: comparing minority and white pharmacies across Michigan. *J Pain.* 2005;6(10):689–699.

76. Morrison RS, Wallenstein S, Natale DK, Senzel RS, Huang LL. "We don't carry that"—failure of pharmacies in predominantly nonwhite neighborhoods to stock opioid analgesics. *N Engl J Med.* 2000;342(14):1023–1026.

77. Fuentes M, Hart-Johnson T, Green CR. The association among neighborhood socioeconomic status, race and chronic pain in black and white older adults. *J Natl Med Assoc.* 2007;99(10):1160–1169.

78. de Wit R, van Dam F, Zandbelt L, et al. A pain education program for chronic cancer pain patients: follow-up results from a randomized controlled trial. *Pain.* 1997;73(1):55–69.

79. Miaskowski C, Dodd M, West C, et al. Randomized clinical trial of the effectiveness of a self-care intervention to improve cancer pain management. *J Clin Oncol.* 2004;22(9):1713–1720.

80. Oliver JW, Kravitz RL, Kaplan SH, Meyers FJ. Individualized patient education and coaching to improve pain control among cancer outpatients. *J Clin Oncol.* 2001;19(8):2206–2212.

81. Syrjala KL, Abrams JR, Polissar NL, et al. Patient training in cancer pain management using integrated print and video materials: a multisite randomized controlled trial. *Pain.* 2008;135(1–2):175–186.

82. Wells N, Hepworth JT, Murphy BA, Wujcik D, Johnson R. Improving cancer pain management through patient and family education. *J Pain Symptom Manage.* 2003;25(4):344–356.

83. Anderson KO, Mendoza TR, Payne R, et al. Pain education for underserved minority cancer patients: a randomized controlled trial. *J Clin Oncol.* 2004;22(24):4918–4925.

84. Smith MY, Duhamel KN, Egert J, Winkel G. Impact of a brief intervention on patient communication and barriers to pain management: results from a randomized controlled trial. *Patient Educ Couns.* 2010;81(1):79–86.

85. Du Pen SL, Du Pen AR, Polissar N, et al. Implementing guidelines for cancer pain management: results of a randomized controlled clinical trial. *J Clin Oncol.* 1999;17(1):361–370.

86. Trowbridge R, Dugan W, Jay SJ, et al. Determining the effectiveness of a clinical-practice intervention in improving the control of pain in outpatients with cancer. *Acad Med.* 1997;72(9):798–800.

87. Lebrecht S, Pierce LJ, Tarr MJ, Tanaka JW. Perceptual other-race training reduces implicit racial bias. *PLoS ONE.* 2009;4(1):e4215.

88. Bates MS, Edwards WT, Anderson KO. Ethnocultural influences on variation in chronic pain perception. *Pain.* 1993;52(1):101–112.

89. Bates MS, Rankin-Hill L. Control, culture and chronic pain. *Soc Sci Med.* 1994;39(5):629–645.

90. Linton JM, Feudtner C. What accounts for differences or disparities in pediatric palliative and end-of-life care? A systematic review focusing on possible multilevel mechanisms. *Pediatrics.* 2008;122(3):574–582.

91. McGrath PJ, Walco GA, Turk DC, et al. Core outcome domains and measures for pediatric acute and chronic/recurrent pain clinical trials: PedIMMPACT recommendations. *J Pain.* 2008;9(9):771–783.

92. Palos G. Cultural heritage: cancer screening and early detection. *Semin Oncol Nurs.* 1994;10(2):104–113.

20

THE PAIN OF CHILDBIRTH

Management Among Culturally Diverse Women

LYNN CLARK CALLISTER, RN, PHD, FAAN
Professor Emerita, Brigham Young University College
of Nursing, Provo, Utah, USA

Key Points
- Childbirth is a significant and often pivotal life event
- Perspectives of childbirth pain vary according to women's sociocultural context.
- Barriers to effective pain management exist and should be overcome.
- Use of the Coping with Labor Algorithm is appropriate for childbirth pain assessment.
- Demonstrating respect and providing essential support for culturally diverse childbearing women will contribute to ensuring quality birth experiences.

The transforming care for childbearing women initiative includes improving the cultural competence of health professionals through promoting cultural shifts in attitudes, suggesting that "childbirth is a meaningful process that can be profoundly transformative for women and families, and not just a clinical event." [1] An anthropologist has noted that "every culture ritualizes birth, as it is one of the most significant rites of passage in the social life of mother and child." [2] Giving birth is a pivotal life event. [3] There is a paucity of literature on the perceptions of the pain of childbirth in culturally diverse women. [4–6]

Pain is culturally bound. [7] Researchers have concluded that "bio-psychosocial influences of culture can alter the development of neural systems, cognitions, and behaviors that affect the sensation of pain, its experience, and its expression." [8]

This chapter focuses on the expression and language of the childbirth pain experience and the meaning of such pain. It also describes how childbirth pain is managed, including cultural practices and the use of spirituality and/or religious observances. Barriers to effective pain management and implications for clinical practice in caring for culturally diverse childbearing women are explicated.

ATTITUDES, PERCEPTIONS AND MEANING: CULTURE AND CHILDBIRTH PAIN

The theoretical model for this chapter focuses on a culture and pain model adapted from the work of Lasch[9] and includes variables such as the woman and significant others, cultural beliefs and behaviors, as well as interactions with and responses to clinicians and healthcare systems (see Figure 20.1).

Few studies have been conducted on culture and pain in childbearing women. In a study of nulliparous Danish and Swedish women, fear of childbirth at 37 weeks gestation was positively correlated with fear at admission to the hospital in active labor.[10] In another study of Dutch women, negative recall of their birth experience three years later was associated with lack of choice for pain relief and being dissatisfied with how the women coped with pain.[11] In Belgian and Dutch women, a sense of personal control buffered the impact of their labor pain.[12]

In a comparative study of pain behaviors in Jewish and Arabic women giving birth, it was noted that behavioral expressions of pain differ. Arabic women were more vocal, crying and screaming, while Jewish women verbalized their pain, moaned, and some women wept.[13]

Perceptions of childbirth pain in culturally diverse women from North and Central America, Scandinavia, the Middle East, the People's Republic of China, and Tonga have been documented.[7,14] Childbirth was perceived as a bittersweet experience, with contrasting word descriptors used by women speaking of their birth experiences as "painful but beautiful," or "exhausting and exhilarating," or "difficult yet empowering."[6]

Data from cross-cultural qualitative studies of Australian, Armenian, Ecuadorian, Chinese, Dutch, Ghanaian, East Indian, and Russian childbearing women also document their perceptions of the pain of childbirth. Giving birth within differing sociocultural contexts with varying healthcare delivery models means that women's experiences are unique and varied globally. Pain may be perceived as an expected part of the mortal experience, or it may be perceived as deserved punishment. Some women view the pain of childbirth as an opportunity for personal growth and character, or pain may be associated with serious complications. Some women may take a fatalistic approach to the pain of childbirth, and others may feel helpless and vulnerable in the face of pain.[14] Narratives and analysis of these studies related to pain perceptions are described.

Armenian Women

Armenian women give birth in hospitals without medication unless they opt to pay privately for facilities where epidural analgesia may be available. Armenian women are often

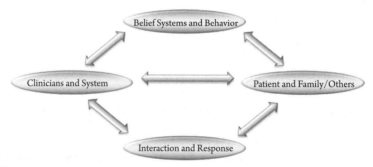

FIGURE 20.1 Culture and pain management model

without their significant others in the birthing room. Pain is an expected part of giving birth. One said, "I was offered painkillers but I refused … At that moment I thought that if this is natural pain and everyone is going through it, then I can do it, too." While the women expected birth to be painful, they sometimes underestimated the intensity of the experience. As one woman described: "I knew that it was going to be painful, but I had no idea that it would be that painful."[15]

Australian Women

In a study of Australian women giving birth in birthing centers and hospitals, birth was viewed as a challenge. While pharmacological methods of pain relief are available, some Australian women choose not to use them. One woman made meaning of giving birth, viewing it as symbolic of managing life challenges. "[Giving birth] makes you more resilient. You know you are able to handle things that you didn't think you could. I think it gives you strength because you know if you can get through that, you can cope with a lot of other things."[16]

One Australian first-time mother described why she decided to have an epidural:

It was just more intense than I thought it would be. Again—what do you expect? You just don't know what to expect in the first place. It was painful—the labor pain was intense and nothing helped. Showering didn't help. Being in the right position didn't help. They told me I was dilated to six centimeters. I thought, "Oh my God." That's when I said, "I can't do this for another four centimeters. I need an epidural." Once the epidural was in, I was a different person. I was much more relaxed. Then I had more excitement that he was coming.[16]

Another Australian woman described being empowered by giving birth. She contrasted her first birth experience with her second birth, which was unmedicated.

[During my first birth with epidural analgesia], I was awake, but I was numb. With my second birth, I experienced full-on labor, and that was just the most amazing experience. Oh my gosh, you think you are going to die. So I'm glad I went through it and I'm amazed that I did it. My body is capable of a lot more pain than I give it credit for! Your body is amazing and is designed to give birth. Mothers all over the world have done it, and I did it![16]

Chinese women

For Chinese childbearing women living in the People's Republic of China (PRC), giving birth may literally be a once in a lifetime experience.[17,18] Cesarean births by maternal request in the PRC are common because women have only one birth and want to avoid the pain of labor. The meaning of the birth experience, however, is not diminished by experiencing pain. One Chinese woman reported:

It was so painful. The nurses didn't give me pain medicine; they just encouraged me to keep going. I was so tired and in so much pain. I didn't think I could handle it. I hurt for a long time. It really was painful. But when the time came to actually push, I just had to use my strength to push and then he just came out. The thing I remember the most was just the moment he came out. I felt like I was amazing—I could give birth to a little child. I had always prepared my heart to have a cesarean section, but that didn't happen. It made me feel really good about myself. (Unpublished data, 2009)

Another Chinese mother reflected on her feelings of self-actualization as she gave birth unmedicated: "It really was painful. I always thought I was someone that was afraid of pain, but I realized that I am actually quite brave." (Unpublished data, 2009)

Dutch Women

In a study of women living in The Netherlands who were among the 33% of Dutch women who give birth unmedicated at home, the focus was on birth as a peak experience, with pain as a difficult but not insurmountable challenge to be overcome. One woman reported that her mother told her, "It will be painful but not impossible." Another woman described her pain experience in retrospect: "I remember the pain. [It was] very strong, intense, and painful. You really get to know your spirit more. The way you act, the way you respond to the pain, the whole process is quite a mirror in a way." Another woman spoke of finding inner strength: "I really went down to my earth … The deep down feelings. You have a lot of strength … I didn't know I had it." A mother spoke of her feelings of personal strength after giving birth: "I did it! I succeeded! I am capable of doing such a thing and I am capable of being calm during the process. I felt so in touch with myself."[19]

Ecuadorian Women

For socially disadvantaged Ecuadorian women giving birth unmedicated in a large public maternity hospital, birth was viewed as a painful but time-limited moment, to be endured in order to obtain the gift of a child.[20] For example, one study participant said: "Endure it because the pains come, but then they are gone and then comes the joy because you have your baby."[20] These women expected pain and were stoic during labor and birth and passively accepted the pain, as was expressed by one young woman: "My mother told me not to scream, not to open your mouth so nothing comes out, because if not, the baby goes inside. The labor [will] get more complicated."[19] These women had what was described as "the physical, emotional and social experience of pregnancy and childbirth characterized by pain, fear, and solitude."[20]

Another Ecuadorian woman described how lack of knowledge and fear added to the traumatic intensity of her birth experience. "I felt like I was going to die. The pains came much stronger. I didn't know what to do. And then I just gave three big pushes and that was it."[21] Ecuadorian childbearing women who immigrate to the United States may exhibit stoicism and passivity during labor and birth, with the expectation of enduring childbirth pain rather than seeking to be medicated.[20]

Ghanaian Women

Ghanaian women perceive pain as an inevitable part of giving birth, noting that there is nothing more painful, even death. Many Ghanaian Christian women believe that childbirth pain is God's will, a punishment for Biblical Eve's disobedience in partaking of the forbidden fruit.[21] They give birth without labor support or pain medication and are encouraged to be stoic. Some maintain their stoicism because they fear crying out may delay the birth and result in a woman being transferred to a higher-level facility with financial consequences for the family. One new mother said: "Whether you cry or not, it doesn't make it any easier, so there's no need for you to cry or shout. You are going to give birth to the child so if there is pain or anything, you don't have to cry: You have to give birth to the child." [22] Another reported: "[The traditional birth attendant] said I should just be quiet and strengthen myself, the baby would soon come out." [22]

Ghanaian women are acutely aware of the risks of maternal and infant morbidity and mortality associated with giving birth in rural Ghana. For example, one woman defined a successful birth as "having my own life and the life of my child." [22] They rely on the strength of their spirituality and religious beliefs to sustain them. Another Ghanaian mother reported: "When I went to the clinic, I climbed [into] the hospital bed and all my thoughts at that place [the birthing room] were that God should help me. 'God, have mercy on me! Oh, help me to delivery safely!' " [22]

East Indian Women

Socially disadvantaged East Indian childbearing women in one qualitative study expressed fears and anxiety about childbirth related to lack of knowledge. One woman said that she had, "so much fear of the unknown and pain. I didn't know what to do." All but one of the study participants gave birth unmedicated because of lack of availability of pain medication. Their labor and birth experiences were influenced by their strong desire to receive the "double blessing" of having a son, and when they learned they had given birth to a daughter, these women expressed deep disappointment. They utilized warm water, massage, and walking to help manage the pain of childbirth. [23]

Russian Women

Russian women give birth in birth houses where they are attended by predominantly female physicians and educated midwives. Some are publicly funded facilities, whereas others are private. Depending on the policies of the birth house and the desires of the couple, the father of the child may or may not attend the birth. Some women report putting religious icons to put under their pillows while laboring. Participants in a qualitative study of Russian women reported that they depended on knowledgable authority figured for advice, perhaps because of the sociopolitical context of Eastern Europe. They listened to the advice of their mothers regarding cultural practices and usually followed them, "just in case." Most of them give birth unmedicated. For some, epidurals were not available; others preferred not having epidural not only because of the cost but also because of concerns about potential effects on their newborn. Kactya expressed a sense of being comforted during labor, "I think it is so important for women during that period to be surrounded by love and care." Svetlana said, "During the contractions I was only thinking, 'is it possible to love the child after this?' But when she was born and lying on my chest, she looked at me. At that time I forgot all the pain." [24]

It should be noted that most cultures have strategies for providing supportive care to childbearing women to help them manage the pain of childbirth, including "birth talk." [26] For example, the author observed the interactions between a Tongan woman experiencing her first labor, her "auntie" (a culturally designated birth companion), and the birthing nurse. As the intensity of labor increased, and the nurse offered the option of epidural analgesia, the "auntie" spoke up for the laboring woman, saying, "No, no. She's young and strong and very capable. She can do it without any drugs." Sure enough, a few moments later, with only two pushes, the young woman gave birth to her 10-pound son unmedicated!

Based on a review of the literature on childbirth and other pain, important assumptions can be made about childbirth pain and culture. [25-31] These are summarized in Table 20.1.

TABLE 20.1 Assumptions About Childbirth Pain and Culture

- Pain is REAL, complex, and intensely personal, with the individual woman the best source of pain information.
- Higher pain intensity is associated with higher levels of anxiety.
- Levels of self efficacy predict labor pain and distress.
- Women who catastrophize experience more intense pain.
- Pain has different meanings.
- Choice of childbirth pain management is dependent on sociocultural factors.
- Pain is a recognized part of giving birth.
- Long-term recall of labor pain is vivid.
- A quality birth experience can occur in the presence of pain.
- Pain is not predictive of satisfaction with giving birth.
- Appropriate pain management should include consideration of multiple complex variables contributing to childbirth pain.

BARRIERS TO EFFECTIVE PAIN MANAGEMENT

Barriers to effective pain management have been identified.[14] These are summarized in Table 20.2.

Clinical Implications

According to standards of clinical care, it is critical to "deliver care in a compassionate manner that preserves patient autonomy, dignity, safety, and rights."[32] This includes the appropriate assessment of childbirth pain.

Childbirth Pain Assessment

When assessing the pain of childbirth, it is important to understand that pain-related behaviors may range from stoicism to expressivity. If a woman is stoic, she may prefer to be left alone, to cope individually without seeking attention or care. She may keep her face "masked" and expressionless. She may worry about being perceived as being weak if she admits that she needs help, or she may deny having any pain. If a woman is expressive, she may feel that the best way to cope with the pain of childbirth is to verbalize her pain

TABLE 20.2 Barriers to Effective Pain Management

- Language difficulties when women lack English proficiency
- Nonverbal cues that may be subject to misinterpretation, such as facial expression, body posture, or activity level
- Culturally or linguistically inappropriate pain assessment tools
- Underreporting of the presence of pain
- Reluctance to use medication for pain management
- Lack of access to pain medication
- Prejudice and discrimination.

TABLE 20.3 Culturally Competent Management of Childbirth Pain

- Understand the woman as a unique person
- Explore the woman's experience with pain
- Utilize an appropriate pain assessment tool
- Perceive pain management from the woman's perspective
- Demonstrate respect for the woman's preferences for pain management
- Promote shared decision making and adapt care to meet the woman's needs and expectations.

by groaning, screaming, crying out loud, or praying. She may also cry and express anxiety about and fear of being left alone.[14]

Most acute care facilities, including birthing units in medical centers, use the Numerical Rating Scale (NRS), a 0 to 10 scale with 0 being "no pain" and 10 being "the worst possible pain."[33] Perinatal nurses recently developed the Coping with Labor Algorithm, which specifically focuses on the pain of childbirth.[34,35] The woman is asked, "How are you coping with labor?" Clues are provided in the algorithm that may indicate that the woman is not coping well, including crying/tearfulness, a tremulous voice, demonstrating the inability to focus or concentrate, manifesting panicked activity during contractions, jitteriness, sweaty, wincing/writhing or clawing/biting behaviors, or tenseness. Conversely, the caregiver may note the following if the woman is coping: she states she is coping, she is engaging in rhythmic activity, she is focusing inward with rhythmic breathing, she is relaxing between contractions, and she is vocalizing (e.g., moaning, counting, or chanting). In the algorithm, suggestions are provided for caregivers to implement depending on whether the woman is coping or not coping. Strategies include ambulation, hydrotherapy, the use of sterile water papules injected in the lower back, positioning such as squatting, acupuncture and self-hypnosis, and warm packs applied to the perineum.

Use of the Coping with Labor Algorithm to assess the pain experience of culturally diverse childbearing women is highly recommended, especially because pain in racially and ethnically diverse women is often undocumented and/or underestimated by healthcare providers.[36] Suggestions for providing culturally competent and effective pain management for childbearing women are summarized in Table 20.3.[14,25,34–36]

The 2010 vision for the care of culturally diverse childbearing women includes care that "respects the values, culture, choices, and preferences of the woman and her family within the context of promoting optimal health outcomes,"[37] with each woman having "access to a full-range of evidence-based, non-pharmacologic and pharmacologic strategies for pain management and relief as appropriate to each birth setting."[37] For culturally diverse childbearing women, having options for pain management with respect and support demonstrated for their choices, the goal is that women will have safe, quality, self-actualizing birth experiences. As stated by Leap and Anderson,[38] "As we birth our children, we birth ourselves."

REFERENCES

1. The Transforming Maternity Care Symposium Steering Committee. Steps toward a high-quality, high-value maternity care system. *Womens Health Issues.* 2010;20:S18–S49.
2. Davis-Floyd R. Afterword. In: Star RB, ed. *The Healing Power of Birth.* Austin, TX: Star Publishing; 1986:287.

3. Callister LC, Khalaf I. Culturally diverse women giving birth: Their stories. In: Selin H, ed. *Childbirth Across Cultures*. New York: Springer; 2009:33–39.

4. Callister LC. Cultural influences on pain perception and behaviors. *Home Health Care Manag Pract*. 2003;15(3):207–211.

5. Callister LC. Pain and celebrating new life. In: Lucas A, ed. *Frontiers in Pain Research*. Happauge, NY: Nova Science; 2006:157–176.

6. Callister LC, Khalaf I, Semenic S, Kartchner R, Vevilainen-Julkunen K. The pain of childbirth: Perceptions of culturally diverse women. *Pain Manag Nurs*. 2003;4(4):145–154.

7. Callister LC. Making meaning: Women's birth narratives. *J Obstet Gynecol Neonatal Nurs*. 2004;33(4):508–518.

8. Giordano J, Engebretson JC, Benedikter R. Culture, subjectivity, and the ethics of patient-centered care. *Camb Q Healthc Ethics*. 2009;18:47–56.

9. Lasch KE. Culture, pain, and culturally sensitive pain care. *Pain Manag*. 2000;1(3)(suppl 1):16–22.

10. Kjaergaard H, Wijam K, Dykes AK, Alehagen S. Fear of childbirth in obstetrically low-risk nulliparous women in Sweden and Denmark. *J Reprod Infant Psychol*. 2008;26(4):340–350.

11. Rijnders M, Baston H, Schoenbeck Y, van der Pal K, Prins M, Green J, Buitendik S. Perinatal factors related to negative or positive recall of birth experiences in women 3 years postpartum in the Netherlands. *Birth*. 2008;35(2):107–116.

12. Christiaens W, Beacke P. Assessment of social psychological determinants of satisfaction with childbirth in a cross-national perspective. BioMedical Center Pregnancy and Childbirth. http://www.biomedcentral.com/1471-2393/7/26

13. Rassin M, Klug E, Nathanzon H, Kan A, Silner D. Cultural differences in child delivery: comparisons between Jewish and Arab women in Israel. *Int Nurs Rev*. 2009;56:123–130.

14. Narayan MC. Culture's effects on pain assessment and management. *Am J Nurs*. 2010;110(4):38–47.

15. Amoros ZU, Callister LC, Sarkisyan K. Giving birth: The voices of American women. *Int Nurs Rev*. 2010;57:135–141.

16. Callister LC, Holt S, Kuhre MW. Giving birth: The voices of Australian women. *J Perinat Neonatal Nurs*. 2010;24(2):128–136.

17. Callister LC, Eads MC, Diehl JSJY. Perceptions of giving birth and adherence to cultural practices in Chinese women. *MCN: Am J Matern Child Nurs*. 2011;36(6):387–394.

18. Kartchner R, Callister LC. Giving birth: The voices of Chinese women. *J Holist Nurs*. 2003;21(2):100–116.

19. Johnson TRS, Callister LC, Beckstrand RL, Freeborn DS. Dutch women's perceptions of childbirth in the Netherlands. *MCN: Am J Matern Child Nurs*. 2007;32(3):170–177.

20. Callister LC, Corbett C, Reed S, Tomao C, Thornton KG. Giving birth: The voices of Ecuadorian women. *J Perinat Neonatal Nurs*. 2010;24(2):146–154.

21. Farnes C, Beckstrand RL, Callister LC. Healer shopping among childbearing women in Ghana, West Africa. *International Nursing Review*. 2011;58:491–497.

22. Wilkinson SE, Callister LC. Giving birth: The voices of Ghanaian women. *Health Care Women Int*. 2010;31(3):201–220.

23. Corbett C, Callister LC. Givinig birth: The voices of women in Tamil, Nadu, India. *MCN: Am J Mat Child Nsg*. 2012;37.

24. Callister LC, Getmanenko N, Garvrish N, Masrakov OE, Zotina NV, Lassetter J, Turkina N. Giving birth: The voices of Russian women. *MCN: Am J Mat Child Nsg*. 2007; 32(1):18–24.

25. Bergstrom L, Richards L., Morse JM, Roberts J. How caregivers manage pain and distress in second-stage labor. *J Midwifery Women's Health*. 2010;55:38–45.

26. Alves B, Zakka T, Teixeira MJ, Siqueira JTT, Siqueira, SRDT . Evaluation of pain before and after vaginal delivery. *Clin Exp Obstet Gynecol*. 2009;36(4):241–244.

27. Biedma Velazquez L, deDiego G, del Rosal S. Analysis of rejection of epidural analgesia during labor in Andalusian women: "The silent sufferer." *Revista de la Sociedad Espanola del Dolor*. 2010;17(1):3–15.

28. Briggs E. Cultural perspectives on pain management. *J Perioper Pract*. 2008;18(11):468–471.

29. Flink IK, Mroczek MZ, Sullivan MJL, Linton SJ. Pain in childbirth and postpartum recovery—The role of catastrophizing. *Eur J Pain.* 2009;13:212–316.

30. Lovering S. Cultural attitudes and beliefs about pain. *J Transcult Nurs.* 2006;17:389–395.

31. Weissman DE, Gordon D, Bidar-Sieflaff S. Cultural aspects of pain management. *J Palliat Med.* 2005;7(5):715–716.

32. Association of Women's Health, Obstetric, and Neonatal Nurses . *Standards for Professional Nursing Practice in the Care of Women and Newborns.* 7th ed. Washington, DC: AWHONN;2009.

33. McCaffery M, Pasero C. *Pain Clinical Manual.* 2nd ed. Philadelphia: Mosby; 1999.

34. Gulliver BG, Fisher J, Roberts L. A new way to assess pain in laboring women: Replacing the rating scale with a "coping" algorithm. *Nurs Womens Health.* 2008;12(5):406–408.

35. Roberts L, Gulliver B, Fisher J, Cloyes KG. The Coping with Labor Algorithm: An alternate pain assessment tool for the laboring woman. *J Midwifery Womens Health.* 2010;55:107–116.

36. Cintron A, Morrison RS. Pain and ethnicity in the United States: A systematic review. *J Palliat Med.* 2006;18(11):1454–1473.

37. The Transforming Maternity Symposium Steering Committee. Steps toward a high-quality, high-value maternity care system. *Womens Health Issues.* 2010;20:S18–S49.

38. Leap N, Anderson T. The role of pain in normal birth and the empowerment of women. In: Downe S, ed. *Normal Childbirth: Evidence and Debate.* Edinburgh: Church Livingstone; 2004:25–39.

WEBSITES

Culture Clues
http://depts.washington.edu/pfes/CultureClues.htm
Cultural Competence Resources for Healthcare Providers
Ethno-Med
http://ethnomed.org
Transcultural C.A.R.E. Associates
http://www.transculturalcare.net

21

GENDER AND ETHNIC DIFFERENCES IN RESPONSES TO PAIN AND ITS TREATMENT

BUREL R. GOODIN, PHD
Post-Doctoral Fellow, Comprehensive Center for
Pain Research, University of Florida College of Dentistry,
Gainesville, Florida, USA

KIMBERLY SIBILLE, PHD
Research Assistant Professor, Department of Community
Dentistry and Behavioral Sciences, University of Florida,
Gainesville, Florida, USA

ROGER B. FILLINGIM, PHD
Professor, Department of Community Dentistry and Behavioral
Sciences, University of Florida College of Dentistry, Gainesville,
Florida, USA

Key Points

- Sex differences in clinical pain have been widely documented, such that women show greater pain prevalence in the general population and are overrepresented in many chronic pain disorders.
- Sex differences in experimental pain responses are consistently reported, with women exhibiting greater sensitivity to pain and diminished pain inhibitory capacity across multiple stimulus modalities.
- Sex differences in responses to pain treatment, especially opioids, have been reported, but the findings are somewhat conflicting.
- Ethnic group differences in pain and pain-related disability have been observed, with the trend indicating greater pain and disability among minority patients compared to non-Hispanic Whites.
- Laboratory studies of ethnic group differences in pain sensitivity generally suggest lower pain tolerances and greater pain ratings in response to suprathreshold stimuli among African Americans compared to non-Hispanic Whites.
- Relatively little information is available regarding interactive influences of sex and ethnicity on pain responses.
- Multiple biopsychosocial mechanisms contribute to sex and ethnic differences in pain.

INTRODUCTION

Responses to pain and its treatment are characterized by considerable interindividual variability, such that identical painful stimuli or equivalent medication regimens will produce vastly different responses in different people.[1,2]. In the clinical setting, we often assume that interindividual variability in pain severity is driven by differences in disease severity or tissue damage. However, substantial evidence suggests poor correspondence between tissue damage and pain. For example, patients undergoing similar surgical procedures report widely disparate pain intensities, which are difficult to explain based on differences in tissue damage.[3-7] Additional evidence of individual differences in pain derives from laboratory studies, in which identical stimuli result in markedly different reports of pain by different subjects.[1] The literature is replete with examples of substantial individual differences in responses to pain treatments. For example, one study reported that the number of 3 mg morphine doses required to achieve postoperative pain relief varied from 1 to 20 across patients.[3] Understanding individual differences is crucial in order to enhance pain diagnosis and treatment by allowing providers to personalize pain medicine based on the sources of this variation. Multiple situational (e.g., transient stress, environmental conditions) and dispositional (e.g., sex/gender, race/ethnicity, genetics) factors contribute to individual differences. This chapter will focus on the contributions of sex/gender and ethnicity to individual differences in pain and responses to pain treatment. These two demographic factors are important as they represent major population groups that show significant differences in pain-related phenotypes. Also, the influences of sex/gender and ethnicity on pain responses are similar in that each is driven by complex interactions among multiple biological, psychological, and sociocultural factors. We first will discuss sex and gender differences in pain and analgesic response, then review ethnic group differences in responses to pain and its treatment. We will then summarize and make recommendations for future research.

SEX AND GENDER DIFFERENCES IN PAIN

Historically, the majority of animal, experimental, and clinical studies examining pain-related outcomes was conducted almost exclusively with male subjects; results were then extrapolated to females. As noted in a recent review, at least 79% of animal studies published in *Pain* over the preceding 10 years included male subjects only, with a mere 8% of studies on female subjects only, and another 4% explicitly designed to test for sex differences (remaining studies did not specify).[8] However, with growing awareness of important biological and psychosocial differences between males and females, research addressing sex and gender differences in pain proliferated. The pain field has moved from debating whether sex differences in pain exist, to recognizing the importance of these differences. Greater research efforts now explore our understanding of the biopsychosocial mechanisms underlying sex and gender differences in pain experience and reactivity and how these differences can inform clinical pain management. However, current clinical translation of research on sex differences in pain remains tenuous. In fact, some posit that awareness of the possible differences between males and females in response to pain is the only clinical application of the present data with no steadfast guidance for particular clinical pain treatment situations.[9] There is still much to learn from studying sex differences in pain, and translating research findings into direct clinical applications is of the utmost importance. Before reviewing the current state of the science regarding pain sex and gender differences, it is important to clarify our use of the terms *sex* and *gender*.

Sex and gender

The terms "sex" and "gender" are often considered equivalent and are used interchangeably; however, these terms have distinct meanings and are not synonymous. According to the Institute of Medicine, sex "refers to the classification of living things, generally as male or female according to their reproductive organs and functions assigned by chromosomal complement." Gender is "a person's self-representation as male or female, or how that person is responded to by social institutions based on the individual's gender presentation. Gender is rooted in biology and shaped by environment and experience."[10] For the purpose of empirical inquiry, if subjects are categorized by anatomical features (chromosomes, reproductive organs), then it is appropriate to describe the study as one of "sex differences." Conversely, if additional measures of masculinity/femininity or gender identity are used to describe subjects, then the designation of "gender differences" is appropriate.[10,11] Despite the conceptual distinction between sex and gender, it is important to recognize in practice that the two constructs are inextricably related. Indeed, some suggest that any statistical analysis of human subjects involving the dichotomous variable sex (male vs. female) is inherently confounded by the social construct of gender.[12] Moreover, gender-related phenotypes are inevitably influenced by the biological processes that comprise sex. For the sake of this chapter, and because most studies to date have classified subjects by sex rather than gender, the terms "sex" and "sex difference" will be used, except when gender is specifically measured.

Sex differences in clinical pain

Several review articles summarize the literature on sex differences in clinical pain,[12–16] and we briefly discuss these below. Sex differences in the prevalence and severity of many chronic pain conditions are well documented.[17–19] Women generally report more severe pain, more frequent bouts of pain, more anatomically diffuse and longer-lasting pain than men with similar disease processes.[14] Further, this sex difference persists even after male and female specific disorders (e.g., male urologic and female gynecologic) are excluded from analyses. Chronic pain states are more prevalent in women than in men from puberty to menopause and beyond.[13,20] To illustrate, a study of 1016 adults enrolled in a health maintenance organization in Seattle, Washington, found that the prevalence of at least 1 of 5 painful conditions (back pain, headache, abdominal pain, chest pain, facial pain) was much higher in women aged 18 to 24 years than in men in the same age group.[20] The prevalence of this sex difference lessened with age but persisted through at least 65 years of age. When the analysis examined people with 3 or more of the pain conditions studied, the sex difference at most ages was even greater. This study is consistent with more recent reports suggesting that women have higher odds than men for developing a number of chronic pain conditions.[21,22] Common chronic pain conditions that are more prevalent in women than in men include migraine,[16] fibromyalgia,[23] irritable bowel syndrome,[24] temporomandibular joint disorder,[25] and pain associated with rheumatic diseases.[26] However, one chronic pain condition, cluster headache, is more prevalent in men.[27] There is little evidence for sex differences in cancer pain; however, it appears that women are at greater risk for neuropathic pain, musculoskeletal pain, and postprocedural pain such as that produced by surgery or other invasive procedures (see reference 14 for an extensive review of this topic).

Sex differences in experimental pain

Older and more recently published articles reviewing laboratory studies of pain perception conclude that noxious stimuli are generally perceived as more painful by women than by men.[12,14,28,29] In particular, women demonstrate lower pain thresholds and tolerances compared with men for pressure pain, electrical pain, ischemic pain, heat pain, and cold pain.[14] Further, a number of investigators have used more dynamic models of pain assessment to evaluate sex differences including temporal summation (e.g., a pain facilitatory process), endogenous pain inhibition (e.g., diffuse noxious inhibitory controls), and tonic pain induced via intramuscular administration of chemical stimuli. These pain assays are arguably more clinically relevant and allow for more sophisticated examinations of central pain processing. Compared to men, women exhibit a more pronounced temporal summation of heat pain[30,31] and mechanical pain,[32] less pronounced inhibitory controls,[33,34] and greater sensitivity to muscle pain induced by injection of hypertonic saline or glutamate.[35,36] Thus, based on a large number of studies using widely varying methodologies, it appears that women exhibit more robust perceptual responses than men to experimental painful stimuli.

Although generally consistent in direction, the magnitudes of sex differences in experimental pain vary across studies, and sex differences in laboratory pain responses are not always statistically significant.[37–39] Further, sex differences may be more apparent when using particular quantitative sensory testing protocols or stimulus modalities. A meta-analysis reported that sex differences in threshold and tolerance measures were largest and most consistently found for pressure pain and electrical stimulation, while smaller and less consistent for thermal pain stimuli.[29] Although variability in the magnitude of sex differences in laboratory pain responses may be attributable to methodological factors such as the characteristics of the pain stimulus, it is important to consider that responses to pain are influenced by a complex interplay of biopsychosocial factors that may vary across sex. The contributions of these biopsychosocial factors to sex differences in experimental and clinical pain are explored below.

Sex differences in pain treatment and analgesic response

Gender bias in pain treatment is receiving increasing attention. A frequently cited study reports that after cardiac surgery, women were more likely than men to be prescribed sedatives, whereas men were more likely to receive analgesics.[40] However, this study failed to examine doses of medications or pain reports, and differences in frequency of opioid administration were quite small between sexes. More recently, investigators reported that women were less likely than men to receive analgesics for abdominal pain in an emergency department setting.[41] However, others reported that women presenting in the emergency room with headache, neck, or back pain were more likely to receive analgesics, due to greater pain among women.[42] Other studies reveal no sex differences in provision of pain medications (see [43] for review). Vignette studies have further examined gender biases in pain treatment. For example, one vignette study reported an interaction between physician and patient sex, such that female physicians "prescribed" higher doses of opioid pain medication for women than men with low back pain, whereas the reverse pattern occurred for male physicians.[44] Recent research using virtual human technology reveals that healthcare providers in training judged female "patients" to have more pain than males.[45,46] Thus, some evidence suggests potential gender biases in pain treatment; however, the findings are mixed and clinical characteristics of the patient and the sex of the provider may influence the magnitude and direction of the effect.

In addition to gender biases in pain treatment, recent research focuses on whether men and women respond differently to pharmacological pain treatment. Sex differences in pharmacokinetics and pharmacodynamics,[47] as well as in mechanisms of pain and analgesia, suggest that medication efficacy and side-effect profiles may differ between men and women. However, recent tests of this assertion provided a mixed picture, particularly regarding opioid analgesia. A meta-analysis of sex differences in opioid analgesia produced the following conclusions: (1) there is no overall sex difference in response to μ-opioids in clinical studies; however, when restricting the analysis to studies of patient-controlled analgesia with morphine, women consume significantly lower amounts of morphine than men; (2) experimental studies indicate increased morphine analgesia in women, though the difference is modest; (3) clinical studies reveal greater analgesic responses for women to mixed action μ/κ agonist-antagonist drugs, and this sex difference is large in magnitude; (4) experimental studies show no sex differences in analgesic responses to mixed action μ/κ agonist-antagonist drugs.[48]

In contrast to research on pharmacological treatments, whether nonpharmacological interventions produce differential effects in men and women has received relatively little attention. Limited clinical research addresses sex differences in outcomes from physical therapy and multidisciplinary treatments. For example, women, but not men, with back pain undergoing cognitive-behavioral treatment with or without physical therapy exhibit improved health-related quality of life.[49] Also among patients with back pain, a conventional physical therapy intervention produced better outcomes for men, but women showed greater pain reduction in response to intensive dynamic back exercises.[49] In contrast, other studies report no sex differences in the effectiveness of rehabilitation treatments for chronic low back pain.[50,51] Multidisciplinary treatment for pain due to temporomandibular disorder was associated with significant decreases in pain over a two-year period in women, but not men.[52] More recently, Keogh and colleagues[53] found that women and men showed comparable initial responses to multidisciplinary pain treatment; however, men maintained their treatment gains over the three-month follow-up period, while women regressed to their pretreatment levels. Some research addresses this issue in the context of experimentally induced pain. Women, but not men, reported lower ratings of cold pressor pain after treadmill exercise, whereas men, but not women, demonstrate reduced pain ratings after playing video games.[54] This limited literature suggests that sex differences exist in responses to nonpharmacological pain treatment, but the findings are inconsistent and additional research is needed.

Biopsychosocial contributors to sex differences in pain response

Many biological, psychological, and sociocultural variables may contribute to pain-related differences between men and women. From a biological perspective, reproductive hormones likely contribute to sex differences in pain.[55] A number of clinical pain conditions vary in their severity across the female menstrual cycle.[56] Also, laboratory studies in humans demonstrate greater pain sensitivity among females during the late luteal (i.e., premenstrual) phase versus the follicular (i.e., postmenstrual) phase of their menstrual cycle; although, the effects are inconsistent across studies and are often small.[57,58] In addition to endogenous hormonal influences, exogenous hormones, especially hormone replacement among postmenopausal women, has been associated with increased risk for clinical pain[59–62] and greater experimental pain sensitivity,[63] with some exceptions.[64] While these findings suggest that estrogen increases pain sensitivity, potential pain inhibitory effects of estrogen have been reported by others. Indeed, cerebral responses to heat pain, particularly in brain regions associated with the affective component of pain, were lower during high versus low estrogen menstrual phases.[65] Moreover, exogenous administration of estrogen was associated with both reduced muscle pain sensitivity and enhanced pain-related brain μ-opioid receptor binding in healthy women,[66] suggesting that estrogen enhances endogenous opioid-mediated pain inhibition. Thus, while gonadal hormones almost certainly influence pain responses, the magnitude and direction of these effects remain unclear, and the precise biological mechanisms whereby sex hormones influence pain responses remain unknown.

In addition to hormonal influences, psychosocial factors contribute to sex differences in pain. From a sociocultural perspective, stereotypic gender roles appear to be associated with experimental pain responses, based on the assumption that traditional feminine roles may encourage reporting pain, while masculine roles discourage pain reporting. There is empirical support for this assumption, as both women and men describe women as more willing to report pain, and this willingness to report pain has accounted for sex differences in experimental pain responses.[31,67] Also, using validated measures of gender roles, masculinity and femininity have been associated with lower and higher pain sensitivity, respectively.[68–72] In addition, identification with gender norms appears to be an important consideration, as men who identify strongly with masculine gender norms have higher pain tolerance than men with low masculine identification.[73] Moreover, male subjects report less pain and exhibit higher thresholds when tested by a female versus male experimenter, while experimenter gender has no influence on pain reporting among female participants.[74] In another study, men again had lower reports of pain and higher thresholds with an attractive female examiner; conversely, women reported more pain and had lower thresholds with attractive male examiners.[75] These data suggest that gender roles can substantially influence pain responses in women and men and contribute to sex differences in laboratory pain studies; however, the importance of gender roles in differential clinical pain response is less clear.

Regarding psychological influences, pain coping is another factor that may contribute to sex differences in pain. Maladaptive pain coping strategies, such as catastrophizing, have been associated with poorer adjustment to clinical pain and higher sensitivity to experimental pain.[76] Women have reported higher levels of pain catastrophizing, and sex differences in catastrophizing were found to mediate sex differences in clinical pain due to osteoarthritis.[77] Edwards and colleagues[38] further examined this issue and found that controlling for negative affect and catastrophizing did not fully explain sex differences in pain threshold or pain tolerance; however, the factors themselves have large effect sizes. In sum, sex differences in pain coping have been widely reported and in some studies have mediated sex differences in pain. Additional discussions of psychosocial contributions to sex differences in pain can be found elsewhere.[14]

ETHNIC GROUP DIFFERENCES IN PAIN

Conceptual issues

The observation of ethnic disparities in the prevalence, severity, and management of clinical pain has driven efforts to understand contributing biological and psychosocial factors. The terms race and ethnicity convey distinct meanings that are important to clarify in pain-related research. In general, the term race refers to a biological designation based on physical features or genetic background and retains residual impressions of discrimination or prejudice.[78,79] From a research perspective, race classification is difficult and provides poorly differentiated demographic information due to the complex biological and cultural integration of individuals. Ethnicity, in contrast, encompasses a broader array of factors to help distinguish heterogeneous groups of people based on similar culture, behaviors, traditions, and beliefs.[80,81] Consistent with the biopsychosocial model, the term ethnicity reflects a more comprehensive array of factors contributing to the experience and expression of pain and is the preferred phrasing in biomedical research.[82,83] Given the historical connotations of race and the more appropriate broadness of the term ethnicity, we will use the latter in describing population groups throughout this chapter. Also, we use the terms African American and non-Hispanic White to refer to these two ethnic groups, except where citing others' work, in which case we use the terms specified by the authors.

Ethnic differences in clinical pain

In the United States, disparities in health status across ethnic groups have been well documented. For example, as indicated by the Centers for Disease Control, a number of diseases and health conditions disproportionally affect ethnic minority groups (e.g., cancer, cardiovascular disease, diabetes, HIV/AIDS, hepatitis).[84,85] Importantly, persistent pain characterizes most of these conditions. Additionally, there is evidence of ethnic disparity in the prevalence of chronic pain conditions such as osteoarthritis (OA). Lawrence and colleagues, in a review of data from three population–based studies, found a greater incidence of radiograph knee osteoarthritis among African Americans (AA) compared to non-Hispanic Whites (NHW).[86] Moreover, numerous studies report greater pain severity and pain-related disability as a result of chronic pain conditions among AA compared to NHW.[87-92] Thus, while not as widely appreciated as in other disease conditions, ethnic disparities in pain exist and merit empirical attention. Below we discuss the nature of these disparities as well as some of the possible contributing factors.

In addition to findings regarding pain prevalence, ethnic differences in clinical pain severity have been reported in both acute and chronic conditions. For instance, following dental procedures, more severe pain was reported by Black American and Latino patients compared to patients of European descent.[93] Tan and colleagues[94] also reported significant ethnic differences in self-reported postoperative pain and morphine usage following an elective lower caesarian section procedure. In this study, Indian Singaporean patients reported the highest mean pain score and morphine consumption over a 24-hour period compared to Chinese or Malaysian patients. Numerous studies have identified ethnic variability in the severity of chronic pain, across multiple clinical conditions, including: AIDS/HIV,[95] cancer pain,[96] back pain,[97] glaucoma,[98] spinal fusion,[99] temporomandibular disorders in children,[100] and OA,[101-104] with most studies reporting greater pain among minority patients, though the absence of ethnic group differences has also been reported.[105,106] Interestingly, in addition to differences in pain severity, ethnic differences have also been noted in symptom presentation. For example, ethnic differences have been observed in site and type of initial symptom presentation in coronary heart disease and acute myocardial infarction.[107,108]

Ethnic differences in experimental pain responses

Research on ethnic differences in laboratory pain extends over a 60-year period, with the incorporation of a wide range of pain assays, and the evaluation of healthy subjects as well as those with clinical pain.[81] Early laboratory findings demonstrated increased pain tolerance on thermal, pressure, and cold pressor measures in Whites compared to other racial/ethnic groups, most often African Americans.[109,110,111] Recent research employing more sophisticated procedures replicates, clarifies, and expands upon these studies. Specifically, the following have emerged: lower thermal pain tolerance in AA compared to NHW;[112] lower thermal, cold pressor, and ischemic pain tolerance in AA compared to NHW;[113,114] and lower cold pressor and thermal pain tolerance in AA and Hispanics compared to NHW.[115] Lower ischemic pain tolerance in AA compared to NHW was also demonstrated in a clinical study[92] and in women with a history of mood disorders.[116] In contrast to the direction of most findings, some studies have reported increased ischemic pain threshold in AA compared to NHW.[113–115]

These studies have generally reported lower pain tolerance, but not pain threshold, among AA compared to NHW. Pain threshold and pain tolerance measures are thought to reflect different dimensions of pain, with threshold capturing the sensory dimension and tolerance reflecting more psychological features.[81] Two studies specifically assessed ethnic group differences in the intensity (sensory) and unpleasantness (affective) of experimentally induced pain.[117] In a study of ethnic differences and thermal pain measures, no group differences emerged for measures of heat pain threshold and heat pain intensity, but AA showed lower heat pain tolerance and reported higher ratings of heat pain unpleasantness compared to NHWs.[112] These findings were replicated in a subsequent study of thermal pain,[118] and interestingly, a similar pattern of ethnic group differences in pain unpleasantness but not pain intensity has been observed in a chronic pain population.[119] These findings provide evidence that ethic group differences in pain responses may be particularly robust for the affective/motivational dimensions of pain.

In addition to traditional self-report measures of laboratory pain sensitivity, ethnic differences have been observed in measures of nociceptive reflexes and central pain-inhibitory mechanisms. In a study of the nociceptive flexion reflex, a measure of a stimulus-driven spinal reflex response, AA demonstrated this reflex at a lower stimulus intensity than NHW.[120] Differences in descending inhibition have also been demonstrated as measured by diffuse noxious inhibitory controls, with NHW demonstrating a more robust pain inhibitory response compared to AA.[121] These results were replicated using different methodology in a subsequent study.[122] In summary, an array of convincing evidence from laboratory pain studies demonstrates ethnic differences, particularly between AA and NHW, in suprathreshold experimental pain responses as well as measures of endogenous pain modulation.

Ethnicity and pain treatment

Multiple studies have addressed whether patients from different ethnic backgrounds receive different treatments for their pain.[123–128] One overarching finding is that opioid analgesics are prescribed less frequently or in lower doses to ethnic minority patients compared to non-Hispanic White patients. These differences have been reported for postoperative pain,[129,130] trauma-related pain,[131,132] and for chronic pain.[133] Encouragingly, some recent studies have shown similar frequencies of opioid use across ethnic groups.[134–136] Multiple factors have been recognized as contributing to the ethnic disparities in the treatment of pain-related conditions, including patient-level, provider-level, and system-level variables. Addressing the medical management discrepancies will require a comprehensive and integrative approach targeting all three entities.[128]

Ethnic group differences in patient preferences regarding pain treatment have also been documented. For example, African Americans undergo total joint arthroplasty at lower rates than non-Hispanic Whites, and part of this disparity is related to patient preferences. AA report lower willingness than Whites to consider joint replacement as a treatment for lower extremity osteoarthritis. This difference is explained, at least in part, by their expectations regarding surgery.[137–139] Specifically, African Americans are less familiar with arthroplasty and they expect the surgery to be more painful and less effective compared to the expectations of Whites.[140,141]

With the increased awareness of ethnic disparities in the provision of pain treatment, there is a growing interest in exploring whether treatment efficacy differs as a function of ethnic group. Clinical studies have indicated significant variability by ethnic group in opioid dose required for pain relief.[94,142,143] In a 20-year review of medical records of cancer patients treated for chronic pain with intramuscular morphine, the dosage necessary for pain relief was substantially lower among Blacks (8 mg) compared to Whites (16 mg).[142] Similarly, in the evaluation of postoperative pain, greater amounts of morphine were required to achieve pain relief among Caucasian patients than African and Asian patients.[143] Other studies of both healthy and clinical populations indicate ethnic differences in morphine pharmaco-dynamics and pharmacokinetics;[144,145] and opioid withdrawal symptoms.[146] Thus, limited clinical evidence demonstrates significant ethnic differences in the treatment response to exogenous opioids; however, additional research is warranted to confirm and explain these findings.

Factors contributing to ethnic differences in pain response

Myriad biopsychosocial factors interactively contribute to ethnic differences in pain-related experiences. Zatzick and Dimsdale[81] provide a comprehensive list of social and cultural variables influencing pain research that also have clinical relevance, such as language, pain-related vocabulary, cultural patterns of pain expression, sex/gender role, age, previous life experience, experimenter sex/ethnicity, and acculturation/assimilation. Additionally, important social and cultural influences include those associated with healthcare provid-ers, the healthcare system, and social policies.[83,147] A number of psychological factors may have contributed to ethnic group differences in pain. For example, Hispanic patients with chronic pain report a more external health-related locus of control style.[148,149] Also, ethnic differences in pain coping are observed in clinical populations and among healthy indi-viduals, with African Americans typically reporting more passive coping strategies, includ-ing catastrophizing and praying/hoping.[150–152] In a study of experimental pain perception, African Americans showed not only higher levels of passive coping but also greater hyper-vigilance.[113] Though receiving less empirical attention, sociocultural factors likely contrib-ute to ethnic group differences in the experience of pain.[153] Zborowski[154] proposed that pain expression is culturally influenced, based on pain-related attitudes that are inherent within cultural groups. Indeed, a recent study found that higher levels of ethnic identifica-tion predicted greater pain sensitivity among African American and Hispanic groups, but not among non-Hispanic Whites.[155] Additional investigation of sociocultural contributions to clinical and experimental pain responses is needed.

From a biological perspective, limited research directly addresses biological contribu-tions to ethnic/racial group differences in pain. Mechlin and colleagues[114] explored the association of stress-induced increases in blood pressure, norepinephrine, and cortisol with experimental pain responses in African Americans and a non-African American group comprised primarily of Caucasians. African Americans showed blunted physiological responses to a laboratory stress protocol, and stress-induced physiological reactivity was associated with reduction of pain responses only in the non-African American participants. Recently, these findings were replicated and extended using additional pain modalities.[156] These researchers also reported that lower resting levels of allopregnanolone, higher corti-sol, and higher beta-endorphin are associated with reduced pain sensitivity among NHWs or non-Hispanic Whites but not African Americans.[157] Thus, neuroendocrine factors may contribute to ethnic/racial group differences in pain perception.

Genetic variations represent another biological factor that could contribute to ethnic group differences in pain-related phenotypes. Abundant evidence implicates genetic fac-tors in pain and analgesic responses,[158–160] and despite considerable genetic similarity across population groups, allele frequencies for many single nucleotide polymorphisms (SNPs) differ substantially across ethnic groups, which may contribute to ethnic differences in health relevant phenotypes.[161–164] While limited pain research directly explores this issue, ethnic differences have been reported in allele frequencies for SNPs on pain-related candidate genes, such as the mu-opioid receptor gene (*OPRM1*) and the catechol-o-methyl-transferase gene (*COMT*).[165,166] These genes have been associated with pain sensitivity[167–169] and morphine requirements;[170,171] therefore, it is plausible that ethnic group differences in allelic frequencies of such pain-related SNPs contribute to differences in pain sensitivity and analgesic responses. Additional research should investigate this possibility.

Interactions between sex/gender and race/ethnicity

The preceding discussion separately addresses the influences of sex and ethnicity on pain responses. However, because both factors exist within all individuals, the interaction of sex and ethnicity is important to consider. One could speculate, for example, that gender-related factors may exert differential influences on pain across ethnic groups due to cultural influences that vary in the extent to which they promote pain expression in women versus men. Unfortunately, little research has directly investigated the interactive influences of sex and ethnicity on pain responses. In a previous study of responses to cold pressor pain, ethnic and sex differences were reported, such that males and Anglo-Saxons showed the greatest pain tolerance.[111] An interaction between sex and ethnicity was also observed, which indicated that the ethnic group difference was significantly larger for males than for females. Interestingly, using the same pain model, Weisse and colleagues[172] demonstrated that experimenter gender differentially influenced pain reports in Black and White subjects. Specifically, Black subjects reported greater cold pressor pain unpleasantness to female versus male experimenters, while White subjects reported similar pain unpleasantness regardless of experimenter gender. Also, female subjects reported greater pain unpleasantness than male subjects only when the experimenter was Black. In a community-based study of orofacial pain, Riley and Gilbert[173] found some evidence of interactions between race and sex, in that only among Whites were women more likely than men to report multiple orofacial pain symptoms. These limited findings suggest that sex and gender may interact with ethnic group to influence pain responses, and the pattern of findings may suggest that sex differences in pain are more robust among Whites. However, given the paucity of evidence available, no firm conclusions should be drawn. Clearly, additional research is warranted to further characterize interactive influences of sex and ethnicity on pain and to delineate the mechanisms whereby these effects occur.

SUMMARY AND FUTURE DIRECTIONS

Sex/gender and ethnicity represent two important factors associated with considerable variability in pain and analgesic responses. These two demographic characteristics are interesting not only because they represent major population groups, but also because each is a proxy for complex and interactive influences of multiple biopsychosocial factors on pain responses. Regarding sex differences, women are at greater risk than men for many forms of clinical pain, and laboratory studies consistently demonstrate significantly greater pain sensitivity among women than men. There is some evidence, albeit inconsistent, that women show greater analgesic responses to some opioids, particularly mixed agonist-antagonist drugs. Regarding ethnic differences, minority patients, specifically African Americans and Hispanics, experience higher levels of pain and disability than non-Hispanic Whites in several clinical populations and these minority groups exhibit greater sensitivity to experimental pain. Numerous studies document biases in pain treatment, such that ethnic minorities and women are at risk for undertreatment of pain. Insufficient information is available to draw conclusions regarding ethnic group differences in analgesic effectiveness or that of nonpharmacologic interventions. Myriad biopsychosocial factors contribute to these sex and ethnic group differences.

Multiple avenues of future research could address gaps in the literature and help advance knowledge regarding sex and ethnic group differences in pain. For example, research designed to determine sex and ethnic group differences in responses to pharmacologic and nonpharmacologic pain treatments could be quite valuable. Moreover, very few studies are sufficiently powered to examine the interactive influences of sex and ethnicity on pain responses, and large-scale studies are needed that permit modeling interactions among these as well as other individual difference factors. Also, it is important to evolve from descriptive studies to those that are designed to elucidate the mechanisms underlying sex and ethnic group differences in pain. Specifically, investigators should incorporate a battery of biological markers and psychosocial measures that can help explicate observed group differences. More widespread recognition of the importance of individual differences in pain, and additional research to illuminate the mechanisms mediating these individual differences, should ultimately lead to more effective pain diagnosis and treatment.

Regarding clinical implications, based on the current available evidence, tailoring pain treatment based on sex or ethnicity is not recommended, and additional research as described above is needed to increase our understanding of the influence of these variables on pain and treatment responses. Given observed biases in pain treatment, clinicians should strive to ensure equitable pain treatment across all population groups. This may require increased efforts to communicate effectively with minority patients and to educate patients regarding the benefits of available pain treatment options. Increased awareness and understanding of sex and ethnic group differences in pain should ultimately help reduce biases and enhance pain diagnosis and treatment for all patients.

REFERENCES

1. Fillingim RB. Individual differences in pain responses. *Curr Rheumatol Rep.* 2005;7:342–347.
2. Nielsen CS, Staud R, Price DD. Individual differences in pain sensitivity: measurement, causation, and consequences. *J Pain.* 2009;10:231–237.
3. Aubrun F, Langeron O, Quesnel C, Coriat P, Riou B. Relationships between measurement of pain using visual analog score and morphine requirements during postoperative intravenous morphine titration. *Anesthesiology.* 2003;98:1415–1421.
4. Bisgaard T, Klarskov B, Rosenberg J, Kehlet H. Characteristics and prediction of early pain after laparoscopic cholecystectomy. *Pain.* 2001;90:261–269.
5. Perkins FM, Kehlet H. Chronic pain as an outcome of surgery. A review of predictive factors. *Anesthesiology.* 2000;93:1123–1133.
6. Uchiyama K, Kawai M, Tani M, Ueno M, Hama T, Yamaue H. Gender differences in postoperative pain after laparoscopic cholecystectomy. *Surg Endosc.* 2006;20:448–451.
7. Werner MU, Duun P, Kehlet H. Prediction of postoperative pain by preoperative nociceptive responses to heat stimulation. *Anesthesiology.* 2004;100:115–119.
8. Mogil JS, Chanda ML. The case for the inclusion of female subjects in basic science studies of pain. *Pain.* 2005;117:1–5.
9. Hurley RW, Adams MC. Sex, gender, and pain: an overview of a complex field. *Anesth Analg.* 2008;107:309–317.

10. Wizemann TM, Pardue MLe. *Exploring The Biological Contributions To Human Health: Does Sex Matter?* Washington, DC: National Academies Press; 2001.

11. Hughes RN. The categorisation of male and female laboratory animals in terms of "gender." *Brain Res Bull.* 2003;60:189–190.

12. Greenspan JD, Craft RM, LeResche L, et al. Studying sex and gender differences in pain and analgesia: A consensus report. *Pain.* 2007;132(suppl 1):S26–S45.

13. Berkley KJ. Sex differences in pain. *Behavioral and Brain Sciences.* 1997;20:371–380.

14. Fillingim RB, King CD, Ribeiro-Dasilva MC, Rahim-Williams B, Riley JL III. Sex, gender, and pain: a review of recent clinical and experimental findings. *J Pain.* 2009;10:447–485.

15. Rollman GB, Lautenbacher S. Sex differences in musculoskeletal pain. *Clin J Pain.* 2001;17:20–24.

16. Unruh AM. Gender variations in clinical pain experience. *Pain.* 1996;65:123–167.

17. Bouhassira D, Lanteri-Minet M, Attal N, Laurent B, Touboul C. Prevalence of chronic pain with neuropathic characteristics in the general population. *Pain.* 2008;136:380–387.

18. Tsang A, von Korff M, Lee S, et al. Common chronic pain conditions in developed and developing countries: gender and age differences and comorbidity with depression-anxiety disorders. *J Pain.* 2008; 9:883–891.

19. Wijnhoven HA, de Vet HC, Picavet HS. Prevalence of musculoskeletal disorders is systematically higher in women than in men. *Clin J Pain.* 2006;22:717–724.

20. Von Korff M, Dworkin SF, LeResche L, Krueger A. An epidemiologic comparison of pain complaints. *Pain.* 1988;32:173–183.

21. Hardt J, Jacobsen C, Goldberg J, Nickel R, Buchwald D. Prevalence of chronic pain in a representative sample in the United States. *Pain Med.* 2008; 9:803–812.

22. Sjogren P, Ekholm O, Peuckmann V, Gronbaek M. Epidemiology of chronic pain in Denmark: an update. *Eur J Pain.* 2009;13:287–292.

23. White KP, Speechley M, Harth M, Ostbye T. The London Fibromyalgia Epidemiology Study: comparing the demographic and clinical characteristics in 100 random community cases of fibromyalgia versus controls. *J Rheumatol.* 1999;26:1577–1585.

24. Shiotani A, Miyanishi T, Takahashi T. Sex differences in irritable bowel syndrome in Japanese university students. *J Gastroenterol.* 2006;41:562–568.

25. Riley JL III, Gilbert GH. Orofacial pain symptoms: an interaction between age and sex. *Pain.* 2001;90:245–256.

26. van Vollenhoven RF. Sex differences in rheumatoid arthritis: more than meets the eye.. *BMC Med.* 2009;7:12:12.

27. Wiesenfeld-Hallin Z. Sex differences in pain perception. *Gend Med.* 2005;2:137–145.

28. Fillingim RB, Maixner W. Gender differences in the responses to noxious stimuli. *Pain Forum.* 1995;4:209–221.

29. Riley JL, Robinson ME, Wise EA, Myers CD, Fillingim RB. Sex differences in the perception of noxious experimental stimuli: a meta-analysis. *Pain.* 1998;74:181–187.

30. Fillingim RB, Maixner W, Kincaid S, Silva S. Sex differences in temporal summation but not sensory-discriminative processing of thermal pain. *Pain.* 1998;75:121–127.

31. Robinson ME, Wise EA, Gagnon C, Fillingim RB, Price DD. Influences of gender role and anxiety on sex differences in temporal summation of pain. *J Pain.* 2004;5:77–82.

32. Sarlani E, Grace EG, Reynolds MA, Greenspan JD. Sex differences in temporal summation of pain and aftersensations following repetitive noxious mechanical stimulation. *Pain.* 2004;109:115–123.

33. Goodin BR, McGuire L, Allshouse M, et al. Associations between catastrophizing and endogenous pain-inhibitory processes: sex differences. *J Pain.* 2009;10:180–190.

34. Popescu A, LeResche L, Truelove EL, Drangsholt MT. Gender differences in pain modulation by diffuse noxious inhibitory controls: a systematic review. *Pain.* 2010;150:309–318.

35. Cairns BE, Wang K, Hu JW, Sessle BJ, Arendt-Nielsen L, Svensson P. The effect of glutamate-evoked masseter muscle pain on the human jaw-stretch reflex differs in men and women. *J Orofac Pain.* 2003;17:317–325.

36. Ge HY, Madeleine P, Arendt-Nielsen L. Gender differences in pain modulation evoked by repeated injections of glutamate into the human trapezius muscle. *Pain.* 2005;113:134–140.

37. Ayesh EE, Jensen TS, Svensson P. Somatosensory function following painful repetitive electrical stimulation of the human temporomandibular joint and skin. *Exp Brain Res.* 2007;179:415–425.

38. Edwards RR, Haythornthwaite JA, Sullivan MJ, Fillingim RB. Catastrophizing as a mediator of sex differences in pain: differential effects for daily pain versus laboratory-induced pain. *Pain.* 2004;111:335–341.

39. Nie H, Arendt-Nielsen L, Andersen H, Graven-Nielsen T. Temporal summation of pain evoked by mechanical stimulation in deep and superficial tissue. *J Pain.* 2005;6:348–355.

40. Calderone KL. The influence of gender on the frequency of pain and sedative medication administered to postoperative patients. *Sex Roles.* 1990;23:713–725.

41. Chen EH, Shofer FS, Dean AJ, et al. Gender disparity in analgesic treatment of emergency department patients with acute abdominal pain. *Acad Emerg Med.* 2008;15:414–418.

42. Raftery KA, Smith-Coggins R, Chen AH. Gender-associated differences in emergency department pain management. *Ann Emerg Med.* 1995;26:414–421.

43. LeResche L. Defining gender disparities in pain management. *Clin Orthop Relat Res.* 2011; 469:1871–1877.

44. Weisse CS, Sorum PC, Sanders KN, Syat BL. Do gender and race affect decisions about pain management? *J Gen Intern Med.* 2001;16:211–217.

45. Hirsh AT, Alqudah AF, Stutts LA, Robinson ME. Virtual human technology: capturing sex, race, and age influences in individual pain decision policies. *Pain.* 2008;140:231–238.

46. Stutts LA, Hirsh AT, George SZ, Robinson ME. Investigating patient characteristics on pain assessment using virtual human technology. *Eur J Pain.* 2010;14:1040–1045.

47. Gandhi M, Aweeka F, Greenblatt RM, Blaschke TF. Sex differences in pharmacokinetics and pharmacodynamics. *Annu Rev Pharmacol Toxicol.* 2004;44:499–523..

48. Niesters M, Dahan A, Kest B, et al. Do sex differences exist in opioid analgesia? A systematic review and meta-analysis of human experimental and clinical studies. *Pain.* 2010;151:61–68.

49. Hansen FR, Bendix T, Skov P, et al. Intensive, dynamic back-muscle exercises, conventional physiotherapy, or placebo-control treatment of low-back pain. A randomized, observer-blind trial. *Spine.* 1993;18:98–108.

50. Kankaanpaa M, Taimela S, Airaksinen O, Hanninen O. The efficacy of active rehabilitation in chronic low back pain. Effect on pain intensity, self-experienced disability, and lumbar fatigability. *Spine.* 1999;24:1034–1042.

51. Mannion AF, Junge A, Taimela S, Muntener M, Lorenzo K, Dvorak J. Active therapy for chronic low back pain: part 3. Factors influencing self-rated disability and its change following therapy. *Spine.* 2001;26:920–929.

52. Krogstad BS, Jokstad A, Dahl BL, Vassend O. The reporting of pain, somatic complaints, and anxiety in a group of patients with TMD before and 2 years after treatment: sex differences. *J Orofacial Pain.* 1996;10:263–269.

53. Keogh E, McCracken LM, Eccleston C. Do men and women differ in their response to interdisciplinary chronic pain management? *Pain.* 2005;114:37–46.

54. Sternberg WF, Bokat C, Kass L, Alboyadjian A, Gracely RH. Sex-dependent components of the analgesia produced by athletic competition. *J Pain.* 2001;2:65–74.

55. Aloisi AM, Bonifazi M. Sex hormones, central nervous system and pain. *Horm Behav.* 2006;50:1–7.

56. Kuba T, Quinones-Jenab V. The role of female gonadal hormones in behavioral sex differences in persistent and chronic pain: clinical versus preclinical studies. *Brain Res Bull.* 2005;66:179–188.

57. Riley JLI, Robinson ME, Wise EA, Price DD. A meta-analytic review of pain perception across the menstrual cycle. *Pain.* 1999;81:225–235.

58. Sherman JJ, LeResche L. Does experimental pain response vary across the menstrual cycle? A methodological review. *Am J Physiol Regul Integr Comp Physiol.* 2006;291:R245–R256.

59. Brynhildsen JO, Bjors E, Skarsgard C, Hammar ML. Is hormone replacement therapy a risk factor for low back pain among postmenopausal women? *Spine*. 1998;23:809–813.

60. Musgrave DS, Vogt MT, Nevitt MC, Cauley JA. Back problems among postmenopausal women taking estrogen replacement therapy. *Spine*. 2001;26:1606–1612.

61. Wise EA, Riley JLI, Robinson ME. Clinical pain perception and hormone replacement therapy in post-menopausal females experiencing orofacial pain. *Clin J Pain*. 2000;16:121–126.

62. LeResche L, Saunders K, Von Korff MR, Barlow W, Dworkin SF. Use of exogenous hormones and risk of temporomandibular disorder pain. *Pain*. 1997;69:153–160.

63. Fillingim RB, Edwards RR. The association of hormone replacement therapy with experimental pain responses in postmenopausal women. *Pain*. 2001;92:229–234.

64. Macfarlane TV, Blinkhorn A, Worthington HV, Davies RM, Macfarlane GJ. Sex hormonal factors and chronic widespread pain: a population study among women. *Rheumatology (Oxford)*. 2002;41:454–457.

65. De LR, Albuquerque RJ, Andersen AH, Carlson CR. Influence of estrogen on brain activation during stimulation with painful heat. *J Oral Maxillofac Surg*. 2006;64:158–166.

66. Smith YR, Stohler CS, Nichols TE, Bueller JA, Koeppe RA, Zubieta JK. Pronociceptive and antinociceptive effects of estradiol through endogenous opioid neurotransmission in women. *J Neurosci*. 2006;26:5777–5785.

67. Robinson ME, Riley JL III, Myers CD, et al. Gender role expectations of pain: relationship to sex differences in pain. *J Pain*. 2001;2:251–257.

68. Myers CD, Robinson ME, Riley JL III, Sheffield D. Sex, gender, and blood pressure: contributions to experimental pain report. *Psychosom Med*. 2001;63:545–550.

69. Myers CD, Tsao JC, Glover DA, Kim SC, Turk N, Zeltzer LK. Sex, gender, and age: contributions to laboratory pain responding in children and adolescents. *J Pain*. 2006;7:556–564.

70. Otto MW, Dougher MJ. Sex differences and personality factors in responsivity to pain. *Percept Mot Skills*. 1985;61:383–390.

71. Sanford SD, Kersh BC, Thorn BE, Rich MA, Ward LC. Psychosocial mediators of sex differences in pain responsivity. *J Pain*. 2002;3:58–64.

72. Thorn BE, Clements KL, Ward LC, et al. Personality factors in the explanation of sex differences in pain catastrophizing and response to experimental pain. *Clin J Pain*. 2004;20:275–282.

73. Pool GJ, Schwegler AF, Theodore BR, Fuchs PN. Role of gender norms and group identification on hypothetical and experimental pain tolerance. *Pain*. 2007;129:122–129.

74. Levine FM, De Simone LL. The effects of experimenter gender on pain report in male and female subjects. *Pain*. 1991;44:69–72.

75. Gijsbers K, Nicholson F. Experimental pain thresholds influenced by sex of experimenter. *Percept Mot Skills*. 2005;101:803–807.

76. Sullivan MJ, Thorn B, Haythornthwaite JA, et al. Theoretical perspectives on the relation between catastrophizing and pain. *Clin J Pain*. 2001;17:52–64.

77. Keefe FJ, Lefebvre JC, Egert JR, Affleck G, Sullivan MJ, Caldwell DS. The relationship of gender to pain, pain behavior, and disability in osteoarthritis patients: the role of catastrophizing. *Pain*. 2000;87:325–334.

78. Chaudhry IB, Neelam K, Duddu V, Husain N. Ethnicity and psychopharmacology. *J Psychopharmacol*. 2008;22:673–680.

79. Edwards CL, Fillingim RB, Keefe FJ. Race, ethnicity and pain: a review. *Pain*. 2001;94:133–137.

80. Dimsdale J. Stalked by the past: The influence of ethnicity on health. *Psychosom Med*. 2000;62:161–170.

81. Zatzick DF, Dimsdale JE. Cultural variations in response to painful stimuli. *Psychosom Med*. 1990;52:544–557.

82. Bhopal R, Rankin J. Concepts and terminology in ethnicity, race and health: be aware of the ongoing debate. *Brit Dent J.*. 1999;186:483–484.

83. Todd KH. Pain assessment and ethnicity. *Ann Emerg Med.* 1996;27:421–423.

84. Racial disparities in nationally notifiable diseases—United States, 2002. *MMWR Morb Mortal Wkly Rep.* 2005;54:9–11.

85. Smedley BD, Stith AY, Nelson ARE. *Unequal Treatment.* Washington, DC: The National Academies Press; 2003.

86. Lawrence RC, Felson DT, Helmick CG, et al. Estimates of the prevalence of arthritis and other rheumatic conditions in the United States. Part II. *Arthritis Rheum.* 2008;58:26–35.

87. Ndao-Brumblay SK, Green CR. Racial differences in the physical and psychosocial health among black and white women with chronic pain. *J Natl Med Assoc.* 2005;97:1369–1377.

88. Riley J, Gilbert G, Heft M. Orofacial pain: racial and sex differences among older adults. *J Public Health Dent.* 2002;62:132–139.

89. Green CR, Baker TA, Smith EM, Sato Y. The effect of race in older adults presenting for chronic pain management: a comparative study of black and white Americans. *J Pain.* 2003;4:82–90.

90. Green CR, Baker TA, Sato Y, Washington TL, Smith EM. Race and chronic pain: A comparative study of young black and white Americans presenting for management. *J Pain.* 2003;4:176–183.

91. McCracken LM, Matthews AK, Tang TS, Cuba SL. A comparison of blacks and whites seeking treatment for chronic pain. *Clin J Pain.* 2001;17:249–255.

92. Edwards RR, Doleys DM, Fillingim RB, Lowery D. Ethnic differences in pain tolerance: clinical implications in a chronic pain population. *Psychosom Med.* 2001;63:316–323.

93. Faucett J, Gordon N, Levine J. Differences in postoperative pain severity among four ethnic groups. *J Pain Symptom Manage* 1994;9:383–389.

94. Tan E, Lim Y, Teo Y, Goh R, Law H, Sia A. Ethnic differences in pain perception and patient-controlled analgesia usage for postoperative pain. *J Pain.* 2008;9:849–855.

95. Breitbart W, McDonald MV, Rosenfeld B, et al. Pain in ambulatory AIDS patients. I: Pain characteristics and medical correlates. *Pain.* 1996;68:315–321.

96. Castel LD, Saville BR, Depuy V, Godley PA, Hartmann KE, Abernethy AP. Racial differences in pain during 1 year among women with metastatic breast cancer: a hazards analysis of interval-censored data. *Cancer.* 2008;112:162–170.

97. Carey TS, Garrett JM. The relation of race to outcomes and the use of health care services for acute low back pain. *Spine.* 2003;28:390–394.

98. Sherwood MB, Garcia-Siekavizza A, Meltzer MI, Hebert A, Burns AF, McGorray S. Glaucoma's impact on quality of life and its relation to clinical indicators. A pilot study [see comments]. *Ophthalmology.* 1998;105:561–566.

99. White SF, Asher MA, Lai SM, Burton DC. Patients' perceptions of overall function, pain, and appearance after primary posterior instrumentation and fusion for idiopathic scoliosis. *Spine.* 1999;24:1693–1699.

100. Widmalm SE, Christiansen RL, Gunn SM, Hawley LM. Prevalence of signs and symptoms of craniomandibular disorders and orofacial parafunction in 4–6-year-old African-American and Caucasian children. *J Oral Rehabil.* 1995;22:87–93.

101. Creamer P, Lethbridge-Cejku M, Hochberg MC. Determinants of pain severity in knee osteoarthritis: effect of demographic and psychosocial variables using 3 pain measures. *J Rheumatol.* 1999;26:1785–1792.

102. Golightly YM, Dominick KL. Racial variations in self-reported osteoarthritis symptom severity among veterans. *Aging Clin Exp Res.* 2005;17:264–269.

103. Ibrahim SA, Burant CJ, Siminoff LA, Stoller EP, Kwoh CK. Self-assessed global quality of life: a comparison between African-American and white older patients with arthritis. *J Clin Epidemiol.* 2002;55:512–517.

104. Shih VC, Song J, Chang RW, Dunlop DD. Racial differences in activities of daily living limitation onset in older adults with arthritis: a national cohort study. *Arch Phys Med Rehabil.* 2005;86:1521–1526.

105. Ang DC, Ibrahim SA, Burant CJ, Kwoh CK. Is there a difference in the perception of symptoms between african americans and whites with osteoarthritis? *J Rheumatol.* 2003;30:1305–1310.

106. Allen KD, Golightly YM, Olsen MK. Pilot study of pain and coping among patients with osteoarthritis: a daily diary analysis. *J Clin Rheumatol.* 2006;12:118–123.

107. Meshack AF, Goff DC, Chan W, et al. Comparison of reported symptoms of acute myocardial infarction in Mexican Americans versus non-Hispanic whites (the Corpus Christi Heart Project). *Am J Cardiol.* 1998;82:1329–1332.

108. Hravnak M, Whittle J, Kelley M, et al. Symptom expression in coronary heart disease and revascularization recommendations for black and white patients. *Res Pract.* 2007;97:1701–1708.

109. Woodrow KM, Friedman GD, Siegelaub AB, Collen MF. Pain tolerance: Differences according to sex and race. *Psychosom Med.* 1972;34:548–556.

110. Chapman WP, Jones CM. Variations in cutaneous and visceral pain sensitivity in normal subjects. *J Clin Invest.* 1944;23:81–91.

111. Walsh NE, Schoenfeld L, Ramamurthy S, Hoffman J. Normative model for cold pressor test. *Am J Phys Med Rehab.* 1989;68:6–11.

112. Edwards RR, Fillingim RB. Ethnic differences in thermal pain responses. *Psychosom Med.* 1999;61:346–354.

113. Campbell CM, Edwards RR, Fillingim RB. Ethnic differences in responses to multiple experimental pain stimuli. *Pain.* 2005;113:20–26.

114. Mechlin MB, Maixner W, Light KC, Fisher JM, Girdler SS. African Americans show alterations in endogenous pain regulatory mechanisms and reduced pain tolerance to experimental pain procedures. *Psychosom Med.* 2005;67:948–956.

115. Rahim-Williams FB, Riley JL III, Herrera D, Campbell CM, Hastie B.A., Fillingim RB. Ethnic identity predicts experimental pain sensitivity in African Americans and Hispanics. *Pain.* 2007;129:177–184.

116. Klatzkin RR, Mechlin B, Bunevicius R, Girdler SS. Race and histories of mood disorders modulate experimental pain tolerance in women. *J Pain.* 2007;8:861–868.

117. Price DD. *Psychological Mechanisms of Pain and Analgesia.* Seattle: IASP Press; 2000.

118. Sheffield D, Biles PL, Orom H, Maixner W, Sheps DS. Race and sex differences in cutaneous pain perception. *Psychosom Med.* 2000;62:517–523.

119. Riley JL, Wade JB, Myers CD, Sheffield D, Papas RK, Price DD. Racial/ethnic differences in the experience of chronic pain. *Pain.* 2002;100:291–298.

120. Campbell C, France C, Robinson M, Logan HL, Geffken G, Fillingim R. Ethnic differences in the nociceptive flexion reflex (NFR). *Pain.* 2008;1334:91–96.

121. Campbell C, France C, Robinson M, Logan H, Geffken G, Fillingim R. Ethnic differences in diffuse noxious inhibitory controls (DNIC). *J Pain.* 2008;9:759–766.

122. Campbell CM. Diffuse noxious inhibitory controls (DNIC) in African Americans, Asian Americans and non-Hispanic whites. [abstract]Campbell CM. *J Pain.* 2008;9:P62.

123. Jimenez N, Seidel K, Martin L. Perioperative analgesic treatment in Latino and non-Latino pediatric patients. *J Health Care Poor Underserved.* 2010;21:229–236.

124. Tamayo-Sarver JH, Hinze SW, Cydulka RK, Baker DW. Racial and ethnic disparities in emergency department analgesic prescription. *Am J Public Health.* 2003;93:2067–2073.

125. Heins JK, Heins A, Grammas M, Costello M, Huang K, Mishra S. Disparities in analgesia and opioid prescribing practices for patients with musculoskeletal pain in the emergency department. *J Emerg Nurs.* 2006;32:219–224.

126. Pletcher MJ, Kertesz SG, Kohn MA, Gonzales R. Trends in opioid prescribing by race/ethnicity for patients seeking care in US emergency departments. *JAMA.* 2008;299:70–78.

127. Ng B, Dimsdale JE, Shragg GP, Deutsch R. Ethnic differences in analgesic consumptoin for postoperative pain. *Psychosomatic Med.* 1996;58:125–129.

128. Green CR, Anderson KO, Baker TA, et al. The unequal burden of pain: confronting racial and ethnic disparities in pain. *Pain Med.* 2003;4:277–294.

129. Ng B, Dimsdale JE, Shragg GP, Deutsch R. Ethnic differences in analgesic consumption for postoperative pain. *Psychosom Med.* 1996;58:125–129.

130. Ng B, Dimsdale JE, Rollnik JD, Shapiro H. The effect of ethnicity on prescriptions for patient-controlled analgesia for post-operative pain. *Pain.* 1996;66:9–12.

131. Todd KH, Deaton C, D'Adamo AP, Goe L. Ethnicity and analgesic practice. *Ann Emerg Med.* 2000;35:11–16.

132. Todd KH, Samaroo N, Hoffman JR. Ethnicity as a risk factor for inadequate emergency department analgesia. *JAMA.* 1993;269:1537–1539.

133. Chen I, Kurz J, Pasanen M, et al. Racial differences in opioid use for chronic nonmalignant pain. *J Gen Intern Med.* 2005;20:593–598.

134. Carey TS, Freburger JK, Holmes GM, et al. Race, care seeking, and utilization for chronic back and neck pain: population perspectives. *J Pain.* 2010;11:343–350.

135. Dobscha SK, Soleck GD, Dickinson KC, et al. Associations between race and ethnicity and treatment for chronic pain in the VA. *J Pain.* 2009;10:1078–1087.

136. Bijur P, Berard A, Esses D, Calderon Y, Gallagher EJ. Race, ethnicity, and management of pain from long-bone fractures: a prospective study of two academic urban emergency departments. *Acad Emerg Med.* 2008;15:589–597.

137. Ang DC, Ibrahim SA, Burant CJ, Siminoff LA, Kent KC. Ethnic differences in the perception of prayer and consideration of joint arthroplasty. *Med Care.* 2002;40:471–476.

138. Ibrahim SA, Siminoff LA, Burant CJ, Kwoh CK. Differences in expectations of outcome mediate African American/white patient differences in "willingness" to consider joint replacement. *Arthritis Rheum.* 2002;46:2429–2435.

139. Ibrahim SA, Siminoff LA, Burant CJ, Kwoh CK. Understanding ethnic differences in the utilization of joint replacement for osteoarthritis: the role of patient-level factors. *Med Care.* 2002;40:44–51.

140. Groeneveld PW, Kwoh CK, Mor MK, et al. Racial differences in expectations of joint replacement surgery outcomes. *Arthritis Rheum.* 2008;59:730–737.

141. Ibrahim SA. Racial variations in the utilization of knee and hip joint replacement: an introduction and review of the most recent literature. *Curr Orthop Pract.* 2010;21:126–131.

142. Kaiko RF, Wallenstein SL, Rogers AG, Houde RW. Sources of variation in analgesic responses in cancer patients with chronic pain receiving morphine. *Pain.* 1983;15:191–200.

143. Dahmani S, Dupont H, Mantz J, Desmonts JM, Keita H. Predictive factors of early morphine requirements in the post-anaesthesia care unit (PACU). *Br J Anaesth.* 2001;87:385–389.

144. Cepeda MS, Farrar JT, Roa JH, et al. Ethnicity influences morphine pharmacokinetics and pharmacodynamics. *Clin Pharmacol Ther.* 2001;70:351–361.

145. Zhou HH, Sheller JR, Nu H, Wood M, Wood AJ. Ethnic differences in response to morphine. *Clin Pharmacol Ther.* 1993;54:507–513.

146. Kosten TR, Rayford BS. Effects of ethnicity on low-dose opiate stabilization. *J Subst Abuse Treat.* 1995;12:111–116.

147. Green CR, Anderson KO, Baker TA, et al. The unequal burden of pain: confronting racial and ethnic disparities in pain. *Pain Med.* 2003;4:277–294.

148. Bates MS, Edwards WT, Anderson KO. Ethnocultural influences on variation in chronic pain perception. *Pain.* 1993;52:101–112.

149. Bates MS, Rankin-Hill L. Control, culture and chronic pain. *Social Science & Medicine.* 1994; 39:629–645.

150. Jordan MS, Lumley MA, Leisen JC. The relationships of cognitive coping and pain control beliefs to pain and adjustment among African-American and Caucasian women with rheumatoid arthritis. *Arthritis Care Res.* 1998;11:80–88.

151. Edwards RR, Moric M, Husfeldt B, Buvanendran A, Ivankovich O. Ethnic similarities and differences in the chronic pain experience: a comparison of african american, Hispanic, and white patients. *Pain Med.* 2005;6:88–98.

152. Hastie BA, Riley JL III, Fillingim RB. Ethnic differences in pain coping: factor structure of the coping strategies questionnaire and coping strategies questionnaire-revised. *J Pain.* 2004;5:304–316.

153. Bates MS. *Biocultural Dimensions of Chronic Pain: Implications for Treatment of Multiethnic Populations*. Albany: State University of New York Press; 1996.

154. Zborowski M. Cultural components in response to pain. *J Soc Issues*. 1952;8:16–30.

155. Rahim-Williams FB, Riley JL III, Herrera D, Campbell CM, Hastie BA, Fillingim RB. Ethnic identity predicts experimental pain sensitivity in African Americans and Hispanics. *Pain*. 2007;129:177–184.

156. Mechlin B, Heymen S, Edwards CL, Girdler SS. Ethnic differences in cardiovascular-somatosensory interactions and in the central processing of noxious stimuli. *Psychophysiology*. 2011;48:762–773.

157. Mechlin B, Morrow AL, Maixner W, Girdler SS. The relationship of allopregnanolone immunoreactivity and HPA-axis measures to experimental pain sensitivity: Evidence for ethnic differences. *Pain*. 2007;131:142–152.

158. Diatchenko L, Nackley AG, Tchivileva IE, Shabalina SA, Maixner W. Genetic architecture of human pain perception. *Trends Genet*. 2007;23:605–613.

159. Fillingim RB, Wallace MR, Herbstman DM, Ribeiro-Dasilva M, Staud R. Genetic contributions to pain: a review of findings in humans. *Oral Dis*. 2008;14:673–682.

160. Max MB, Stewart WF. The molecular epidemiology of pain: a new discipline for drug discovery. *Nat Rev Drug Discov*. 2008;7:647–658.

161. Gower BA, Fernandez JR, Beasley TM, Shriver MD, Goran MI. Using genetic admixture to explain racial differences in insulin-related phenotypes. *Diabetes*. 2003;52:1047–1051.

162. Mountain JL, Risch N. Assessing genetic contributions to phenotypic differences among "racial" and "ethnic" groups. *Nat Genet*. 2004;36:S48–S53.

163. Shriver MD. Ethnic variation as a key to the biology of human disease. *Ann Intern Med*. 1997;127:401–403.

164. Shriver MD, Kennedy GC, Parra EJ, et al. The genomic distribution of population substructure in four populations using 8,525 autosomal SNPs. *Hum Genomics*. 2004;1:274–286.

165. Gelernter J, Kranzler H, Cubells J. Genetics of two mu opioid receptor gene (OPRM1) exon I polymorphisms: population studies, and allele frequencies in alcohol- and drug-dependent subjects. *Mol Psychiatry*. 1999;4:476–483.

166. Kunugi H, Nanko S, Ueki A et al. High and low activity alleles of catechol-O-methyltransferase gene: ethnic difference and possible association with Parkinson's disease. *Neurosci Lett*. 1997;221:202–204.

167. Fillingim RB, Kaplan L, Staud R, et al. The A118G single nucleotide polymorphism of the mu-opioid receptor gene (OPRM1) is associated with pressure pain sensitivity in humans. *J Pain*. 2005;6:159–167.

168. Lotsch J, Stuck B, Hummel T. The human mu-opioid receptor gene polymorphism 118A > G decreases cortical activation in response to specific nociceptive stimulation. *Behav Neurosci*. 2006;120:1218–1224.

169. Shabalina SA, Zaykin DV, Gris P, et al. Expansion of the Human mu-Opioid Receptor Gene Architecture: Novel Functional Variants. *Hum Mol Genet*. 2009;18:1037–1051.

170. Chou WY, Yang LC, Lu HF, et al. Association of mu-opioid receptor gene polymorphism (A118G) with variations in morphine consumption for analgesia after total knee arthroplasty. *Acta Anaesthesiol Scand*. 2006;50:787–792.

171. Chou WY, Wang CH, Liu PH, Liu CC, Tseng CC, Jawan B. Human opioid receptor A118G polymorphism affects intravenous patient-controlled analgesia morphine consumption after total abdominal hysterectomy. *Anesthesiology*. 2006;105:334–337.

172. Weisse CS, Foster KK, Fisher EA. The influence of experimenter gender and race on pain reporting: does racial or gender concordance matter? *Pain Med*. 2005;6:80–87.

173. Riley JL III, Gilbert GH. Racial differences in orofacial pain. *J Pain*. 2002;3:284–291.

22

PAIN MANAGEMENT AMONG CHINESE-AMERICAN CANCER PATIENTS

LARA DHINGRA, PHD
Co-Chief, Research Division, Department of Pain Medicine and Palliative Care, Beth Israel Medical Center, New York, New York, USA *and* Assistant Professor, Departments of Neurology and Psychiatry and Behavioral Sciences, Albert Einstein College of Medicine, Bronx, New York, USA

GRACIETE LO, MA
Pre-Doctoral Fellow, Department of Pain Medicine and Palliative Care, Beth Israel Medical Center, New York, New York, USA *and* Department of Psychology, Fordham University, Bronx, New York, USA

JOHN TSOI, LMSW
Project Director, Asian Family Caregiver Program, Department of Pain Medicine and Palliative Care, Asian Services Center, Beth Israel Medical Center, New York, New York, USA

VICTOR T. CHANG, MD
Hematology/Oncology Service, New Jersey Veterans Affairs Health Care System East Orange, East Orange, New Jersey, USA

Key Points
- Chinese-American immigrants with cancer may be at high risk for poorly controlled cancer pain.
- While the prevalence of cancer pain in Chinese populations in Hong Kong, China, and Taiwan is comparable to rates observed in studies with non-Chinese populations, few studies have addressed cancer pain among Chinese immigrants in the United States.
- Traditional Chinese responses to pain may reflect passive coping strategies, leading to underreporting and underassessment of pain. Healthcare professionals can

use translated validated symptom assessment scales, and address educational, linguistic, and cultural barriers to discussing pain and cancer.

- Chinese patients are often fearful of the potential for opioid addiction and adverse effects.
- Understanding family-related influences and caregiver burden are important factors in the development and implementation of cancer pain treatment programs.
- Chinese individuals often believe in the beneficial effects of Traditional Chinese Medicine treatments on health maintenance, pain control, and chronic disease management.
- Despite much heterogeneity in cultural beliefs among Chinese patients, it may be helpful to express general understanding of Chinese concepts when speaking with the patient and family. This will immediately provide common ground, assist in establishing rapport, and provide a safe space to discuss otherwise sensitive topics, such as complementary and alternative medical therapies, and different concepts and beliefs about pain.

INTRODUCTION

Chinese Americans are the largest Asian subgroup (3.3 million)[1] in the United States, comprising a diverse and rapidly changing population. Many (21%) are recent immigrants[1] who suffer a disproportionately high burden of mortality for specific cancers, including nasopharyngeal, liver, and stomach cancer.[2] Because Chinese-American immigrants often present with advanced illness,[2] have low levels of acculturation,[1] are medically underserved[1] and economically disadvantaged,[1] they are at high risk for poorly controlled pain.[20] This chapter discusses the epidemiology of cancer-pain management among Chinese Americans, a population underrepresented to date in pain research, and presents data from an ongoing study of cancer pain with Chinese patients in New York City.[21] We address concepts of pain within Chinese culture that may influence the pain experience and identify potential barriers to pain treatment.[3] We conclude with practice recommendations to facilitate culturally relevant pain treatment.

EPIDEMIOLOGY OF CANCER PAIN AMONG CHINESE AMERICANS

Cancer-related disparities

Emerging data on cancer incidence for Asian-American subgroups show that Chinese Americans have high rates of nasopharyngeal and stomach cancers, with six times the rate of liver cancer compared to Caucasians.[2,4] One study in New York City documented mortality rates from nasopharyngeal cancer that were 12 times higher for Chinese women, and 20 times higher for Chinese men than Caucasians.[5] Data from the Surveillance, Epidemiology, and End Results Program showed that prostate, colorectal, and lung cancer are the top three causes of death among Chinese men, with liver cancer mortality rates exceeding that of all other Asian and white groups except Vietnamese and Koreans.[2] Despite evidence of these disparities, the prevalence and burden of cancer-related symptoms in Chinese Americans is largely unknown.

Prevalence of cancer pain

Numerous studies have identified the prevalence of cancer pain and symptoms in Chinese populations abroad, including Hong Kong, China, and Taiwan. This prevalence is 38–42%

in newly diagnosed patients,[3, 6, 7] 48–83% in those with advanced cancer,[3,8–11] and up to 88% in patients nearing the end of life.[11,12,13] While comparisons are difficult to make because of methodological differences among studies, these rates from Chinese samples in Asia are similar to non-Chinese samples in the United States. Some studies of Chinese patients in Asia have found that pain intensity is generally higher than in Western populations,[14,15] whereas others document similar distributions of pain severity.[16–18]

In contrast, there are far fewer studies of cancer pain among Chinese-American populations. For example, a survey of 50 cancer patients in California observed that the prevalence of current pain was 83.3% and that 28% reported worst pain > 7 on a 0 to 10 scale.[19] Research has been facilitated in recent years by the development of validated Chinese language instruments. We recently utilized these instruments in a study aimed at assessing the prevalence and correlates of cancer pain in a sample of economically disadvantaged Chinese-American cancer patients treated in a community-based oncology setting in New York City.[20] In this study ("Identifying the epidemiology of chronic malignant pain among ethnic Chinese patients treated in a multi-culturally diverse community setting"; PI: Lara Dhingra, PhD), a consecutive sample of 312 ethnic Chinese patients in a community-based oncology practice was screened, and 178 (57%) reported frequent or persistent pain. The most prevalent cancers were gastrointestinal (28%), lung (22%), and breast (21%), with 44% who had metastatic disease. The mean worst pain severity on a 0 to 10 scale was 4.7 (SD = 2.4), with 28% of patients rating their worst pain *greater than* 7 out of 10. Although 38% used opioids and 47% used non-opioids, 46% reported "little" or "no" pain relief from these medications. In multiple regression analyses, worst pain was positively associated with acculturation to the English language and opioid therapy, and pain-related distress was positively associated with opioid therapy.[20] We are currently conducting an intervention to improve the quality of pain management for this population ("Symptom control in underserved Chinese patients"; PI: Lara Dhingra, PhD).[21] Further, we will clarify the association between linguistic acculturation and pain intensity, which may be hypothesized to result from other modifying variables not evaluated in our prior study, including willingness to express pain, family-related influences, and cultural beliefs about pain.[21]

Human suffering, psychological distress, and disability

Undertreated pain has serious consequences for patients' health status,[22] and psychological distress may amplify pain severity and disability.[23] Preliminary analyses from our study in Chinese-American patients showed that higher levels of worst pain intensity were significantly associated with greater global symptom distress, greater psychological morbidity, and poorer physical, emotional, social, and functional well-being.[24] Consistent with these findings, studies in Asia confirm that higher levels of pain intensity and pain interference are associated with greater psychological distress among cancer patients.[8,25,26] While these studies have identified the burden of cancer pain and its association with human suffering, they have not elucidated the role of culturally specific factors. In the next sections, we review these potential influences and their relevance to pain in the Chinese-American population.

CULTURAL AND SOCIOCONTEXTUAL FACTORS

Sociocultural attitudes and beliefs

Culture is, in part, defined by the shared history among individuals or members of a specific group. According to Chinese tradition, during The Three Kingdoms period (AD 225–265),

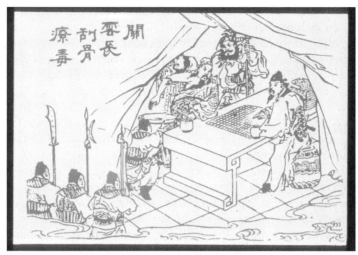

FIGURE 22.1 General Kuan Yu Playing Chess While His Wound is Treated (Wang, S. *A Hundred Pictures of Guan Gong*, Guangzhou, Lingnan Fine Arts Publishing House, 1996. p.73.)

the eminent physician Hua Tuo developed an analgesic potion called *mafeisan* (a mixture of herbal extracts) that he used perioperatively. His patient, General Kuan Yu, was wounded by a poisoned arrow. In this story, Kuan Yu drank the potion and played chess as his bone was scraped clean by Hua Tuo while his attendants fainted[27] (Figure 22.1). Medical scholars believe that this is the first documented use of anesthesia during surgery.[28] According to the text, General Kuan Yu maintains his poise and does not betray the slightest sign of pain. The implicit message is that the ideal patient does not complain of pain and the ideal physician prescribes effective pain medication.

Confucianism, Buddhism, and Taoism may also be central to shaping how some Chinese Americans view and experience pain. According to Confucianism, the ability to empathize with someone in pain verifies one's humanity.[29] Confucian teachings encourage an individual's efforts to control, confine, and manage distress through inner adaptation to pain, while discouraging outward expressions of pain. In this way, hardships are a trial to be endured to promote personal growth and development.[30] A second important concept emphasizes moderation in conduct and behavior. The direct effect of this is that Chinese tend to be less expressive than Caucasians, and this should be accounted for when assessing patients. In contrast to Buddhist beliefs about pain's origins, which are described in the next section, pain is not associated with sin or evil.[31]

Since the third century AD, Buddhist teachings have had a prominent influence on Chinese society. According to Buddhism, pain, sorrow, turmoil, and suffering are fundamental experiences in human life and serve to deepen an individual's understanding of the transient and impermanent nature of worldly objects, ideas, and emotions. There is an implicit belief that pain is a punishment for earlier deeds, even those from previous existences. According to Buddhist teachings, if an individual can detach from pain and not become psychologically distressed by it, then the individual can attain higher levels of being.[32,33]

In addition, Traditional Chinese Medicine (TCM) incorporates a combination of various Chinese schools of thought, including Taoism, and is distinctive for its emphasis on *qi*, or "energy theory." Health represents the manifestation of these energy fields interacting within the body. Pain is a result of *qi* disharmonies and imbalances in the body.[32] A TCM clinician would not treat headaches by focusing on the superficial, timely relief of pain symptoms, but instead, target the underlying cause with its deeper roots elsewhere. Thus, a Chinese patient who believes that pain is caused by a *yin yang* imbalance of the body may seek treatment with TCM or acupuncture to unblock the meridians and repair the imbalance. Another example is the preference for noninvasive natural methods of pain management. Chinese individuals often believe that TCM techniques help regulate and strengthen the body and facilitate recovery from cancer and cancer treatments. Thus, patients may regard Western pain interventions as a temporary suppression of the pain, but not an effective long-term strategy or "cure".[34] In addition to beliefs about the effects of TCM on health, some patients may hold longstanding folk and superstitious beliefs that demons and ghosts can cause illnesses, and cause pain.[35]

The aversion to opioids as medications in Chinese culture may also in part be explained through an understanding of recent Chinese historical perspectives. In the 1800s, opium addiction was an epidemic in China. The First (1839–42) and Second (1856–60) Opium Wars were fought between Britain and China over attempts by China to restrict illegal British imports of opium into China. China lost both wars, leading to a century of "unequal treaties" between China and Western countries from the Chinese national perspective, and an estimated 20 million addicts in 1949 when the People's Republic of China was established.[36] Even though illicit drug abuse was significantly reduced by the 1950s, the stigma of addiction remains a part of Chinese culture.[37] Even now, opioid consumption for medical purposes in several countries, including the United States, far outweighs that of China.[38]

Coping styles and pain

According to norms within Chinese culture, the display of negative affect, even in response to pain, could be regarded as disruptive to social harmony. Previous research shows that the predominant coping strategies exhibited among Chinese are generally more passive than active. This "passive-prosocial" coping strategy dominates traditional Chinese culture.[39] Emphasis on avoiding conflict may be apparent when a patient is reluctant to challenge or question a physician's recommendation about treatment in order to avoid being perceived as improper or disrespectful toward an authority figure.[40]

Passive coping diverges from the paradigm in Western culture. While Western cultures value active coping styles and problem-solving, this coping style may not be accepted by Chinese patients. Accordingly, He and Liu[41] found that the presence of a problem-focused coping style was not significantly associated with better quality of life in a sample of Chinese patients with nasopharyngeal carcinoma. Efforts to promote active coping efforts and behaviors (e.g., assertiveness, engaging with physicians and healthcare providers) may require educating patients and their families about the value and appropriateness of these approaches.

Pain, spirituality, and coping behaviors

Spirituality is associated with potential health benefits and may have great relevance to the Chinese population with cancer pain, yet few studies have examined the association between spirituality and health among those of Asian descent in the United States. A review[3] of cancer pain in Chinese patients showed that while 11 empirical studies reported on the patients' religious affiliation, religious variables were not evaluated in the context of cancer pain experiences (e.g., severity, mood, adjustment, irrational thoughts or meaning). While qualitative research has explored spiritual concerns among Asian cancer patients with pain,[42-46] we know of no existing published quantitative studies. This dearth of research may be attributed to several factors. First, few religion/spirituality measures have been translated and validated with Chinese-speaking populations. Second, most existing scales of religious/ spiritual coping are formulated within a monotheistic or Judeo-Christian framework, with items that may lack relevance for Chinese who do not follow these specific beliefs and practices. In our ongoing research, we use the "Daily Spiritual Experiences Scale," which was translated and validated with a Chinese sample from Hong Kong.[47] This scale does not reference specific institutional or organizational religious beliefs or activities and has been successfully used with individuals from different ethnic and religious backgrounds.[47–50] In summary, there are potential shortcomings to applying Western measurements of adaptive coping (e.g., active) and spirituality (e.g., monotheistic) to Chinese patients and pain experience.

POTENTIAL BARRIERS TO PAIN ASSESSMENT AND TREATMENT

Pain measurement

An important obstacle to pain assessment and treatment in the Chinese population has been a lack of translated and validated measurement tools for symptoms. The recent development of several culturally relevant instruments addresses this barrier. For example, the "Brief Pain Inventory-Chinese" (BPI-C), which evaluates pain intensity and pain-related interference, has been translated and validated in Chinese medical populations.[15,51] Similarly, the "Memorial Symptom Assessment Scale" and the "Memorial Symptom Assessment Short Form-Chinese" have been translated and validated with Chinese populations.[52,53] These measures evaluate symptom frequency, severity, and symptom-related distress (e.g., fatigue, pain, sleep disturbance, and gastrointestinal symptoms) in the past week, and enable comparisons with symptom data published in the research literature. Another useful tool is the "M.D. Anderson Symptom Inventory" (MDASI), a 19-item self-report measure on common symptoms (e.g., pain, fatigue) across cancer diagnoses and treatments, which also assesses symptom interference with daily life.[54] The MDASI has been translated into traditional and simplified Chinese characters and psychometrically validated with Taiwanese and Chinese cancer patients.[55,56]

Acculturation, linguistic, and communication barriers

Acculturation and language differences may pose formidable barriers to pain assessment and treatment. For example, a recent qualitative study using focus groups with elderly Chinese-American immigrants showed that problems communicating with healthcare providers were among the most profound barriers to disease self-management and health literacy in this group.[57] Another cross-sectional study of cancer pain in a community sample showed that lower acculturation and greater depressive symptoms were the most potent correlates of barriers to pain management.[58]

Shame and stigma

Studies in Chinese populations have shown that sociocultural and spiritual variables may also act as barriers to pain expression and management among patients. In Chinese culture, cancer is a taboo subject.[45] The open discussion of cancer is inhibited or discouraged, and euphemisms are used.[34] As a result of these attitudes, some patients with cancer may feel stigmatized or ashamed of their illness and refuse to talk openly about their symptoms.

Because of the potential stigma, distress, and other social consequences associated with cancer, some Chinese patients, especially elderly patients, may not be informed by their healthcare providers or family members that they have a diagnosis of cancer. In contrast to Western principles valuing autonomy and truth-telling, Chinese consider these practices cruel. In a study of 112 Taiwanese cancer patients, 79% were informed of their diagnosis, a rate lower than in non-Chinese samples. Patients not informed of their diagnosis tended to be older and had lower educational levels. However, patients informed of their diagnosis had lower levels of pain intensity and pain-related interference and higher levels of satisfaction with pain management.[59]

Stoicism and fatalism

Stoicism may hinder the ability of cancer patients to express pain to healthcare providers.[32] Perceptions of cancer are likely to reinforce patients' openness or stoicism, and compromise their willingness to communicate pain despite symptom distress. Confucian and Buddhist elements of Chinese culture favor a non-complaining attitude towards pain. Regarding fatalism, patients may believe their illness is predestined and immutable. Religious fatalism involves beliefs that pain should be endured for spiritual purposes, and thereby not carried into the next life.[60] Cancer-specific fatalism pertains to beliefs and perceptions that pain is an inevitable part of cancer and attempts to control it are futile.[60,61] Fatalism may also affect pain expression and treatment. One study showed that Taiwanese cancer inpatients who reported more cancer-specific fatalistic beliefs reported more barriers to pain management than medically similar cohorts in the United States and Puerto Rico.[62] Further, patients who reported more cancer-specific fatalistic beliefs also had more fears that pain represented a sign that their cancer was progressing, more pain-related functional interference, and used fewer pain medications.[62]

Traditional Chinese Medicine

As described earlier, Chinese-American patients may have strong preferences for TCM treatment modalities.[63] In our study, 36% of patients reported using complementary and alternative medicine (CAM) therapies for cancer pain.[20] One study in Chinese and Vietnamese immigrants showed that many used TCM prior to seeing a Western healthcare provider. Despite a willingness to discuss this with their healthcare providers, many patients did not wish to disclose their TCM use because they were concerned that their healthcare providers would react negatively based on previous experience.[64] This suggests that healthcare providers should ask about the use of TCM and facilitate open communication.

Caregiver burden

When a patient is affected by cancer, a family member frequently serves as the primary caregiver, especially if the patient is elderly. One study showed that medically ill Chinese patients often feared that they would become a burden to family members.[65] Such perceptions may enhance psychological distress[66] and are associated with severe decrements in health-related quality of life.[65] Fears of burdening family members could cause some elderly patients to minimize their pain symptoms. Glajchen and colleagues have translated "The Brief Assessment Scale for Caregivers" (BASC[67]), a 14-item measure of caregiver distress and burden in a clinical setting for use in Chinese populations (the BASC-Chinese[68]). They found that respondents with higher scores for two subscales: Negative Personal Impact (e.g., on caregivers' emotional health or quality of life) and Concern about the Loved One (e.g., caregivers' concerns or distress about the patient's illness, pain, or discomfort) had much higher distress rates (20% and 71%, respectively) than respondents with lower scores.[68]

Family-related influences

Family relationships are considered paramount in Chinese culture, and family members often play a key role in patients' healthcare and decision-making.[69] In one study, 15% of patients reported reticence to report pain because they feared how their family would perceive them, and had greater fears of addiction than those who had little or no hesitancy.[69] Caregivers' fears about patients' addiction to analgesics are associated with patient-related barriers to pain management.[60] Similar findings have been observed in non-Chinese samples.[70]

Medication adherence

Treatment adherence is a multifactorial outcome, and data from Asian studies show that patient-related concerns about analgesic use are positively associated with pain medication nonadherence.[71] Edrington et al[58] found that the most common barriers to cancer-pain management were related to analgesic use, including concerns about tolerance, dosing times, and addiction. These findings are consistent with studies from Taiwan.[60,71,72] Chinese cancer patients who were hesitant to use analgesics had greater concerns about addiction and side effects than patients who were not hesitant.[73] Patients with access to education about pain medications and a greater understanding of pain medications were more likely to adhere to their analgesic regimens.[74] When healthcare providers and pharmacists provided Chinese translations of pain prescriptions to patients, self-efficacy for analgesic use was significantly improved.[75] Chang et al[72] showed that a pain education program can be used to improve analgesic adherence by decreasing misconceptions and concerns about using analgesics and reporting pain. These findings suggest the need to understand better the factors that contribute to both limited knowledge of treatment and adherence with prescribed opioid therapy.

Additional factors

Barriers to pain management among Chinese-American patients are consistent with other ethnic or underserved groups. These include potential system-related factors such as limited access to care or treatment providers, lack of medical insurance or underinsurance, and lack of linguistic or culturally relevant pain management services.[76] Further, provider-related barriers may include lack of education or competency in pain assessment and management, fears about the risks of opioid misuse and abuse, reluctance to prescribe opioids, and physicians' personal bias and beliefs regarding racial/ethnic minority patients.[77-79]

RECOMMENDATIONS FOR CULTURALLY-RELEVANT TREATMENT

Vignettes of cancer pain

When pain practitioners conduct assessments and manage pain in Chinese patients, the family is usually involved in the process of medical decision-making. If the patient or family refuses the recommended strategy or treatment plan, pain practitioners should strive to determine their rationale. In our experience, open-ended communication is essential to achieving a balance between medical needs and culturally specific concerns. A recent study in Chinese cancer patients identified perception of the right dose, prompt delivery of medications, comprehensible explanations, and consistency of explanations by healthcare providers as important contributors to patient satisfaction.[80]

Thus, a pain management plan for Chinese patients should be flexible and negotiable, especially if the patient is also using CAM therapies. Practitioners should make sure they are aware of such alternative treatments by directly asking about them as some patients may not volunteer this information on their own. We offer the following practical suggestions to pain practitioners:

1. It may be helpful to express some interest, understanding, or general knowledge of Chinese concepts when speaking with the patient and family. This will immediately provide common ground, assist in establishing rapport with the patient, and provide a safe space to bring up otherwise awkward topics, such as the use of CAM therapies, and different perceptions and beliefs about pain.
2. Whenever possible, validate and legitimize pain control as a medical goal, in the larger context of reducing suffering. Pain practitioners are advised to present pain interventions as ways of enabling the patient to function, as a social goal to enable the patient to fulfill his or her role in the family and larger society, and as a way for the family to care for the patient.
3. Acknowledge the potential for treatment-related side effects and reassure patients and family members that follow-up care will address these issues in a flexible way based on patient and family-perceived concerns.
4. Provide clear, concrete, and written instructions about when to take medications, and translated educational materials (if available).
5. Recognize that there is a significant degree of heterogeneity in cultural beliefs among Chinese patients and their families.
6. Understand that Chinese patients' satisfaction with pain management is not based solely on their actual pain relief but their perception of pain management practices.[80]

We present four clinical vignettes to illustrate these suggestions.

CASE STUDIES

Case 1   **Pain Communication**
Background and History   Mrs. Chan is a 68-year-old Chinese woman with metastatic lung cancer. She completed radiation therapy and is undergoing chemotherapy. Even though she emigrated from southern China to the United States more than 30 years ago, she speaks only Cantonese. Her two adult children were raised in the United States, and recently noticed that their mother grimaces and rubs her back repeatedly. Mrs. Chan admitted to having frequent back pain, especially when she exerts herself or when she lies down. At this visit, her children inform you in English that their mother is in severe pain.
Clinical Commentary: Mrs. Chan is at high risk of having epidural cord compression, a potentially catastrophic

complication of metastatic cancer. The physician feels obliged to conduct a work-up and start appropriate treatment, including possible admission to the hospital.

Segments of Dialogue **Physician**: *Your children told me that you're in a lot of pain. How are you feeling today?*

Mrs. Chan *(via medical interpreter): I have some discomfort. It's nothing. I can tolerate it.*

Physician: *Can you tell me how the pain affects your ability to walk or to sleep at night?*

Mrs. Chan *(via interpreter): You are such a kind and considerate doctor. Everything is OK.*

Physician: *I would like to examine you, and we may need to do some tests.*

Mrs. Chan *(via interpreter): No more tests. They are very tiring for me.*

Physician: *Your children seem to be very concerned about your pain. Would you like me to prescribe some medication to help with the pain?*

Mrs. Chan: *No, I don't want to depend on pain medication. I don't want to get addicted.*

Her children *(in English): It's so frustrating that mom doesn't tell you how much pain she's in. She's also been buying and taking these herbal pills she buys in China. They tell her that it will cure cancer, and she's spent over $800 already! Can you please talk her out of it?*

Assessment/Interpretation *Because Chinese patients may hesitate to report their pain*
& *to their physician spontaneously, it is important to ask them*
Practice *about pain in a straightforward manner. Moreover, it is not*
Recommendations *uncommon for Chinese patients, especially elderly patients, to downplay their level of pain and distress. Thus, when assessing pain, asking the question in multiple ways may elicit more accurate assessment. Nonverbal cues and pain behaviors are important to note. Concrete questions that elicit close-ended answers are useful, such as "How many hours each day are you in bed because of pain?"*

Outcome *The physician highlighted the importance of these additional tests and explained their purpose and provided more details about the procedures (both invasive and noninvasive) while assessing her pain with the interpreter's help. The physician discussed with Mrs. Chan her intentions of using "herbal pills" from China and explained the risks of using both treatments at the same time. Lastly, the physician asked Mrs. Chan if she would like information about her medical condition to be communicated directly to her, or to her children. The physician then met with her adult children, and asked them how they would prefer this alarming news to be presented to their mother.*

Case 2

Background and History

Family's Role in Treatment Decision-making

Mrs. Pan is a 75-year-old Mandarin-speaking Chinese widow with terminal liver cancer who is hospitalized. She immigrated to the United States and worked as a seamstress before retiring. She is alert and lucid, but bed bound. On the "Wong-Baker FACES Pain Rating Scale,"[81] Mrs. Pan rated her pain as a "9" out of "10" in the past day. She is visibly distressed, has difficulty swallowing pills, and reports that she is experiencing episodic abdominal pain that keeps her awake when she turns on her side. The patient has two adult daughters and one son, all of whom were born in China. Her daughters are bilingual and work in the health field, while her son lives in Washington, D.C. and works in a Chinese restaurant. He has been staying in New York City for the past week.

Clinical commentary: The patient most likely has hepatic distention syndrome, where the liver capsule is distended and causes chronic and breakthrough pain.

The pain specialist (non-Chinese speaking) plans to provide patient-controlled analgesia (PCA) for pain relief and discusses this with Mrs. Pan via a medical interpreter. However, the patient expresses a preference for her son, who speaks only Mandarin, to make this decision on her behalf.

The doctor met with the son:

Segments of Dialogue

Pain Specialist: *Since your mother is experiencing a lot of pain from the cancer, we would like to put in a PCA pump to control the pain in a more flexible way. It is important that the PCA be controlled by your mother. While you may feel tempted to help by pressing the control button, your mother should be the only one to press the button. She is alert and quite able to do this.*

Son: *OK. (Continues to smile and nod, remains silent.)*

Later that day, the PCA pump was found to have been pressed by the son.

*Assessment /
Interpretation &
Practice Recommendations*

Patients and caregivers' cultural norms and values may differ from those of their healthcare professionals.

Healthcare professionals should be aware that even if a patient or family members nods, it does not indicate that she or he agrees with, or understands your treatment plan or explanation. It is customary for Chinese Americans to shy away from saying "no" in order to avoid offending others, especially those perceived to be in a position of authority. The key is to explore their understanding of material presented and ensure it is accurate.

Medical decision-making in Chinese traditional culture is oriented towards family-based decision-making processes. The highest role in the family hierarchy is usually held by the father or the eldest son.

Outcome	*The son's action of pressing the PCA button tapped into larger concerns and fears that his mother would die in severe pain. He is conflicted about watching his mother in pain and having to balance her perceived inadequate pain relief with the doctor's instructions. His perception that she was suffering led to the uncovering of larger unanswered questions about her end-of-life care. The team realized that the son had felt responsible for his family since his father died. These cultural beliefs, compounded by the expectation of his sisters that he should make the important healthcare decisions, were a burden to him. During a family meeting, all members were informed about Advance Directives, and they agreed to discuss this with their mother.*
Case 3	**Patient's Refusal to Use Analgesic Therapies for Cancer-Pain Treatment**
Background and History	*Mr. Chen is a 52-year-old man with nasopharyngeal cancer undergoing his fifth week of radiotherapy. Mr. Chen is from southern China, and although he speaks English he prefers to speak Fujianese. He lives alone, but has a relative nearby. He resides in a one-bedroom apartment on the sixth floor of a walk-up building, but he has dyspnea climbing the stairs. He has had extremely severe throat pain but refuses to take pain medications. He uses only alternative Chinese herbal medicine and cupping for pain, leaving some dark red scratches on his body. He arrives at his oncologist's office for a visit.*
	Clinical commentary: The patient most likely has radiation-related mucositis, a potentially severe pain syndrome that resolves after treatment is completed.
Segments of Dialogue	**Mr. Chen**: *Pain is only a symptom, not a disease. The treatment of pain will only delay the treatment of the disease by my daily qigong. The best treatment is to be patient, not anxious, and rest quietly to allow the qi to circulate properly.*
	Oncologist: *There are many effective analgesics that we can give you to help your pain.*
	Mr. Chen: *I don't want to cause trouble for my relative because he has to assist me to go see a doctor. In addition, all Western medications are too strong and very risky. I had a friend who had cancer and took those pain medications you talk about and he died. They have a negative effect on the brain's natural function. I know these medicines are addicting.*
Assessment / Interpretation & Practice Recommendations	*Similar to non-Chinese patients, Chinese patients may believe that all pain medications are highly addictive. Mr. Chen is enduring and living with pain because he is worried about becoming a burden to his relative.*
	It is useful to address Chinese cultural beliefs and incorporate them into the treatment plan. The addition of CAM therapies for pain treatment should be closely monitored because some traditional Chinese herbs can cause toxicity from poisonous compounds or heavy metals, are adulterated

with Western medications, or may have dangerous drug interactions.[82,83]

Healthcare professionals should convey to Asian patients and family caregivers that there is no shame involved with having their pain treated safely and effectively with opioids. Potential concerns should be addressed.

Outcome

Mr. Chen's oncologist and nurse explained the benefits and risks of taking opioids and asked Mr. Chen about his own beliefs regarding opioid treatments. This was an opportunity to correct misconceptions. His nurse explained that the treatment of pain does not interfere with his cancer treatment. To motivate him to consider Western symptom-control treatments, the oncologist then discussed how improving his pain and his dyspnea would reduce his difficulty climbing the stairs. The oncologist was respectful of Mr. Chen's preference for qigong and encouraged him to consider using both Eastern and Western approaches for the treatment of pain.

Case 4

Background and History

Truth-telling in the Context of Cancer and Cancer Pain

Mr. Wang is a 75-year-old Chinese man with a right lung mass that was noted on a routine chest X-ray nine months ago. His family did not want the patient to be informed and insisted that the patient be told he had pneumonia. He is now admitted from his doctor's office with progressively severe right-chest pain and dyspnea. On exam, he is unable to sit up because of pain, and has to lie down. Computed tomography of the chest shows an enormous mass invading the right chest wall and partially compressing the right mainstem bronchus. Mr. Wang wants to know why his pneumonia is getting worse after he took the antibiotics and what can be done to relieve the pain.

Clinical commentary: Chest wall invasion by lung cancer is a severe pain syndrome that may require an epidural infusion of opioid analgesics.

Segments of Dialogue

The Eldest Daughter: *I don't agree that you should tell my father about his health problems getting worse. He should not be told that he is dying or told about hospice. It is too cruel. My dad is already suffering, it is unnecessary to burden him any further.*

Physician: *According to our regulations, we must tell your father about his medical condition and treatment plan because he is capable of making his own decisions.*

Assessment/
Interpretation &
Practice
Recommendations

Before confronting the family caregivers about the patient's role in his/her own decision-making, in this case pain management, healthcare providers should first consider several important factors within a Chinese family.

Cancer can be an unspeakable diagnosis in some Chinese families. "Truth-telling" signifies the withdrawal of hope, and hope is central to the adult daughter. She may also feel out of control and helpless, and may need additional information on this subject matter, along with supportive counseling.

Outcome

Maintaining peace within the family is often a key priority in order for the family caregiver to realize the ultimate goal of harmony. Family caregivers are usually open to accepting outside help if they realize that it can help reduce their loved-one's burden or level of stress.

Finally, it is important to elicit, understand, and fulfill the patient's wishes, even indirectly. The patient may want to express many thoughts and feelings to his/her family members, discuss plans for the future, or engage in valued activities, which can help bring peace to the patient. It can be a very valuable time for the patient and family. Healthcare professionals can suggest specific strategies to family members for delivering information about diagnosis, prognosis, and treatment decisions and enable a family conference and provide appropriate follow-up counseling to patients and family caregivers.

Conducting the Family Meeting:

The healthcare professional was able to conduct a family meeting, which included a medical interpreter. During this meeting, the physician directly asked the patient in the presence of the family, "How much do you want to know about what is going on with your medical condition or do you want to authorize the family to make your decisions?" The patient wanted to know about his condition. A multidisciplinary team was mobilized after delivery of the bad news. Psychotherapy with family caregiver support, music therapy, and pastoral counseling were all provided to ameliorate distress with good results.

Clinical Commentary: In the case that no agreement between the family and patient can be made, the recommended course is to refer to an institution's ethics committee if the dilemma may pose violation of the patient's best interests.

ACKNOWLEDGMENTS

We wish to thank Mr. Jack Chen and Mr. Jae Shin for their assistance with literature reviews and references; Dr. Myra Glajchen for her contribution on caregiver burden; Dr. Kin Lam, Dr. William Cheung, Dr. Theresa Shao, Dr. Zujun Li and the Asian Services Center at Beth Israel Medical Center for their collaboration on research; and the cancer patients who have assisted us by participating in our protocols. This work was supported by the American Cancer Society, RSG 117416-RSGT-09–201–01-PC and the United States Cancer Pain Relief Committee.

REFERENCES

1. US Census Bureau. American Community Survey 5-year Selected Population Tables: United States. Washington, DC: US Census Bureau; 2010. http://factfinder.census.gov. Accessed June 2012.
2. Miller BA, Chu KC, Hankey BF, Ries LAG. Cancer incidence and mortality patterns among specific Asian and Pacific Islander populations in the U.S. *Cancer Causes and Control.* 2008;19(3):227–256.
3. Edrington J, Miaskowski C, Dodd M, Wong C, Padilla G. A review of the literature on the pain experience of Chinese patients with cancer. *Cancer Nurs.* 2007;30(5):335–346.

4. McCracken M, Olsen M, Chen MS Jr, et al. Cancer incidence, mortality, and associated risk factors among Asian Americans of Chinese, Filipino, Vietnamese, Korean, and Japanese ethnicities. *CA Cancer J Clin.* 2007;57(4):190–205.

5. Stellman S, Wang Q. Cancer mortality in Chinese immigrants to New York City. Comparison with Chinese in Tianjin and with United States-born whites. *Cancer.* 1994;73(4):1270–1275.

6. Ger LP, Ho ST, Wang JJ, Cherng CH. The prevalence and severity of cancer pain: A study of newly-diagnosed cancer patients in Taiwan. *J Pain Symptom Manage.* 1998;15(5):285–293.

7. Yan H, Sellick K. Symptoms, psychological distress, social support, and quality of life of Chinese patients newly diagnosed with gastrointestinal cancer. *Cancer Nurs.* 2004;27(5):389–399.

8. Hsu TH, Lu MS, Tsou TS, Lin CC. The relationship of pain, uncertainty, and hope in Taiwanese lung cancer patients. *J Pain Symptom Manage.* 2003;26(3):835–842.

9. Liu Z, Lian Z, Zhou W, et al. National survey on prevalence of cancer pain. *Chin Med Sci J.* 2001;16(3):175–178.

10. Sze F, Chung T, Wong E, Lam K, Lo R, Woo J. Pain in Chinese cancer patients under palliative care. *Palliat Med.* 1998;12(4):271–277.

11. Wang XS, Li TD, Yu SY, Gu WP, Xu GW. China: Status of pain and palliative care. *J Pain Symptom Manage.* 2002;24(2):177–179.

12. Chiu TY, Hu WY, Chen CY. Prevalence and severity of symptoms in terminal cancer patients: A study in Taiwan. *Support Care Cancer.* 2000;8(4):311–313.

13. Tsai JS, Wu CH, Chiu TY, Hu WY, Chen CY. Symptom patterns of advanced cancer patients in a palliative care unit. *Palliat Med.* 2006;20(6):617–622.

14. Cleeland CS, Nakamura Y, Mendoza TR, Edwards KR, Douglas J, Serlin RC. Dimensions of the impact of cancer pain in a four country sample: New information from multidimensional scaling. *Pain.* 1996;67:267–273.

15. Wang XS, Mendoza TR, Gao SZ, Cleeland CS. The Chinese version of the Brief Pain Inventory (BPI-C): Its development and use in a study of cancer pain. *Pain.* 1996;67(2–3):407–416.

16. Glover J, Dibble SL, Dodd MJ, Miaskowski C. Mood states of oncology outpatients: Does pain make a difference? *J Pain Symptom Manage.* 1995;10(2):120–128.

17. Lin CC. Applying the American Pain Society's QA standards to evaluate the quality of pain management among surgical, oncology, and hospice inpatients in Taiwan. *Pain.* 2000;87(1):43–49.

18. Ward SE, Gordon D. Application of the American Pain Society quality assurance standards. *Pain.* 1994;56(3):299–306.

19. Edrington J, Sun A, Wong C, et al. A pilot study of relationships among pain characteristics, mood disturbances, and acculturation in a community sample of Chinese American patients with cancer. *Oncol Nurs Forum.* 2010;37:172–181.

20. Dhingra L, Lam K, Homel P, et al. Pain in community-dwelling Chinese American cancer patients: Demographic and medical correlates. *Oncologist.* 2011;16(4):523–533.

21. Dhingra L, Thakker D, Lo G, Lam K, Chen J, Chang V, et al. Symptom control in underserved Chinese American cancer patients. *J Pain.* 2011;12(4)(suppl):P29.

22. Balducci L. Supportive care of elderly patients with cancer. *Support Cancer Ther.* 2005;2(4):225–228.

23. Turk D, Sist T, Okifuji A, Miner M, Florio G, Harrison P, et al. Adaptation to metastatic cancer pain, regional/local cancer pain and non-cancer pain: Role of psychological and behavioral factors. *Pain.* 1998;74(2–3):247–256.

24. Dhingra L, Lam K, Homel P, et al. Prevalence of pain and symptoms among ethnic Chinese cancer patients treated in a community cancer setting. *J Pain.* 2009;10(4): S7.

25. Sze F, Wong E, Lo R, Woo J. Do pain and disability differ in depressed cancer patients? *Palliat Med.* 2000;14(1):11–17.

26. Lin CC, Lai YL, Ward SE. Effect of cancer pain on performance status, mood states, and level of hope among Taiwanese cancer patients. *J Pain Symptom Manage.* 2003;25(1):29–37.

27. Lo KC, Hegel RE, Brewitt-Taylor CH . *Romance of the Three Kingdoms.* Boston, MA: Tuttle Publishing; 2002.

28. Golub RM. The cover. The physician Hua Tuo scraping the bone of Guan Yu to treat an arrow wound. *JAMA*. 2009;302(12):1262–1263.

29. Chan W. Idealistic Confucianism: Mencius. 2A:6. In: Chan, Wing-tsit, ed. *A Source Book in Chinese Philosophy*. Princeton NJ: Princeton University Press; 1963:49–83.

30. Chan W. Idealistic Confucianism: Mencius. 6B:15. In: Chan, Wing-tsit, ed. *A Source Book in Chinese Philosophy*. Princeton NJ: Princeton University Press; 1963:78.

31. Tu WM. A Chinese perspective on pain. *Acta Neurochir Suppl (Wien)*. 1987;38:147–151.

32. Chen LM, Miaskowski C, Dodd M, Pantilat S. Concepts within the Chinese culture that influence the cancer pain experience. *Cancer Nurs*. 2008;31(2):103–108.

33. Smith-Toner M. How Buddhism influences pain control choices. *Nursing*. 2003;33(4):17.

34. Im EO, Liu Y, Kim YH, Chee W. Asian American cancer patients' pain experience. *Cancer Nurs*. 2008;31(3):E17–E23.

35. von Glahn R. Plague demons and epidemic gods. *The Sinister Way: The Divine and Demonic in Chinese Religious Culture*. Los Angeles, CA: University of California Press; 2004.

36. Brook T, Wakabayashi BT, eds. *Opium Regimes: China, Britain and Japan 1839–1952*. Los Angeles, CA: University of California Press; 2000:5–7.

37. Liu W, Luo A, Liu H. Overcoming the barriers in pain control: An update of pain management in China. *Eur J Pain Suppl*. 2007;1(1):10–13.

38. International Narcotics Control Board. Levels of consumption of narcotic drugs: Average consumption of narcotic drugs, in defined daily doses for statistical purposes per million inhabitants per day. 2008.http://www.incb.org/pdf/NAR_Stat_tables/Table_XIV_1_SDDD_consumption.pdf. Accessed February 2011.

39. Hsu WY, Chen MC, Wang TH, Sun SH. Coping strategies in Chinese social context. *Asian J Soc Psychol*. 2008;11(2):150–162.

40. Chen YC. Chinese values, health and nursing. *J Adv Nurs*. 2001;36(2):270–273.

41. He G, Liu S. Quality of life and coping styles in Chinese nasopharyngeal cancer patients after hospitalization. *Cancer Nurs*. 2005;28(3):179–186.

42. Chan CWH, Molassiotis A, Yam BMC, Chan SJ, Lam CSW. Traveling through the cancer trajectory: Social support perceived by women with gynaecologic cancer in Hong Kong. *Cancer Nurs*. 2001;24(5):387–394.

43. Chung JW, Wong TK, Yang JC. The lens model: Assessment of cancer pain in a Chinese context. *Cancer Nurs*. 2000;23(6):454–461.

44. Kawa M, Kayama M, Maeyama E, et al. Distress of inpatients with terminal cancer in Japanese palliative care units: From the viewpoint of spirituality. *Support Care Cancer*. 2003;11(7):481–490.

45. Lui CW, Ip D, Chui WH. Ethnic experience of cancer: A qualitative study of Chinese-Australians in Brisbane, Queensland. *Soc Work Health Care*. 2009;48(1):14–37.

46. Simpson P. Hong Kong families and breast cancer: Beliefs and adaptation strategies. *Psychooncology*. 2005;14(8):671–683.

47. Ng SM, Fong TCT, Tsui EYL, Au-Yeung FSW, Law SKW. Validation of the Chinese version of Underwood's Daily Spiritual Experience Scale—Transcending cultural boundaries? *Int J Behav Med*. 2009;16:91–97.

48. Dean M. *Islam and Psychosocial Wellness in an Afghan Refugee Community*. [dissertation]. Bentley, Western Australia, Australia: Curtin University; 2007.

49. Fowler DN, Hill HM. Social support and spirituality as culturally relevant factors in coping among African American women survivors of partner abuse. *Violence Against Women*. 2004;10(11):1267–1282.

50. Mayoral EG, Underwood LG, Laca FA, Mejía JC. Validation of the Spanish version of Underwood's Daily Spiritual Experience Scale in Mexico. *Int J Hisp Psychol*. In press.

51. Ger LP, Ho ST, Sun WZ, Wang MS, Cleeland CS. Validation of the Brief Pain Inventory in a Taiwanese population. *J Pain Symptom Manage*. 1999;18(5):316–322.

52. Cheng KK, Wong EM, Ling WM, Chan CW, Thompson DR. Measuring the symptom experience of Chinese cancer patients: A validation of the Chinese version of the Memorial Symptom Assessment Scale. *J Pain Symptom Manage*. 2009;37(1):44–57.

53. Lam WW, Law CC, Fu YT, Wong KH, Chang VT, Fielding R. New insights in symptom assessment: The Chinese versions of the Memorial Symptom Assessment Scale Short Form (MSAS-SF) and the Condensed MSAS (CMSAS). *J Pain Symptom Manage.* 2008;36(6):584–595.

54. Cleeland CS, Mendoza TR, Wang XS, et al. Assessing symptom distress in cancer: The M. D. Anderson Symptom Inventory. *Cancer.* 2000;89:1634–1646.

55. Lin CC, Chang AP, Cleeland CS, Mendoza TR, Wang XS. Taiwanese version of the M. D. Anderson symptom inventory: Symptom assessment in cancer patients. *J Pain Symptom Manage.* 2007;33(2):180–188.

56. Wang XS, Wang Y, Guo H, Mendoza TR, Hao XS, Cleeland CS. Chinese version of the M. D. Anderson Symptom Inventory: Validation and application of symptom measurement in cancer patients. *Cancer.* 2004;101(8):1890–1901.

57. Wang J, Matthews JT. Chronic disease self-management: Views among older adults of Chinese descent. *Geriatr Nurs.* 2010;31(2):86–94.

58. Edrington J, Sun A, Wong C, et al. Barriers to pain management in a community sample of Chinese American patients with cancer. *J Pain Symptom Manage.* 2009;37(4):665–675.

59. Lin CC. Disclosure of the cancer diagnosis as it relates to the quality of pain management among patients with cancer pain in Taiwan. *J Pain Symptom Manage.* 1999;18(5):331–337.

60. Lin C. Barriers to the analgesic management of cancer pain: A comparison of attitudes of Taiwanese patients and their family caregivers. *Pain.* 2000;88(1):7–14.

61. Wills BS, Wootton YS. Concerns and misconceptions about pain among Hong Kong Chinese patients with cancer. *Cancer Nurs.* 1999;22(6):408–413.

62. Wang K, Ho S, Ger L, Wang J, Cherng C, Lin C. Patient barriers to cancer pain management: From the viewpoint of the cancer patients receiving analgesics in a teaching hospital of Taiwan. *Acta Anaesthesiol Sin.* 1997;35(4):201–208.

63. Wong-Kim E, Merighi JR. Complementary and alternative medicine for pain management in U.S and foreign-born Chinese women with breast cancer. *J Health Care Poor Underserved.* Nov 2007;18(suppl 4):118–29.

64. Ngo-Metzger Q, Massagli MP, Clarridge BR, et al. Linguistic and cultural barriers to care: Perspectives of Chinese and Vietnamese immigrants. *J Gen Intern Med.* 2003;18(1):44–52.

65. Tang ST, Liu TW, Tsai CM, Wang CH, Chang GC, Liu LN. Patient awareness of prognosis, patient-family caregiver congruence on the preferred place of death, and caregiving burden of families contribute to the quality of life for terminally ill cancer patients in Taiwan. *Psychooncology.* 2008;17(12):1202–1209.

66. Akechi T, Okuyama T, Sugawara Y, Nakano T, Shima Y, Uchitomi Y. Major depression, adjustment disorders, and post-traumatic stress disorder in terminally ill cancer patients: Associated and predictive factors. *J Clin Oncol.* 2004;22(10):1957–1965.

67. Glajchen M, Kornblith A, Homel P, Fraidin L, Mauskop A, Portenoy RK. Development of a brief assessment scale for caregivers of the medically ill. *J Pain Symptom Manage.* 2005;29(3):245–254.

68. Homel P, Glajchen M, Tsoi J, Chan S, Chan S, Portenoy RK. Measuring caregiver burden in the Chinese-speaking community. Poster presented at: Annual Meeting of the American Psychological Association; 2010; San Diego, CA.

69. Lin CC, Wang P, Lai YL, Lin CL, Tsai SL, Chen TT. Identifying attitudinal barriers to family management of cancer pain in palliative care in Taiwan. *Palliat Med.* 2000;14(6):463–470.

70. Ward SE, Berry PE, Misiewicz H. Concerns about analgesics among patients and family caregivers in a hospice setting. *Res Nurs Health.* 1996;19(3):205–211.

71. Lin CC, Ward S. Patient-related barriers to cancer pain management in Taiwan. *Cancer Nurs.* 1995;18:16–22.

72. Chang MC, Chang YC, Chiou JF, Tsou TS, Lin CC. Overcoming patient-related barriers to cancer pain management for home care patients. A pilot study. *Cancer Nurs.* 2002;25(6):470–476.

73. Chung T, French P, Chan S. Patient-related barriers to cancer pain management in a palliative care setting in Hong Kong. *Cancer Nurs.* 1999;22(3):196–203.

74. Lai YH, Keefe F, Sun WZ, et al. Relationship between pain-specific beliefs and adherence to analgesic regimens in Taiwanese cancer patients: A preliminary study. *J Pain Symptom Manage.* 2002;24(4):415–423.

75. Liang SY, Yates P, Edwards H, Tsay SL. Factors influencing opioid-taking self-efficacy and analgesic adherence in Taiwanese outpatients with cancer. *Psychooncology.* 2008;17(11):1100–1107.

76. Anderson KO, Green CR, Payne R. Racial and ethnic disparities in pain: Causes and consequences of unequal care. *J Pain.* 2009;10(12):1187–1204.

77. Anderson K, Mendoza T, Valero V, et al. Minority cancer patients and their providers: Pain management attitudes and practice. *Cancer.* 2000;88(8):1929–1938.

78. Anderson K, Richman S, Hurley J, et al. Cancer pain management among underserved minority outpatients: Perceived needs and barriers to optimal control. *Cancer.* 2002;94(8):2295–2304.

79. Von Roenn J, Cleeland C, Gonin R, Hatfield A, Pandya K. Physician attitudes and practice in cancer pain management. A survey from the Eastern Cooperative Oncology Group. *Ann Intern Med.* 1993;119(2):121–126.

80. Tang ST, Tang WR, Liu TW, Lin CP, Chen JS. What really matters in pain management for terminally ill cancer patients in Taiwan. *J Palliat Care.* Autumn 2010 ;26(3):151–158.

81. Wong DL, Hockenberry-Eaton M, Wilson D, Winkelstein ML, Schwartz P. *Wong's Essentials of Pediatric Nursing.* 6th ed. St. Louis, MO: C.V. Mosby Co; 2001:1301.

82. Chiu J, Yau T, Epstein RJ. Complications of traditional Chinese/herbal medicines (TCM) – A guide for perplexed oncologists and other cancer caregivers. *Support Care Cancer.* 2009;17:231–240.

83. Ko RJ. A U.S. perspective on the adverse reactions from traditional Chinese medicines. *J Chin Med Assoc.* 2004;67:109–116.

23

PAIN AND AGING: MANAGING PAIN IN AN ETHNICALLY DIVERSE POPULATION

CIELITO C. REYES-GIBBY, DRPH, MSN
Associate Professor, Department of Emergency Medicine,
The University of Texas MD Anderson Cancer Center,
Houston, Texas, USA

GUADALUPE R. PALOS, DRPH
Office of Cancer Survivorship, The University
of Texas MD Anderson Cancer Center, Houston,
Texas, USA

Key Points

- Although the age-related pattern of pain is unclear, studies suggest that older adults are at higher risk for pain.
- Evidence suggests that older adults who are members of diverse ethnic, cultural, or racial minority groups face a disproportionate burden of receiving inadequate management of pain.
- A better understanding of the cultural context and the interplay of different worldviews (social, cultural, and medical) of the pain experience can lead to the optimal practice of pain management.
- Age-related physiologic decline, cognitive impairment, psychological distress, and the lack of a social network are important considerations in pain assessment, treatment, and management.
- New advances in the delivery of immediate-release opioids and the use of complementary and alternative therapies are important considerations in pain management.
- Studies of pain, aging, and ethnicity are mainly descriptive and do not examine the extent of the interaction between aging and ethnicity as it relates to pain assessment and treatment.

INTRODUCTION

Maintaining optimal physical function and psychological health is a major goal for older adults their families, and their healthcare providers. Yet physical and psychological functioning in aging adults may be impaired by comorbid conditions, such as arthritis, diabetes, or cancer. These conditions often cause pain and other debilitating symptoms such as depression, fatigue, and sleep disturbances. The combination of these symptoms might be particularly detrimental to an older person's quality of life.

Research suggests that older persons and those belonging to diverse ethnic, cultural, or racial minority groups are more likely to receive inadequate management of persistent and acute pain. Projected increases in the number of older persons and in ethnic diversity[1-3] reflect the need to understand the challenges of providing effective pain management to older patients from various ethnic and cultural backgrounds.

EPIDEMIOLOGY OF PAIN

The United States is undergoing dramatic demographic shifts that will have profound implications for pain management practice. These shifts include an increased number of older persons and growth in the ethnic and racial heterogeneity of this group.[1-3] Demographic projections indicate these trends will continue over the next four decades.

Multiple factors contribute to the increase in older persons, including advances in medical care that prolong longevity, increased awareness and participation in the prevention and early detection of chronic diseases, and the aging of the "baby boomers," born between 1946 and 1964. From a global demographic perspective, the United States is considered a young nation, because older adults account for only 13% of its population. In comparison, Japan has the highest percentage (22%) of older adults, and in most European countries, such as Italy and Germany, 20% of the population are older adults.[1,2] According to a report from the Federal Interagency Forum on Aging-Related Statistics Centers, global demographic projections indicate that by 2050, the number of people age 100 years and older will increase 15-fold to 2.2 million worldwide.[3] These projections may not apply to developing or underdeveloped countries with higher poverty rates, poorer health status, and less access to medical care.[2]

Another demographic trend that will affect pain management practice is the growing ethnic and racial diversity of older adults. By 2050, more than 42% of older adults in the United States will belong to an ethnic or racial minority group.[1] According to a report by Vincent and Velkoff, there will be an increase in the older Hispanic group and in the group of older adults who are a race other than white. Additionally, the ethnic and racial composition of each age group will vary.[2] For example, the 65 years and older group will be more racially diverse than the 85 years and older group. The US Census Bureau's global demographic projections indicate that the elderly population, 65 years and older, will triple in size by the year 2050.[4] In fact, aging among the worldwide population will be expected to grow at a progressively higher rate for higher ages. Therefore, understanding the unique needs of older adults from diverse ethnic and racial backgrounds is critical for providing effective pain management services.[5,6]

Pain in aging populations

Although pain is not a normal condition of the aging process, several community-based studies of pain suggest that pain prevalence increases from the early adult years to approximately age 60[7,8] and thereafter reaches a plateau and may even decline in extreme old age.[7,8] It is generally accepted that increased pathological load is an overriding factor in the increased pain complaints that come with advancing age,[9] as older adults are at greater risk for diseases that cause pain, such as arthritis and cancer. Patients older than 60 years have twice the incidence of painful conditions as younger patients[8] and older patients are less likely to receive adequate analgesic treatment.[10] Furthermore, older adults tend to be less likely to complain of pain;[11] some accept pain as an expected consequence of aging, whereas others have concerns about not being heard, being labeled a "bad patient," or becoming overly dependent on others or on analgesics. Factors such as other medical problems, cognitive and sensory impairment, and depression might also contribute to the underreporting of pain in older adults.

We reviewed the literature (Table 23.1, Panel A) and found that from 11% to 60% of general adult populations suffer from chronic pain.[12–30] Because definitions of pain and the measures for assessing it are neither uniform nor standard (i.e., no gold standard exists) and because pain conditions are heterogeneous (i.e., nociceptive versus neuropathic), the estimates of pain prevalence vary widely. Other factors that contribute to the wide variation in results include, but are not limited to, the heterogeneity of disease conditions (e.g., low back pain, psychological disorders versus musculoskeletal conditions, etc); and the types of settings in which the studies were conducted.

Left untreated, pain adversely affects function and daily activity. A study of patients in Africa, Asia, Europe, and the Americas suggested that individuals with persistent pain were more likely to experience severe activity limitations than those without persistent pain (odds ratio, 1.63; 95% confidence interval, 1.41–1.89).[31] Among individuals in the United States with abdominal pain, more than 65% reported some activity limitations.[32] In the United Kingdom, Thomas and colleagues found that up to 66% of people age 50 years and older in North Staffordshire had pain in the previous four weeks and that reports of pain that interfered with daily life increased with age: among women, 32% in the 50–59 age group and 50% in the 80+ age group and among men, 33% in the 50–59 age group and 41% in the 80+ age group.[33]

In a 1993 population-based household survey, as many as 20% of US adults age 70 years and older in the general population reported having significant pain that resulted in activity limitations.[34] The adverse impact of pain is not limited to function. Individuals with chronic pain have up to a four-fold increase in the incidence of psychological disorders when compared with those without chronic pain.[31,35,36] Some researchers have suggested that pain is predictive of the development of depression,[37] whereas others have found that depression has either a causal or mediating effect on pain. One study in particular found a strong correlation between pain severity and depression in older patients but a weak and insignificant correlation between the two in younger patients.[38] Although the causal relationship between depression and pain remains debatable, at least in primary care settings, studies have shown that symptoms such as pain are in fact associated with depressive disorders or psychological distress and anxiety in aging populations.[39–41]

Pain in racial and ethnic minorities

Race and ethnicity are defined either by ancestry and combinations of physical characteristics or as social and sociopolitical constructs that include self-identity and culture. A number of definitions of race and ethnicity exist, especially in multicultural societies. For example, in the United States, the five racial categories are American Indian or Alaska native, Asian,

TABLE 23.1 **Panel A:** Population-based Studies Of Chronic Pain

Author	Country	Study Design	Setting	Age Range (Years)	Number of Subjects	Data collection methods Pain Assessment Tools	Pain Prevalence (Type)	Age-related Findings
Andersson(11)	Sweden	Cross-sectional	Two primary health care districts, rural areas	25–74	1625	Mailed questionnaire	55.0% and 49.0% (chronic)	Prevalence of pain increased by age up to 50–59 years for both genders and then slowly decreased
Bergman et al.(12)	Sweden	Cross-sectional	West coast of Sweden, community-based	20–74	2425	Mailed questionnaire	23.9% (CRP) 11.4% (CWP)	Odds ratio (OR) for CWP showed a systematic increasing gradient with age and was highest in the age group 59–74 yrs (OR 6.36, 95% CI 3.85–10.50) vs age group 20–34 yrs
Blyth et al.(13)	Australia	Cross-sectional	Nationwide, community-based	≥16	17,543	Computer-assisted telephone interview	17.1% male, 20.0% female	For males, prevalence peaked at 27.0% in the 65–69 year age group and for females, prevalence peaked at 31.0% in the oldest age group (80–84 years)

(continued)

TABLE 23.1 **Panel A:** (Continued)

Author	Country	Study Design	Setting	Age Range (Years)	Number of Subjects	Data collection methods Pain Assessment Tools	Pain Prevalence (Type)	Age-related Findings
Blyth et al.(14)	Australia	Cross-sectional	Northern Sydney, community-based	≥18	2092	Telephone survey	22.1% (chronic)	Prevalence was highest in the 70 years and over age group for men (26%; 95% CI, 18%–35%) and the 60–69 year age group for women (36%; 95% CI, 27%–46%)
Breivik et al.(15)	Fifteen European countries* and Israel	Cross-sectional	Community-based	>18	46,394	Screening questionnaire	19.0% (chronic; half reported having received inadequate treatment	Those below 40 years of age appeared to suffer less, whereas the 41–60 age group appeared to be more likely than others to suffer from chronic pain
Cassidy et al.(16)	Canada	Cross-sectional	Nationwide, community based	20–69	1131	SHBPS	28.4% (low back pain)	There was little variation in the estimates over age groups
Catala et al. (17)	Spain	Cross-sectional	Nationwide, general population	18–95	5000	Telephone survey	29.6% (pain day before interview) 43.2% (week before interview)	Frequency of pain increased with age, reaching 42.6% for people older than 65 years

Author	Country	Study design	Setting/population	Age	N	Instrument	Prevalence	Findings
Chrubasik et al. (18)	Germany	Cross-sectional	Regierungsbezirk Karlsruhe County, general population	18–80	1304	Mailed survey	47.0% (unduly prolonged pain)	Increasing age, obesity, and being female pre-disposed to the reporting of pain
Croft et al. (19)	England	Cross-sectional	North England, general population,	≥18	2034	Mailed survey	11.2% (chronic widespread pain)	????
Elliot et al. (20)	United Kingdom	Cross-sectional	Grampian region, sample of patients from 29 general practice/primary care facilities	≥25	3605	Chronic Pain Grade questionnaire	50.4% (chronic), 16.0% (back), and 15.8% (arthritis)	Proportion of chronic pain significantly increased with age from 31.7% for the youngest age-group to 62.0% for the oldest age-group.
Eriksen et al. (21)	Denmark	Cross-sectional	Nationwide, random sample, patients without cancer	≥16	10,066	SF-36	16.0% male, 21.0% female (chronic)	Prevalence of chronic pain increased with increasing age. Persons >/=67 years had 3.9 higher odds of suffering from chronic pain than persons in the age group 16–24 years.
Hassan et al. (22)	Saudi Arabia	Cross-sectional	Ten regional health care centers		100		41.0% (neuropathic), 59.0% (nociceptive)	?????

(continued)

TABLE 23.1 **Panel A:** (Continued)

Author	Country	Study Design	Setting	Age Range (Years)	Number of Subjects	Data collection methods Pain Assessment Tools	Pain Prevalence (Type)	Age-related Findings
Moulin et al. (23)	Canada	Cross-sectional	Nationwide, random samples and patients prescribed pain medication	≥18	2012	Telephone survey	29.0% (chronic, not cancer-related)	Mean age of respondents with pain was higher than those without pain (47.7 vs 42.7 years) and the prevalence of pain increased with older age groups.
Ng et al. (24)	China	Cross-sectional	Hong Kong, random sample	≥18	1051	Telephone interview	10.8% (chronic)	Two risk factors were identified: the female gender (O.R. 1.5, 95% C.I. 1.0–2.3) and age greater than 60 (O.R. 2.2, 95% C.I. 1.3–3.6).
Rustoen et al. (25)	Norway	Cross-sectional	Nationwide, general population	18–91	1912	Mailed questionnaire	24.4% (chronic)	A greater proportion of women, older individuals, those who were receiving a pension, those who were divorced or separated, and those with less education were in the chronic pain group.

Study	Country	Design	Setting	Age	N	Instrument	Prevalence	Findings
Saastamoinen et al. (26)	Finland	Cross-sectional	Helsinki, city employees	40, 45, 50, 55, and 60	6010	Chronic Pain Grade questionnaire	24.0% male, 29.0% female (chronic)	Those with older age, lower education and occupational class appear to be at excess risk for chronic pain, especially for disabling chronic pain.
Taylor(27)	New Zealand	Cross-sectional	North Island, general population	≥18	329	Mailed questionnaire	40.0%–60% musculoskeletal	Prevalence of MSK pain ranged from 40.0% (women aged less than 40 years) to 66.7% (women aged older than 65 years).
Torrance et al. (28)	United Kingdom	Cross-sectional	Aberdeen, Leeds, and London; random samples generated by six family practices	≥18	3120	S-LANSS	48.0% (chronic)	Pain of predominantly neuropathic origin was independently associated with older age, gender, employment (being unable to work), and lower educational attainment.
Yu et al. (29)	Taiwan	Cross-sectional	Taipei City, multiple-stage random sampling technique	≥65	219	Interview	42.0% (chronic)	????

Abbreviations: CRP, chronic regional pain; CWP, chronic widespread pain; SHBPS, Saskatchewan Health and Back Pain Survey; SF-36, Short-Form-36; S-LANSS, Leeds Assessment of Neuropathic Symptoms and Signs score; MSK, musculoskeletal.

*The 15 European countries were Finland, Norway, Sweden, France, Belgium, Spain, Italy, Poland, Ireland, Denmark, The Netherlands, United Kingdom, Switzerland, Austria, and Germany.

TABLE 23.1 **Panel B:** Population-based Studies of Chronic Pain in Ethnic Minorities

Author	Ethnicity	Age	Study Design	Study Sample Size	Pain Assessment Tool	Type of pain	Pain Outcome	Other Findings
Bernabei et al. (10)	White / African American / Hispanic / Asian / American Indian	≥ 65	Cross-sectional	13625	Patients' reports and observation	Cancer pain	13% of patients aged 85+ received strong opiates while 38% of patients aged 65–74 received opiates	Cancer pains among elderly minority patients frequently go untreated
Huang et al. (44)	White/African American/ Hispanic	45–80	Cross-sectional	44	Focus groups	Urogenital pain	66% reported dryness, 41% reported soreness, 41% reported pain/ discomfort during sexual intercourse, and 36% reported itching	Many reluctant to seek treatment, lack of focus on treatments for pain in female populations
Leveille et al. (46)	Black/Non-black	≥ 65	Cross-sectional	990 (female only)	Rating of pain on a scale of 0–10	Foot pain	Chronic and severe pain reported by 14% of the women	22% of the study population was receiving help with ADL (Activities of Daily Living)
McIlvane et al.(45)	African Americans/ Whites	45–90	Cross-sectional	175 (female only)	Questionnaires	Arthritis pain/ stress	African Americans reported having more functional impairment and lower arthritis stress than Whites	

Author	Ethnic group	Age	Study design	Sample size	Method	Pain type	Results	Conclusion
Palmer et al. (42)	South Asians	18–75	Cross-sectional	7668	Questionnaires translated into the patient's native language	Musculoskeletal pain	21% widespread pain in South Asian groups and 9% in European groups	Excess musculoskeletal pain is related to patients of South Asian culture
Riley et al, (47)	Black/White	≥ 65	Cross-sectional	1636	Questionnaires	Orofacial pain	37.6% of black females, 47.2% of white females, 49.3% of white males, and 62.7% of black males visited a healthcare provider	Financial constraints have greater impact on elderly blacks in receiving pain treatment than whites
Woodrow et al. (43)	White/Black/Oriental ["Asian"?]	≤ 20–70+	Cross-sectional	41119	AMS examination	Induced pain	Pain tolerance decreased with age, and was higher in males than in females	Whites are better able to withstand pain than blacks, who are better able to withstand pain than Asians"

SD= standard deviation

black or African American, native Hawaiian or other Pacific Islander, and white. Each race can be further categorized into two ethnic groups: Hispanic or Latino and not Hispanic or Latino. In the United Kingdom, the Office for National Statistics defines ethnicity as a rich balance of ancestry, religion, culture, nationality, language, region, etc. Although the Office for National Statistics suggests that there is no consensus on what defines an ethnic group because of the subjective, multifaceted, and changing nature of ethnic identification, it did develop ethnic classifications for the 2001 Census. Interestingly, these classifications varied slightly for Scotland and Northern Ireland as compared to England and Wales. To date, *race* and *ethnicity* are poorly defined terms that serve as flawed surrogates for multiple environmental and genetic factors in disease causation, including ancestral geographic origins, socioeconomic status, education, and access to health care. Research must move beyond the use of these weak and imperfect proxy relationships, i.e., discount self-identified race or ethnicity as a variable correlated with health, to better define the more proximate factors that influence health.[42]

Our review of the literature using the terms *aging, pain,* and *ethnicity* showed that certain ethnic minority groups are more likely to experience pain and the adverse impact of pain (Table 23.1, Panel B).[43–48] In a study from the United Kingdom, a greater proportion of South Asians reported widespread pain than white Europeans.[43] In studies of chronic pain conditions in the United States, African Americans and other ethnic minority groups consistently reported greater pain severity and disability than did those in other racial and ethnic groups.[49,50] A recent study of a nationally representative sample of adults in the United States showed that Hispanics and whites reported lower rates of activity impairment resulting from pain than did African Americans.[51] More African Americans than whites and Latinos reported activity impairment as a result of pain, a result that approached statistical significance at mild levels of pain severity.[51]

Studies of acute and postoperative pain have shown that minority patients are at higher risk than whites for undertreatment of pain.[49, 52, 53] Studies of cancer patients have also suggested that ethnic minority groups are at higher risk for severe pain and for undertreatment of pain.[54,55] Many studies have argued that in general, the association between race/ethnicity and poor health outcomes is largely a result of poor socioeconomic conditions among racial and ethnic minorities.[56–58] However, an Institute of Medicine report[58] suggested that in the United States, factors such as stereotyping and bias on the part of healthcare providers, lack of clinical appropriateness of care, and persistent racial and ethnic discrimination are among the reasons for racial and ethnic disparities in health care.

Influence of cultural, social and health care systems perspectives on pain

The function of pain varies according to cultural, social, and healthcare system perspectives. Models that address the interaction of these perspectives on the pain experience include the biocultural model[59] and the health systems explanatory model.[60] The first model is the biocultural model of pain perception, which suggests differences in patients' cultural worldviews may affect their experiences of pain.[59] The biocultural model focuses on the influence that cultural factors have on the chronic pain experience. It suggests that attitudes, expectations, behavior, and expression of pain are transmitted by one's cultural group. The model evolves from social learning, social comparison, and neurophysiology theories. Most important, the originators of this model recommend that pain assessment must be conducted within the individual's cultural background and that culturally appropriate pain management programs increase the likelihood of achieving optimal pain relief for the patient.

Another model is the healthcare systems explanatory approach, which suggests three distinct sociocultural "worlds" exist within a healthcare system.[60] These "worlds" or perspectives have the potential to influence a provider's treatment plan for an individual's pain, as well as how the individual perceives their pain experience and their expectations of pain management. The first world is the social support world, which consists of the patient's family (nuclear and extended), friends, community leaders, and spiritual advisors. Clinicians know that the level of approval and support from the family, larger community, and faith community heavily influences a person's response to pain. The second world is the individual's cultural background, which serves as a guide for behavior, practices, and values. For example, studies have shown that there are differences among cultural groups regarding pain behavior, expression, or preferences for pain management.[53,54,60,61] The third world, or perspective, focuses on the patient's perceptions of the health care received for their pain management. These perceptions may be influenced by the patient's acceptance of modern medicine versus more traditional medical beliefs and practices. Many Western societies have modern and scientific medical systems that value patients' autonomy in making decisions about treatment. In contrast, some ethnic groups value the family's input when making these types of decisions. Patients from diverse ethnic or cultural backgrounds may even have their own folk-healing practices and treatment for pain. Often time, healthcare providers in a biomedical healthcare system may have their own views or even biases about alternative treatments for pain. Patients who use alternative pain management treatments may be reluctant to share this information with providers if they sense their provider may be biased about the use of folk-healing practices for pain management. A better understanding of the interaction of these sociocultural perspectives and their influence on the pain experience may contribute to better pain management outcomes.

KEY ISSUES IN CHRONIC PAIN CARE FOR OLDER ADULTS

Pain management practitioners and researchers have long used the terms *chronic pain* and *persistent pain* interchangeably. However, the American Geriatric Society recommends using the term *persistent pain* instead of *chronic pain* when working with the older population.[4] The American Geriatric Society believes there is less stigma associated with this term, a perspective with which many older adults agree. *Persistent pain* is defined as a condition that lasts for a long period and is not always linked with a well-defined disease condition.[62] In this chapter, the terms chronic pain and persistent pain are used interchangeably.

Age-related physiologic decline

Chronic pain in older adults stems from various sources and leads to various types of pain syndromes (Table 23.3). The aging process is accompanied by physiologic decline and changes that place older adults at higher risk for developing multiple conditions that should be considered in pain treatment and management.[63,64] Vital organs such as the heart, lungs, and brain are affected, as are the urinary, immune, and endocrine systems.[63-64] The aging process is also accompanied by decreased muscle strength and mass and declining rates of gastric emptying and absorption.[64,65]

It has been reported that aging is also accompanied by neurobiological changes, including reduced myelination, axonal atrophy, and altered electrophysiology, all of which place older adults at higher risk for pain.[63,65] Although these changes are not linear with age, the degree of neuronal regeneration following injury decreases with increasing age. Others have proposed that differences in endogenous pain modulation by central pain-inhibitory

TABLE 23.2 Common Health Conditions and Types of Pain in Older Adults

Health Condition	Type of Pain	Cause	Description
Psychological disorders or existential suffering	Psychogenic	Psychological or physical disorder	Fear, depression, anxiety, or stress
Central nervous system or peripheral neuropathy from diabetes, neuralgia, phantom limb pain, post-mastectomy pain, complex regional pain syndrome	Neuropathic	Stems from damage to the nerve(s)	Burning, tingling, shooting, numbing, hypersensitivity and hard to localize
Musculoskeletal conditions including rheumatoid arthritis, osteoarthritis, myofascial disorders, visceral or ischemic pain	Nociceptive	Result of injury to tissues or muscles	Aching, sharp, dull, throbbing, and generally localized
Headaches (recurrent) and cancer	Mixed or unspecified	Combination of neuropathic and nociceptive pain	

63–65, 67, 68

TABLE.23.3 Age-Related Changes Affecting Pain Management in Older Adults

Heart	Decreased heart rate and cardiac output
	Increased systolic blood pressure
Lung	Decline in vital capacity and expiratory volume; Increased residual volume
Brain	Loss of nerve cells and synapses
	Increased atrophy and widening sulci
Renal/Hepatic	Decrease in glomerular filtration rate
	Reduced elimination of agents metabolized by liver
Immune System	Decrease in cytokines (IL-2, IgC and IgA)
	Altered T-cell function;
	Increase in memory cells and cytokines (IL-6, IL-1B)
Endocrine System	Reduction in estrogen and testosterone production

5, 6, 64, 67, 68

mechanisms and decreasing inhibition of pain signals may help explain the influence of aging on pain.[63,65] Research continue to explore age-related differences in pain sensitivity (i.e., threshold and tolerance) and endogenous pain modulation.

The prevalence of pain associated with common chronic or comorbid conditions in the older population is estimated at 39% (diabetes), 37% (hypertension), 41% (cardiovascular disease), 60% (arthritis), 34% (cancer), and 44% (lung disease) and is even higher for older minority adults.[34,64] The use of medications used to treat comorbid conditions may interact with classes of medications or adjuvant drugs used for pain management, thereby resulting in an increased risk for interactions and adverse effects. Examples of these types of drugs include antidepressants (tricyclic or selective serotonin reuptake inhibitors), anticonvulsants (e.g., gabapentin), corticosteroids, muscle relaxants, and benzodiazepines.[64,66–68]

Overall, clinical pain management in aging populations can be complex and challenging. Although pain in general is multifactorial, the complexity of pain management in older populations is compounded by factors such as the effects of aging on pain perception and processing, multiple comorbidities, and general physiological decline.

Cognitive impairment

As populations age and advances in medical care continue to be made, a growing proportion of individuals can expect to live well into their eighth and even ninth decades. This extended life span comes with the increased likelihood of both cognitive impairment and pain. Thus, the techniques for assessing and managing pain must be a central priority when treating cognitively impaired older persons.[69,70] Few studies have focused on the preference for the type of assessment scale to use in cognitively impaired older adults of specific ethnic or racial groups.[70,71] One such study found that cognitively impaired Hispanic and African-American older adults preferred the Faces Pain Scale; the investigators surmised that this preference was based on the impact of culture on pain expression in these groups.[72] Clinicians may need to be reminded that assessment scales such as the numerical or visual analog scale may not be appropriate for cognitively impaired adults.[71] Elderly patients with dementia may also have difficulty with these scales, commonly because of decreased memory, poor orientation, and compromised visual and spatial skills.[73] Verbal communication between a clinician and patient may be limited when a patient is cognitively impaired. Nonverbal signs of pain in cognitively impaired patients include grimacing, tightening of muscles, or lack of appetite.[71,73] Thus, assessment of verbal and nonverbal cues is critical in managing pain in cognitively impaired elders.

Psychological issues

Older adults face a multitude of psychosocial issues. In general, they must cope with common grief and loss responses related to their mortality, finances, role changes within their families, and changes in their cognitive and physical abilities. Several studies have documented the association between pain and depressive disorders, psychological distress, and anxiety in aging populations.[34,39–41,51,74] Therefore, screening and further diagnostic evaluation of patients for symptoms such as distress, anxiety, or depression should be facilitated. Several methods of assessment, including single-item interviews (e.g., "Have you been depressed most of the time for the past two weeks?") or multiple-item scales such as the Beck Depression Inventory-13 may be very useful.[75] Key symptoms may include hopelessness, excessive guilt, worthlessness, and suicidal ideation.

Social network

Older adults frequently face social isolation, and widowhood is the most common cause. For many, this translates into a lack of a social network that could provide support in navigating the complex world of pain management. Identifying a person who can function as a "pain navigator" is a key component of effective pain care. A pain navigator may be recommended as part of the follow-up services provided by the pain management team.[76] For example, a social worker or case manager might help the patient transition from the hospital to the community by identifying self-help pain resources or advocacy groups in the patient's immediate community or by compiling a list of neighborhood pharmacies that provide opioids and other medications used as adjuvant therapy in pain management. For older patients whose primary language may differ from that of the healthcare provider, it is critical to have a pain navigator who speaks the patient's primary language when pain treatment plans and regimens are being explained. Nowadays, pain management teams routinely include interpreters. The patient navigator model has been quite successful in linking older adults and groups who are unfamiliar with the healthcare system to the appropriate services in their community.[76]

New routes to deliver pain medicine

Many older adults might not be aware that recent technological advances have changed the manner in which pain medications are delivered. In the past, most available opioids had to be administered every three to four hours. The short half-life of these drugs resulted in many limitations, including poor patient compliance and inadequate pain relief. Now novel delivery systems, including sustained release and continuous infusion, are available.[73–75] Even more encouraging are the advances made in the delivery of immediate-release opioids, including transmucosally and buccally delivered fentanyl.[77–80] In addition, morphine is now available for acute pain via an intranasal delivery system, which allows the medication to be quickly absorbed through the nasal mucous membranes.[80]

Treating pain in other ways

Many older adults who are individuals living with chronic pain often seek treatment that does not include the use of medications. A variety of methods may be used, including nonpharmacological, alternative, or complementary methods.[81] Pain is a complex, multidimensional, and subjective experience. Therefore, a combination of pain medications and nonpharmacological treatment methods should be made available. Many individuals may use traditional or folk remedies to obtain pain relief or to deal with the side effects of their pain medications. The majority of these remedies may be harmless, but a few may lead to harmful outcomes when combined with stronger pain or adjuvant medications. Thus, careful and detailed assessment of current pain treatment practices is needed in this population.

SUMMARY AND FUTURE DIRECTIONS

While studies have suggested that older adults who are also ethnic or racial minorities face a disproportionate burden of acquiring adequate pain management, these studies are mainly descriptive and fail to examine the extent of the interaction between aging and ethnicity as it relates to pain assessment and treatment. Aging and ethnicity are nonmodifiable factors. Therefore, the goal of clinicians should be to provide equitable and individualized pain treatment and management. Future studies should further explore the influence of the patient-provider relationship; stereotyping, biases, and prejudicial practices in pain assessment and treatment; and the influence of health policy and healthcare system factors. Laboratory studies that examine neurobiological changes associated with aging, age-related differences in pain modulation, differential expression of pain-related genes among ethnic and racial groups, and pharmacogenetics hold promise for individualized pain treatment and management.

REFERENCES

1. Vincent GR, Velkoff VA. The next four decades, the older population in the United States: 2010–2050. Washington,DC: U.S. Census Bureau; 2010. Report No.: P25–1138.
2. Centers for Disease Control. Older Americans 2010 key indicators of well-being. 2010.
3. Administration on Aging. A profile of older Americans:2009. Washington, DC: U.S. Department of Heatth and Human Services; 2009.
4. International Programs Center PDUCB. Global population profile: 2002. Washington, DC: US Government Printing Office; 2004. Report No.: PASA HRN-P-00-97-00016-00.
5. American Geriatrics Society. Pharmacological management of persistent pain in older persons. *Journal of American Geriatric Society* 2009;57(8):1331–1346.
6. Chapman S. Managing pain in the older person. *Nurs Stand* 2010;25(11):35–39.
7. Crook J, Rideout E, Browne G. The prevalence of pain complaints in a general population. *Pain* 1984;18(3):299–314.
8. Helme RD, Gibson SJ. The epidemiology of pain in elderly people. *Clin Geriatr Med* 2001;17(3):417–431.
9. Ferrell BA, Ferrell BR, Osterweil D. Pain in the nursing home. *J Am Geriatr Soc* 1990;38(4):409–414.
10. Weiner DK. Improving pain management for older adults: an urgent agenda for the educator, investigator, and practitioner. *Pain* 2002;97(1–2):1–4.
11. Bernabei R, Gambassi G, Lapane K et al. Management of pain in elderly patients with cancer. SAGE Study Group. Systematic Assessment of Geriatric Drug Use via Epidemiology. *JAMA* 1998;279(23):1877–1882.
12. Andersson HI. The epidemiology of chronic pain in a Swedish rural area. *Qual Life Res* 1994;3 Suppl 1:S19–S26.
13. Bergman S, Herrstrom P, Hogstrom K, Petersson IF, Svensson B, Jacobsson LT. Chronic musculoskeletal pain, prevalence rates, and sociodemographic associations in a Swedish population study. *J Rheumatol* 2001;28(6):1369–1377.
14. Blyth FM, March LM, Brnabic AJ, Jorm LR, Williamson M, Cousins MJ. Chronic pain in Australia: a prevalence study. *Pain* 2001;89(2–3):127–134.
15. Blyth FM, March LM, Cousins MJ. Chronic pain-related disability and use of analgesia and health services in a Sydney community. *Med J Aust* 2003;179(2):84–87.
16. Breivik H, ollett B, entafridda V, ohen R, allacher D. Survey of chronic pain in Europe: Prevalence, impact on daily life, and treatment. *European Journal of Pain* 2006;10(4):287–333.
17. Cassidy JD, Carroll LJ, Cote P. The Saskatchewan health and back pain survey. The prevalence of low back pain and related disability in Saskatchewan adults. *Spine (Phila Pa 1976)* 1998;23(17):1860–1866.
18. Catala E, Reig E, Artes M, Aliaga L, Lopez JS, Segu JL. Prevalence of pain in the Spanish population: telephone survey in 5000 homes. *Eur J Pain* 2002;6(2):133–140.
19. Chrubasik S, Junck H, Zappe HA, Stutzke O. A survey on pain complaints and health care utilization in a German population sample. *Eur J Anaesthesiol* 1998;15(4):397–408.
20. Croft P, Rigby AS, Boswell R, Schollum J, Silman A. The prevalence of chronic widespread pain in the general population. *J Rheumatol* 1993;20(4):710–713.
21. Elliott AM, Smith BH, Penny KI, Smith WC, Chambers WA. The epidemiology of chronic pain in the community. *Lancet* 1999;354(9186):1248–1252.
22. Eriksen J, Jensen MK, Sjogren P, Ekholm O, Rasmussen NK. Epidemiology of chronic non-malignant pain in Denmark. *Pain* 2003;106(3):221–228.
23. Ng KF, Tsui SL, Chan WS. Prevalence of common chronic pain in Hong Kong adults. *Clin J Pain* 2002;18(5):275–281.

24. Rustoen T, Wahl AK, Hanestad BR, Lerdal A, Paul S, Miaskowski C. Prevalence and characteristics of chronic pain in the general Norwegian population. *Eur J Pain* 2004;8(6):555–565.

25. Saastamoinen P, Leino-Arjas P, Laaksonen M, Lahelma E. Socio-economic differences in the prevalence of acute, chronic and disabling chronic pain among ageing employees. *Pain* 2005;114(3):364–371.

26. Torrance N, Smith BH, Bennett MI, Lee AJ. The epidemiology of chronic pain of predominantly neuropathic origin. Results from a general population survey. *J Pain* 2006;7(4):281–289.

27. Yu HY, Tang FI, Kuo BI, Yu S. Prevalence, interference, and risk factors for chronic pain among Taiwanese community older people. *Pain Manag Nurs* 2006;7(1):2–11.

28. Hassan AE, Saleh HA, Baroudy YM et al. Prevalence of neuropathic pain among patients suffering from chronic low back pain in Saudi Arabia. *Saudi Medical Journal* 2004;25(12):1986–1990.

29. Moulin DE, Clark AJ, Speechley M, Morley-Forster PK. Chronic pain in Canada—prevalence, treatment, impact and the role of opioid analgesia. *Pain Res Manag* 2002;7(4):179–184.

30. Taylor WJ. The frequency and impact of musculoskeletal pain in the adult New Zealand general population. *Ann Rheum Dis* 2005;64:548.

31. Gureje O, Von KM, Simon GE, Gater R. Persistent pain and well-being: a World Health Organization Study in Primary Care. *JAMA* 1998;280(2):147–151.

32. Sandler RS, Stewart WF, Liberman JN, Ricci JA, Zorich NL. Abdominal pain, bloating, and diarrhea in the United States: prevalence and impact. *Dig Dis Sci* 2000;45(6):1166–1171.

33. Thomas E, Peat G, Harris L, Wilkie R, Croft PR. The prevalence of pain and pain interference in a general population of older adults: cross-sectional findings from the North Staffordshire Osteoarthritis Project (NorStOP). *Pain* 2004;110(1–2):361–368.

34. Reyes-Gibby CC, Aday L, Cleeland C. Impact of pain on self-rated health in the community-dwelling older adults. *Pain* 2002;95(1–2):75–82.

35. Magni G, Rigatti-Luchini S, Fracca F, Merskey H. Suicidality in chronic abdominal pain: an analysis of the Hispanic Health and Nutrition Examination Survey (HHANES). *Pain* 1998;76(1–2):137–144.

36. Magni G, Caldieron C, Rigatti-Luchini S, Merskey H. Chronic musculoskeletal pain and depressive symptoms in the general population. An analysis of the 1st National Health and Nutrition Examination Survey data. *Pain* 1990;43(3):299–307.

37. Magni G, Moreschi C, Rigatti-Luchini S, Merskey H. Prospective study on the relationship between depressive symptoms and chronic musculoskeletal pain. *Pain* 1994;56(3):289–297.

38. Turk DC, Okifuji A, Scharff L. Chronic pain and depression: role of perceived impact and perceived control in different age cohorts. *Pain* 1995;61(1):93–101.

39. McWilliams LA, Goodwin RD, Cox BJ. Depression and anxiety associated with three pain conditions: results from a nationally representative sample. *Pain* 2004;111(1–2):77–83.

40. Ohayon MM. Specific characteristics of the pain/depression association in the general population. *J Clin Psychiatry* 2004;65 Suppl 12:5–9.

41. Onder G, Landi F, Gambassi G et al. Association between pain and depression among older adults in Europe: results from the Aged in Home Care (AdHOC) project: a cross-sectional study. *J Clin Psychiatry* 2005;66(8):982–988.

42. Collins FS. What we do and don't know about "race", "ethnicity", genetics and health at the dawn of the genome era. *Nat Genet* 2004;36(11 Suppl):S13–S15.

43. Palmer B, Macfarlane G, Afzal C, Esmail A, Silman A, Lunt M. Acculturation and the prevalence of pain amongst South Asian minority ethnic groups in the UK. *Rheumatology (Oxford)* 2007;46(6):1009–1014.

44. Woodrow KM, Friedman GD, Siegelaub AB, Collen MF. Pain tolerance: differences according to age, sex and race. *Psychosom Med* 1972;34(6):548–556.

45. Huang AJ, Luft J, Grady D, Kuppermann M. The day-to-day impact of urogenital aging: perspectives from racially/ethnically diverse women. *J Gen Intern Med* 2010;25(1):45–51.

46. McIlvane JM, Baker TA, Mingo CA. Racial differences in arthritis-related stress, chronic life stress, and depressive symptoms among women with arthritis: a contextual perspective. *J Gerontol B Psychol Sci Soc Sci* 2008;63(5):S320–S327.

47. Leveille SG. Musculoskeletal aging. *Curr Opin Rheumatol* 2004;16(2):114–118.

48. Riley JL, III, Wade JB, Myers CD, Sheffield D, Papas RK, Price DD. Racial/ethnic differences in the experience of chronic pain. *Pain* 2002;100(3):291–298.

49. Green CR, Anderson KO, Baker TA et al. The unequal burden of pain: confronting racial and ethnic disparities in pain. *Pain Med* 2003;4(3):277–294.

50. Green CR, Baker TA, Sato Y, Washington TL, Smith EM. Race and chronic pain: A comparative study of young black and white Americans presenting for management. *J Pain* 2003;4(4):176–183.

51. Reyes-Gibby CC, Aday LA, Todd KH, Cleeland CS, Anderson KO. Pain in aging community-dwelling adults in the United States: non-Hispanic whites, non-Hispanic blacks, and Hispanics. *J Pain* 2007;8(1):75–84.

52. Ezenwa MO, Ameringer S, Ward SE, Serlin RC. Racial and ethnic disparities in pain management in the United States. *J Nurs Scholarsh* 2006;38(3):225–233.

53. Green C, Todd KH, Lebovits A, Francis M. Disparities in pain: ethical issues. *Pain Med* 2006;7(6):530–533.

54. Anderson KO, Richman SP, Hurley J et al. Cancer pain management among underserved minority outpatients: perceived needs and barriers to optimal control. *Cancer* 2002;94(8):2295–2304.

55. Anderson KO, Mendoza TR, Payne R et al. Pain education for underserved minority cancer patients: a randomized controlled trial. *J Clin Oncol* 2004;22(24):4918–4925.

56. Aday LA. Access to what? For whom? *Health Manage Q* 1990;12(4):18–22.

57. Aday LA. Equity, accessibility, and ethical issues: is the U.S. health care reform debate asking the right questions? *Am Behav Sci* 1993;36(6):724–740.

58. Institute of Medicine. *Crossing the quality chasm.* 2001 ed. Washington, DC: National Academies Press; 2003.

59. Bates MS. Ethnicity and pain: a biocultural model. *Soc Sci Med* 1987;24(1):47–50.

60. Kleinman A. Concepts and a model for the comparison of medical systems as cultural systems. *Soc Sci Med* 1978;12(2B):85–95.

61. Juarez G, Ferrell B, Borneman T. Cultural considerations in education for cancer pain management. *J Cancer Educ* 1999;14(3):168–173.

62. Hadjistavropoulos T, Herr K, Turk D, et al. An interdisciplinary expert consensus statement on assessment of pain in older persons. *Clin J Pain* 2007;23(23 (Suppl.)):S1–S43.

63. McCarberg B., Cole BE. *Pain in the older person. In: Biobehavioral approaches to pain*, editor.New York: Springer; 2009. 195–218.

64. Fine PG. Chronic pain management in older adults: special considerations. *J Pain Symptom Manage* 2009;38(2 Suppl):S4–S14.

65. Davis MP, Srivastava M. Demographics, assessment and management of pain in the elderly. *Drugs Aging* 2003;20(1):23–57.

66. Catananti C, Gambassi G. Pain assessment in the elderly. *Surg Oncol* 2010;19(3):140–148.

67. Wynne H. Drug metabolism and ageing. *J Br Menopause Soc* 2005;11(2):51–56.

68. Bruckenthal P, Reid MC, Reisner L. Special issues in the management of chronic pain in older adults. *Pain Med* 2009;10 Suppl 2:S67–S78.

69. Catananti C, Gambassi G. Pain assessment in the elderly. *Surg Oncol* 2010;19(3):140–148.

70. Parmelee PA. Pain in cognitively impaired older persons. *Clin Geriatr Med* 1996;12(3):473–487.

71. Stolee P, Hillier LM, Esbaugh J, Bol N, McKellar L, Gauthier N. Instruments for the assessment of pain in older persons with cognitive impairment. *J Am Geriatr Soc* 2005;53(2):319–326.

72. Taylor LJ, Herr K. Pain intensity assessment: a comparison of selected pain intensity scales for use in cognitively intact and cognitively impaired African American older adults. *Pain Manag Nurs* 2003;4(2):87–95.

73. Ware LJ, Epps CD, Herr K, Packard A. Evaluation of the Revised Faces Pain Scale, Verbal Descriptor Scale, Numeric Rating Scale, and Iowa Pain Thermometer in older minority adults. *Pain Manag Nurs* 2006;7(3):117–125.

74. Smedley BD, Stith AY, Nelson AR, Institute of Medicine (, Committee on Understanding and Eliminating Racial and Ethnic Disparities in Health Care. *Unequal treatment confronting racial and ethnic disparities in health care.* Washington, DC: National Academy Press; 2003.

75. Scogin F, Beutler L, Corbishley A, Hamblin D. Reliability and validity of the short form Beck Depression Inventory with older adults. *J Clin Psychol* 1988;44(6):853–857.

76. Palos GR, Hare M. Patients, family caregivers and patient navigators: A partnership approach. *Cancer* 2011;117(15 Suppl):3592–3602.

77. Rhiner M, Palos G, Termini M. Managing breakthrough pain: a clinical review with three case studies using oral transmucosal fentanyl citrate. *Clin J Oncol Nurs* 2004;8(5):507–512.

78. Fine PG, Narayana A, Passik SD. Treatment of breakthrough pain with fentanyl buccal tablet in opioid-tolerant patients with chronic pain: appropriate patient selection and management. *Pain Med* 2010;11(7):1024–1036.

79. de Leon-Casasola OA. Current developments in opioid therapy for management of cancer pain. *Clin J Pain* 2008;24 Suppl 10:S3–S7.

80. Devillier P, Grassin-Delyle S, Naline E, Buenestado A, Blouquit-Laye S, Advenier C. [Intranasal delivery of systemic drugs: a new route for opioid drugs]. *Therapie* 2010;65(5):475–481.

81. Pan CX, Morrison RS, Ness J, Fugh-Berman A, Leipzig RM. Complementary and alternative medicine in the management of pain, dyspnea, and nausea and vomiting near the end of life. A systematic review. *J Pain Symptom Manage* 2000;20(5):374–387.

82. Jablonski AM, DuPen AR, Ersek M. The use of algorithms in assessing and managing persistent pain in older adults. *Am J Nurs* 2011;111(3):34–43.

83. International Association for the Study of Pain. Classification of chronic pain: descriptions of chronic pain syndromes and definitions of pain terms. *Pain* 1986;3(Suppl):S1–S226.

84. Reisner L. Pharmacological management of persistent pain in older persons. *J Pain* 2011;12(3 Suppl 1): S21–S29.

24

OLDER AFRICAN-AMERICANS

Managing Pain among the Underserved and Most Vulnerable Populations

CARMEN R. GREEN, MD
Professor of Anesthesiology, Obstetrics & Gynecology,
and Health Management & Policy, *and* Director,
Health Disparities Research Program,
Michigan Institute for Clinical & Health Research,
Ann Arbor, Michigan, USA

MYTHILI PRABHU, MD
Department of Obstetrics and Gynecology, University
of Michigan Medical School, Ann Arbor, Michigan, USA

Key Points

- Ethnic differences in clinical pain are widely documented. Older ethnic minority adults have increased pain and pain severity.
- Ethnic differences in pain assessment and treatment are well recognized. Older ethnic minority adults are at risk for decreased access to pain treatment and decreased quality of care.
- Ethnic differences in the negative health sequelae due to pain such as pain-related disability are known, with greater pain and increased disability among older ethnic minority adults.
- Ethnic differences in coping and pain coping are described for older ethnic minority adults.
- Little information is available regarding interactive influences of gender and ethnicity on the pain experience in older ethnic minority adults.
- Older ethnic minority adults are at risk for suboptimal pain care and quality, and variability in clinical decision-making for acute, chronic, and cancer pain.
- Multiple biopsychosocial mechanisms contribute to ethnic differences in pain among older adults.

INTRODUCTION

According to 2000 US census data, 12.4% of the United States population is currently ≥ 65 years old (59% women and 29% minority.[1,2] By 2030, 20% of the United States will be >65 years old (>60% women and 50% minority).[1,3] This translates to an estimated 71.5 million people >65 years old, 137 million ethnic minorities (e.g., African Americans, Hispanics, and Native Americans), and 185 million women, in the United States.[4,5] The United States will become the most multi-ethnic, multi-generational nation ever seen.[6–9] In 2050, an 81% increase in Caucasian-American older adults and a 217% increase in ethnic minority older adults is expected, and minority older adults will increase to 40% of the US older population by 2050.[3,10,11] Ethnic minority populations are at significant risk for health status and healthcare disparities.[10] Despite lower survival rates, the relative growth of ethnic minority older adults makes aging a women's and minority health issue.[12]

Sociodemographic factors (i.e., age, ethnicity, gender, and class) will play a significant role in determining health and well-being while influencing healthcare quality.[13–16] Although health and healthcare-related disparities based upon age, gender, and socioeconomic status (SES) are well described, the literature discussing disparities in health and the healthcare experience has rarely addressed the quality of pain care or the impact pain has on overall health and well-being for ethnic minority older adults.[13,17–32] All in all, the health and healthcare disparities literature has focused primarily on a few chronic disease states, such as cardiovascular disease, cancer, diabetes, osteoarthritis, and obesity that are also associated with aging and can contribute to pain states.[33–38] Yet, the literature documents variability and disparities in pain care based upon ethnicity and gender across several painful conditions (e.g., osteoarthritis, sickle cell anemia, fibromyalgia, lupus), types of pain (i.e., acute, cancer, and chronic pain), and treatment settings (e.g., ambulatory, inpatient).[17,39–53] In general, ethnic minority patients (i.e., African Americans, Hispanic Americans, Native Americans), lower socioeconomic status individuals, and women (across the life span) receive lesser quality pain care when compared to Caucasian men.[45] Considering predicted shifts in the US population, the increasing prevalence of pain, as well as its impact on ethnic minority American older adults, is critically important to consider.[54,55]

Consistent with emerging policy discussions positioning pain relief as a human rights issue, this chapter will focus on the overall health and well-being of ethnic minority older adults. Background information and a platform for discussing the role ethnicity, age, gender, and class have on pain care for an increasingly aging and diversifying society will be provided. Lastly, this chapter will focus on disparities in pain care.

DO HEALTHCARE DISPARITIES MATTER?

The importance of health and healthcare disparities across a full spectrum of disease states and treatments has attracted attention from all branches of government at the local, state, and federal level as well as the public and private sector.[37,38] Several definitions for health disparities exist, such as, "...differences in the incidence, prevalence, mortality, and burden of diseases and other adverse health conditions that exist among specific population groups...."[56] Others define disparities as ethnic differences in the quality of health care that are not due to access-related factors, clinical needs, preferences, or appropriateness of interventions. Implicit in all definitions is disadvantage and increased disease burden for those negatively impacted.[57]

The United States Congress charged the Institute of Medicine (IOM) with assessing healthcare inequities and disparities in the delivery of healthcare services. It confirmed disparities throughout the healthcare system, including for acute and chronic conditions, as well as clinician variability in decision making.[37,38,58] Although pain management was one of the clinical areas where disparities exist, the discussions regarding pain were limited to a few pages and did not address chronic pain.

Legislation designed to address health and healthcare disparities has just begun to focus on understanding, reducing, and eliminating disparities in pain care (e.g., the National Pain Care Policy Act of 2009; H.R. 2994). The Department of Health and Human Services has sponsored many research initiatives attempting to understand, reduce, and eliminate health disparities and to address the needs of older adults.[59] However, pain is often missing from other well publicized public health agendas as is the differential impact pain may have on ethnic minorities, vulnerable populations, and older adults.[60-65] An emerging literature has begun to highlight differences in pain perception as well as disparities in pain care for ethnic minorities for all types of pain and across all settings.[45,66-70] However, less than one percent of NIH research dollars are directed toward primary pain research.[45,66-68,70,71]

THE IMPACT OF PAIN ON OVERALL HEALTH AND WELL-BEING

The World Health Organization defines health as a state of complete physical, social, and emotional well-being and not merely the absence of disease and infirmities.[72,73] Chronic pain (nonmalignant or benign pain lasting for six months or more) is the third largest global health problem.[74-77] Whether pain is viewed as a symptom or as a disease state, it is a major threat to physical, social, emotional, and economic health and well-being.[7,15,27,28,32,45,70,78,79] Pain is a neglected part of medicine despite its threat to public health, causing tremendous suffering, and increasing disability and healthcare utilization.[15,27,28,70,80-84] Nearly 50% of older adults meet criteria for chronic pain (a several-fold increase over young adults).[31] Although the National Institutes of Health (NIH) pain consortium's 2008 exploratory workshop emphasized the critical need for research focusing on pain in older adults, its impact on ethnic minorities was missing from the National Institute on Aging (NIA) deliberations.[79]

Older adults with chronic pain often experience concomitant depression, anxiety, post-traumatic stress disorder (PTSD), sleep disturbance, fatigue, and decreased physical functioning.[27,28,85-89] Pain may also lead them to withdraw from their societal roles, leading to impaired family and social relationships while also diminishing health and quality of life (QOL).[89-93] From a life course perspective, aging is a nonstatic and contextual process where life transitions and trajectories are shaped by historical, social, cultural, and temporal contexts.[94] The cumulative effects of positive (e.g., wealth, positive social support) and negative (e.g., diminished social support) life experiences as well as the timing and duration of these effects impact overall health and well-being. These positive and negative exposures over the life course may contribute to differences in health and well-being.[95] Thus, structural inequalities across the life course can compound and may disproportionately impact minorities and women (especially ethnic minority older adults).[38] Consistent with accelerated aging, African Americans and minority women also experience many chronic illnesses (e.g., diabetes, cancer) associated with chronic pain at an earlier age than Caucasian Americans.[85,86] Thus, age, ethnicity, and gender are important factors in preserving health and wellness and promoting healthy aging. However, the literature focusing on these populations primarily has focused on fairly homogeneous younger populations and not on ethnic minority older adults.[68]

Pain complaints increase with aging. Aging and increased survivorship from chronic illnesses such as cancer, diabetes, and trauma has yielded an increase in pain. Thus, the prevalence of pain will increase and progressively impact the United States' collective health. Chronic pain most often accompanies musculoskeletal conditions (e.g., osteoarthritis), physical disability, and functional limitations due to muscle disuse, weakness, and atrophy.[2,28] For older adults, the most common way they cope with pain is by restricting their activities, leading to increased dependence and isolation. Family members, often respond with overprotective behavior or denial.[96-101] Being a woman and having less social support from caregivers and family members are both risk factors for increasing psychological morbidity.[45,99,100,102-104] Sleep disturbance, depression, anxiety and PTSD symptoms are also associated with chronic pain and are more prevalent than in the general population.[45,105-111]

Chronic pain often coexists with other medical conditions associated with aging, such as osteoarthritis, Parkinson's disease, and depression.[108-111] Pain complaints are the most frequent cause of disability (>700 million lost workdays) and the second leading cause for all physician visits in the United States (>$100 billion in annual healthcare expenditures).[76-78,112-115] Americans spend an additional $40 billion a year on chronic pain medications and aides.[116-120] Indeed without necessary improvements in the quality of chronic pain management, the increasing prevalence of chronic pain will have devastating socioeconomic and health ramifications as our society ages and diversifies. Thus, the societal implications of chronic pain are staggering when medical advances and aging baby boomers (i.e., those born between 1946 and 1964) are considered. Total expenditures on health amount to more than 16% of the nation's gross national product, with most provided to older adults with chronic illnesses such as chronic pain.[70,121,122,123-126] Older adults use more healthcare resources (e.g., prescription pain medicines and procedures) than younger adults while also being at risk for suboptimal pain care.[97,116,127,128] Between 2005 and 2030, the number of hip replacements is expected to grow by 174%, to 572,000 procedures annually by 2030 while the number of knee replacements is projected to grow 673% to 3.48 million procedures annually.[129]

Coping with pain

The most striking feature of gender-based, as well as age and ethnically based, differences in pain perception and response is that multiple variables are cooperatively and competitively operative. This variability is influenced by a complex interaction of individual factors (e.g., biological, psychological, social, and cultural). People with the same disease activity may report differences in pain intensity and its impact on their lives.[130-133] Differences in pain-care beliefs, coping, comorbidities, and social roles may also predispose certain individuals toward multiple actions that maximize rather than minimize threats to bodily integrity or societal dangers that may amplify or exacerbate chronic pain.[134,135]

Altogether, differences in pain response have been attributed to sociodemographic characteristics, disease status, culture, past experiences, response bias, and experimental setting.[136-140] Differences in resource availability, coping styles, and psychological, social, and physical health may influence chronic pain while predisposing either an adaptive or ineffective response to pain.[141-146] Folkman described coping as "a person's cognitive and behavioral efforts to manage the internal and external demands of the person-environment transaction that is appraised as taxing or exceeding the person's resources."[147] Older adults with chronic pain may have attitudes, beliefs, and coping strategies that impact outcomes.[148,149] For example, older adults with chronic illnesses may not communicate pain complaints to their physicians fearing that pain means their illness has progressed or believing that it is a natural part of aging.[150] The literature also reveals differences based upon ethnicity, with ethnic minority persons less likely to share their pain complaints.

Differences in pain perception and response have been attributed to differences in coping styles.[15,151-155] Maladaptive coping (e.g., catastrophizing, repression) and poor adjustment (e.g., poor information-seeking, passivity) are important contributors to diminished health and quality of life.[148,149,156,157] Thus, both coping skills and social learning influence a person's ability to tolerate pain.[158,159] Patient coping styles, attitudes, and experiences may influence their healthcare preferences, information-seeking, and decision-making.[150] For instance, passive coping and catastrophizing is detrimental to successfully coping with a pain problem.[160]

Age, gender, ethnicity, and class also influence coping, as well as an individual's health and well-being. Women are more likely to seek support and use social coping strategies when dealing with stress than men. They also tend to use a wider variety of coping strategies, healthcare services, and social support services. African Americans tend to use religious coping (e.g., participating in worship), wishful thinking, and social support systems differently than Caucasians. For example, African Americans often describe stoicism and believe pain is inevitable, but also fear reporting pain because their family and friends may not understand. These factors also influence pain measurement and response to pain.[15,151-155,161-164] African Americans are more likely to seek support and use social coping strategies when dealing with stress.[165,166] The association between John Henryism (a pattern of actively coping with stressors by working increasingly harder against potentially insurmountable obstacles) and hypertension and bodily pain were described in a general population of older African Americans.[167-169] This coping style is consistent with the attitudes of African-Americans with chronic pain who tend to believe ethnicity affected the health care and pain care they received.[150] Thus, there are potentially important and unique considerations for improving health care and optimizing pain care as more minorities and women age.[170,171] Overall, African Americans with chronic pain report significantly more suffering due to pain, less ability to control their pain symptoms, and more impairment in their sleep due to pain than Caucasians regardless of age or gender.[85,172] There are also differences based upon age, with older African Americans reporting more ability to cope with pain than younger African Americans, or younger and older Caucasians.[86]

[left off here]There may also be greater complexity in the social roles of older adults (e.g., caregiving for relatives or non-relatives) that may impact coping.[159,173,174] Over the past 30 years, the proportion of children raised by grandparents has dramatically increase (>40%).[175] In Detroit, 8.2% of grandparents live with their grandchildren; of those 44.1% were responsible for their grandchildren (a rate of 250% above the national average).[175] The literature shows increased morbidity and mortality for caregivers yet the chronic pain literature fails to explore this when examining health outcomes.[174,176-180] Since social roles are generally conceptualized as stressor, social roles and satisfaction with these roles are important considerations in the ability to adapt to the stress associated with any chronic illness such as chronic pain. Thus, differences in social support, coping styles, and attitudes may contribute to how an individual experiences and lives with pain. Thus, new models addressing the unique characteristic of an increasingly diverse and aging population in the context of chronic pain are critically important for health research and healthcare planning.

Pain assessment

Despite scientific advances yielding increased longevity and the ability to alleviate suffering, ethnic minority Americans have not uniformly benefited.[45,70] Overall, the advancements in technology allowing an individual to survive significant and life-threatening trauma that would have previously ended in death a decade ago, may now be associated with persistent and chronic pain.[27] Thus, the epidemiology of pain is changing with significant public health, individual, and societal effects.[70,181] Ethnic minority older adults are an understudied population at increased risk for decreased health and healthcare quality. Nearly 100 million Americans have pain with ethnic minorities, women, older adults, and lower SES individuals disproportionately experiencing increased pain severity and disability.[116,127,182,183] More specifically, nearly 50 percent of older Americans currently live with pain interfering with successful aging and their ability to independently navigate their environments.[116] When compared to Caucasian older adults, ethnic minority older adults are more likely to rate their health as poor while also reporting increased pain and disability.[44,45,85,86] Considering the impact of accelerated aging in ethnic minorities, pain (especially chronic pain) may further worsen their health. Thus, those at the most risk for suboptimal healthcare—impoverished ethnic minority older adults—are particularly vulnerable to diminished health when they have pain.

The cornerstone for quality pain care is assessment.[47,46,150] Optimizing pain assessment can be problematic since pain is a subjective experience, and there are no objective measures. The pain experience varies substantially at the individual level while being influenced by sex, hormones, age, and culture.[184,185] Patients with the same disease activity may report differences in pain intensity and its impact on their lives. Both ethnic minorities and women respond differently to a painful stimulus than Caucasian men. Ethnicity, increasing age, and female gender may substantially increase the risk for physical and psychological impairment and disability due to pain.[45] In addition, clinician assessment of a patient's pain is also subjective and often discordant with the patient's pain report.[50] These are important considerations since older adults, ethnic minority Americans, and women often report increased pain and negative sequelae associated with pain while being at increased risk for poor pain assessment and under-treatment of their pain complaints. We showed poor pain assessment and unequal pain treatment with African-Americans and women adversely impacted in several studies.[45] All in all, the literature reveals unequal pain care in all clinical settings with clinician variability in decision-making complicating therapy for women and ethnic minorities.[45] In addition, African-Americans are more likely to use the emergency department for pain care, and are less likely to be referred for specialty pain care.[38,150]

Biological, physiological, and social mechanisms may explain part of the observed differences in vulnerability to pain. Differences in pain and suffering experiences, culturally imposed factors, pain care beliefs, and gender and social roles may predispose certain individuals toward actions that exacerbate rather than minimize threats such as pain. Disability, depression, and pain intensity often complicate chronic pain assessment and management. In a study evaluating ethnicity, age and gender influences among black and white clusters of chronic pain patients (*i.e.,* chronic pain syndrome, good pain control, and disability with mild pain syndrome), important ethnic and age related variability in pain symptom severity when patients presented with similar physical, emotional, and pain characteristics were revealed.[186] African-Americans and younger adults experiencing chronic pain were more likely to present with chronic pain syndrome. African-Americans present with "chronic pain syndrome" or disability with mild syndrome reported higher disability then their Caucasian-American counterparts. [186] Older patients and women within the good pain control reported lower level of pain and depression. Older patients presenting with a disability with mild syndrome also reported lower pain and depression. Despite similar physical, emotional and pain characteristics, we confirmed the response to chronic pain differs based upon ethnicity and age. Overall, these findings show ethnic minority Americans experience more disease burden than their Caucasian counterparts.

Very few studies have described the impact of chronic pain on health in ethnically diverse populations across the life span. In a series of studies using 7,000 African-American and Caucasian-American men and women with chronic pain across the life span, important and persistent differences were found in health based upon ethnicity.[186,187] Overall, African-Americans reported significantly more co-morbidities, higher pain scores, increased pain severity, more suffering, and less control of pain then Caucasians across the life span, regardless of gender. African-Americans also reported increased physical disability [i.e., impairment in activities of daily living due to pain (e.g., sexual, self-care, occupation, family life)], and more problems with sleep (i.e., difficulty falling asleep, difficulty staying asleep). Regardless of age and gender, emotional health was also severely impacted by chronic pain in African-Americans. African-Americans were also significantly more depressed (moderate to severe depression) and had more symptoms consistent with post-traumatic stress disorder (PTSD) and anxiety than Caucasians. Beyond ethnic and gender differences in the pain experience, intra-ethnic differences also exist.[188] For instance, younger African-Americans and Caucasians experience more morbidity and disability than their older counterparts with chronic pain suggesting potential differences in coping and a generation gap in pain. These findings may reflect poor pain assessment, inadequate pain treatment, over reporting differenced or some combination of all of the above. Lastly, most individuals with mental health disorders do not receive treatment while ethnic minorities and socioeconomically disadvantaged individuals are often reluctant to seek treatment. Thus, it follows that the adverse sequelae associated with pain are more likely to decrease their overall health and well-being while further diminishing their quality of life.

As previously mentioned, although the gold standard for pain assessment is patient report, clinician estimates of patient's pain intensity are often lower than the patient's report.[116] How ethnicity, gender, and age influence pain management seeking behavior is unknown. What is known is that there is disturbing variability in how the pain complaints of ethnic minorities, older adults, women, and impoverished individuals are assessed and managed.[44,46,47] Complementing or complicating the process is patient behavior, communication styles, clinician-patient communication, and stereotyping. There are often differences in the way older adults, women, and ethnic minorities communicate their pain complaints regardless of socioeconomic status.[116] These communication difficulties are especially problematic if there is also a language barrier. All increase the likelihood of miscommunication and poor communication as well as the patient's pain complaints being discounted, especially when their gender or ethnicity is not the same as their clinician's.[189] In addition, most measures used to assess pain lack cultural and linguistic sensitivity while failing to account for patient's literacy, and health literacy, in particular.

Treating pain

The major and most important building block for quality pain care and physician pain management decision-making is optimizing pain assessment. Yet, this is a neglected topic in most medical, nursing, dental and pharmacy school curricula, further leading to suboptimal pain assessment and treatment.[44,46,47,81,190] A study in Michigan revealed nearly 30% of physicians reported they had not received any medical school, residency, or continuing medical education directed at assessing and managing pain.[44,46,47,191] Thus, it is not surprising that physicians and healthcare professionals are ill-equipped to assess and treat pain. In addition, clinician knowledge and education, healthcare system factors, trust, legal factors, and clinician variability in decision-making influences how well pain is assessed and treated.

The prevalence of chronic pain will increase as Americans live longer.[116,162] The literature documents the benefits of optimizing pain management yet 40% of people in the
United States reported significant acute postoperative pain following surgery and 70% of
people die with unrelieved pain world wide.[192–196] Only 25% of people with chronic pain
are receiving appropriate treatment.[197–202] The literature focusing on assessing and treating chronic pain in later life, older women, and older ethnic minorities is lacking, limiting
the ability to translate results to needed improvements in healthcare quality. There is a
dearth of studies specifically addressing the multi-dimensional impact of chronic pain
in the lives of older ethnic minority adults.[85,86,187] Despite guidelines for managing pain,
physicians are ill-quipped to assess and treat chronic pain due to limited knowledge and
education.[46,47,150,161,163,192–194,196,203–206]

Chronic pain profoundly affects morbidity, mortality, and healthcare expenditures.[182,207,208] An important consideration is that few guidelines specifically address the
differential impact pain has on ethnic minorities, women, and the socioeconomically
disadvantaged individual [193] There is also clear evidence that underserved and vulnerable
populations suffer disproportionately from all types of pain than Caucasians. Thus, a significant pain care gap exists with older ethnic minorities at particular risk for poor pain care.
Bernabei's study of African-Americans and Caucasian older nursing home residents with
cancer found that African-Americans were less likely to have their pain score assessed and
documented in their medical charts.[209] African-Americans were also 63% more likely than
Caucasians to receive no pain medications. Even when African-Americans reported daily
pain (40%), 25% received no analgesics.

Although pain is ubiquitous, healthcare providers are not knowledgeable or satisfied
with the pain care they provide. Physicians express confidence in their pain management
with little knowledge and varying goals for pain relief based upon the type of pain. [44,46,
47] Physicians report lower goals and less satisfaction with their chronic pain management
while providing lesser quality pain care when compared to acute and cancer pain. This is an
important consideration since physicians reported seeing a higher percentage of chronic
pain patients. Ethnicity, age, gender, and class seems to also play a role in how physicians
make their decisions for similar pain problems. Thus, they may be less likely to hear or
respond to chronic pain complaints contributing to sub-optimal care.[210] Altogether these
findings suggest treatment disparities lead to increased disability due to chronic pain.

Sub-optimal pain management leads to poorer health status and quality of life. In a
chronic pain sample, African-Americans believed they should have been referred to a pain
center sooner, reported decreased access to healthcare overall, and believed ethnicity
influenced pain care.[150] Several studies show minorities with cancer pain received significantly less potent analgesics than those recommended by the World Health Organization
(WHO).[39–41] In settings with predominantly ethnic minority patients, most were under
treated using WHO standards. Anderson showed physicians under estimated pain severity for the majority of the Hispanic-American and African-American patients.[39–41] Overall,
ethnic minority patients reported more pain, less pain relief, and were less likely to be adequately assessed for all types of pain and in all settings than Caucasian patients. Physicians
gender and ethnicity also affect pain management decision-making.[48–50,162] Male primary
care physicians prescribed better treatment (e.g., referral to a pain specialist) for men than
for women. Another study examined breakthrough pain (pain flares interrupting well controlled baseline pain) in an ethnically diverse sample with advanced cancer documented
shortcomings in assessing and treating break through pain. Women and minorities
reported increased breakthrough pain and worse health and quality of life.[211,212] Another
study revealed that 20% of diverse cancer survivors experienced cancer related chronic

pain with women and minorities disproportionately impacted. Regardless of pain type, the literature continues to suggest women and ethnic minorities receive lesser quality pain care. Thus, although cultural competency is part of the medical school curriculum, translating the principles of cultural competence into clinical practice is much more problematic.

Health System Related Barriers

Health system related variables such as reduced access to medical care, health insurance, low SES, and low neighborhood SES (nSES) influence health and quality of life as well as the ability to cope with pain.[26] For instance, Green showed minorities, low income individuals, and elders faced structural barriers to obtaining prescription opioid analgesics in their local pharmacies even when their pain was assessed and treated.[213] All in all, ethnic minorities face additional barriers to adequate pain management.

Pain care in the United States is plagued by misinformation, poor clinician and patient education, problematic access to specialists, and physician variability in pain management decision-making.[181,214] While health insurance coverage provides access to medical care it does not ensure equal health or quality health care delivery.[125,126] Ethnic minorities are also more likely to be uninsured, underinsured, and lack a physician or a usual source of medical care. Individuals without health insurance coverage or a primary care physician are more likely to use emergency departments for care and have less access to specialty care. Even when ethnic minorities have a primary care physician and health insurance, they may experience more difficulty in securing referrals to specialty physicians from their primary care physician. Since there is a close association between ethnicity and income; rising co-pays for healthcare services tend to impact ethnic minorities disproportionately more than whites. These finding are consistent with literature that showed African-Americans had increased difficulty paying for healthcare, were more likely to use the emergency room, and chronic pain was major reason for financial problems than Caucasians.[150] Overall, ethnic minorities have less access to pain management specialists, receive less pain medication, and are at risk for under-treatment of their pain complaints while also having an increased disease burden for many co-morbid conditions associated with pain (*e. g.,* diabetes, cancer).

Pain care beliefs may also present barriers to quality pain care in a study looking at access to a tertiary care pain center. African-Americans and women believed good patients avoid talking about pain, pain medications could not really control pain, and ethnicity, culture, and gender affected access to health and pain care.[150] These findings point to differences in trust and problematic communication while begging the question whether the origin of these perceptions and attitudes is due in part to their previous healthcare experiences. Thus, as mentioned earlier in this chapter, differences in social support, coping styles, and attitudes contribute to how an individual experiences and lives with pain. They may also represent barriers that need to be addressed in order to improve the quality of pain care.

Living in a resource-poor neighborhood impacted older African-Americans more so than older Caucasians and contributes to negative consequences of chronic pain in older African-Americans.[26] A study examining low neighborhood SES (nSES) and ethnicity found blacks experienced more affective pain, disability for obligatory domains (life support, self-care), and mood disorder symptoms than whites (relationship mediated by lower nSES). A complex relationship between ethnicity, nSES and the health of older adults with chronic pain depends upon the health dimension studied. Increasing nSES is associated with decreasing negative chronic pain outcomes for both blacks and whites. Another study assessed attitudes regarding health, pain and finances in 582 community-dwelling older African-Americans (i.e., > 60 years old) living in greater metropolitan Detroit who attended an annual heath reception. Most (53%) reported often being troubled with pain during the last year with the majority (82.5%) describing their pain as moderate to severe. When compared to those without pain, older African-Americans with pain reported their health had worsened (28.6% vs. 14.1; *p<.001*), trouble paying their bills (41% vs. 28%, *p* = .002), difficulty paying for housing (23% vs. 13%, *p* =.003), having to choose between health care and food (19% vs. 7%, *p* = .001), having to decrease spending on prescription drugs (33% vs. 25%, *p* = .05), and being a victim of fraud (15% vs. 5%; *p* =.001). Overall, older blacks with pain had greater economic consequences and diminished health than those without pain. Thus, age, ethnicity and nSES are important considerations when examining chronic pain's impact and barriers to quality pain care.[215]

In a study looking at access to pain medicine across Michigan, pharmacies located in minority neighborhoods were less likely to carry opioid analgesics than those in non-minority neighborhoods. [213,216] Green revealed important structural barriers when minorities (regardless of income), low-income Caucasians, and older adults had increased difficulty getting their opioid analgesic prescriptions filled in their local pharmacies. Even at higher incomes, African-Americans have decreased access to specialty care (including pain care and pharmacies) in their local communities than low income Caucasians. Thus, poor pain assessment, inadequate pain treatment, and decreased ability to obtain pain medications (even when medications are prescribed and income is controlled for) complicate quality pain management for ethnic minorities, in particular, thereby impairing their overall health and well-being.

CONCLUSIONS

Pain profoundly affects morbidity, mortality, quality of life, and healthcare expenditures. The potential implications of poorly treated pain are devastating for the individual and the financial cost to society is staggering. Therefore, ensuring optimal pain management is critically important form a public health perspective. There is evidence that pain (especially chronic pain) has unique health implications based upon race and ethnicity, gender, age, and class that are often overlooked. Longitudinal and prospective studies examining the long-term effects of pain on overall health and well-being in an ethnically diverse population across the life span are necessary. Appropriate cultural and linguistic interventions must be developed to ensure quality pain assessment and management such that ethnic disparities in pain care are reduced and eliminated. The role of healthcare provider variability in pain management decision-making as well as healthcare system factors must be examined. In a climate where there is increasing attention regarding patient safety, inadequate pain assessment and treatment must also be viewed as a quality of care issue. By improving pain care in the underserved and most vulnerable populations, the quality of care will be improved for all.[217] Overall, adequate pain relief is a human rights and social justice issue and there remains much more to do to improve the quality of pain care for all.[217]

ACKNOWLEDGMENTS

The authors thank the Michigan-Pain Outcomes Study Team (M-POST) for their ongoing support.

REFERENCES

1. U.S. Census Bureau. Population Profile of the United States. 2000.
2. Helme RD, Gibson SJ. The epidemiology of pain in elderly people. *Clinical Geriatrist Medicine.* Aug 2001;17(3):417–431.

3. U.S. Census Bureau. *Census Bureau Projects Tripling of Hispanic and Asian Populations in 50 Years; Non-Hispanic Whites May Drop To Half of Total Population.* 2004; http://www.census.gov/Press-Release/www/releases/archives/population/001720.html. Accessed December 9, 2009.

4. U.S. Department of Commerce. Minority population growth: 1995 to 2050. In: Agency MB, ed. Washington, DC;1999:1–8.

5. U.S. Census Bureau. U.S. Population Projections. 2008; http://www.census.gov/population/www/projections/projectionsagesex.html. Accessed September 25, 2009.

6. Centers for Disease Control and Prevention and The Merck Company Foundation. *The State of Aging and Health in America 2007.* Whitehouse Station, NJ: The Merck Company Foundation; 2007

7. Farrell MJ. Pain and aging. *American Pain Society Bulletin.* 2000;10(4):8–12.

8. Anderson GF, Hussey PS. Population aging: A comparison among industrialized countries. *Health Aff (Millwood).* May-Jun 2000;19(3):191–203.

9. Institute of Medicine. *Retooling for an Aging America: Building the Health Care Workforce.* Washington, DC: The National Academies Press; 2001.

10. Projected Population by Single Year of Age, Sex, Race, and Hispanic Origin for the United States: July 1, 2000 to July 1, 2050 (NP2008_D1) 2008. http://www.aoa.gov/AoARoot/Aging_Statistics/future_growth/future_growth.aspx#hispanic. Accessed June 10, 2010.

11. Burke G, Hsiao K. Older women of color and the challenge of regulating cultural competence. *Clearinghouse Review Journal of Poverty Law and Policy.* May-June 2009;43(1–2):27–36.

12. U. S. Census Bureau. Interim State Projections of Population for Five-Year Age Groups and Selected Age Groups by Sex: July 1, 2004 to 2030. 2005. http://www.aoa.gov/AoARoot/Aging_Statistics/future_growth/future_growth.aspx. Accessed June 10, 2010.

13. Mayberry RM, Mili F, Ofili E. Racial and ethnic differences in ccess to medical care. *Med Care Res Rev.* 2000;57(suppl 1):108–145.

14. Institute of Medicine. *Crossing the Quality Chasm: A New Health System for the 21st Century.* Washington, DC: National Academies Press; 2001.

15. Helme R, Gibson S. Chapter 8: Pain in older people. In: Crombie IK, ed. *Epidemiology of Pain.* Seattle: IASP Press; 1999:103–112.

16. Mayberry RM, Mili F, Vaid I, et al. *Racial and Ethnic Differences in Access to Medical Care: A Synthesis of the Literature:* Menlo Park, CA: The Henry J. Kaiser Family Foundation, Morehouse Medical Treatment Effectiveness Center (MMEDTEC); 1999.

17. Lurie N. Addressing health disparities: Where should we start? *Health Serv Res.* 2002;37(5):1125–1127.

18. Clancy CM, Massion CT. American women's health care. A patchwork quilt with gaps. *JAMA.* 1992;268(14):1918–1920.

19. Mustard CA, Kaufert P, Kozyrskyj A, Mayer T. Sex Differences in the Use of Health Care Services. *N Engl J Med.* 1998;338(23):1678–1683.

20. Haas J. The cost of being a woman. *N Engl J Med.* 1998;338(23):1694–1695.

21. Waidmann TA, Rajan S. Race and ethnic disparities in health care access and utilization: an examination of state variation. *Med Care Res Rev.* 2000;57(suppl 1):55–84.

22. Whelan CT, Jin L, Meltzer D. Pain and satisfaction with pain control in hospitalized medical patients: no such thing as low risk. *Arch Intern Med.* Jan 26 2004;164(2):175–180.

23. Gallagher RM, Verma S. Managing pain and comorbid depression: a public health challenge. *Semin Clin Neuropsychiatry.* 1999;4(3):203–220.

24. Gallagher RM. Primary Care and Pain Medicine. A Community Solution to the Public Health Problem of Chronic Pain. *Med Clin North Am.* 1999;83(3):555–583, v.

25. Fishman SM, Gallagher RM, Carr DB, Sullivan LW. The case for pain medicine. *Pain Med.* Sep 2004;5(3):281–286.

26. Fuentes M, Hart-Johnson T, Green CR. The Association among Neighborhood Socioeconomic Status, Race and Chronic Pain in Black and White Older Adults. *J Natl Med Assoc.* October 2007;99(10):1160–1169.

27. Crombie IK, Croft PR, Linton SJ, LeResche L, VonKorff M. *Epidemiology of Pain*. Seattle: IASP Press; 1999.

28. Crombie IK, Davies HT, Macrae WA. The epidemiology of chronic pain: time for new directions. *Pain*. 1994;57(1):1–3.

29. LeResche L. Gender differences in pain: epidemiologic perspectives. *Pain Forum*. 1995; 4(4):228–230.

30. LeResche L. Gender considerations in the epidemiology of chronic pain. In: Crombie IK, Croft PR, Linton SJ, LeResche L, VonKorff M, eds. *Epidemiology of Pain*. Seattle: IASP Press; 1999:43–51.

31. LeResche L. *Epidemiologic Perspectives on Sex Differences in Pain*. Vol 17. Seattle: International Association of the Study of Pain; 2000.

32. IASP Special Interest Group on Sex, Gender, and Pain,. *Sex, Gender, and Pain*. Vol 10. Siena, Italy: IASP Press; 2000.

33. Baquet CR, Hammond C, Commiskey P, Brooks S, Mullins CD. Health Disparities Research—A Model for Conducting Research on Cancer Disparities: Characterization and Reduction. *J Assoc Acad Minor Phys*. 2002;13(2):33–40.

34. Caldwell J, Hart-Johnson T, Green CR. Body mass index and quality of life: examining blacks and whites with chronic pain. *J Pain*. Sep 15 2009;10(1):60–67.

35. Institute of Medicine. *Goal to Eliminate Health Care Disparities: Guidance for the National Healthcare Disparities Report*. Washington, DC: National Academies Press; 2002.

36. Egede LE, Zheng D, Simpson K. Comorbid depression is associated with increased health care use and expenditures in individuals with diabetes. *Diabetes Care*. Mar 2002;25(3):464–470.

37. Institute of Medicine. *The Unequal Burden of Cancer: An Assessment of NIH Research and Programs for Ethnic Minorities and the Medically Underserved*. Washington, DC: National Academies Press; 1999.

38. Institute of Medicine. *Unequal Treatment: Confronting Racial and Ethnic Disparities in Health Care*. Washington, DC: The National Academies Press; 2002.

39. Anderson KO, Mendoza TR, Payne R, et al. Pain education for underserved minority cancer patients: a randomized controlled trial. *J Clin Oncol*. Dec 15 2004;22(24):4918–4925.

40. Anderson KO, Mendoza TR, Valero V, et al. Minority cancer patients and their providers: pain management attitudes and practice. *Cancer*. Apr 15 2000;88(8):1929–1938.

41. Anderson KO, Richman SP, Hurley J, et al. Cancer pain management among underserved minority outpatients: perceived needs and barriers to optimal control. *Cancer*. Apr 15 2002;94(8):2295–2304.

42. Todd KH. Influence of ethnicity on emergency department pain management. *Emerg Med (Fremantle)*. Sep 2001;13(3):274–278.

43. Todd KH, Deaton C, D'Adamo AP, Goe L. Ethnicity and analgesic practice. *Ann Emerg Med*. Jan 2000;35(1):11–16.

44. Green CR, Wheeler JR. Physician variability in the management of acute postoperative and cancer pain: A quantitative analysis of the Michigan experience. *Pain Med*. 2003;4(1):8–20.

45. Green CR, Anderson KO, Baker TA, et al. The unequal burden of pain: confronting racial and ethnic disparities in pain. *Pain Med*. 2003;4(3):277–294.

46. Green CR, Wheeler JR, LaPorte F, Marchant B, Guerrero E. How well is chronic pain managed? Who does it well? *Pain Med*. 2002;3(1):56–65.

47. Green CR, Wheeler JR, Marchant B, LaPorte F, Guerrero E. Analysis of the physician variable in pain management. *Pain Med*. 2001;2(4):317–327.

48. Weisse CS, Foster KK, Fisher EA. The influence of experimenter gender and race on pain reporting: Does racial or gender concordance matter? *Pain Med*. 2005;6(1):80–87.

49. Weisse CS, Sorum PC, Dominguez RE. The influence of gender and race on physicians' pain management decisions. *J Pain*. Nov 2003;4(9):505–510.

50. Weisse CS, Sorum PC, Sanders KN, Syat BL. Do gender and race affect decisions about pain management? *J Gen Internal Med*. 2001;16(4):211–217.

51. Lurie N. Health disparities—less talk, more action. *N Engl J Med*. Aug 18 2005;353(7):727–729.

52. Lurie N, Jung M, Lavizzo-Mourey R. Disparities and quality improvement: Federal policy levers. *Health Affairs*. 2005;24(2):354–364.

53. Lurie N, Margolis KL, McGovern PG, Mink PJ, Slater JS. Why do patients of female physicians have higher rates of breast and cervical cancer screening? *J Gen Intern Med*. Jan 1997;12(1):34–43.

54. Juarez G, Ferrell B, Borneman T. Influence of culture on cancer pain management in Hispanic patients. *Cancer Pract*. Sep-Oct 1998;6(5):262–269.

55. Bates M, Edwards WT, Anderson KO. Ethnocultural influences on variation in chronic pain perception. *Pain*. 1993;52:101–112.

56. National Cancer Institute. Health Disparities Defined. http://crchd.cancer.gov/disparities/defined. html. Accessed July 19, 2012.

57. Sohler N, Walmsley PJ, Lubetkin E, Geiger HJ. *Equal Treatment: An Annotated Bibliography of Studies on Race and Ethnic Disparities in Healthcare, Their Cause, and Related Issues*. New York, NY: Physicians for Human Rights; 2003.

58. Smedley BD. Expanding the frame of understanding health disparities: from a focus on health systems to social and economic systems. *Health Educ Behav*. Aug 2006;33(4):538–541.

59. U.S. Department of Health and Human Services. *Healthy People 2010: Understanding and Improving Health*. Washington, DC: Department of Health and Human Services, Government Printing Office; 2000.

60. AHRQ AfHRaQ. *Health Care for Minority Women*. Rockville, MD: Agency for Healthcare Research and Quality; 2006.

61. AHRQ AfHRaQ. *Reducing Ethnic and Racial Inequities in Health Care: AHRQ Resources for Research*. Rockville, MD: Agency for Healthcare Research and Quality; 2001.

62. AHRQ AfHRaQ. *National Healthcare Quality Report, 2004b*. Rockville, MD: Agency for Healthcare Research and Quality; 2004.

63. AHRQ AfHRaQ. *National Healthcare Disparities Report, 2004a*. Rockville, MD: Agency for Healthcare Research and Quality; 2004.

64. Frist WH. Shattuck Lecture: health care in the 21st century. *N Engl J Med*. Jan 20 2005; 352(3):267–272.

65. Nerenz DR, Bonham VL, Green-Weir R, Joseph C, Gunter M. Eliminating racial/ethnic disparities in health care: Can health plans generate reports? *Health Aff (Millwood)*. May-Jun 2002;21(3):259–263.

66. Bradshaw DH, Nakamura Y, Chapman CR. National Institutes of Health grant awards for pain, nausea, and dyspnea research: an assessment of funding patterns in 2003. *J Pain*. May 2005;6(5):275–276.

67. Fillingim RB, Edwards RR, Powell T. The relationship of sex and clinical pain to experimental pain responses. *Pain*. 1999;83(3):419–425.

68. Fillingim RB. Sex, gender, and pain: Women and Men Really are Different. *Curr Rev Pain*. 2000;4(1):24–30.

69. Abramson J, Starfield B. The effect of conflict of interest on biomedical research and clinical practice guidelines: Can we trust the evidence in evidence-based medicine? *J Am Board Fam Pract*. Sep 1 2005;18(5):414–418.

70. Green CR. The healthcare bubble through the lens of pain research, practice, and policy: advice to the new President and Congress [editorial]. *J Pain*. 2008;9(12):1071–1073.

71. Edwards CL, Fillingim RB, Keefe F. Race, ethnicity and pain. *Pain*. 2001;94(2):133–137.

72. Pearl JD. Cancer pain management: still a public health issue. *Am Soc Anesthesiol*. 1998;62:17.

73. Breslow L. A Quantitative Approach to the World Health Organization Definition of Health: Physical, Mental and Social Well-Being. *Int J Epidemiol*. 1972;1(4):347–355.

74. Gunn CC. Chronic Pain: Time for epidemiology. *J R Soc Med*. 1996;89(8):479–480.

75. Moore R, Brodsgarrd I. *Cross Cultural Investigations of Pain Epidemiology of Pain*. Seattle: International Association for the Study of Pain; 1999.

76. Ferrell BR, Dean GE. Ethical issues in pain management at home. *J Palliat Care*. Autumn 1994;10(3):67–72.

77. Ferrell BR, Griffith H. Cost issues related to pain management: report from the Cancer Pain Panel of the Agency for Health Care Policy and Research. *J Pain Symptom Manage.* 1994;9(4):221–234.

78. Stewart WF, Ricci JA, Chee E, Morganstein D, Lipton R. Lost productive time and cost due to common pain conditions in the US workforce. *JAMA.* Nov 12 2003;290(18):2443–2454.

79. NIH Pain Consortium. Mechanisms of Management of Pain in the Elderly: Workshop Executive Summary. 2008; http://painconsortium.nih.gov/NIAPainWorkshopSummary.html. Accessed July 20, 2012.

80. Brennan F, Carr DB, Cousins M. Pain management: a fundamental human right. *Anesth Analg.* Jul 2007;105(1):205–221.

81. International Association for the Study of Pain. Task Force on Professional Education. *Core Curriculum for Professional Education in Pain.* 2nd ed. Seattle: International Association for the Study of Pain (IASP); 1995.

82. Skevington SM. Investigating the relationship between pain and discomfort and quality of life, using the WHOQOL. *Pain.* Jun 1998;76(3):395–406.

83. Cleeland CS. The impact of pain on the patient with cancer. *Cancer.* 1984;54(suppl 11):2635–2641.

84. Gibson S, Kart B, Corran TM, Farrell MJ, Helme RD. Pain in older persons. *Disabil Rehabil.* 1994;16:127–139.

85. Green CR, Baker TA, Sato Y, Washington TL, Smith EM. Race and chronic pain: A comparative study of young black and white Americans presenting for management. *J Pain.* May 2003;4(4):176–183.

86. Green CR, Baker TA, Smith EM, Sato Y. The effect of race in older adults presenting for chronic pain management: A comparative study of black and white Americans. *J Pain.* Mar 2003;4(2):82–90.

87. Scher AI, Stewart WF, Lipton RB. Epidemiology of migraine and headache: A meta-analytic approach. In: Crombie IK, ed. *Epidemiology of Pain.* Seattle: IASP Press; 1999:159–170.

88. Schmader KE. Epidemiology and impact on quality of life of postherpetic neuralgia and painful diabetic neuropathy. *Clin J Pain.* 2002;18:350–354.

89. Kulich RJ, Mencher P, Bertrand C, Maciewicz R. Comorbidity of post-traumatic stress disorder and chronic pain: implications for clinical and forensic Assessment. *Curr Rev Pain.* 2000;4(1):36–48.

90. Feine JS, Lund JP. An assessment of the efficacy of physical therapy and physical modalities for the control of chronic musculoskeletal pain. *Pain.* May 1997;71(1):5–23.

91. Call-Schmidt TA, Richardson SJ. Prevalence of sleep disturbance and its relationship to pain in adults with chronic pain. *Pain Manag Nurs.* Sep 2003;4(3):124–133.

92. Buchwald D, Goldberg J, Noonan C, Beals J, Manson S, Team A-S. Relationship between post-traumatic stress disorder and pain in two American Indian tribes. *Pain Med.* 2005;6(1):72–79.

93. Menefee LA, Frank ED, Doghramji K, et al. Self-reported sleep quality and quality of life for individuals with chronic pain conditions. *Clin J Pain.* 2000;16(4):290–297.

94. Bengtson VL, Burgess EO, Parrott TM. Theory, explanation, and a third generation of theoretical development in social gerontology. *J Gerontol B Psychol Sci Soc Sci.* Mar 1997;52(2):S72–S88.

95. Hertzman C. The life-course contribution to ethnic disparities in health. In: Anderson NB, Bulatao RA, Cohen B, eds. *Critical Perspectives on Racial and Ethnic Differences in Health in Late Life.* Washington, DC: The National Academies Press; 2004:145–170.

96. Roy R, ed *Chronic Pain in Old Age. An Integrated Biopsychosocial Perspective.* Toronto: University of Toronto, Inc.; 1995.

97. Roberto KA. Chronic pain in the lives of older women. *J Am Med Womens Assoc.* 1997;52(3):127–131.

98. Jakobsson U, Klevsgard R, Westergren A, Hallberg IR. Old people in pain: a comparative study. *J Pain Symptom Manage.* 2003;26(1):625–636.

99. Dew MA, Kormos RL, DiMartini AF, et al. Prevalence and risk of depression and anxiety-related disorders during the first three years after heart transplantation. *Psychosomatics.* 2001;42(4):300–313.

100. Jarrett M, Heitkemper M, Cain KC, et al. The relationship between psychological distress and gastrointestinal symptoms in women with irritable bowel syndrome. *Nurs Res.* 1998;47(3):154–161.

101. Jarrett M, Heitkemper M, Cain KC, Burr RL, Hertig V. Sleep disturbance influences gastrointestinal symptoms in women with irritable bowel syndrome. *Dig Dis Sci.* 2000;45(5):952–959.

102. Weir R, Browne G, Tunks E, Gafni A, Roberts J. Gender differences in psychosocial adjustment to chronic pain and expenditures for health care services used. *Clin J Pain.* 1996;12(4):277–290.

103. Lichtenberg PA, Chapleski EE, Youngblade LM. The effect of depression on functional abilities among Great Lakes indians. *J Appl Gerontol.* 1997;16:235–248.

104. Arfken CL, Lichtenberg PA, Tancer M. Cognitive impairment and depression predict mortality in medically ill older adults. *J GerontolA. Med Sci..* 1999;54A:M152–M156.

105. Gilbar O, Bazak Y, Harel Y. Gender, primary headache, and psychological distress. *Headache.* 1998;38(1):31–34.

106. Bolton JE, Christensen MN. Back pain distribution patterns: relationship to subjective measures of pain severity and disability. *J Manipulative Physiol Ther.* 1994;17(4):211–218.

107. Bolton JE. Psychological distress and disability in back pain patients: evidence of sex differences. *J Psychosom Res.* 1994;38(8):849–858.

108. Macfarlane GJ. Chronic widespread pain and fibromyalgia: Should reports of increased mortality influence management? *Curr Rheumatol Rep.* Oct 2005;7(5):339–341.

109. Macfarlane GJ, Jones GT, Knekt P, et al. Is the report of widespread body pain associated with long-term increased mortality? Data from the Mini-Finland Health Survey. *Rheumatology (Oxford).* May 2007;46(5):805–807.

110. Michaud K, Wolfe F. Comorbidities in rheumatoid arthritis. *Best Pract Res Clin Rheumatol.* Oct 2007;21(5):885–906.

111. Mantyselka PT, Turunen JH, Ahonen RS, Kumpusalo EA. Chronic pain and poor self-rated health. *JAMA.* Nov 12 2003;290(18):2435–2442.

112. Clark JD. Chronic Pain Prevalence and Analgesic prescribing in a general medical population. *J Pain Symptom Manage.* 2002 2002;23(2):131–137.

113. Ferrell BR, Jacox A, Miaskowski C, Paice JA, Hester NO. Cancer pain guidelines: now that we have them, what do we do? *Oncol Nurs Forum.* Aug 1994;21(7):1229–1231.

114. Ferrell BR, Rhiner M. Managing cancer pain—a three-step approach. *Nursing.* Jul 1994;24(7): 57–59.

115. Ferrell BR, Rhiner M, Shapiro B, Strause L. The family experience of cancer pain management in children. *Cancer Pract.* Nov-Dec 1994;2(6):441–446.

116. Levitt SH, Kempen PM. Managing pain in elderly patients. *JAMA.* 1999;281(7):605; discussion 606.

117. Canine C. Pain, profit, and sweet relief. *Worth* March, 1997:79–82, 151–157.

118. Lethbridge-Cejku M, Schiller JS, Bernad lL. Summary health statistics for U.S. adults: National Health Interview Survey. *Vital Health Stat 10.* Jul 2004(222):1–151.

119. American FactFinder. Census 2000 Summary File. 2000; http://factfinder.census.gov/home/saff/main.html?_lang=en. Accessed March 31, 2004.

120. Pleis JR, Schiller JS, Benson V. Summary health statistics for U.S. adults: National Health Interview Survey, 2000. *Vital Health Stat 10.* Dec 2003(215):1–132.

121. Reinhardt UE. Is there hope for the uninsured? *Health Aff (Millwood).* Aug 27 2003; (Jul-Dec 2003):W3–376–W373–390.

122. Thorpe KE. The rise in health care spending and what to do about it. *Health Aff (Millwood).* Nov 2005;24(6):1436–1445.

123. Thorpe KE, Florence CS, Howard DH, Joski P. The impact of obesity on rising medical spending. *Health Aff (Millwood).* Jul-Dec 2004;Suppl Web Exclusives:W4–480–486.

124. Thorpe KE, Florence CS, Joski P. Which medical conditions account for the rise in health care spending? *Health Aff (Millwood).* Jul-Dec 2004;Suppl Web Exclusives:W4–437–445.

125. Institute of Medicine. *Coverage Matters: Insurance and Health Care.* Washington, DC: National Academies Press; 2001.

126. Institute of Medicine. *Care Without Coverage: Too Little, Too Late.* Washington, DC: National Academies Press; 2002.

127. Pilowsky I, Crettenden I, Townley M. Sleep disturbance in pain clinic patients. *Pain.* 1985; 23:27–33.

128. Wilcox S, Brenes GA, Levine D, Sevick MA, Shumaker SA, Craven T. Factors Related to Sleep Disturbance in Older Adults Experiencing Knee Pain with Radiographic Evidence of Knee Osteoarthritis. *J Am Geriatr Soc.* 2000;48:1241–1251.

129. Kurtz S, Ong K, Lau E, Mowat F, Halpern M. Projections of primary and revision hip and knee arthroplasty in the United States from 2005 to 2030. *J Bone Joint Surg Am.* 2007 Apr;89(4):780–785.

130. Melzack R, Wall PD. Pain mechanisms: a new theory. *Science.* 1965;150(699):971–979.

131. Haefner HK, Khoshnevisan MH, Bachman JE, Flowe-Valencia HD, Green CR, Reed BD. Use of the McGill Pain Questionnaire to compare women with vulvar pain, pelvic pain and headaches. *J Reprod Med.* 2000;45(8):665–671.

132. Loeser JD, Melzack R. Pain: an overview. *Lancet.* May 8 1999;353(9164):1607–1609.

133. Geisser ME, Roth RS, Bachman JE, Eckert TA. The relationship between symptoms of post-traumatic stress disorder and pain, affective disturbance and disability among patients with accident and non-accident related pain. *Pain.* Aug 1996;66(2–3):207–214.

134. Rollman GB, Lautenbacher S. Sex differences in musculoskeletal pain. *Clin J Pain.* 2001;17(1): 20–24.

135. Rollman G. Sex makes a difference: experimental and clinical pain responses. *Clin J Pain.* 2003; 19(4):204–207.

136. Edwards RR, Fillingim RB. Age-associated differences in responses to noxious stimuli. *J Gerontol A, Biol Sci Med Sci.* 2001;56(3):M180–M185.

137. Mudrick NR. Predictors of disability among midlife men and women: differences by severity of impairment. *J Community Health.* 1988;13(2):70–84.

138. Unruh AM. Gender variations in clinical pain experience. *Pain.* 1996;65(2–3):123–167.

139. Unruh AM, Ritchie J, Merskey H. Does gender affect appraisal of pain and pain coping strategies? *Clin J Pain.* 1999;15(1):31–40.

140. Khasar SG, Isenberg WM, Miao FJ, Gear RW, Green PG, Levine JD. Gender and gonadal hormone effects on vagal modulation of tonic nociception. *J Pain.* 2001;2(2):91–100.

141. Edwards RR, Fillingim RB. Ethnic differences in thermal pain responses. *Psychosom Med.* 1999;61(3): 346–354.

142. Edwards RR, Fillingim RB, Yamauchi S, et al. Effects of gender and acute dental pain on thermal pain responses. *Clin J Pain.* 1999;15(3):233–237.

143. Drossman DA, Leserman J, Li Z, Keefe F, Hu YJ, Toomey TC. Effects of coping on health outcome among women with gastrointestinal disorders. *Psychosom Med.* 2000;62(3):309–317.

144. Berkley KJ. Sex differences in pain. *Behav Brain Sci.* 1997;20(3):371–380; discussion 435–513.

145. Klapow JC, Slater MA, Patterson TL, et al. Psychosocial factors discriminate multidimensional clinical groups of chronic low back pain patients. *Pain.* 1995;62(3):349–535.

146. Olden KW, Drossman DA. Psychologic and psychiatric aspects of gastrointestinal disease. *Med Clin North Am.* 2000;84(5):1313–1327.

147. Folkman S, Lazarus RS, Dunkel-Schetter C, DeLongis A, Gruen RJ. Dynamics of a stressful encounter: cognitive appraisal, coping, and encounter outcomes. *J Pers Soc Psychol.* 1986;50(5): 992–1003.

148. Geisser ME, Roth RS, Theisen ME, Robinson TE, Riley III TL. Negative affect, self-report of depressive symptoms, and clinical depression: relation to the experience of chronic pain. *Clin J Pain.* 2000;16(2):110–120.

149. Gracely RH, Geisser ME, Giesecke T, et al. Pain catastrophizing and neural responses to pain among persons with fibromyalgia. *Brain.* 2004;127(Pt 4):835–843.

150. Green CR, Baker TA, Ndao-Brumblay SK. Patient attitudes regarding healthcare utilization and referral: a descriptive comparison in African- and Caucasian Americans with chronic pain. *J Natl Med Assoc.* Jan 2004;96(1):31–42.

151. Spitzer A, Bar-Tal Y, Golander H. The moderating effect of demographic variables on coping effectiveness. *J Adv Nurs.* 1995;22(3):578–585.

152. Gil KM. Coping with sickle cell disease pain. *Soc Behav Med.* 1989;11(2):49–57.

153. Hasenbring M, Marienfeld G, Kuhlendahl D, Soyka D. Risk factors of chronicity in lumbar disc patients. A prospective investigation of biologic, psychologic, and social predictors of therapy outcome. *Spine.* 1994;19(24):2759–2765.

154. Herr KA, Mobily PR, Wallace RB, Chung Y. Leg pain in the rural Iowa 65+ population. Prevalence, related factors, and association with functional status. *Clin J Pain.* 1991;7(2):114–121.

155. Herr KA, Mobily PR. Complexities of pain assessment in the elderly. Clinical considerations. *J Gerontol Nurs.* 1991;17(4):12–19.

156. Green C, Flowe-Valencia H, Rosenblum L, Tait A. Do physical and sexual abuse differentially affect chronic pain states in women? *J Pain Symptom Manage.* 1999;18(6):420–426.

157. Green CR, Flowe-Valencia H, Rosenblum L, Tait AR. The role of childhood and adulthood abuse among women presenting for chronic pain management. *Clin J Pain.* 2001;17:359–364.

158. Davis DA, Luecken LJ, Zautra AJ. Are reports of childhood abuse related to the experience of chronic pain in adulthood? A meta-analytic review of the literature. *Clin J Pain.* Sep-Oct 2005;21(5):398–405.

159. Chadiha LA, Adams P, Biegel DE, Auslander W, Gutierrez L. Empowering African American women informal caregivers: a literature synthesis and practice strategies. *Soc Work.* Jan 2004;49(1):97–108.

160. Roth RS, Geisser ME, Bates R. The relation of post-traumatic stress symptoms to depression and pain in patients with accident-related chronic pain. *J Pain.* Jul 2008;9(7):588–596.

161. Greenwald BD, Narcessian EJ, Pomeranz BA. Assessment of physiatrists' knowledge and perspectives on the use of opioids: review of basic concepts for managing chronic pain. *Am J Phys Med Rehabil.* 1999;78(5):408–415.

162. Levy S, Dowling P, Boult L, Monroe A, McQuade W. The effect of physician and patient gender on preventive medicine practices in patients older than fifty [see comments]. *Family Med.* 1992;24(1):58–61.

163. Weinstein SM, Laux LF, Thornby JI, et al. Physicians' attitudes toward pain and the use of opioid analgesics: results of a survey from the Texas Cancer Pain Initiative. *South Med J.* 2000;93(5):479–487.

164. Pappagallo M, Heinberg LJ. Ethical issues in the management of chronic nonmalignant pain. *Semin Neurol.* 1997;17(3):203–211.

165. Affleck G, Urrows S, Tennen H, Higgins P. Daily coping with pain from rheumatoid arthritis: patterns and correlates. *Pain.* 1992;51(2):221–229.

166. Hobfoll SE, Dunahoo CL, Ben-Porath Y, Monnier J. Gender and coping: the dual-axis model of coping. *Am J Community Psychol.* 1994;22(1):49–82.

167. James SA, Hartnett SA, Kalsbeek WD. John Henryism and blood pressure differences among black men. *J Behav Med.* 1983;6(3):259–278.

168. James SA, Keenan NL, Strogatz DS. Socioeconomic status, John Henryism and blood pressure in black adults: The Pitt County Study. *Am J Epidemiol.* Jan 1 1992;135(1):59–67.

169. James SA, Strogatz DS, Wing SB, Ramsey DL. Socioeconomic status, John Henryism, and hypertension in blacks and whites. *Am J Epidemiol.* Oct 1987;126(4):664–673.

170. Chirieac MC. Pain, depression, and social resources in elderly women. Paper presented at: 129th Annual Meeting of American Public Health Association; October 2001 ; Atlanta, GA.

171. Jackson-Triche ME, Greer Sullivan J, Wells KB, Rogers W, Camp P, Mazel R. Depression and health-related quality of life in ethnic minorities seeking care in general medical settings. *J Affect Disord.* 2000;58(2):89–97.

172. McCracken LM, Matthews AK, Tang TS, Cuba SL. A comparison of blacks and whites seeking treatment for chronic pain. *Clin J Pain.* Sep 2001;17(3):249–255.

173. Dilworth-Anderson P, Williams IC, Gibson BE. Issues of race, ethnicity, and culture in caregiving research: a 20-year review (1980–2000). *Gerontologist.* Apr 2002;42(2):237–272.

174. Burton LM. Black grandparents rearing children of drug-addicted parents: stressors, outcomes, and social service needs. *Gerontologist.* Dec 1992;32(6):744–751.

175. Simmons TaD, Jane Lawler. Grandparents living with grandchildren: 2000; 2003:1–10. http://www.census.gov/prod/2003pubs/c2kbr-31.pdf. Accessed July 20, 2012.

176. Dubowitz H, Sawyer RJ. School behavior of children in kinship care. *Child Abuse Negl.* Nov 1994;18(11):899–911.

177. Minkler M, Roe KM, Price M. The physical and emotional health of grandmothers raising grandchildren in the crack cocaine epidemic. *Gerontologist.* Dec 1992;32(6):752–761.

178. Ross MET, Aday LA. Stress and coping in African American grandparents who are raising their grandchildren. *J Fam Issues.* 2006;27(7):753–761.

179. Edwards OW. Living with grandma: a grandfamily study. *School Psychol Int.* 2003;24(2):204–217.

180. Smith GC, Palmieri PA. Risk of psychological difficulties among children raised by custodial grandparents. *Psychiatr Serv.* Oct 2007;58(10):1303–1310.

181. Bonham VL. Race, ethnicity, and pain treatment: striving to understand the causes and solutions to the disparities in pain treatment. *J Law Med Ethics.* 2001;29(1):52–68.

182. Schlenk EA, Erlen JA, Dunbar-Jacob J, et al. Health-related quality of life in chronic disorders: a comparison across studies using the MOS SF-36. *Qual Life Res.* 1998;7(1):57–65.

183. Flor H, Turk DC, Scholz OB. Impact of chronic pain on the spouse: marital, emotional and physical consequences. *J Psychosom Res.* 1987;31(1):63–71.

184. Edwards R, Augustson EM, Fillingim R. Sex-specific effects of pain-related anxiety on adjustment to chronic pain. *Clin J Pain.* 2000;16(1):46–53.

185. Fillingim RB, Edwards RR, Powell T. Sex-dependent effects of reported familial pain history on recent pain complaints and experimental pain responses. *Pain.* 2000;86(1–2):87–94.

186. Green CR, Ndao-Brumblay SK, Nagrant AM, Baker TA, Rothman E. Race, age, and gender influences among clusters of African American and white patients with chronic pain. *J Pain.* Apr 2004;5(3):171–182.

187. Ndao-Brumblay SK, Green CR. Racial differences in the physical and psychosocial health among black and white women with chronic pain. *J Natl Med Assoc.* Oct 2005;97(10):1369–1377.

188. Baker TA, Green CR. Intrarace differences among black and white americans presenting for chronic pain management: the influence of age, physical health, and psychosocial factors. *Pain Med.* Jan-Feb 2005;6(1):29–38.

189. Green CR. Unequal burdens and unheard voices: Whose pain? Whose narratives? In: Carr DB, Loeser JD, Morris DB, eds. *Narrative, Pain, and Suffering, Progress in Pain Research and Management.* Vol 34. Seattle: IASP Press; 2005:195–214.

190. International Association for the Study of Pain. Task Force on Professional Education. Postoperative Pain. In: Fields HL, ed. *Core Curriculum for Professional Education In Pain.* 2nd ed. Seattle: IASP Press; 1995:99–101.

191. Todd K, Samaroo N, Hoffman J. Ethnicity as a risk factor in inadequate emergency department analgesia. *JAMA.* 1993;269(12):1537–1539.

192. Carr DB, Jacox A, Chapman CR. *Acute Pain Management: Operative or Medical Procedures and Trauma: Clinical Practice Guideline No. 1.* Rockville, MD: U.S. Public Health Service, Agency for Health Care Policy and Research; 1992.

193. Payne R. Pain management in sickle cell disease. Rationale and techniques. *Ann N Y Acad Sci.* 1989;565(1):189–206.

194. Carr DB, Miaskowski C, Dedrick SC, Williams GR. Management of perioperative pain in hospitalized patients: A national survey. *J Clin Anesth.* 1998;10(1):77–85.

195. Carr TD, Lemanek KL, Armstrong FD. Pain and fear ratings: clinical implications of age and gender differences. *J Pain Symptom Manage.* 1998;15(5):305–313.

196. Rose VL. Guidelines from the American Geriatric Society Target Management of Chronic Pain in Older Persons. *Am Fam Physician.* 1998;58(5):1213–1214, 1217.

197. Whitten CF, Kirkland J. Unmet needs of parents of and individuals with sickle cell anemia. Pediatric Research 1970;4:475 (Abstract).

198. Miaskowski C, Crews J, Ready LB, Paul SM, Ginsberg B. Anesthesia-based pain services improve the quality of postoperative pain management. *Pain.* 1999;80(1–2):23–29.

199. Fowler FJ Jr, Cleary PD, Magaziner J, Patrick DL, Benjamin KL. Methodological issues in measuring patient-reported outcomes: the agenda of the Work Group on Outcomes Assessment. *Med Care.* 1994;32(suppl 7):JS65–JS76.

200. Zambrana RE, Kelly MA, Raskin IE. *Patient Outcomes and Medical Effectiveness Research: An Annotated Bibliography Related to Race, Ethnicity, and Clinical Condition (January 1987–January 1994).* Rockville, MD: U.S. Department of Health and Human Services Public Health Service Agency for Health Care Policy and Research;1994.

201. Stryer D, Tunis S, Hubbard H, Clancy C. The outcomes of outcomes and effectiveness research: impacts and lessons from the first decade. *Health Serv Res.* 2000;35(5 Pt 1):977–993.

202. Stryer DB, Weinick RM, Clancy CM. Reducing racial and ethnic disparities in health care. *Health Serv Res.* 2002;37(5):XV–XXVI.

203. Weinstein MC, Siegel JE, Gold MR, Kamlet MS, Russell LB. Recommendations of the Panel on Cost-effectiveness in Health and Medicine. *JAMA.* 1996;276(15):1253–1258.

204. Greenwald BD, Narcessian EJ. Opioids for managing patients with chronic pain: community pharmacists' perspectives and concerns. *J Pain Symptom Manage.* 1999;17(5):369–375.

205. Weinstein SM, Laux LF, Thornby JI, et al. Medical students' attitudes toward pain and the use of opioid analgesics: implications for changing medical school curriculum. *South Med J.* 2000;93(5):472–478.

206. Jacox A, Carr DB, Payne R. New clinical-practice guidelines for the management of pain in patients with cancer. *N Engl J Med.* Mar 3 1994;330(9):651–655.

207. Ferrell BR, Grant M, Funk B, Garcia N, Otis-Green S, Schaffner ML. Quality of Life in Breast Cancer. *Cancer Pract.* 1996;4(6):331–340.

208. Wang S, Fuh J, Lu S, Juang K. Quality of life differs among headache diagnoses: analysis of SF-36 Survey in 901 headache patients. *Pain.* 2001;89(2–3):285–292.

209. Bernabei R, Gambassi G, Lapane K, et al. Management of pain in elderly patients with cancer. SAGE Study Group. Systematic assessment of geriatric drug use via epidemiology. *JAMA.* 1998;279(23):1877–1882.

210. Tait RC, Chibnall JT. Factor structure of the pain disability index in workers compensation claimants with low back injuries. *Arch Phys Med Rehabil.* Jun 2005;86(6):1141–1146.

211. Montague L, Green CR. Cancer and breakthrough pain's impact on a diverse population. *Pain Med.* 2009;10(3):549–561.

212. Green CR, Montague L, Hart-Johnson T. Consistent and breakthrough pain in diverse advanced cancer patients: a longitudinal examination. *J Pain Symptom Manage.* 2009;37(5):831–847.

213. Morrison RS, Wallenstein S, Natale DK, Senzel RS, Huang LL. "We don't carry that"—failure of pharmacies in predominantly nonwhite neighborhoods to stock opioid analgesics. *N Engl J Med.* 2000;342(14):1023–1026.

214. Bonham VL, Sellers SL, Gallagher TH, et al. Physicians' attitudes toward race, genetics, and clinical medicine. *Genet Med.* Apr 2009;11(4):279–286.

215. Hart-Johnson TA, Green CR. Physical and psychosocial health in older women with chronic pain: comparing clusters of clinical and nonclinical samples. *Pain Med.* Feb 23 2010;11(4):564–574.

216. Green CR, Ndao-Brumblay SK, West B, Washington T. Differences in prescription opioid analgesic availability: comparing minority and white pharmacies across Michigan. *J Pain.* 2005;6(10):689–699.

217. Green C, Todd KH, Lebovits A, Francis M. Disparities in pain: ethical issues. *Pain Med.* 2006;7(6):530–533.

Pharmacogenomics and Analgesic Drugs

25

INSENSITIVITY TO PAIN

Lessons from Recent Genetics Advances

NANCY MERNER, PHD
Post-Doctoral Fellow, Centre of Excellence in
Neurosciences, University of Montréal, Centre Hospitalier
de l'Université de Montréal, Montréal, Québec, Canada

PATRICK A. DION, PHD
Scientific Coordinator, Centre of Excellence in Neurosciences,
University of Montréal, Centre Hospitalier de l'Université de
Montréal and Assistant Researcher, Departments of Pathology and
Cellular Biology, University of Montréal, Montréal, Québec, Canada

ANNA SZUTO, MSC
Genetic Counsellor, Centre of Excellence in Neurosciences,
University of Montréal, Centre Hospitalier de l'Université de
Montréal, Montréal, Québec, Canada

GUY A. ROULEAU, MD, PHD, FRCPC
Director, Centre of Excellence in Neurosciences, University of
Montréal, Centre Hospitalier de l'Université de Montréal; Director,
Ste-Justine Hospital Research Center; and Professor, Department
of Medicine, University of Montréal, Montréal, Québec, Canada

Key Points
- Congenital absence of pain sensation is a rare phenotype.
- Historically, the terms insensitivity and indifference to pain were used interchangeably but over time they acquired distinct meanings; insensitivity is defined as a failure to receive and perceive a stimulus in the presence of a neuropathy, and indifference as a lack of concern or reaction to a nociceptive stimulus received without the presence of neuropathy.
- Hereditary sensory and autonomic neuropathies (HSANs), peripheral neuropathies associated with nociception defects and relative degrees of autonomic dysfunction, are divided into five subtypes based on pattern of dysfunction, age of onset, inheritance pattern, and additional clinical features.
- The distinct roles of HSAN and CIP (congenital indifference to pain) causative proteins thus far identified support the phenotypic differences between these disorders.

- Proteins encoded by genes mutated in HSAN appear to be linked to various forms of intracellular and endocytic signalling routes, however many causative genes remain to be identified.
- Future research is needed to improve our still very incomplete understanding of the different mechanisms involved.

INTRODUCTION

Inherited peripheral neuropathies are clinically and genetically heterogeneous with over 30 causative genes associated to these disorders. The present chapter will not discuss all of these neuropathies; it will address only those that have been associated primarily with nociception defects and relative degrees of autonomic dysfunction for which a causative gene has been identified. Nociception, the ability to feel pain following the stimulation of a sensory receptor, is physiologically a four-step process: transduction, transmission, modulation, and perception.

Congenital absence of pain sensation is a rare phenotype that includes a spectrum of abnormal responses; early reports termed these "congenital general pure analgesia,"[1] "congenital universal insensitiveness to pain,"[2] "congenital universal indifference to pain,"[3] and "congenital absence of pain."[4] Historically, the terms insensitivity and indifference were used interchangeably but over time they acquired distinct meanings.[5,6] In the 1970s, insensitivity was defined as a failure to receive and perceive a stimulus, and indifference as a lack of concern or reaction to a stimulus received;[5] another criteria that further discriminated insensitivity and indifference has been the presence or absence of a neuropathy. Insensitivity to pain is often observed with a neuropathy while indifference to pain is not.[6–9]

No specific therapies are yet available but genetic research into these disorders has revolutionized our understanding of the peripheral nervous system and opened the field for the development of rational approaches to therapy. Several hereditary syndromes that involve complete or almost complete insensitivity to pain have been discovered and are listed in the Online Mendelian Inheritance in Man database (http://www.omim.org/).

Some of these conditions are associated with significant morbidity and while the identification of a causal mutation does not currently influence the therapeutic approach, couples with a family history can benefit from genetic counseling where issues such as recurrence risk and disease prevention via carrier screening and prenatal diagnosis or preimplantation genetic diagnosis can be explored. Indeed, advances in the molecular characterization of genes involved in peripheral neuropathic disorders affecting nociception allows for genetic testing in the clinical setting for several conditions. This has had an impact on diagnosis, which is critical to providing a family with accurate genetic counselling and reproductive options.

HEREDITARY SENSORY AND AUTONOMIC NEUROPATHIES (HSANS)

The hereditary sensory and autonomic neuropathies are rare but a number of genes have been identified (Table 25.1). Autonomic abnormalities are often minimal and motor involvement is rarely present. The sensory loss can lead to severe complications, including recurrent injuries, ulcerations, osteomyelitis, and amputations. There are currently five types of HSANs, differing in pattern of dysfunction, age of onset, inheritance pattern, and additional clinical features.[6] Individuals with indifference to pain have painless injuries but otherwise no additional sensory dysfunctions.[10] As proposed in the late 1900's [5,8] the disease mechanisms, which can now be postulated through recent genetic advances, implicate disrupted sensory pathways in HSANs (such as NGF/TrkA signalling) that are intact in individuals showing indifference to pain.

TABLE 25.1 The clinical aspects and causative genes of HSAN

HSAN type	OMIM	Inheritance pattern	Clinical description	Gene Name	OMIM	Reference
1	162400	AD	Adult onset that begins with loss of pain and temperature sensation in the lower extremities. It is progressive, and touch and pressure may deteriorate over time. Autonomic involvement is absent or weak. Ulcers on the extremities are common, which may lead to amputation and painless injuries.	SPTLC1	605712	Nicholson et al 1996. Dawkins et al 2001. Bejaoui et al 2001.
2	201300, 613115	AR	Early childhood onset with primarily distal sensory loss, affecting the lower limbs most severely. Abnormalities in the sensation of discriminative touch and pressure are most common. Pain insensitivity is observed but at varying levels; complete loss is possible. The lack of pain perception results in ulcerations, self-mutilations, painless fractures, and joint injuries.	(HSAN2A) WNK1/HSN2 isoform (HSAN2B) FAM134B	605232 613114	Lafreniere et al 2004. Shekarabi et al 2008 Kurth et al 2009
3	223900	AR	Infant onset characterized by a loss of pain and temperature sensation with extensive autonomic dysfunction. Autonomic disturbances include the inability to secrete tears, excessive sweating, and vasomotor and cardiovascular perturbations. Self- mutilation is less common than in other types of HSANs. Lifespan of an HSAN3 patient is greatly reduced.	IKBKAP	603722	Blumenfeld et al 1993. Slaugenhaupt et al 2001. Anderson et al 2001.

(continued)

TABLE 25.1 (Continued)

HSAN type	OMIM	Inheritance pattern	Clinical description	Gene Name	OMIM	Reference
4	256800	AR	A very rare HSAN that involves both pain insensitivity and autonomic defects, which is described as congenital insensitivity to pain with anhidrosis (inability to perspire). Onset is either during infancy or in early childhood. The sensation of pain is abnormal, but touch and pressure are unaffected. Painless injuries and self- mutilations are frequent.	NTRK1	191315	Indo et al 1996.
5	608654	AR	A childhood onset of pain and temperature insensitivity that results in painless burns, fractures, and ulcerations. No other sensory components are affected and variable autonomic deficits have been noted, ranging from no autonomic dysfunction, to a case involving skin blotching, decreased sweating, and episodes of increased body temperature.	NGFβ	162030	Einarsdottir et al 2004.

HEREDITARY SENSORY AUTONOMIC NEUROPATHY TYPE I (HSAN1) [MIM #162400]

Serine palmitoyltransferase long chain base subunit 1 (SPTLC1; MIM *605712). HSAN1 is a dominantly inherited sensorimotor axonal neuropathy with onset in the first or second decades of life. The presenting features of HSAN1 cases included lightning pains, painless skin injuries and ulceration, distal sensory loss to sharp, hot, and cold sensation, with loss of distal reflexes and distal muscle wasting. Nerve conduction velocities are consistent with an axonal neuropathy, particularly of the lower limbs. *SPTLC1* encodes the first of three long chain base subunits (LCB1) of serine palmitoyltransferase (SPT), which is a catalyst of the first and rate-limiting step of *de novo* sphingolipid synthesis.[11] In 2001, mutations in *SPTLC1* were shown to cause HSAN1 (Table 25.1), following the locus identification and refinement by studying four Australian families.[12–15] Three different mutations, p.C133Y, p.C133W, and p.V144D, were originally detected[14,15] and there are currently five *SPTLC1* mutations associated with HSAN1; more recently S331F and A352V mutations have been reported but their pathogenicity has not been be confirmed.[16–18]

It was initially believed that HSAN1 mutations enhanced SPT activity, but the opposite has now been repeatedly shown.[15,18–23] Nevertheless, HSAN1 is not simply explained by the loss of SPT activity. Transgenic SPTLC1^{C133W} mice, which develop a small fiber neuropathy, show a significant decrease in SPT activity but no reduction in total sphingolipid levels,[22,24] also heterozygous *SPTLC1* and *SPTLC2* knock-out mice do not develop a neuropathy despite having reduced SPT expression and activity.[23,25] In fact, the mechanism underlying HSAN1 seems related to the accumulation of two neurotoxic sphingolipids.[23] Two *SPTLC1* mutations, p.C133W and p.C133Y, have been shown to cause a shift in the substrate specificity of SPT from serine to alanine and, to a lesser degree, glycine. Consequently, two sphingolipid metabolites, deoxy-SA and deoxymethyl-SA, also called deoxysphingolipid bases (DSBs), are formed. Neither of the latter have a hydroxyl group in C_1, which prevents their conversion to more complex phospho- or glycol-sphingolipids, and their degradation.[23] Increased DSB levels in neuronal dorsal root ganglion cultures interfere with the formation of neurites by decreasing the number and length of growing neurites, and retracting the existing ones. Under these conditions the cytoskeleton of neurites is affected due to retraction of neurofilaments.[23] The tissue specificity of the HSAN1 phenotype can be explained by comparing DSB levels in tissues of transgenic SPTLC1^{C133W} mice compared to control wild-type mice. Some tissues (e.g., plasma, sciatic nerve, and testis) of SPTLC1^{C133W} mice present elevated DSB levels, by comparison to wild-type animals, while, others like brain and spinal cord, have normal DSB levels in both mutant and wild-type animals; something fitting with the pathology because the central nervous system is not disturbed in HSAN1.[22] These findings suggest the possibility of DSB dosage as a diagnostic tool (or disease biomarker) and of therapeutic avenues aiming to reduce the levels of these neurotoxic metabolites.

HEREDITARY SENSORY AUTONOMIC NEUROPATHY TYPE II (HSAN2) [MIM #201300]

Protein kinase with-no-lysine(K)-1 (WNK1; MIM *605232). HSAN2 is an early-onset autosomal recessive disorder characterized by loss of perception to pain, touch, and heat due to a loss of peripheral sensory nerves. There is a marked reduction in the number of myelinated fibers due to Wallerian-like axonal degeneration, as well as segmental demyelination, most likely secondary to axonal changes. In 2008, mutations in a newly identified nervous system-specific isoform of *WNK1* were determined to cause HSAN2 (Table 25.1).[26] Previously, an open reading frame called *HSN2*, which was thought to be an independent intragenic gene of *WNK1*, was recognized as being causal.[27] This open reading frame was identified after a genome-wide scan of two HSAN2 Newfoundland families and the observation of a homozygous haplotype of 1.2 Mb around *D12S352*; two French-Canadian families also showed linkage to this locus.[27] Sequencing of all known positional candidates revealed no pathogenic variant. However, a search of conserved expressed sequence tags between mice and humans identified a novel unannotated 434 amino acid ORF located within intron 8 of *WNK1* and it was shown to contain three different truncating mutations.[27] Subsequent sequencing of this *HSN2* ORF in a French family later only revealed a heterozygous variant (c.639delA, p.Arg214fsX215) and so the entire coding sequence of *WNK1* was screened and shown to contain a second mutation (c.1584_1585delAG, p.Asp531fsX547) in exon 6; HSN2 was thus revealed to be an exon of WNK1. This is the only report of compound heterozygous mutations in HSAN2.[26] A careful examination of *HSN2* structure and expression in mouse showed that it was in fact a nervous system-specific exon of *WNK1* expressed in sensory and nociceptive components.[26] At least twelve mutations have been reported to cause HSAN2.[26–32]

WNK1 is a serine-threonine kinase without the well-conserved lysine residue in its catalytic domain.[33–35] This kinase is widely expressed, including in the nervous system and it is deemed to be critical during development because knocking it down in mice embryos is lethal.[34,36] WNK1 mutations were first reported to cause pseudohypoaldosteronism type II [MIM#145260], which involves kidney failure. While the kidney specific isoform of WNK1, which lacks a large portion of the catalytic domain, was extensively investigated, little is known about the role of other WNK1 isoforms in the nervous system, thus the recent identification of a nervous system-specific isoform (WNK1/HSN2) is interesting.[26,37] WNK1 had nonetheless been shown to control the proliferation and migration of neural progenitor cells, as well as neurite outgrowth. Given that WNK1 is essentially observed in the neuronal cell body, while WNK1/HSN2 is present in both the cell body and axons,[26] it may be that WNK1/HSN2 is involved in endosomal trafficking and axonal maintenance.

WNK1 also interacts with LINGO-1, a transmembrane protein known to control axon growth by mediating the activity of myelin inhibitors through a tripartite receptor complex with Nogo-66 receptor (NgR) and p75 (or TROY).[38] LINGO-1 does not, however, always coexist within that complex as it was shown to be regulated by NGF and inhibit myelination of TrkA-positive dorsal root ganglia.[39,40] Hence, additional signalling of LINGO-1 may explain the axon degeneration observed in HSAN2. WNK1 is also involved in the regulation of ion channels, in particular TRPV4, a vanilloid receptor involved in thermal and mechanical nociception.[35,41]

Family with sequence similarity to 134 member B (FAM134B; MIM *613114). Following the examination of a consanguineous, Saudi Arabian family with impaired nociception and ulcerations of the hands and feet, *FAM134B* was reported to be a second HSAN2 gene (Table 25.1).[42] Genome-wide homozygosity mapping identified a 3 Mb candidate locus at 5p15.1 and follow-up sequencing of positional candidates revealed a homozygous *FAM134B* truncating mutation (p.S309X) in affected individuals. Screening a cohort of additional HSAN individuals identified three additional *FAM134B* mutations: a deletion, nonsense, and splicing mutation.[42] FAM134B (also known as JK1) was previously known to be over-expressed in esophageal squamous cell carcinoma cell lines and tumors, and as a result, was shown to increase cell proliferation in mouse fibroblasts and HEK293 cells.[43] FAM134B was also shown to be a *cis*-Golgi protein that when knocked down leads to structural alterations of this compartment and triggers apoptosis in primary dorsal roots ganglia cultures.[42]

HEREDITARY SENSORY AUTONOMIC NEUROPATHY TYPE III (HSAN3) [MIM #223900]

Kinase complex-associated protein (IKAP; MIM *603722). HSAN3 (Table 25.1) is an autosomal recessive disorder occurring almost exclusively among Ashkenazi Jews. In 1993, affected individuals from such families were studied to search for the HSAN3 gene.[44] Common features included alacrima, absence of lingual fungiform papillae with impaired taste, vasomotor instability, hypoactive or absent deep tendon reflexes, and relative indifference to pain and temperature. Ultimately, this effort enabled the identification of a major Ashkenazi Jewish disease haplotype on chromosome 9q31, and two additional minor haplotypes.[44,45] *IKBKAP*, which encodes the protein IKAP, was then identified as the causal gene by two independent groups.[45,46] Each of the individuals with the c.2507+6T>C or p.R696P mutations was found to have the polymorphic DNA markers associated with the major or minor haplotypes, respectively.[47] The *IKBKAP* mutation of the major Ashkenazi Jewish haplotype is 6 bp into intron 20 and has a tissue-specific splicing effect.[45,46] The mutations underlying the other HSAN3 minor haplotypes were determined to be p.R696P and p.P914L.[45,48] The latter was the first mutation reported among non-Ashkenazi Jews.[48] Only three *IKBKAP* variants have been reported and the splicing variant is estimated to account for 99.5% of all HSAN3 chromosomes.[48] Furthermore, the identification of two founder mutations (c.2204+6T>C and p.R696P) having a combined carrier rate of 1/31 among Ashkenazi Jews, accounts for over 99% of disease alleles, leading to practice guidelines recommending carrier screening for familial dysautonomia (among other conditions) to all Ashkenazi Jews who are pregnant or considering pregnancy. These guidelines have been widely implemented and well-received by the community.[49]

IKAP is a well-conserved protein that belongs to an unknown protein family and shows no domain homology to predict its function. IKAP localizes to both the nucleus and cytosol. Nuclear IKAP is involved in RNA polymerase-II-mediated transcriptional elongation; hence it has also been termed elongator protein-1 (ELP1) and it forms a complex with ELP2 and ELP3. In the cytosol IKAP has been suggested to be involved in Jun N-terminal kinase (JNK)-mediated stress signalling, exocytosis, tRNA modification, and actin cytoskeleton organization during cell migration.[50–53] shRNA and siRNA directed against IKAP leads to a severe deficit in cell adhesion and migration that was rescued by wild-type IKAP but not HSAN3 IKAP mutants.[53] IKAP interacts with several cytosolic proteins involved in cell migration, including filamin A, dynein heavy chain, ubiquitin-specific processing protease USP9X, and the non-receptor tyrosine kinase BMX.[53] Therefore, it has been proposed that loss of function *IKBKAP* mutations disrupt neural migration and cause HSAN3.[54] While a detailed mechanism still awaits clarification, two very different explanations have been proposed as to how IKAP regulates cell migration: via transcriptional regulation and via cytosolic interactions.[54]

HEREDITARY SENSORY AUTONOMIC NEUROPATHY TYPE IV (HSAN4) [MIM #256800]

The neurotrophin receptor (NTR/TrkA; MIM *191315). HSAN4 also is referred to as congenital insensitivity to pain with anhidrosis (CIPA). Mutations in *NTRK1*, which encodes the TrkA receptor protein, were shown to cause HSAN4 (Table 25.1),[55] a very rare autosomal recessive disorder.[56,57] In 1996, Indo and coworkers screened HSAN4 patients, all of whom had consanguineous parents, for mutations in three candidate genes (*NTRK1*, *NGF*, and *p75*), identifying three distinct *NTRK1* variants (a deletion, splice, and missense mutation).[55] Since then, over 40 different and unclustered *NTRK1* mutations have been reported. TrkA is one of three tyrosine kinases from the Trk receptor family, which are activated by one or more neurotrophins. NGF specifically activates TrkA.[58–62] The activation of TrkA triggers its dimerization and phosphorylation, which in turns activates different signalling pathways.[59,63,64]

HEREDITARY SENSORY AUTONOMIC NEUROPATHY TYPE V (HSAN5) [MIM #608654]

***Nerve growth factor* β *subunit (NGFβ; MIM *162030)*.** Affected individuals suffer from a severe loss of deep pain perception that prevents them from feeling pain originating in bone fractures and joints; heat perception is also impaired. In 2004, homozygosity mapping identified a locus (1p11.2-p13.2, ~8.3 Mb) and homozygous mutation (c.661C>T; p.R100W in the mature protein) in *NGFβ* that are shown to underlie HSAN5 (Table 25.1).[65] NGF is a glycoprotein with three subunits α_2, β, and γ_2. α–NGF is not known to be active, β-NGF (encoded by *NGFβ*) is responsible for all of the biological properties, and γ-NGF has a specific protease function that processes the NGF precursor to its mature form.[66] The initial synthesized protein is termed pro-NGF and requires cleavage to produce the carboxyl-terminus mature protein.[67] NGF was originally identified as a factor stimulating the growth of nerve processes and thus believed to be important in development.[68,69] The p.R100W mutation reported in HSAN5 was shown to inhibit the neuron-like differentiation of rat PC12 cells, commonly used cell lines that can differentiate into neurons, and to affect normal NGF processing and secretion of the mature form. Cells expressing the mutant NGF mainly expressed pro-NGF.[70] In vitro binding assays were also used to determine if the p.R100W mutation affected the binding of either pro–NGF or its mature form to TrkA and p75. Only binding of the mature NGF to p75 was disrupted, thus suggesting p75 may play a role in loss of pain sensation as well as the ability to sense temperature changes in limbs.[59,71]

The association between NGF and nociception is intriguing, as a timeline of NGF functions indicates that NGF, during development, is vital for the survival of pain receptors or sensory neurons known as nociceptors.[72] Late in development, up to postnatal day 2, it has been shown that removing NGF results in the selective loss of nociceptors[73,74] and later between postnatal days 4 and 11, the absence of NGF generally results in a change in nociceptor phenotype. For example, C-fiber nociceptors become less sensitive to intense heat.[75] Continuing into adulthood, NGF affects the sensitization of nociceptors.[72,76] Furthermore when a tissue is damaged or inflamed, NGF expression is up-regulated, the protein is released from damaged cells where it acts as an inflammatory mediator that activates nociceptors by binding to their surface receptors (TrkA and/or p75) and initiating signalling cascades (PKA and/or MAPK pathways). This ultimately increases sensitivity and excitability of nociceptors by enhancing pro-nociceptive receptors and ion channels (e.g., TRPV1 and $Na_v1.8$).[71,76] It remains unclear which NGF receptor(s) and signalling cascade(s) mediate(s) this sensitization. A general consensus deems that TrkA is the NGF receptor activated during this process; however, it has also been suggested that the p75 NTR contributes.[59] How TrkA and p75 act independently or together during this process remains to be determined.

CHARCOT-MARIE-TOOTH DISEASE TYPE 2B (CMT2B) [MIM #600882]

Ras-associated protein (RAB7; MIM *602298). The most common feature of CMT2B is distal sensory loss affecting all modalities that often results in foot calluses and poorly healing ulcers, which can lead to osteomyelitis and autoamputation. Motor and sensory nerve conduction velocities (NCVs) are normal or moderately decreased, suggesting axonal degeneration. *RAB7* is the causative gene for CMT2B [MIM#600882].[77] CMTs (also known as a hereditary motor and sensory neuropathy; HMSN) are traditionally divided into two classes. Type 1 (CMT1) is a demyelinating neuropathy and CMT2 an axonal neuropathy.[78] Over 25 CMT genes have been identified.[79,80] CMT2 can be inherited in both an autosomal recessive and dominant pattern, the latter being more common, and is genetically heterogeneous. For the identification of the first autosomal dominant locus (*CMT2A*), only three out of the six CMT2 families studied were linked to the novel locus.[81] In 1995, the *CMT2B* locus was identified by studying an American family that did not link to *CMT2A*; this new locus extended over 30 cM on chromosome3q13–22.[82] This region was reduced to 2.5 cM, in 2003, and screening three candidate genes identified *RAB7* as the causative gene.[77] To date, four missense mutations have been identified.[77,83,84] Sensory abnormalities and ulcerations are the most prominent clinical features in CMT2B, therefore it was suggested in 2006 that CMT2B be included in the HSAN-spectrum.[85]

RAB7 is a small GTPase found on late endosomes' membrane-bound compartments that are associated with the sorting of intracellular material before it reaches its final destination or its trafficking of degradative lysosomes.[86–89] It is ubiquitously expressed but plays a specific role in neuronal transport pathways.[90,91] Intracellular membrane trafficking is an essential process in all eukaryotic cells, but it is particularly critical at synaptic terminals, in which a large number of specific ion channels, scaffolding molecules, and a variety of signal transduction modulators have to be precisely targeted to ensure proper synaptic function. RAB7 was reported to form a complex with NGF/TrkA and control the trafficking and signalling of NGF/TrkA endosomes.[91] More precisely, a dominant negative Rab7 mutant (p.T22N) was shown to trigger TrkA accumulation and increased signalling (e.g., MAPK), and neurite outgrowth.[91] However, CMT2B-causing Rab7 mutants actually inhibit neurite outgrowth.[92] The biological properties of these mutants have been studied and GTP hydrolysis is altered because of a guanine nucleotide decreased dissociation, which results in the accumulation of active GTP-bound Rab7.[93,94] Why mutant Rab7 hydrolysis selectively affects peripheral cells, and axon regeneration is only affected later in life, remains to be elucidated; this may be due to a cell-specific effector protein(s). The second to third decade age of onset indicates that CMT2B *Rab7* mutations do not impair development.

AUTOSOMAL RECESSIVE MUTILATING SENSORY NEUROPATHY WITH SPASTIC PARAPLEGIA [MIM #256840]

Cytosolic chaperonin-containing TPCP1 subunit 5 (CCT5; MIM *610150). Affected individuals have distal sensory loss for all modalities in the upper and lower limbs, particularly in the feet. Although the progression of spasticity is slow, the sensory neuropathy is rapidly progressive and severe. Electrophysiologic studies show normal or mildly decreased motor nerve conduction velocities consistent with a sensory axonal neuropathy. Mutations in *CCT5* cause an autosomal recessive mutilating sensory neuropathy with spastic paraplegia. CCT is a group II chaperonin and consists of two back-to-back octameric rings that contain subunits α, β, γ, δ, ε, ζ, η and θ.[95] The main role of CCT is to promote folding of newly synthesized polypeptides, and it is well-known for its involvement in the processing of actin and tubulin.[96,97] However, it is important to note that additional CCT interacting proteins have been identified and that these potentially link CCT to many cellular processes.[98,99] Similarly to HSAN1, mutilating ulcerations on hands and feet were first described; however, it was determined that affected individuals also had spastic paraplegia features.[100] A consanguineous Moroccan family was studied to identify the gene, but this recessive disorder is very rare as only a few patients in the world have been described.[100–102] A genome-wide scan was performed and positive LOD (logarithm of the odds) scores were observed for only three markers on chromosome 5. A fine-mapping effort first identified a 25 cM genetic interval delineated by *DS52054* and *D5S648*.[101] Subsequently, *CCT5*, a positional candidate that encodes the epsilon subunit of the cytosolic chaperonin-containing t-complex peptide-1 (CCT complex), was screened because mutations in *Cct4*, which encodes the delta subunit of the CTT complex, cause mutilating sensory neuropathy in mice;[103] the disease causing variant was reported to be p.H147R.[104]

CONGENITAL INDIFFERENCE TO PAIN (CIP)

Individuals with indifference to pain have painless injuries but otherwise normal sensory functions. While pain sensations are not normally perceived by these individuals, they are nonetheless aware of the existence of painful stimuli perceived by others, but they lack the affective-motivational component of pain. However, they have normal nerve fibers, nerve conduction velocities, and intact axon reflex upon subcutaneous histamine injections. These are all distinguishing features of indifference to pain.[10] Both autosomal dominant and recessive inheritance of indifference to pain are genetically transmitted. Nonetheless, only a few examples of autosomal dominant inheritance have actually been reported.[8,105,106] To date, no gene(s) has been identified for autosomal dominant cases. Autosomal recessive indifference to pain (CIP) is also rare. Fewer than 30 cases have been reported worldwide.[10]

CONGENITAL AUTOSOMAL RECESSIVE INDIFFERENCE TO PAIN [MIM #243000]

Sodium channel voltage-gated type-IX α subunit (SCN9A or NAV1.7; MIM *603415).
Individuals with congenital indifference to pain have painless injuries beginning in infancy but otherwise possess normal sensory modalities. Perception of passive movement, joint position, and vibration are normal, as are tactile thresholds and light-touch perception. Reflexes and autonomic responses are also normal. For the identification of the first and only causal congenital insensitivity to pain (CIP) gene, three Pakistani families with six affected children were studied.[107] A genome-wide scan identified an 11.7 Mb region of homozygosity on chromosome 2q24 that was noted only in affected individuals. Fine-mapping determined that each family had a different disease haplotype corresponding to distinct mutations. There were 50 genes in the disease region and bioinformatics predicted *SCN9A*, the gene encoding the α-subunit of the tetrodotoxin-sensitive voltage-gated sodium channel (also known as Na(v)1.7) to be the best candidate. Sequencing revealed three different homozygous mutations, all of which were determined to cause loss of function.[107] Since then, SCN9A loss-of-function mutations have been detected worldwide (e.g., Canada and Israel).[10,108,109] Altogether, this suggests that Na(v)1.7 is essential for pain regulation. Na(v)1.7 has also been associated with two other pain disorders: erythromelalgia (IEM) and paroxysmal extreme pain disorder (PEPD), where distinct gain of function mutations have

been detected.[110] Interestingly, a recent report demonstrated that loss-of-function muta-tions in *SCN9A* also cause a general loss of smell in these CIP patients.[111] The loss of both these major senses provides a mechanistic link between these two sensory modalities.

CONCLUSIONS

Sensory pathways historically have been considered defective for insensitivity to pain[5,8] and, at present, most proteins encoded by genes mutated in HSANs or HSAN-like pheno-types appear to be linked to various forms of intracellular signalling or transmission (e.g., sphingolipids, kinase signal transduction, and growth factor). Furthermore, both RAB7 and SPTLC1 have a function in endocytotic membrane trafficking. It is noteworthy that amid these signalling routes, four causative proteins (WNK1, TrkA, β-NGF, and RAB7) are directly, or indirectly, linked to the NGF/TrkA endocytic pathway, which is critically important in the development and function of nociceptive neurons, and also dependent upon retrograde transport through signaling endosomes.[112] By opposition, the only CIP for which a defective protein has thus far been identified revealed it to be an ion channel disorder; interestingly various nociceptor ion channels (e.g., TRPV1 and $Na_v1.81$) are in fact enhanced by NGF signalling.[71,76]

The emerging role of proteins, thus far established for these disorders, somehow offers the first opportunity of appreciating the phenotypic differences between CIP and HSANs. In 1970, the first distinction between insensitivity and indifference to pain was made by Jewesbury as it was postulated that insensitivity to pain is a failure to receive and perceive a stimulus, and indifference to pain is a lack of concern or reaction to a stimulus received.[5] This early assumption is congruent with current molecular findings as most of the disease causative genes identified thus are involved in signalling, except for the CIP causative gene, *SCN9A,* which is a voltage-gated sodium channel that acts more at the perception level.

Rotthier et al recently carried out a systematic mutation screen of genes causing HSAN and CMT2B (*IKAP* was not screened because their cohort did not contain patients with familial dysautonomia) in 100 familial and isolated HSAN patients, and established a muta-tion frequency of 19%;[16] thus clearly demonstrating that additional HSAN genes must exist. The mechanisms now known to cause peripheral neuropathies associated with nociception defect should be kept in mind as future mutational screening efforts focused on candidate genes will be performed.

High-throughput next-generation sequencing technologies are now making it possible to screen increasingly larger and unbiased set of genes for the discovery of novel causative genes;[113] it is particularly crucial to focus on re-sequencing high-value genomic regions or "target-enriched" protein-coding exons (exomes). Since 2010, the use of exome sequencing has snowballed and over ten disease causative genes were identified for rare diseases that have a recessive mode of inheritance like HSANs. There is no doubt this exome sequencing approach, or whole genome sequencing (when it becomes more affordable), will help to identify some of the remaining causative genes in patients who received diagnosis compat-ible with any subtypes of HSAN, CIP, or other rare neuropathies associated with nocicep-tion deficits.

Current insights into the molecular basis of disease processes associated with nocicep-tion defects, such as HSAN and CIP, may also be helpful in prioritizing the validation of sequencing variants that will be identified after sequencing exomes of affected families. Nonetheless, even if signalling and endocytic pathways represent emerging mechanistic themes in peripheral neuropathies associated with nociception defects, other or unknown cellular dysfunctions will likely be identified when an unbiased approach is used.

Also, as it stands, costs of diagnostic testing in a clinical setting currently oblige clinicians to adopt a selective approach to molecular testing, leaving many families with an undetermined cause of disease. As the costs of sequencing technologies continue to fall and the technology improves, it will allow for a single comprehensive genetic testing of every gene associated with nociception disorders. Furthermore, as molecular and clinical characterization of disease causing mutations continues to expand, this will contribute to a better understanding of genotype-phenotype correlations with regards to age of onset, phenotypic variability, severity, and prognosis of the various disease subtypes.

Although the genetic developments discussed in this chapter have not yet translated into treatments capable of correcting HSANs or CIPs, they have nonetheless increased our comprehension of the molecular mechanisms that underlie pain perception and transmission pathways, while suggesting avenues of investigation for these future treatments. Because the deregulation of several cellular processes underlies the neuropathies, cocktails of nociception regulating agents that target different pathways may one day offer the hope of treating some of these. From a clinical perspective, genetically diagnosed individuals might be more likely to benefit from early therapeutic intervention.

REFERENCES

1. Dearborn G. A case of congenital general pure analgesia. *J Nerv Ment Dis.* 1932;75:612–615.
2. Ford FR, Wilkins L. Congenital universal insensitiveness to pain. *Bull John Hopkins Hosp.* 1938;62:448–466.
3. Boyd DA Jr, Nie LW. Congenital universal indifference to pain. *Arch Neurol Psychiatry.* 1949;61(4):402–412.
4. Winkelmann RK, Lambert EH, Hayles AB. Congenital absence of pain. Report of a case and experimental studies. *Arch Dermatol.* 1962;85:325–339.
5. Jewesbury ECO, ed. *Congenital Indifference to Pain.* Amsterdam: Elsevier; 1970. Vincken P, Bruyn G, eds. *Handbook of Clinical Neurology*; No. 8.
6. Dyck PJ, Mellinger JF, Reagan TJ, et al. Not "indifference to pain" but varieties of hereditary sensory and autonomic neuropathy. *Brain.* 1983;106 (Pt 2):373–390.
7. Klein CJ, Sinnreich M, Dyck PJ. Indifference rather than insensitivity to pain. *Ann Neurol.* 2003;53(3):417–418; author reply 418–419.
8. Landrieu P, Said G, Allaire C. Dominantly transmitted congenital indifference to pain. *Ann Neurol.* 1990;27(5):574–578.
9. Nagasako EM, Oaklander AL, Dworkin RH. Congenital insensitivity to pain: an update. *Pain.* 2003;101(3):213–219.
10. Goldberg YP, MacFarlane J, MacDonald ML, et al. Loss-of-function mutations in the Nav1.7 gene underlie congenital indifference to pain in multiple human populations. *Clin Genet.* 2007;71(4):311–319.
11. Hanada K. Serine palmitoyltransferase, a key enzyme of sphingolipid metabolism. *Biochim Biophys Acta.* 2003;1632(1–3):16–30.
12. Nicholson GA, Dawkins JL, Blair IP, et al. The gene for hereditary sensory neuropathy type I (HSN-I) maps to chromosome 9q22.1-q22.3. *Nat Genet.* 1996;13(1):101–104.
13. Blair IP, Dawkins JL, Nicholson GA. Fine mapping of the hereditary sensory neuropathy type I locus on chromosome 9q22.1≥q22.3: exclusion of GAS1 and XPA. *Cytogenet Cell Genet.* 1997;78(2):140–144.
14. Bejaoui K, Wu C, Scheffler MD, et al. SPTLC1 is mutated in hereditary sensory neuropathy, type 1. *Nat Genet.* 2001;27(3):261–262.
15. Dawkins JL, Hulme DJ, Brahmbhatt SB, Auer-Grumbach M, Nicholson GA. Mutations in SPTLC1, encoding serine palmitoyltransferase, long chain base subunit-1, cause hereditary sensory neuropathy type I. *Nat Genet.* 2001;27(3):309–312.

16. Rotthier A, Baets J, De Vriendt E, et al. Genes for hereditary sensory and autonomic neuropathies: a genotype-phenotype correlation. *Brain.* 2009;132(Pt 10):2699–2711.

17. Verhoeven K, Coen K, De Vriendt E, et al. SPTLC1 mutation in twin sisters with hereditary sensory neuropathy type I. *Neurology.* 2004;62(6):1001–1002.

18. Hornemann T, Penno A, Richard S, et al. A systematic comparison of all mutations in hereditary sensory neuropathy type I (HSAN I) reveals that the G387A mutation is not disease associated. *Neurogenetics.* 2009;10(2):135–143.

19. Bejaoui K, Uchida Y, Yasuda S, et al. Hereditary sensory neuropathy type 1 mutations confer dominant negative effects on serine palmitoyltransferase, critical for sphingolipid synthesis. *J Clin Invest.* 2002;110(9):1301–1308.

20. Dedov VN, Dedova IV, Merrill AH Jr, Nicholson GA. Activity of partially inhibited serine palmitoyltransferase is sufficient for normal sphingolipid metabolism and viability of HSN1 patient cells. *Biochim Biophys Acta.* 2004;1688(2):168–175.

21. Gable K, Han G, Monaghan E, et al. Mutations in the yeast LCB1 and LCB2 genes, including those corresponding to the hereditary sensory neuropathy type I mutations, dominantly inactivate serine palmitoyltransferase. *J Biol Chem.* 2002;277(12):10194–10200.

22. Eichler FS, Hornemann T, McCampbell A, et al. Overexpression of the wild-type SPT1 subunit lowers desoxysphingolipid levels and rescues the phenotype of HSAN1. *J Neurosci.* 2009;29(46):14646–14651.

23. Penno A, Reilly MM, Houlden H, et al. Hereditary sensory neuropathy type 1 is caused by the accumulation of two neurotoxic sphingolipids. *J Biol Chem.* 2010;285(15):11178–11187.

24. McCampbell A, Truong D, Broom DC, et al. Mutant SPTLC1 dominantly inhibits serine palmitoyltransferase activity in vivo and confers an age-dependent neuropathy. *Hum Mol Genet.* 2005;14(22):3507–3521.

25. Hojjati MR, Li Z, Jiang XC. Serine palmitoyl-CoA transferase (SPT) deficiency and sphingolipid levels in mice. *Biochim Biophys Acta.* 2005;1737(1):44–51.

26. Shekarabi M, Girard N, Riviere JB, et al. Mutations in the nervous system—specific HSN2 exon of WNK1 cause hereditary sensory neuropathy type II. *J Clin Invest.* 2008;118(7):2496–2505.

27. Lafreniere RG, MacDonald ML, Dube MP, et al. Identification of a novel gene (HSN2) causing hereditary sensory and autonomic neuropathy type II through the Study of Canadian Genetic Isolates. *Am J Hum Genet.* 2004;74(5):1064–1073.

28. Cho HJ, Kim BJ, Suh YL, An JY, Ki CS. Novel mutation in the HSN2 gene in a Korean patient with hereditary sensory and autonomic neuropathy type 2. *J Hum Genet.* 2006;51(10):905–908.

29. Coen K, Pareyson D, Auer-Grumbach M, et al. Novel mutations in the HSN2 gene causing hereditary sensory and autonomic neuropathy type II. *Neurology.* 2006;66(5):748–751.

30. Riviere JB, Verlaan DJ, Shekarabi M, et al. A mutation in the HSN2 gene causes sensory neuropathy type II in a Lebanese family. *Ann Neurol.* 2004;56(4):572–575.

31. Roddier K, Thomas T, Marleau G, et al. Two mutations in the HSN2 gene explain the high prevalence of HSAN2 in French Canadians. *Neurology.* 2005;64(10):1762–1767.

32. Takagi M, Ozawa T, Hara K, et al. New HSN2 mutation in Japanese patient with hereditary sensory and autonomic neuropathy type 2. *Neurology.* 2006;66(8):1251–1252.

33. Hanks SK, Quinn AM, Hunter T. The protein kinase family: conserved features and deduced phylogeny of the catalytic domains. *Science.* 1988;241(4861):42–52.

34. Xu B, English JM, Wilsbacher JL, Stippec S, Goldsmith EJ, Cobb MH. WNK1, a novel mammalian serine/threonine protein kinase lacking the catalytic lysine in subdomain II. *J Biol Chem.* 2000;275(22):16795–16801.

35. Huang CL, Cha SK, Wang HR, Xie J, Cobb MH. WNKs: protein kinases with a unique kinase domain. *Exp Mol Med.* 2007;39(5):565–573.

36. Zambrowicz BP, Abuin A, Ramirez-Solis R, et al. Wnk1 kinase deficiency lowers blood pressure in mice: a gene-trap screen to identify potential targets for therapeutic intervention. *Proc Natl Acad Sci U S A.* 2003;100(24):14109–14114.

37. Delaloy C, Lu J, Houot AM, et al. Multiple promoters in the WNK1 gene: one controls expression of a kidney-specific kinase-defective isoform. *Mol Cell Biol.* 2003;23(24):9208–9221.

38. Zhang Z, Xu X, Zhang Y, Zhou J, Yu Z, He C. LINGO-1 interacts with WNK1 to regulate nogo-induced inhibition of neurite extension. *J Biol Chem.* 2009;284(23):15717–15728.

39. Llorens F, Gil V, Iraola S, et al. Developmental analysis of Lingo-1/Lern1 protein expression in the mouse brain: interaction of its intracellular domain with Myt1l. *Dev Neurobiol.* 2008;68(4):521–541.

40. Lee X, Yang Z, Shao Z, et al. NGF regulates the expression of axonal LINGO-1 to inhibit oligodendrocyte differentiation and myelination. *J Neurosci.* 2007;27(1):220–225.

41. Fu Y, Subramanya A, Rozansky D, Cohen DM. WNK kinases influence TRPV4 channel function and localization. *Am J Physiol Renal Physiol.* 2006;290(6):F1305–F1314.

42. Kurth I, Pamminger T, Hennings JC, et al. Mutations in FAM134B, encoding a newly identified Golgi protein, cause severe sensory and autonomic neuropathy. *Nat Genet.* 2009;41(11):1179–1181.

43. Tang WK, Chui CH, Fatima S, et al. Oncogenic properties of a novel gene JK-1 located in chromosome 5p and its overexpression in human esophageal squamous cell carcinoma. *Int J Mol Med.* 2007;19(6):915–923.

44. Blumenfeld A, Slaugenhaupt SA, Axelrod FB, et al. Localization of the gene for familial dysautonomia on chromosome 9 and definition of DNA markers for genetic diagnosis. *Nat Genet.* 1993;4(2):160–164.

45. Slaugenhaupt SA, Blumenfeld A, Gill SP, et al. Tissue-specific expression of a splicing mutation in the IKBKAP gene causes familial dysautonomia. *Am J Hum Genet.* 2001;68(3):598–605.

46. Anderson SL, Coli R, Daly IW, et al. Familial dysautonomia is caused by mutations of the IKAP gene. *Am J Hum Genet.* 2001;68(3):753–758.

47. Blumenfeld A, Slaugenhaupt SA, Liebert CB, et al. Precise genetic mapping and haplotype analysis of the familial dysautonomia gene on human chromosome 9q31. *Am J Hum Genet.* 1999;64(4):1110–1118.

48. Leyne M, Mull J, Gill SP, et al. Identification of the first non-Jewish mutation in familial Dysautonomia. *Am J Med Genet A.* 2003;118A(4):305–308.

49. Gross SJ, Pletcher BA, Monaghan KG. Carrier screening in individuals of Ashkenazi Jewish descent. *Genet Med.* 2008;10(1):54–56.

50. Holmberg C, Katz S, Lerdrup M, et al. A novel specific role for I kappa B kinase complex-associated protein in cytosolic stress signaling. *J Biol Chem.* 2002;277(35):31918–31928.

51. Rahl PB, Chen CZ, Collins RN. Elp1p, the yeast homolog of the FD disease syndrome protein, negatively regulates exocytosis independently of transcriptional elongation. *Mol Cell.* 2005;17(6):841–853.

52. Esberg A, Huang B, Johansson MJ, Bystrom AS. Elevated levels of two tRNA species bypass the requirement for elongator complex in transcription and exocytosis. *Mol Cell.* 2006;24(1):139–148.

53. Johansen LD, Naumanen T, Knudsen A, et al. IKAP localizes to membrane ruffles with filamin A and regulates actin cytoskeleton organization and cell migration. *J Cell Sci.* 2008;121(Pt 6):854–864.

54. Naumanen T, Johansen LD, Coffey ET, Kallunki T. Loss-of-function of IKAP/ELP1: could neuronal migration defect underlie familial dysautonomia? *Cell Adh Migr.* 2008;2(4):236–239.

55. Indo Y, Tsuruta M, Hayashida Y, et al. Mutations in the TRKA/NGF receptor gene in patients with congenital insensitivity to pain with anhidrosis. *Nat Genet.* 1996;13(4):485–488.

56. Swanson AG. Congenital insensitivity to pain with anhidrosis. A unique syndrome in two male siblings. *Arch Neurol.* 1963;8:299–306.

57. Swanson AG, Buchan GC, Alvord EC Jr. Anatomic changes in congenital insensitivity to pain. absence of small primary sensory neurons in ganglia, roots, and Lissauer's tract. *Arch Neurol.* 1965;12:12–18.

58. Huang EJ, Reichardt LF. Trk receptors: roles in neuronal signal transduction. *Annu Rev Biochem.* 2003;72:609–642.

59. Nicol GD, Vasko MR. Unraveling the story of NGF-mediated sensitization of nociceptive sensory neurons: ON or OFF the Trks? *Mol Interv.* 2007;7(1):26–41.

60. Niewiadomska G, Mietelska-Porowska A, Mazurkiewicz M. The cholinergic system, nerve growth factor and the cytoskeleton. *Behav Brain Res.* 2011;221(2):515–526.

61. Ultsch MH, Wiesmann C, Simmons LC, et al. Crystal structures of the neurotrophin-binding domain of TrkA, TrkB and TrkC. *J Mol Biol.* 1999;290(1):149–159.

62. Peleshok J, Saragovi HU. Functional mimetics of neurotrophins and their receptors. *Biochem Soc Trans.* 2006;34(Pt 4):612–617.

63. Pezet S, McMahon SB. Neurotrophins: mediators and modulators of pain. *Annu Rev Neurosci.* 2006;29:507–538.

64. Moises T, Dreier A, Flohr S, et al. Tracking TrkA's trafficking: NGF receptor trafficking controls NGF receptor signaling. *Mol Neurobiol.* 2007;35(2):151–159.

65. Einarsdottir E, Carlsson A, Minde J, et al. A mutation in the nerve growth factor beta gene (NGFB) causes loss of pain perception. *Hum Mol Genet.* 2004;13(8):799–805.

66. Sofroniew MV, Howe CL, Mobley WC. Nerve growth factor signaling, neuroprotection, and neural repair. *Annu Rev Neurosci.* 2001;24:1217–1281.

67. Hempstead BL. Commentary: Regulating proNGF action: multiple targets for therapeutic intervention. *Neurotox Res.* 2009;16(3):255–260.

68. Cowan WM. Viktor Hamburger and Rita Levi-Montalcini: the path to the discovery of nerve growth factor. *Annu Rev Neurosci.* 2001;24:551–600.

69. Levi-Montalcini R. Effects of mouse tumor transplantation on the nervous system. *Ann N Y Acad Sci.* 1952;55(2):330–344.

70. Larsson E, Kuma R, Norberg A, Minde J, Holmberg M. Nerve growth factor R221W responsible for insensitivity to pain is defectively processed and accumulates as proNGF. *Neurobiol Dis.* 2009;33(2):221–228.

71. Covaceuszach S, Capsoni S, Marinelli S, et al. In vitro receptor binding properties of a "painless" NGF mutein, linked to hereditary sensory autonomic neuropathy type V. *Biochem Biophys Res Commun.* 2010;391(1):824–829.

72. Petruska JC, Mendell LM. The many functions of nerve growth factor: multiple actions on nociceptors. *Neurosci Lett.* 2004;361(1–3):168–171.

73. Lewin GR, Mendell LM. Nerve growth factor and nociception. *Trends Neurosci.* 1993; 16(9):353–359.

74. Molliver DC, Wright DE, Leitner ML, et al. IB4-binding DRG neurons switch from NGF to GDNF dependence in early postnatal life. *Neuron.* 1997;19(4):849–861.

75. Lewin GR, Mendell LM. Regulation of cutaneous C-fiber heat nociceptors by nerve growth factor in the developing rat. *J Neurophysiol.* 1994;71(3):941–949.

76. Cheng JK, Ji RR. Intracellular signaling in primary sensory neurons and persistent pain. *Neurochem Res.* 2008;33(10):1970–1978.

77. Verhoeven K, De Jonghe P, Coen K, et al. Mutations in the small GTP-ase late endosomal protein RAB7 cause Charcot-Marie-Tooth type 2B neuropathy. *Am J Hum Genet.* 2003;72(3):722–727.

78. Reilly MM. Sorting out the inherited neuropathies. *Pract Neurol.* 2007;7(2):93–105.

79. Pareyson D, Marchesi C. Diagnosis, natural history, and management of Charcot-Marie-Tooth disease. *Lancet Neurol.* 2009;8(7):654–667.

80. Szigeti K, Lupski JR. Charcot-Marie-Tooth disease. *Eur J Hum Genet.* 2009;17(6):703–710.

81. Ben Othmane K, Middleton LT, Loprest LJ, et al. Localization of a gene (CMT2A) for autosomal dominant Charcot-Marie-Tooth disease type 2 to chromosome 1p and evidence of genetic heterogeneity. *Genomics.* 1993;17(2):370–375.

82. Kwon JM, Elliott JL, Yee WC, et al. Assignment of a second Charcot-Marie-Tooth type II locus to chromosome 3q. *Am J Hum Genet.* 1995;57(4):853–858.

83. Houlden H, King RH, Muddle JR, et al. A novel RAB7 mutation associated with ulcero-mutilating neuropathy. *Ann Neurol.* 2004;56(4):586–590.

84. Meggouh F, Bienfait HM, Weterman MA, de Visser M, Baas F. Charcot-Marie-Tooth disease due to a de novo mutation of the RAB7 gene. *Neurology.* 2006;67(8):1476–1478.

85. Verpoorten N, De Jonghe P, Timmerman V. Disease mechanisms in hereditary sensory and autonomic neuropathies. *Neurobiol Dis.* 2006;21(2):247–255.

86. Feng Y, Press B, Wandinger-Ness A. Rab 7: an important regulator of late endocytic membrane traffic. *J Cell Biol.* 1995;131(6 Pt 1):1435–1452.

87. Lebrand C, Corti M, Goodson H, et al. Late endosome motility depends on lipids via the small GTPase Rab7. *EMBO J.* 2002;21(6):1289–1300.

88. Mukhopadhyay A, Funato K, Stahl PD. Rab7 regulates transport from early to late endocytic compartments in Xenopus oocytes. *J Biol Chem.* 1997;272(20):13055–13059.

89. Vitelli R, Santillo M, Lattero D, et al. Role of the small GTPase Rab7 in the late endocytic pathway. *J Biol Chem.* 1997;272(7):4391–4397.

90. Deinhardt K, Salinas S, Verastegui C, et al. Rab5 and Rab7 control endocytic sorting along the axonal retrograde transport pathway. *Neuron.* 2006;52(2):293–305.

91. Saxena S, Bucci C, Weis J, Kruttgen A. The small GTPase Rab7 controls the endosomal trafficking and neuritogenic signaling of the nerve growth factor receptor TrkA. *J Neurosci.* 2005;25(47):10930–10940.

92. Cogli L, Progida C, Lecci R, Bramato R, Kruttgen A, Bucci C. CMT2B-associated Rab7 mutants inhibit neurite outgrowth. *Acta Neuropathol.* 2010;120(4):491–501.

93. McCray BA, Skordalakes E, Taylor JP. Disease mutations in Rab7 result in unregulated nucleotide exchange and inappropriate activation. *Hum Mol Genet.* 2010;19(6):1033–1047.

94. Spinosa MR, Progida C, De Luca A, Colucci AM, Alifano P, Bucci C. Functional characterization of Rab7 mutant proteins associated with Charcot-Marie-Tooth type 2B disease. *J Neurosci.* 2008;28(7):1640–1648.

95. Liou AK, Willison KR. Elucidation of the subunit orientation in CCT (chaperonin containing TCP1) from the subunit composition of CCT micro-complexes. *EMBO J.* 1997;16(14):4311–4316.

96. Brackley KI, Grantham J. Subunits of the chaperonin CCT interact with F-actin and influence cell shape and cytoskeletal assembly. *Exp Cell Res.* 2010;316(4):543–553.

97. Thulasiraman V, Yang CF, Frydman J. In vivo newly translated polypeptides are sequestered in a protected folding environment. *EMBO J.* 1999;18(1):85–95.

98. Dekker C, Stirling PC, McCormack EA, et al. The interaction network of the chaperonin CCT. *EMBO J.* 2008;27(13):1827–1839.

99. Yam AY, Xia Y, Lin HT, Burlingame A, Gerstein M, Frydman J. Defining the TRiC/CCT interactome links chaperonin function to stabilization of newly made proteins with complex topologies. *Nat Struct Mol Biol.* 2008;15(12):1255–1262.

100. Cavanagh NP, Eames RA, Galvin RJ, Brett EM, Kelly RE. Hereditary sensory neuropathy with spastic paraplegia. *Brain.* 1979;102(1):79–94.

101. Bouhouche A, Benomar A, Bouslam N, Ouazzani R, Chkili T, Yahyaoui M. Autosomal recessive mutilating sensory neuropathy with spastic paraplegia maps to chromosome 5p15.31–14.1. *Eur J Hum Genet.* 2006;14(2):249–252.

102. Thomas PK, Misra VP, King RH, et al. Autosomal recessive hereditary sensory neuropathy with spastic paraplegia. *Brain.* 1994;117(Pt 4):651–659.

103. Lee MJ, Stephenson DA, Groves MJ, et al. Hereditary sensory neuropathy is caused by a mutation in the delta subunit of the cytosolic chaperonin-containing t-complex peptide-1 (Cct4) gene. *Hum Mol Genet.* 2003;12(15):1917–1925.

104. Bouhouche A, Benomar A, Bouslam N, Chkili T, Yahyaoui M. Mutation in the epsilon subunit of the cytosolic chaperonin-containing t-complex peptide-1 (Cct5) gene causes autosomal recessive mutilating sensory neuropathy with spastic paraplegia. *J Med Genet.* 2006;43(5):441–443.

105. Ervin FR, Sternbach RA. Hereditary insensitivity to pain. *Trans Am Neurol Assoc.* 1960;85:70–74.

106. Comings DE, Amromin GD. Autosomal dominant insensitivity to pain with hyperplastic myelinopathy and autosomal dominant indifference to pain. *Neurology.* 1974;24(9):838–848.

107. Cox JJ, Reimann F, Nicholas AK, et al. An SCN9A channelopathy causes congenital inability to experience pain. *Nature.* 2006;444(7121):894–898.

108. Ahmad S, Dahllund L, Eriksson AB, et al. A stop codon mutation in SCN9A causes lack of pain sensation. *Hum Mol Genet.* 2007;16(17):2114–2121.

109. Cox JJ, Sheynin J, Shorer Z, et al. Congenital insensitivity to pain: novel SCN9A missense and in-frame deletion mutations. *Hum Mutat.* 2010;31(9):E1670–686.

110. Lampert A, O'Reilly AO, Reeh P, Leffler A. Sodium channelopathies and pain. *Pflugers Arch.* 2010;460(2):249–263.
111. Weiss J, Pyrski M, Jacobi E, et al. Loss-of-function mutations in sodium channel Nav1.7 cause anosmia. *Nature.* 2011;472(7342):186–190.
112. Verhoeven K, Timmerman V, Mauko B, Pieber TR, De Jonghe P, Auer-Grumbach M. Recent advances in hereditary sensory and autonomic neuropathies. *Curr Opin Neurol.* 2006;19(5):474–480.
113. Ng SB, Buckingham KJ, Lee C, et al. Exome sequencing identifies the cause of a mendelian disorder. *Nat Genet.* 2010;42(1):30–35.

/// 26 /// OPIOID REQUIREMENTS AND
RESPONSES IN ASIANS

ANNA LEE, PHD
Professor, Department of Anaesthesia and Intensive Care,
The Chinese University of Hong Kong, Prince of Wales Hospital,
Shatin, NT, Hong Kong, China

SIMON K. C. CHAN, MBBS
Clinical Associate Professor (Honorary), Department of
Anaesthesia and Intensive Care, The Chinese University
of Hong Kong, Shatin, NT, Hong Kong, China

TONY GIN, MD
Professor and Chairman, Department of Anaesthesia and
Intensive Care, The Chinese University of Hong Kong, Shatin,
NT, Hong Kong, China

Key Points

- Numerous gene polymorphisms have been examined for their effect on opioid pharmacokinetics and pharmacodynamics.
- Ethnic differences in the frequency of polymorphisms may lead to corresponding differences in overall opioid responses and requirements between ethnic groups.
- Polymorphisms affecting the metabolism of codeine, tramadol, and fentanyl lead to decreased analgesia or altered drug requirements.
- Individuals homozygous for wild-type A118 (AA genotype) of the opioid receptor gene μ_1 (OPRM1) gene have less pain, require less morphine or fentanyl, and are at greater risk of opioid related side effects
- The risk of chronic postoperative pain appears to be lower in patients carrying minor alleles for single-nucleotide polymorphisms in GTP cyclohydrolase 1 (GCH1), catechol-O-methyltransferase (COMT) and β-arrestin2 genes.
- Most polymorphisms appear to have little implication for clinical pain management practice.

INTRODUCTION

Adequate pain management is essential for reducing morbidity and mortality, and improving the patient's quality of life and patient satisfaction. Opioids are extensively used for the treatment of various pain conditions, with large intersubject variations in dosage requirements and clinical responses. It has been shown that Caucasians require more morphine for analgesia than do Asians and Africans.[1] Apart from ethnicity, many factors influence the management of pain.[2] These include the patient's past experience, intensity of pain, expression of pain, cultural influences, their relationship to healthcare professionals, and pharmacogenetics.[2] In a study on the relationship between ethnicity and analgesia, it can be difficult to ascertain which of these factors have a major influence, and this may confound comparison of analgesic requirements between studies, especially when the results are conflicting. Since our review,[2] many advances in the field of opioid pharmacogenomics have occurred. These have enabled a better understanding of opioid requirements in different ethnic groups.

Pharmacogenomics is the study of how genes influence a patient's response to drug therapy.[3] Theoretically, from an understanding of pharmacogenomic variability, clinicians can begin to consider tailoring individual drug regimens for susceptible patients; this concept is known as "personalized medicine."[4] The potential benefits of "personalized medicine" include increased drug efficacy, prevention of drug toxicity, elimination of costly and ineffective drug alternatives, and decreased healthcare utilization.[5]

Polymorphism is a term that is usually applied to a variation in DNA sequence that occurs in more than 1% of the population.[5] The most common type of variation is the single-nucleotide polymorphism, a "point mutation" or position at which two alternative nucleotides occur.[5] Currently, over 3,000 single-nucleotide polymorphisms in 314 genes are linked to the biological pathways that may influence pain sensitivity and/or psychological state associated with pain.[6] The majority of the data have been derived from transgenic animal models, but data from human studies are becoming more widely available. Given the broad biological functions of these single-nucleotide polymorphisms, it is likely that patients who carry the variant genes would have different responses to pain and analgesic treatment. Table 26.1 illustrates the differences in the ratio of wild-type (common) to minor (variant) allele between Asians and Caucasians for common genes outlined later in this chapter.

The most dramatic clinical example is the effect of variations in cytochrome P450 2D6 (CYP2D6), the enzyme that must metabolize codeine to morphine before any analgesia occurs. There are about 100 variants of the CYP2D6 gene,[7] and even though the frequency of alleles may be different across ethnic groups, more important clinically is how these variants affect the phenotype; whether subjects are poor metabolizers, intermediate metabolizers, extensive metabolizers, or ultra-rapid metabolizers of a particular substrate. The variant CYP2D6*4 has no activity and does not metabolize codeine to morphine. In Caucasians, CYP2D6*4 has a frequency of 20% to 25%, and is responsible for 70% to 90% of all poor metabolizers due to the presence of two nonfunctional (null) alleles.[8] These subjects experience much less or even no analgesic effect after receiving codeine. In contrast, CYP2D6*4 is only present in 1% of Chinese.[8] Overall, 10% of Caucasians are poor metabolizers, but only 1% of Asians are poor metabolizers.[8] Thus one could expect that as a group, Caucasians would have included more subjects with little or no analgesic effect after codeine.

However, there is another variant, CYP2D6*10 that produces modest metabolism of codeine to morphine. In Asians, it occurs at a frequency of 35% to 55% and is the most common allele causing reduced metabolism of codeine to morphine, while in Caucasians, CYP2D6*10 occurs at a low frequency of about 2%.[8] Consequently, many Chinese would have reduced conversion of codeine to morphine due to the high frequency of the CYPD6*10, and this may manifest as decreased analgesia (compared to the Caucasian extensive metabolizers).[7]

TABLE 26.1 Allele frequency (%) in Asian and Caucasians from the HapMap database[15]*

Identity of single-nucleotide polymorphism*	Han Chinese in Beijing, China		Japanese in Tokyo, Japan		Utah residents with Northern and Western European ancestry from the CEPH collection	
	Wild-type allele	Minor allele	Wild-type allele	Minor allele	Wild-type allele	Minor allele
CYP2D6*10 rs1065852 [C/T]	54.3	45.7	54.3	45.7	77.5	22.5
UGT2B7 gene rs7439366 [T/C]	27.8	72.2	31.8	68.2	50.8	49.2
ABCB1/MDR1 gene rs1045642 [C/T]	62.6	37.4	54.9	45.1	42.9	57.1
OPRMI gene rs1799971 [A/G]	63.9	36.1	53.1	46.9	84.5	15.5
COMT1 gene rs4680 [G/A]	71.2	28.8	71.0	29.0	52.2	47.8
B-arrestin2 gene rs1045280 [T/C]	83.3	16.7	88.1	11.9	68.1	31.9
GCH1 gene rs4411417 [T/C]	58.9	41.1	58.0	42.0	78.9	21.1
TRPV1 rs8065080 [C/T]	56.6	43.4	70.4	29.6	35.8	64.2
TRPA1 rs11988795 [C/T]	44.3	55.7	44.3	55.7	86.1	13.9

*HapMap data, phases I+II+III release #28 (NCBI build 36, dbSNP b126) (accessed http://hapmap.ncbi.nlm.nih.gov/cgi-perl/gbrowse/hapmap28_B36/, on April 4th 2011).
Single-nucleotide polymorphism alleles are in brackets, where [Allele$_1$ = wild-type/Allele$_2$ = minor].

This chapter focuses on both acute and chronic pain (persistent pain beyond three months) after surgery in patients of Asian origin who have been treated with intravenous patient-controlled opioid analgesia. All studies reviewed in this chapter involved the use of intravenous patient-controlled analgesia (IV PCA) using morphine, fentanyl, or tramadol (a synthetic opioid). By restricting studies to the IV PCA technique, potential confounders are reduced because the between-subject variability in the demand for opioids from healthcare staff is eliminated and better quantitative data are obtained. We review the opioid requirements and responses of patients with polymorphisms of metabolizing enzymes and transporters that alter the pharmacokinetics of opioids, and polymorphisms of opioid receptors and opioid signalers that alter the pharmacodynamics. This genetic variation may contribute to the diverse opioid pharmacology (Figure 26.1). The implications for altered dose regimen and drug interactions with traditional Chinese herbal medicines are briefly discussed.

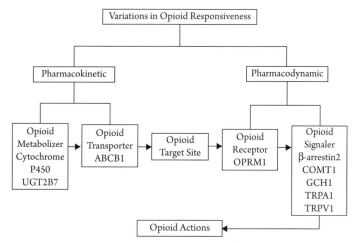

FIGURE 26.1 Variations in opioid responsiveness from polymorphisms identified from pharmaco-genetics studies in Asian patients undergoing surgery. Adapted from Smith[39] with permission.

PHARMACOKINETICS—CHANGES IN BIOTRANSFORMATION

Tramadol

All opioid drugs are substantially metabolized by the cytochrome P450 system. The analgesic effect of tramadol is dependent on its major metabolite O-desmethyl tramadol (weak μ receptor agonist) that is produced by CYP2D6 enzyme activity.[9,10] In a study of 63 Chinese patients undergoing gastrectomy, patients homozygous for CYP2D6*10 (intermediate metabolizers) had significantly higher (~12%) total consumption of tramadol than patients without or heterozygous for CYP2D6*10.[9] However, there were no differences in pain scores or in the incidence of opioid-related nausea and vomiting across the genotypes.[9] Given the clinically insignificant findings and recent evidence in healthy Chinese subjects,[11] we believe that genotyping for CYP2D6*10 alone is currently insufficient to predict tramadol disposition and usage[11] in individual surgical patients.

Tramadol Characteristics
- Tramadol is metabolized by CYP2D6 to O-desmethyl tramadol, which is a weak μ receptor agonist and largely responsible for the analgesic effect.
- Individuals with CYP2D6*10 alleles (intermediate metabolizers) reported higher total consumption of tramadol than patients with the wild-type.
- No impact of CYP2D6*10 polymorphism on pain perception and risk of adverse effects of tramadol.

Fentanyl

In contrast to tramadol, fentanyl is inactivated by CYP3A4 enzyme.[10] The frequency of the CYP3A4*1G variant allele in Chinese patients ranged from 23%[12] to 27%,[13] with the variant homozygote (*1G/*1G) occurring in 4%[12] to 6%[13] of the Chinese population. The variant homozygote (*1G/*1G) was associated with lower CYP3A4 enzyme activity than the other genotypes (*1/*1 and *1/*1G).[13] This may explain the higher plasma fentanyl concentrations found in the variant homozygote (28 ± 10 ng/ml) compared to the wild-type homozygote (13 ± 7 ng/ml) and variant heterozygote (17 ± 9 ng/ml) at 30 minutes after induction of anesthesia.[12] While there were no differences across genotypes in pain scores, patients homozygous for CYP3A4*1G required approximately 35%[12] to 65%[13] less fentanyl during the first 24 hours after surgery than patients carrying the wild-type allele (*1/*1) or the heterozygous (*1/*1G) allele.[13] There were no differences in the incidence of opioid-related side effects across genotypes in either study.[12,13] These findings suggest that patients homozygous for the *1G/*1G variant were more sensitive to fentanyl, required less drug to achieve the same level of pain control,[12,13] and were less likely to need rescue tramadol for pain control than other patients carrying the other genotypes.[12]

Fentanyl Characteristics
- Fentanyl is metabolized and inactivated by CYP3A4.
- Individuals with variant homozygote (*1G/*1G) have lower CYP3A4 enzyme activity.
- Individuals with variant homozygous (*1G/*1G) are more sensitive to fentanyl and require less drug to achieve the same level of analgesia.
- No impact of CYP3A4 polymorphism on risk of fentanyl-related adverse effects

Morphine

Morphine-6-glucuronide (an active metabolite) and morphine-3-glucuronide (a major inactive metabolite) are formed from the metabolism of morphine by uridine diphosphate-glucuronosyltransferase 2B7 (UGT2B7).[14] The frequency of the variant homozygote (CC) UGT2B7 is more common in Asians (41% to 47%) than Caucasians (22%).[15] In a study of 74 Caucasian patients undergoing colorectal surgery, there was no difference between genotypes in the cumulative 24-hour dose of morphine used and in the incidence of postoperative nausea and vomiting requiring ondansetron treatment.[14] In contrast, Sawyer et al's study of 99 patients (68 Caucasian, 27 African ancestry, 2 Hispanic and 2 Asians) receiving patient-controlled analgesia showed that morphine-6-glucuronide/morphine ratio was significantly lower in patients carrying the homozygous C allele (0.59) than heterozygotes (0.81) and homozygous T allele (1.0).[16] Due to the scarcity of studies in the Asian population, and the fact that the results from the two studies differed, the significance of UGT2B7 polymorphism on morphine metabolism is unclear.

Morphine Characteristics
- Morphine is metabolized by uridine diphosphate-glucuronosyltransferase 2B7 (UGT2B7) to form 2 major metabolites: morphine-6-gluronide (active) and morphine-3-glucuronide (inactive).
- Impact of UGT2B7 polymorphism on pain perception and risk of adverse effects of morphine is unclear.

PHARMACOKINETICS—CHANGES IN OPIOID DISTRIBUTION

The ATP-binding cassette B1 (ABCB1)/multiple drug resistance 1 (MDR1) gene encodes the expression of an efflux transporter, P-glycoprotein, in the brain that is responsible for the active transport of opioids (endogenous or exogenous) from the brain into the circulation.[17] Therefore, genetic variations of ABCB1 that reduce efflux of morphine from the central nervous system could enhance its analgesic efficacy.[18] The most common ABCB1 genetic polymorphism investigated is the C3435T single-nucleotide polymorphism. The frequency for wild-type allele in Asians ranged from 56%[18] to 61%.[17] The two Chinese studies mentioned above found no difference in the morphine consumption in the first 24 to 48 hours after surgery, pain scores, or incidence of opioid-related side effects among the C3435T genotypes.[17,18] In contrast, the incidence of postoperative nausea and vomiting during the first 2 hours after surgery was lower in South Korean patients with the variant homozygote (22%) than patients carrying the C allele (53%) when given an infusion of remifentanil and intravenous ondansetron injection intraoperatively.[19] The authors concluded that ABCB1 C3435T single-nucleotide polymorphism may be a clinical predictor of the responsiveness for ondansetron for early prevention of opioid-related nausea and vomiting after surgery.[19]

Patients carrying the homozygous TT allele were at higher risk of chronic pain at 3 months after cesarean section compared to patients carrying the homozygous CC allele.[18] Notably, patients carrying the homozygous TT allele had significantly longer wound pain (52 days) than patients carrying the C allele (43 days).[18] In comparison, the risk of severe chronic pain (pain score ≥5 out of 10 on a visual analogue scale) at 6 months after major abdominal surgery was similar between the wild (6%) and variant (14%) alleles.[17] These findings suggest that ABCB1 C3435T single-nucleotide polymorphism is not associated with variations in opioid requirements in the acute postoperative period, but may have a role in chronic pain after surgery. The role of ABCB1 C3435T single-nucleotide polymorphism on opioid-related side effects is less clear.

PHARMACODYNAMICS—CHANGES IN OPIOID RECEPTOR INTERACTIONS

The μ-opioid receptor is the principal binding site for opioid drugs and acts via inhibitory G-proteins to initiate a cascade of complex neuromodulatory processes resulting in analgesia.[4] One of the most studied single-nucleotide polymorphisms is a substitution, A118G, in the opioid receptor gene μ_1 (OPRM1). Specifically, a substitution at nucleotide position 118 results in a change in amino acid residue (from asparagine to aspartic acid) at position 40 from the N-terminus of the μ opioid receptor, leading to a loss of extracellular sites for N-glycosylation.[20]

All pharmacogenetic studies of the opioid receptor gene μ_1 in Asian surgical patients (Tables 26.2 and 26.3) were conducted prospectively, except one.[21] The frequency of the 118G homozygous in Asians ranged from 11%[22] to 23%.[23] The effect of G allele on pain scores, morphine consumption (Table 26.2), and fentanyl requirements (Table 26.3) for postoperative pain management and side effects are described in more detail in the following section. Two studies by Chou et al[22,23] failed to observe the Hardy-Weinberg equilibrium, suggesting that a possible genotyping error has occurred. Interestingly, a recent study showed that more patients carrying the G allele (15%) requested non-opioid analgesics than those with the wild-type allele (7%).[17]

Morphine

The larger studies[24,25] suggest that patients homozygous for A118 had lower pain scores than patient homozygous for G118. After adjustment for demographic variables, duration of surgery, medical insurance class, and previous cesarean delivery differences, each additional copy of the G allele increased pain scores (0 to 100 on the visual analog scale) by 0.51 units.[24] The inclusion of the opioid receptor gene μ_1 polymorphism variable into a multivariate regression model explained an additional 0.98% of the total variation in pain scores (2.28% for the model with the opioid receptor gene μ_1 polymorphism variable versus

TABLE 26.2 Summary of clinical studies evaluating the effect of A118G in opioid receptor µ1 (OPRM1) gene on patient-controlled analgesia with morphine

Author, year	Subjects	Frequency of genotypes	Clinical pain model	Analgesic effect of G Allele	Opioid-related side effects
Chou et al, 2006 [23]	80 Chinese women	AA (53.7%) AG (23.8%) GG (22.5%)	Acute pain after gynecological surgery	Patients with GG genotype had 19% higher morphine consumption than patients with AA genotype during first 24 hours after surgery; no difference at 48 hours. No difference in pain scores between genotypes in the first 48 hours.	No difference in nausea, vomiting, or sedation scores in first 24 hours.
Chou et al, 2006a [22]	120 Chinese males and females	AA (61.7%) AG (27.5%) GG (10.8%)	Acute pain after knee arthroplasty	Patients with GG genotype had 33% and 39% higher morphine consumption than patients with AA and AG genotype during first 48 hours after surgery. No difference in pain scores between genotypes in the first 48 hours.	No difference in incidence of nausea (mild/moderate), vomiting, headache, respiratory depression, pruritus, or other side effects.
Sia et al, 2008 [24]	588 Chinese women	AA (46.3%) AG (40.0%) GG (13.7%)	Acute pain after cesarean section	Patients with GG genotype had 37% higher morphine consumption than patients with AA genotype during first 24 hours after surgery. Patients with GG genotype had 24% higher pain scores than patients with AA genotype over the first 24 hours after surgery.	AA group had the highest incidence of nausea (10%) compared to the AG (6%) and GG (1%) groups. No difference in the incidence of vomiting, pruritus, and respiratory or central nervous system depression.
Tan et al, 2009 [25]	994 (620 Chinese, 241 Malays, 137 Indians)	AA (39.1%) AG (43.8%) GG (17.1%)	Acute pain after cesarean section	Patients with GG genotype had higher morphine consumption than patients with AA and AG genotypes (43% and 14%, respectively) during first 24 hours after surgery. Compared to patients with GG or AG genotypes, patients with AA genotype had the lowest pain scores.	Compared to patients with GG genotype, patients with AA genotype had highest nausea scores and mean episodes of vomiting.
Meng 2010 [17]	142 Chinese males and females	AA (40.4%) AG (44.9%) GG (14.6%)	Acute pain after abdominal surgery	Morphine consumption was significantly higher in patients with G allele (29%) than patients with AA genotype in the first 24 hours. However, pain scores were similar among patients with different genotypes.	Patients with GG genotype had lower incidence and milder opioid-related side effects than patients with AA and AG genotypes.

TABLE 26.3 Summary of clinical studies evaluating the effect of A118G in opioid receptor μ1 (OPRM1) gene on fentanyl

Author, year	Subjects	Frequency of genotypes	Clinical pain model	Analgesic effect of G Allele	Opioid-related side effects
Hayashida et al, 2008 [21]	138 Japanese males and females	AA (29.7%) AG (50.7%) GG (19.6%)	Acute pain after abdominal surgery. Opioids and NSAIDs[a] were converted to systemic fentanyl equivalent doses.	Total opioid requirements required in the first 24 hours were greater in patients with GG genotype than patients with AA and AG genotypes. Total postoperative analgesia requirements in the first 24 hours were also greater in patients with GG genotype than patients with AA and AG genotypes (17% and 19%, respectively). No difference in pain scores among genotypes.	No data collected.
Fukuda et al, 2009 [37]	280 Japanese males and females	AA (30.7%) AG (51.1%) GG (18.2%)	Acute pain after orofacial cosmetic surgery	No difference in total fentanyl consumption in the first 24 hours or pain scores across genotypes.	No data collected.
Zhang et al, 2010 [38]	174 Chinese women	AA (49.4%), AG (38.5%), GG (12.1%)	Acute pain after gynecological surgery	Patients with GG genotype had 25% and 19% higher fentanyl consumption than patients with AA and AG genotypes during first 24 hours after surgery. No difference in pain scores at rest across genotypes in the first 24 hours.	No difference in the incidence of nausea and vomiting or in sedation scores.

[a] NSAIDs = nonsteroidal anti-inflammatory drugs.

1.30% for the model without opioid receptor gene μ_1 polymorphism variable).[24] This suggests that opioid receptor gene μ_1 polymorphism plays a relatively minor role in the perception of pain.

All studies in Table 26.2 reported a significant difference in morphine consumption between patients with the G allele and the wild-type allele. The results suggest that Chinese patients who were homozygous for G118 required approximately 20% to 40% more morphine in the first 24 hours to achieve adequate pain relief compared with patients homozygous for A118.

However, the differences between genotypes in morphine consumption disappeared at 48 hours after surgery.[17] At 6 months after major abdominal surgery, there were similar risks of chronic pain and severe chronic pain between the wild-type and minor alleles (Table 26.4).[17]

Most studies in Table 26.2 failed to show morphine-related adverse events, likely due to insufficient statistical power. However, Tan et al's study of 1000 women showed that patients homozygous for A118 were more likely to experience mild morphine-related nausea and vomiting events than patients with the G allele.[25] In a Taiwanese study of 212 women given epidural morphine for postoperative pain management after cesarean delivery, women with A allele (95%) were more likely to develop moderate to severe pruritus than women homozygous for G118 (5%).[26] These studies suggest that the G allele may provide protective effects against morphine-related side effects despite the need for higher morphine usage.

- Individuals homozygous for wild-type A118 of opioid receptor gene μ_1 require 20% to 40% less morphine to achieve adequate pain relief in the first 24 hours after surgery.
- Individuals homozygous for wild-type A118 of opioid receptor gene μ_1 are at greater risk of morphine-related adverse effects.

Fentanyl

The effect of opioid receptor gene μ_1 polymorphism on fentanyl requirements and responses is less clear as there are fewer published studies in Asian patients (Table 26.3). Patients homozygous for G118 require up to 20% more fentanyl to achieve adequate pain relief compared with patients homozygous for A118 in the early postoperative period, without an increased risk of fentanyl-related side effects. Younger age was associated with greater postoperative fentanyl requirements, accounting for 7.8% of the variance.

In summary, patients homozygous for G118 required more opioids to achieve adequate pain relief compared to other genotypes without an increased risk of opioid-related side effects. However, the contribution of opioid receptor gene μ_1 polymorphism to explaining opioid consumption appears to be minor. Our conclusions are consistent with the findings from a meta-analysis of eight studies[27] that showed a weak association of increased opioid dosage requirements and less nausea in patients homozygous for G118 in a diverse European and Asian clinical population. The frequency of homozygous G118 in Caucasians and Asian populations is 2%[15] and 12% to 23%[15], respectively.

PHARMACODYNAMICS—CHANGES IN OPIOID SIGNALING PATHWAYS

Several genes regulate neurotransmission in pain pathways. Intuitively, variations in these genes may enhance or suppress the nociceptive pathways and predispose or prevent patients developing chronic postsurgical pain.[17]

TABLE 26.4 Genotype effects of opioid receptor gene μ1 (OPRM1), β-arrestin2, catechol-O-methyltransferase (COMT), GTP cyclohydrolase1 (GCH1) and transient receptor potential (TRPV1, TRPA1) genes on the incidence of chronic postoperative pain at 6 months after surgery in 228 Chinese patients.[17] Patients with at least one minor allele were classified as minor allele.

Identity of Single-nucleotide polymorphisms	Patients with chronic postoperative pain (n)				Patients with severe chronic postoperative pain (n)			
	Wild-type	Minor allele	Odds ratio (95%CI)	P value	Wild-type	Minor allele	Odds ratio (95%CI)	P value
Opioid receptor gene μ1 gene rs1799971 [A/G]	31	58	1.42 (0.82 – 2.46)	0.21	6	14	1.61 (0.60 – 4.36)	0.35
B-arrestin2 gene rs1045280 [T/C]	61	28	0.55 (0.32 – 0.97)	0.04	16	4	0.35 (0.11 – 1.08)	0.07
COMT1 gene rs4680 [G/A]	58	31	0.54 (0.31 – 0.94)	0.03	13	7	0.67 (0.26 – 1.74)	0.41
GCH1 gene rs4411417 [T/C]	46	42	0.51 (0.30 – 0.88)	0.02	13	7	0.36 (0.14 – 0.94)	0.04
TRPV1 gene rs8065080 [C/T]	28	61	1.18 (0.67 – 2.08)	0.58	7	13	0.94 (0.36 – 2.45)	0.89
TRPA1 gene rs11988795 [C/T]	21	66	1.64 (0.90 – 3.01)	0.11	5	15	1.34 (0.47 – 3.85)	0.59

β-arrestin2

β-arrestin is a regulatory protein involved in the desensitization of opioid receptors after prolonged exposure to opioid agonist drugs.[10] A mutation in the β-arrestin2 gene could dampen this response, leading to a greater analgesic effect from opioids.[17] A common β-arrestin2 genetic polymorphism investigated is the T8622C single-nucleotide polymorphism. The frequencies for homozygous wild-type allele and homozygous minor allele for T8622C in a Chinese surgical population were 63% and 6%, respectively.[17]

Although the total IV PCA morphine consumption and pain scores were similar among patients with different genotypes, patients with homozygous minor allele had more mild opioid-related symptoms than other genotypes after surgery.[17] Patients with the minor allele had a lower risk of chronic pain at 6 months after abdominal surgery than patients with the wild-type allele but the risk of severe chronic pain at 6 months was similar[17] (Table 26.4). Further studies are required to define the role of β-arrestin2 on the development of chronic pain.

- β-arrestin desensitizes opioid receptors after prolonged exposure to opioids.
- β-arrestin2 gene polymorphism at T8622C does not appear to affect pain perception or opioid consumption.
- Individuals homozygous for minor C allele have milder opioid-related adverse effects.
- Individuals carrying minor C allele may be at lower risk of chronic pain after surgery..

Catechol-O-methyltransferase (COMT)

COMT regulates the metabolism of catecholamine and mutations in the COMT gene can affect the perception of pain.[4] Polymorphism in COMT1 gene increases the sensitivity of opioid receptor.[17] A common polymorphism in the COMT1 gene is the G472A single-nucleotide polymorphism (rs4680) with the frequencies for homozygous wild-type allele and homozygous minor allele in Chinese patients of 58% and 9%, respectively.[17] In Caucasians, the corresponding frequencies for homozygous GG and homozygous AA alleles are 29% and 25%, respectively.[15]

There was no difference in the total IV PCA morphine consumption, pain scores, incidence, and severity of opioid-related side effects between G472A genotypes.[17] These findings are consistent with the lack of association between COMT G472A single-nucleotide polymorphism and acute pain found in a recent study of Caucasian patients undergoing third molar surgery.[28] Chinese patients with the minor allele had a lower risk of chronic pain at 6 months after abdominal surgery compared to wild-type allele but there was no difference in the risk of severe chronic pain between genotypes (Table 26.4).[17] These findings suggest that COMT1 G472A single-nucleotide polymorphism does not play a role in acute pain, but may have some influence in the development of chronic pain after surgery.

- Catechol-O-methyltransferase 1 gene polymorphism increases the sensitivity of opioid receptor.
- Catechol-O-methyltransferase 1 gene polymorphism at G472A does not appear to affect pain perception, opioid requirement or risk of opioid-related adverse effects.
- Individuals carrying minor A allele may be at lower risk of chronic pain after surgery.

GTP cyclohydrolase 1 (GCH1)

Polymorphisms affecting the enzyme GCH1 lead to a reduction in the synthesis of tetrahydrobiopterin (BH_4), an essential cofactor in the production of monoamine neurotransmitters and nitric oxide.[17] Decreases in these neurotransmitters in the pain pathways would lead to reduced inflammatory response in sensory neurons.[17] The frequencies of the homozygous wild-type allele and homozygous minor allele for GCH1 (rs4411417[T/C] in a Chinese surgical population were 41% and 12%, respectively.[17]

Chinese patients with minor allele for GCH1 (rs4411417 [T/C] had a lower risk of chronic pain at 6 months after abdominal surgery compared with wild-type allele (Table 26.4).[17] The same association was also found for the risk of severe chronic pain (pain score ≥5 of 10 on a visual analogue scale) in patients with the minor allele compared with those carrying the wild-type allele (Table 26.4).[17] In Caucasian patients undergoing surgical diskectomy, patients with the homozygous minor allele for GCH1 (rs4411417) had lower persistent leg pain scores than wild-type allele over the first year after surgery.[29] Thus GCH1 gene polymorphism plays a preventive role in the development of chronic pain after surgery.

- GTP cyclohydrolase 1 gene polymorphism (rs4411417 [T/C]) decreases neurotransmitters in the pain pathways, leading to reduced inflammatory response in sensory neurons.
- Individuals with minor C allele are at lower risk of chronic pain after surgery.

Transient receptor potential (TRP)

The transient receptor potential cation channels TRPV1 and TRPA1 affect the sensitivity of nociceptors.[17] By downregulation of TRPV1 and TRPA1 expression in the afferent nerve terminals, the release of nitric oxide dependent nociceptive mediators is reduced.[17] The frequencies of the homozygous wild-type allele and homozygous minor allele for TRPV1 (rs8065080 [C/T]) single-nucleotide polymorphism in Chinese patients were 33% and 16%, respectively.[17] The corresponding frequencies for TRPV1 homozygous CC and TT alleles in Caucasians are 12% and 40%, respectively.[15] For TRPA1 (rs11988795 [C/T]) single-nucleotide polymorphism, the frequencies of the homozygous wild-type allele and homozygous minor allele in Chinese patients were 30% and 19%, respectively.[17] The corresponding frequencies for TRPA1 homozygous CC and TT alleles in Caucasians are not yet available.[15]

There were no differences across TRPV1 or TRPA1 genotypes for the risk of chronic pain at 6 months after abdominal surgery in Chinese patients (Table 26.4).[17] It is unclear whether this finding is one of no association, or that the study was underpowered to detect a difference. More studies are needed to clarify the role of TRP on chronic pain after surgery in the Asian clinical setting.

- Transient receptor potential cation channels TRPV1 and TRPA1 affect the sensitivity of nociceptors.
- Unclear role of transient receptor potential cation channels on risk of chronic pain after surgery

COMPARISONS WITHIN ASIAN GROUP DIFFERENCES

Most of the studies reviewed in this chapter focused on the overarching and diverse Asian ethnic category. In a study of Singaporean women undergoing cesarean section, there were significant differences in pain scores and PCA morphine consumption between-Asian ethnic groups.[30] The pain scores for Indians were 56% higher than the scores for Chinese and 33% higher than Malays.[30] This corresponded to Indians requiring 105% higher morphine consumption than Chinese and 53% higher than Malays.[30] However, there were no differences in nausea, vomiting, or pruritus scores between Chinese, Indians, and Malays groups.[30] The findings suggest that it is important for clinicians to appreciate that pain perception and subsequent opioid consumption varies among major Asian ethnic groups.

In a related study involving Chinese, Indians, and Malays, the opioid receptor gene μ_1 A118G polymorphism was significantly associated with morphine consumption in Chinese patients, with every additional copy of the G allele resulting in an average increase in morphine consumption by 0.025 mg/kg in the first 24 hours after surgery.[25] Probably due to small sample sizes in the Malay and Indian groups, the association of increased morphine consumption with every additional copy of the G allele was not statistically significant.[25] These findings suggest that genotyping for opioid receptor gene $\mu1$ A118G in Chinese patients will only predict minor variations in opioid consumption.

DOSAGE ADJUSTMENT BASED ON OPIOID POLYMORPHISM

In most individuals, the experience of pain probably results from a complex interaction between several genetic variants involved in different steps of neuronal processing of nociceptive information, with additional contributions of other genetic or psychosocial factors.[31] In Caucasians, preliminary recommendations for dose adaptations based on opioid receptor gene $\mu1$, COMT1 and melanocortin-1 receptor (MCR1) variants have been proposed.[10] However, there have been no gene association studies assessing joint effects of genetic variants on opioid responsiveness in Asian patients. Moreover, given that the genetic effects appears to be small in Asian patients using multivariable analyses, the incorporation of genotyping information for tailoring opioid dose recommendations before surgery is premature at this time.

DRUG INTERACTIONS WITH TRADITIONAL CHINESE HERBAL MEDICINES

The use of traditional Chinese herbal medicines is highly prevalent in Asian countries[32,33] before surgery.[34,35] However, there is a lack of evidence on the importance of the interactions between opioid polymorphism and traditional Chinese herbal medicine. Panax ginseng was widely used before surgery in one study[35] and has been found to be associated with a high inhibition of CYP450 isozymes in vitro.[36] The implication of this finding is that individuals who are poor metabolizers may be at risk of increased plasma concentrations of opioids and also at a higher risk of developing opioid-related adverse effects. Despite this theoretical risk, no clinical cases have been reported.

CONCLUSION

Numerous gene polymorphisms contribute to changes in opioid disposition and effects in Asian surgical patients. However, the exact molecular consequences of most functional variants are not known.[31] Apart from the well-known metabolism of codeine to morphine, most of the genetic variants have small or no effects on acute pain and analgesia. The GTP cyclohydrolase 1, catechol-O-methyltransferase and β-arrestin2 genes may identify patients at risk of chronic pain after surgery, but further studies are required to confirm these associations. The interaction between opioid polymorphism and traditional Chinese medicines is theoretically possible, but its clinical significance has yet to be determined. To examine the effects of genetic variants in the Asian populations, well-designed cohorts with adequate power are needed. In the foreseeable future, pharmacogenomics could be incorporated into the clinical pain management practice.

REFERENCES

1. Dahmani S, Dupont H, Mantz J, Desmonts JM, Keita H. Predictive factors of early morphine requirements in the post-anaesthesia care unit (PACU). *Br J Anaesth.* 2001;87:385–389.
2. Lee A, Gin T, Oh TE. Opioid requirements and responses in Asians. *Anaesth Intensive Care.* 1997;25:665–670.
3. Jannetto PJ, Bratanow NC. Utilization of pharmacogenomics and therapeutic drug monitoring for opioid pain management. *Pharmacogenomics.* 2009;10:1157–1167.
4. Searle R, Hopkins PM. Pharmacogenomic variability and anaesthesia. *Br J Anaesth.* 2009;103:14–25.
5. Palmer SN, Giesecke NM, Body SC, Shernan SK, Fox AA, Collard CD. Pharmacogenetics of anesthetic and analgesic agents. *Anesthesiology.* 2005;102:663–671.
6. Lacroix-Fralish ML, Ledoux JB, Mogil JS. The Pain Genes Database: An interactive web browser of pain-related transgenic knockout studies. *Pain.* 2007;131:3–4.
7. Somogyi AA, Barratt DT, Coller JK. Pharmacogenetics of opioids. *Clin Pharmacol Ther.* 2007;81:429–444.
8. Zhou SF. Polymorphism of human cytochrome P450 2D6 and its clinical significance: Part I. *Clin Pharmacokinet.* 2009;48:689–723.
9. Wang G, Zhang H, He F, Fang X. Effect of the CYP2D6*10 C188T polymorphism on postoperative tramadol analgesia in a Chinese population. *Eur J Clin Pharmacol.* 2006;62:927–931.
10. Argoff CE. Clinical implications of opioid pharmacogenetics. *Clin J Pain.* 2010;26(suppl 10):S16–S20.
11. Li Q, Wang R, Guo Y, Wen S, Xu L, Wang S. Relationship of CYP2D6 genetic polymorphisms and the pharmacokinetics of tramadol in Chinese volunteers. *J Clin Pharm Ther.* 2010;35:239–247.
12. Yuan R, Zhang X, Deng Q, Wu Y, Xiang G. Impact of CYP3A4*1G polymorphism on metabolism of fentanyl in Chinese patients undergoing lower abdominal surgery. *Clin Chim Acta.* 2011;412:755–760.
13. Zhang W, Chang YZ, Kan QC, et al. CYP3A4*1G genetic polymorphism influences CYP3A activity and response to fentanyl in Chinese gynecologic patients. *Eur J Clin Pharmacol.* 2010;66:61–66.
14. Coulbault L, Beaussier M, Verstuyft C, et al. Environmental and genetic factors associated with morphine response in the postoperative period. *Clin Pharmacol Ther.* 2006;79:316–324.
15. The International HapMap Project. *Nature.* 2003;426:789–796.
16. Sawyer MB, Innocenti F, Das S, et al. A pharmacogenetic study of uridine diphosphate-glucuronosyltransferase 2B7 in patients receiving morphine. *Clin Pharmacol Ther.* 2003;73:566–574.
17. Meng Z. *Genetic Determinants of Postoperative Pain.* Hong Kong: The Chinese University of Hong Kong; 2010.
18. Sia AT, Sng BL, Lim EC, Law H, Tan EC. The influence of ATP-binding cassette sub-family B member -1 (ABCB1) genetic polymorphisms on acute and chronic pain after intrathecal morphine for caesarean section: a prospective cohort study. *Int J Obstet Anesth.* 2010;19:254–260.
19. Choi EM, Lee MG, Lee SH, Choi KW, Choi SH. Association of ABCB1 polymorphisms with the efficacy of ondansetron for postoperative nausea and vomiting. *Anaesthesia.* 2010;65:996–1000.
20. Kadiev E, Patel V, Rad P, et al. Role of pharmacogenetics in variable response to drugs: focus on opioids. *Expert Opin Drug Metab Toxicol.* 2008;4:77–91.
21. Hayashida M, Nagashima M, Satoh Y, et al. Analgesic requirements after major abdominal surgery are associated with OPRM1 gene polymorphism genotype and haplotype. *Pharmacogenomics.* 2008;9:1605–1616.
22. Chou WY, Yang LC, Lu HF, et al. Association of mu-opioid receptor gene polymorphism (A118G) with variations in morphine consumption for analgesia after total knee arthroplasty. *Acta Anaesthesiol Scand.* 2006;50:787–792.

23. Chou WY, Wang CH, Liu PH, Liu CC, Tseng CC, Jawan B. Human opioid receptor A118G polymorphism affects intravenous patient-controlled analgesia morphine consumption after total abdominal hysterectomy. *Anesthesiology*. 2006;105:334–337.

24. Sia AT, Lim Y, Lim EC, et al. A118G single nucleotide polymorphism of human mu-opioid receptor gene influences pain perception and patient-controlled intravenous morphine consumption after intrathecal morphine for postcesarean analgesia. *Anesthesiology*. 2008;109:520–526.

25. Tan EC, Lim EC, Teo YY, Lim Y, Law HY, Sia AT. Ethnicity and OPRM variant independently predict pain perception and patient-controlled analgesia usage for post-operative pain. *Mol Pain*. 2009;5:32.

26. Tsai FF, Fan SZ, Yang YM, Chien KL, Su YN, Chen LK. Human opioid mu-receptor A118G polymorphism may protect against central pruritus by epidural morphine for post-cesarean analgesia. *Acta Anaesthesiol Scand*. 2010;54:1265–1269.

27. Walter C, Lotsch J. Meta-analysis of the relevance of the OPRM1 118A>G genetic variant for pain treatment. *Pain*. 2009;146:270–275.

28. Lee PJ, Delaney P, Keogh J, Sleeman D, Shorten GD. Catecholamine-o-methyltransferase polymorphisms are associated with postoperative pain intensity. *Clin J Pain*. 2011;27:93–101.

29. Tegeder I, Costigan M, Griffin RS, et al. GTP cyclohydrolase and tetrahydrobiopterin regulate pain sensitivity and persistence. *Nat Med*. 2006;12:1269–1277.

30. Tan EC, Lim Y, Teo YY, Goh R, Law HY, Sia AT. Ethnic differences in pain perception and patient-controlled analgesia usage for postoperative pain. *J Pain*. 2008;9:849–855.

31. Lotsch J, Geisslinger G. Current evidence for a modulation of nociception by human genetic polymorphisms. *Pain*. 2007;132:18–22.

32. Chen LC, Wang BR, Chou YC, Tien JH. Drug utilization pattern of Chinese herbal medicines in a general hospital in Taiwan. *Pharmacoepidemiol Drug Saf*. 2005;14:651–657.

33. Lim MK, Sadarangani P, Chan HL, Heng JY. Complementary and alternative medicine use in multiracial Singapore. *Complement Ther Med*. 2005;13:16–24.

34. Lee A, Chui PT, Aun CS, Lau AS, Gin T. Incidence and risk of adverse perioperative events among surgical patients taking traditional Chinese herbal medicines. *Anesthesiology*. 2006;105:454–461.

35. Critchley LAH, Chen DQ, Lee A, Thomas GN, Tomlinson B. A survey of Chinese herbal medicine intake amongst preoperative patients in Hong Kong. *Anaesth Intensive Care*. 2005;33:506–513.

36. Foster BC, Vandenhoek S, Tang R, Budzinski JW, Krantis A, Li KY. Effect of several Chinese natural health products of human cytochrome P450 metabolism. *J Pharm Pharm Sci*. 2002;5:185–189.

37. Fukuda K, Hayashida M, Ide S, et al. Association between OPRM1 gene polymorphisms and fentanyl sensitivity in patients undergoing painful cosmetic surgery. *Pain*. 2009;147:194–201.

38. Zhang W, Chang YZ, Kan QC, et al. Association of human micro-opioid receptor gene polymorphism A118G with fentanyl analgesia consumption in Chinese gynaecological patients. *Anaesthesia*. 2010;65:130–135.

39. Smith HS. Variations in opioid responsiveness. *Pain Physician*. 2008;11:237–248.

27

ETHNICITY AND
PSYCHOPHARMACOTHERAPY
IN PAIN

KEH-MING LIN, MD, MPH

Professor Emeritus of Psychiatry, University of California
Los Angeles, Los Angeles, California, USA; 2008–2009
Fellow, Center for Advanced Study in the Behavioral
Science at Stanford (CASBS); Diplomate, American Board
of Psychiatry and Neurology; Distinguished Life-Time
Fellow, American Psychiatric Association

Key Points

- Psychotropics (antidepressants, antipsychotics, mood stabilizers, sedatives, and anxiolytics) are commonly used in patients suffering from pain problems, but as adjunct medications and for the treatment of comorbid psychiatric conditions.
- Patients' responses to psychotropics are influenced by their instrumental (intrinsic) as well as symbolic effects.
- On the instrumental side, the effects of medications are determined by pharmacokinetics (drug disposition and fate in the body) as well as pharmacodynamics (drug effects on therapeutic targets, such as receptors and transporters).
- Both genetic and environmental (e.g., diet and herbal intake) factors influence pharmacokinetic as well as pharmcodynamic processes.
- For the optimal care of pain patients, it is crucial that clinicians take these factors into consideration.

INTRODUCTION

Psychotropics, especially antidepressants, antipsychotics (neuroleptics) and anticonvulsants, have been widely used as "adjuvants," frequently prescribed along with analgesics to "boost" the latter's clinical effects. Such effects have been demonstrated in a number of well-designed studies examining therapeutic efficacy, particularly with regard to the combined use of antidepressants.[1–3] In addition to serving as adjuvants, psychotropics also are widely used in pain patients for a number of other reasons: (1) severe and/or persistent pain affects daily functioning and mental status; (2) pain frequently disturbs sleep, leading to widespread use of hypnotics; (3) underlying pathology such as cancer, HIV infection, or diabetic neuropathy may be life threatening or chronically progressive, eliciting severe psychological responses including depression and anxiety. Comorbidity thus is extremely high between pain conditions and various psychiatric disorders, leading to even more frequent combined use of analgesics and psychotropics.

As clinicians increasingly work with patients from diverse cultural and ethnic backgrounds, knowledge and understanding of the effect of these factors on determining the choice, dosing, and side effect profiles of these medications would seem increasingly crucial in clinical attempts to bring the best care possible to the majority of patients whose pain is a prominent component of their suffering.

THE CULTURAL CONTEXT OF PSYCHOPHARMACOTHERAPY

Contrary to commonly held assumptions, pharmacotherapeutic effects do not take place in a vacuum, and "one size does not fit all."[4] Although mechanisms responsible for such variations are not yet completely understood, it is safe to say that they result from the interplay among genetic, environmental, and cultural factors, and that one's ancestral origin, sociodemographic background, lifestyle, beliefs, and relationship with clinicians all impinge on the individual to determine her or his medication response.[5,6] As shown in Figures 27.1 and 27.2, virtually all these factors are significantly influenced by culture and ethnicity. On the genetic side, patterns of genetic polymorphisms, often with substantial ethnic variations, exist in a large number of genes encoding drug metabolizing enzymes as well as receptors, transporters, and other targets of pharmaceutical agents. The expression of these genes, in turn, is often significantly modified by a large number of environmental factors, including diet and exposure to various substances (e.g., tobacco, herbal preparations). Even more importantly, similar to any form of intervention, the success of pharmacotherapy depends on the participation of the patient and those in his or her social networks. The "symbolic" dimension of medication prescription and use is typically more powerful than its "instrumental" effects. Discrepancies in expectations and beliefs between patients and clinicians, unless elicited and acknowledged, often lead to therapeutic failure.

Clinicians' contributions

Clinicians' perception and conceptualization of patients' problems can be significantly influenced by prevailing stereotypes related to patients' cultural/ethnic backgrounds.[7]

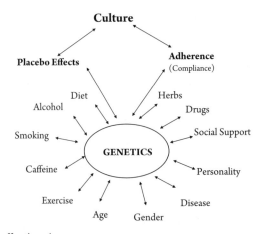

FIGURE 27.1 Factors affecting drug

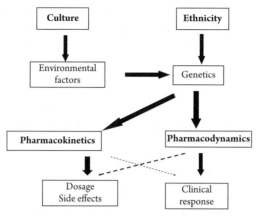

FIGURE 27.2 Factors determining pharmacological response

Studies demonstrated that case vignettes identical in every other aspect were neverthe-less given significantly more severe diagnoses if the cases were identified as being of ethnic minority origin. For example, African-American psychiatric patients are more likely to be given a diagnosis of schizophrenia as compared to their Caucasian counterparts.[8] The use of structured interviews helped to dissipate such discrepancies.[9] Such biases may also be responsible for the pervasive use of higher doses of neuroleptics and depot neuroleptics in treating African-American patients, irrespective of diagnosis.[10] In turn, such "overtreat-ment" might contribute towards the significantly higher rate of tardive dyskinesia observed in African-Americans.[11]

ADHERENCE

Nonadherence is highly prevalent with psychotropic medications as well as other drugs for chronic medical conditions requiring long-term pharmacotherapy.[12] On top of "tangible" var-iables including sociodemographics, financial burden, transportation, and medication side effects, patients' beliefs and expectations loom large in determining adherence, and interven-tion strategies embedded in such contexts significantly enhance treatment adherence.[12–14]

Cross-cultural clinical encounters are laden with pitfalls for mis-understanding aris-ing from mis-matches in the conceptualization of and goals for medical treatment, leading to delayed help-seeking as well as premature termination of treatment in ethnic minority groups.[15] Programs aimed at bridging cultural gaps have been shown to improve treatment retention and outcome significantly.[10,16–18] Culturally shaped beliefs not only influence patients' therapeutic responses, but also their perception and interpretation of side effects. For example, in a study conducted in Hong Kong, Chinese bipolar patients treated with lithium rarely complained of "missing the highs," and "loss of creativity," and regarded poly-dipsia, polyuria, and weight gain as evidence that the medicine was working.[19] They were, however, far more concerned about perceptions of lethargy, drowsiness, and poor memory, as compared with their Caucasian counterparts. Such findings highlight the importance of culturally based beliefs and expectations in determining how physical and psychological experiences associated with drug treatment and responses are perceived and interpreted.

Expectation (placebo) effects

The power of placebo effects makes randomized, blinded study design with placebo control essential in modern clinical trials.[20] In the majority of these trials, placebo responses account for a larger proportion of the improvement than that attributable to the "specific" effect of the therapeutic agent.[21] To the extent that placebo effects are associated with expectations regarding the safety and effectiveness of treatment offered, they are significantly shaped by patients' cultural backgrounds as well as personal experiences. By distorting communication and diminishing trust, gaps in illness constructs between clinicians and patients diminish the "symbolic" ("placebo") aspects of therapeutic effects.[22,23] In clinical encounters where patients' cultural and personal backgrounds diverge significantly from those of the professionals caring for them, such gaps are further aggravated. Unless such discrepancies are routinely assessed, interventions are not likely to lead to therapeutic effects, no matter how "biologically powerful" the therapeutic armamentaria are. This is not just an issue for patients with limited previous exposure to modern medical culture and practices (e.g., illiterate refugees growing up in remote rural areas of the world), but often also is the case for those seemingly highly "Westernized" or "assimilated." The tenacity of traditional beliefs regarding health, illness, and pathway to recovery often takes healthcare professionals by surprise. For example, in contemporary Asian countries, as well as in Asian-American communities, "traditional" medical theories and practices thrive side by side with "Western" medical care systems.[24–26] Patients with full access to modern biomedical approaches continue to hold deeply ingrained traditional beliefs, such as the importance of maintaining a dynamic balance between "coldness" and "hotness," or between "Yin" and "Yang,"[27,28] as well as awareness of the concept of Qi or Chi (vital energy).

Attributes as innocuous as the size, shape, and color of the "pills," as well as their trade names, may inadvertently trigger culturally shaped beliefs and associations, thereby significantly enhancing or diminishing the expectation effects. For example, red-colored pills might be seen as capable of enhancing the "hot" element, and might be regarded as less effective in the treatment of conditions perceived as a result of excessive "hotness" (e.g., fever, anxiety state, or mania). Significant ethnic differences in response to placebo pills in different colors also have been reported, with white capsules achieving more analgesic but less stimulating effects than black capsules in Caucasian subjects, and the reverse for African Americans.[29]

The concomitant use of alternative/indigenous treatment and healing methods

As mentioned above, the worldwide ascendancy of modern "cosmopolitan" ("Western") medicine has not replaced traditional or "indigenous" medical and healing systems.[24–26] Instead, "alternative" traditions (e.g., Chinese medicine and Ayurvedic medicine) continue to evolve and remain salient. Multiple medical and healing traditions and treatment modalities coexist in all societies, and patients often utilize these services simultaneously or sequentially, frequently without informing their physicians. This phenomenon has long been observed in "non-Western" countries as well as among ethnic minority populations in the United States.[24,26,30,31] With the resurgent interest in and popularity of "complementary and alternative medicine" in Europe and North America,[32] it has become increasingly clear that a wide range of "nonconventional" treatment and healing options also are commonly utilized in these societies, and clinicians can ill afford to neglect such practices, even with patients who come from "mainstream" backgrounds.

"Biological" aspects of psychotropic responses

Although numerous reports of significant cross-national and cross-ethnic variations in psychotropic responses have been reported for over half a century,[33] the biological underpinnings for such variations have remained obscure until recently. Fortunately, advances in the field of pharmacokinetics, pharmacodynamics and pharmacogenomics have converged to delineate mechanisms that are responsible for such variations. A large number of genes affecting drug responses have been identified, including those determining the fate and disposition of drugs (pharmacokinetic) and those mediating the response of intended therapeutic targets (pharmacodynamics). In these studies, ethnicity has been identified as a significant factor in determining the distribution of polymorphisms affecting the function of these genes. At the same time, the expression of these genes is often strongly influenced by environmental factors. Together these mechanisms are responsible for interindividual as well as cross-ethnic variations in drug responses. As an example, an early study comparing the pharmacokinetics of haloperidol between Asian and Caucasian subjects demonstrated not only significant ethnic variations in serum haloperidol concentrations, but also substantive interindividual differences with each of the comparison groups[34] (Figure 27.3).

Genetic polymorphism of genes encoding "drug-metabolizing enzymes"

Of the four factors (absorption, distribution, metabolism, and excretion) that together determine the fate and disposition of most drugs, variability in the process of metabolism is most substantial and usually is the reason for interindividual and cross-ethnic variation in drug responses.[4–6,35] Among the drug-metabolizing enzymes, cytochrome P-450 enzymes (CYPs) have been most extensively studied, perhaps because they often control the rate-limiting steps in the metabolism of most psychotropics, including antidepressants, anxiolytics, antipsychotics, and anticonvulsants.

Different forms ("genetic polymorphisms") of each of the CYPs genes[35] lead to large variations in their activities. As a dramatic example, more than 50 "versions" of the CYP2D6 genes have been identified, whose effects on the gene's activity range from inactivation and impairment to acceleration.[36,37] Most of these "genotypes" are unevenly distributed across ethnicity, and some only exist in specific populations. For example, CYP2D6*4, encoding defective proteins, is common only found in Caucasians (25%). Those who are homozygotic (possessing two defective genes) are extremely sensitive to drugs metabolized by this enzyme, and are classified as poor metabolizers (PMs). Instead of CYP2D6*4, extremely high frequencies of CYP2D6*17 and CYP2D6*10 exist in those with African and Asian

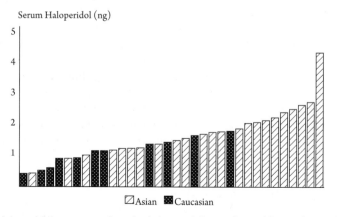

FIGURE 27.3 Haloperidol concentrations in Asian and Caucasian subjects after a single dose of 0.5 mg im Haloperidol

ancestral backgrounds, respectively.[38,39] Both of these alleles are associated with lower enzyme activities and slower metabolism (SMs) of CYP2D6 substrates, and may be in part responsible for previous findings of slower pharmacokinetic profiles and lower therapeutic dose ranges of psychotropics observed in Asians and African Americans.[5,33] Mexican Americans have very low rates of any of these "impairing" mutations, leading to increased overall CYP2D6 activity and possibly faster metabolism of drugs metabolized by this enzyme.[40]

At the other extreme, people possessing more than two copies of the CYP2D6 genes due to gene duplication or multiplication are more effective in "handling" drugs dependent on the enzyme for metabolism, and are classified as "ultra-rapid" metabolizers (UMs). The frequency of UMs is remarkably high among Arabs (19%), Ethiopians (29%), Ethiopian Jews (18%), Sephardic Jews (13%), Italians (8%), and southern Iberians (5%–9%), but rare in northern European and Asian populations. UM patients are likely to fail to respond to usual doses of medications biotransformed by CYP2D6 (including many antidepressants and antipsychotics often co-administered with pain medications), since they typically fail to achieve therapeutic levels unless treated with extremely high doses of these same drugs.[41–44]

CYP2C19 represents another dramatic example of the existence of both cross-ethnic and interindividual variations in drug metabolism. This enzyme is involved in the metabolism of commonly used psychotropics such as diazepam and tertiary tricyclic antidepressants, as well as citalopram. Using S-mephenytoin as the probe, earlier studies demonstrated that up to 20% of East Asians (Chinese, Japanese, and Koreans) are PMs, in contrast to a significantly lower rate of 3%–5% in Caucasians.[45] After the gene for the enzyme had been identified and sequenced, it became clear that such enzyme deficiency is caused by two unique mutations (CYP2C19*2 and CYP2C19*3). While *2 can be found in all ethnic groups, *3 appears to be specific to those with Eastern Asian origins. The presence of *3, together with a higher rate of *2, are responsible for the higher rate of PM among Asians, as well as their often increased sensitivity in the clinical setting to drugs such as diazepam.[46]

"Non-biological" factors affecting the expression of drug-metabolizing enzymes

In addition to genetic endowment, a large number of nongenetic factors also significantly influence gene expression. These include nutrients (components of diet), various plant products, pharmaceutical agents, and other chemicals. Prominent examples include the following:

1. Asian Indians and Africans residing in their native countries were found to metabolize drugs including theophylline, antipyrine, and clomipramine at a significantly slower rate than their Caucasian counterparts. However, immigrants from these "non-Western" regions who subsequently moved to Europe and changed their dietary intake from a low-protein to a high-protein diet metabolized these medications at a rate comparable to Caucasian Europeans.[47–49] Mechanisms responsible for these phenomena were obscure until the identification of the cytochrome P-450 enzyme CYP1A2, as well as its pivotal role in the metabolism of the drugs mentioned above. CYP1A2 also metabolizes clozapine, olanzapine, and tricyclic antidepressants. Its activity is induced by a protein-rich diet, leading to the accelerated degradation of substances metabolized through this route. Other inducers of CYP1A2 include constituents of tobacco (not nicotine, but numerous polycyclic aromatic hydrocarbons

generated in the process of smoking), certain vegetables (e.g., Brussels sprouts, broccoli) and char-grilled meat.[50,51]

2. The activity of CYP3A4, responsible for the metabolism of a large number of medications including most psychotropics, as well as immuno-suppressants, anticancer, and anticholesterol agents, also shows remarkable inter-ethnic variations. Asian Indians,[52-54] East Asians,[55,56] and Mexicans[57-60] have been shown to have lower CYP3A4 activity, whereas African Americans[61] and African Blacks[62] may possess slightly higher CYP3A4 activity, as compared to Caucasians. Although genetic factors may play a small part in such cross-ethnic variations, the main reason for differential CYP3A4 activities, both between individuals and across ethnic/cultural groups, appears to be dietary. CYP3A4 and related enzymes represent a major component of the human body's defense against potentially harmful substances ("xenobiotics"), which has evolved over the millennia to detect and destroy toxic substances produced by plants for the purpose of their own survival.[63] For such a system to work, it has to be highly responsive to environmental "cues." Exposure to trace amounts of certain substances could serve as "alarms" triggering increased production of CYP3A4.[64] A prominent example is the inducing effect of St. John's wort on CYP3A4,[65] at times causing treatment failure in patients receiving concurrent antiviral medications.[66] Similar effects have been observed with a number of traditional Chinese medicines and other herbal drugs.[67-70] Conversely, grape fruit juice, red wine, certain citric fruits, and vegetables containing quercetin and a number of herbs exert strong inhibitory effects on the enzyme,[71-75] lowering the blood level of antiviral drugs as well as psychotropics such as nefazodone and alprazolam by several fold, if taken concurrently.

These examples demonstrate the importance of environmental factors in substantially modifying the activity of drug-metabolizing enzymes. Patients from different ethnic/cultural backgrounds live divergent lifestyles, and are likely to be exposed to unique substances, including unique herbs, which may exert strong effects on the expression and activity of drug metabolizing enzymes. What we currently know about such influences represents only the tip of the iceberg. This issue may be even more salient with ethnic minority and other non-Western populations.

Genetic polymorphism of genes encoding receptors, transporters, or other therapeutic targets

Monoamines including dopamine (DA), serotonin (5-HT), and norepinephrine (NE) have been implicated in the pathogenesis of psychiatric disorders including schizophrenia and major depression. They also often are the targets of psychotropics. For example, selective serotonin re-uptake inhibitors (SSRIs) are believed to exert their antidepressant effects through the 5-HT system. Similarly, the continuing viability of the "dopamine hypothesis" highlights the importance of the dopaminergic system in the pathogenesis and treatment of schizophrenia. Many of the genes controlling the function of these crucial systems are highly polymorphic, and the pattern of these polymorphisms varies significantly across ethnicity. For example, patients possessing a long variant (l) in the promoter region of the serotonin transporter gene (5-HTT) are significantly more likely to have favorable SSRI treatment response, as compared to those possessing the short allele (s).[76] However, the frequency of the l allele varies significantly across ethnicity, ranging from 20% in East Asians to 70% in African Americans. It remains unclear whether the putative effect of the l allele on SSRI responses also holds true with East Asians.[77] Similarly, DRD2 TaqIA restriction fragment length polymorphism (RFLP) affects the receptor's response to neuroleptics, and may be associated with the risk for alcoholism.[78] The frequency of this allele varies significantly, ranging from 9% in Yemenite Jews to 75% in Muskoke Creek Amerindians.[79]

The synthesis and catabolism of the catecholamines are controlled by a number of enzymes including tryptophan hydroxylase, tyrosine hydroxylase, catechol-*O*-methyltransferase (COMT), and the monoamine oxidases (MAO). Interestingly, all of these enzymes are highly polymorphic. For example, COMT activity has long been known to have a trimodal distribution.[80] Recent studies demonstrate that the reduction of its activity is caused by a single nucleotide mutation whose allele frequency is approximately 26% in African Americans, 18% in Asians, and 50% in Caucasians. Higher COMT activity leads to accelerated metabolism of levodopa. Reflecting this, a higher percentage of Asians have been found to be poor responders to levodopa.[81]

INTERACTIONS BETWEEN ANALGESICS AND PSYCHOTROPICS

Most of the psychotropics, especially benzodiazepines and other anxiolytics, but also most neuroleptics and antidepressants, have significant sedative and central suppressant effects. When used in combination with narcotic analgesics, the additive effects could lead to significant or even life-threatening adverse results. Zhou and associates[82] reported that although morphine was metabolized at a similar rate between Chinese and Caucasians, the medicine led to a greater depression in ventilation and blood pressure in the latter group. In another study,[83] Amerindians showed significantly higher degrees of ventilatory suppression, despite having lower levels of morphine-6-glucuronide, the active metabolite of morphine responsible for its CNS effects. Such ethnic pharmacodynamic variations may further influence therapeutic outcomes when psychotropics are co-administered.

On the pharmacokinetic side, psychotropics and analgesics often share the same metabolic pathways, and thus have the potential of interacting with each other through these routes.[84] A number of narcotics, including codeine and hydrocodone are inert prodrugs dependent on CYP2D6 for conversion into their active forms,[85] and are not likely to have analgesic effects with patients either possessing defective CYP2D6 genes or those who are concurrently being treated with CYP2D6 inhibitors (e.g., bupropion, fluoxetine, paroxetine). Conversely, celecoxib has been shown to inhibit CYP2D6, and may accentuate the effects of psychotropics dependent on this enzyme for their elimination.[86] As a potent inhibitor of CYP1A2, Rofecoxib is likely to affect the metabolism of psychotropics such as amitriptyline and olanzapine.[87] Similarly, since most of the nonsteroid anti-inflammatory drugs (NSAIDs) are substrates of CYP2C9,[88] psychotropics (e.g., fluoxetine) capable of inhibiting this enzyme could lead to unexpected side effects of the former.

Lastly, acetaminophen has been implicated in hepatic failure in alcoholic patients. Persistent alcohol intake induces the activity of CYP2E1, which converts acetaminophen into *N*-acetyl-*p*-benzo-quinone imine (NAPQI), a toxic metabolite.[89] East Asians are more likely (20%–29%) to possess an allele (CYP2E1c2) conferring higher enzyme activities,[90] which might render them even more susceptible to such an interaction effect.

Summary and future research directions

This brief survey serves to highlight the significance as well as the complexity of issues surrounding the influence of cultural and ethnic forces on psychotropic and analgesic responses. Taken together, the literature reviewed clearly demonstrates the importance of these factors in psychopharmacotherapy. At the same time, it is equally important that any findings regarding ethnic variations in pharmacological responses not be interpreted stereotypically. In this regard, it is useful to keep in mind that almost all ethnic and cultural contrasts are superimposed on usually very substantial interindividual variations. This is true not only in regard to biological traits such as the ones reviewed above, but equally (or even more) so with regard to "cultural" and psychosocial variables. Stereotypic interpretations of cultural and ethnic differences in either psychological or biological characteristics are not only misleading but also potentially divisive and dangerous.

In interpreting biological diversity, both within and across populations, one should not lose sight of the fact that biological systems are dynamic rather than static, and the expression of genetic predisposition is constantly modified by environmental influences.

Progress in the research on P-450 enzymes and other drug metabolizing enzymes in the past three decades has led to the development of a number of laboratory procedures that could be used for determining the activity of these enzymes as well as polymorphisms of the genes encoding these enzymes. In addition, emergent data also suggest that some of the polymorphisms of genes encoding neurotransmitter transporters and/or receptors might also predict treatment outcome. Thus, it appears that technology may be in place for researchers to systematically test the utility of these procedures in the clinical settings. It is likely that progress in this direction will eventually lead to the development of a panel of tests that will pave the way for our pursuit of the holy grail of "individualized medicine."[4,91,92]

Along with these exciting developments in the field of pharmacogenomics, there are even more urgent needs to promote research on "nonbiological" issues impinging upon pharmacological responses, including the development of culturally informed and effective approaches to minimize "nonadherence," strategies for optimizing expectation ("placebo") effects in divergent cultural groups, and efforts to reduce the effect of stereotyping in clinicians working with patients from different sociocultural backgrounds. Such an integrative approach should enable us to delineate crucial elements for optimal pharmacotherapeutic practices that take both cultural and biological diversity into consideration in the tailoring of treatment for individual patients.

REFERENCES

1. Kung F, Gibson SJ, Helme RD. Factors associated with analgesic and psychotropic medications use by community-dwelling older people with chronic pain. *Aus NZ J Public Health*. 1999;23(5):471–474.
2. Sharp J, Keefe B. Psychiatry in chronic pain: a review and update. *Curr Psychiatry Rep*. 2005;7(3):213–219.
3. Breitbart W. Psychotropic adjuvant analgesics for pain in cancer and AIDS. *Psychooncology*. 1998;7(4):333–345.
4. Chen CH, Chen CY, Lin KM. Ethnopsychopharmacology, *Int Rev Psychiatry*. 2008;20(5):452–459.
5. Lin KM, Poland RE, Nakasaki G. *Psychopharmacology and Psychobiology of Ethnicity*. Washington, DC: American Psychiatric Press; 1993.
6. Kalow W, Ozdemir V, Tang BK, et al. The science of pharmacological variability: an essay. *Clin Pharmacol Ther*. 1999;66(5):445–447.
7. Mezzich JE, Kleinman A, Fabrega H, et al. *Culture and Psychiatric Diagnosis*. Washington DC: American Psychiatric Press; 1995.
8. Lopez SR. Patient variable biases in clinical judgment: Conceptual overview and methodological considerations. *Psychol Bull*. 1989;106:184–203.
9. Adebimpe VR. Overview: White norms and psychiatric diagnosis of Black patients. *Am J Psychiatry*. 1981;138:279–285.

10. Price N, Glazer WM, Morgenstern H. Race and the use of fluphenazine decanoate. *Am J Psychiatry.* 1985; 142:1491–1492.

11. Sramek J, Roy S, Ahrens T, et al. Prevalence of tardive dyskinesia among three ethnic groups of chronic psychiatric patients. *Hosp Community Psychiatry.* 1991;42:590–592.

12. Becker M, Maiman L. Strategies for enhancing patient compliance. *J Community Health.* 1980;6:113–135.

13. Julius RJ, Novitsky MA Jr, Dubin WR. Medication adherence: a review of the literature and implications for clinical practice. *J Psychiatr Pract.* 2009;15(1):34–44.

14. Mitchell AJ. Adherence behaviour with psychotropic medication is a form of self-medication. *Med Hypotheses.* 2007;68(1):12–21.

15. Sue S. Community mental health services to minority groups: some optimism, some pessimism. *Am Psychol.* 1977;32:616–624.

16. Acosta FX, Yamamoto J, Evans LA. *Effective Psychotherapy for Low-income and Minority Patients.* New York: Plenum Press; 1982.

17. Kinzie JD, Leung P, Boehnlein J, et al. Tricyclic antidepressant plasma levels in Indochinese refugees: Clinical implication. *J Nerv Ment Dis.* 1987;175:480–485.

18. Gillis L, Trollip D, Jakoet A, et al. Non-compliance with psychotropic medication. *S Afr Med J.* 1987;72:602–606.

19. Lee S, Wing YK, Wong KC. Knowledge and compliance towards lithium therapy among Chinese psychiatric patients in Hong Kong. *Aust NZ J Psychiatry.* 1992;26:444–449.

20. Jadad AR, Enkin MW. *Randomized Controlled Trials: Questions, Answers, and Musings.* Malden, MA: Blackwell Pub. References; 2007.

21. Swartzman LC, Burkell J. Expectations and the placebo effect in clinical drug trials: why we should not turn a blind eye to unblinding, and other cautionary notes. *Clin Pharmacol Ther.* 1998;64(1):1–7.

22. Kleinman A. *Rethinking Psychiatry: From Cultural Category to Personal Experience.* New York: Free Press; 1998.

23. Scott RA. *Miracle Cures: Saints, Pilgrimage, and the Healing Powers of Belief.* Berkeley: University of California Press; 2010.

24. Daley TC. Beliefs about treatment of mental health problems among Cambodian American children and parents. *Soc Sci Med.* 2005;61(11):2384–2395.

25. Lin KM, Demonteverde L, Nuccio I. Religion, healing and mental health among Filipino-Americans. *Intl J Ment Health.* 1990;19(3):40–44.

26. Pickwell SM. Multilevel healing pursuits of Cambodian refugees. *J Immigr Health.* 1999;1(3):165–179.

27. Castro, FG, Furth P, Karlow H. The health beliefs of Mexican, Mexican-American and Anglo-American women. *Hisp J Behav Sci.* 1994;6:365–383.

28. Lin KM. Traditional Chinese medical beliefs and their relevance for mental illness and psychiatry. In: Kleinman S, Lin TY, eds. *Normal and Abnormal Behavior in Chinese Culture.* Dordrecht, The Netherlands: Reidel Publishing Company; 1981.

29. Buckalew LW, Coffield K. Drug expectations associated with perceptual characteristics: ethnic factors. *Percept Mot Skills.* 1982;55:915–918.

30. Kleinman A. *Patients and Healers in the Context of Culture.* Berkeley: University of California Press; 1980.

31. Lin KM, Cheung F. Mental health issues for Asian Americans, *Psychiatry Serv.* 1999;50(6):774–780.

32. Eisenberg DM, Davis RB, Ettner SL, et al. Trends in alternative medicine use in the United States, 1990–1997: results of a follow-up national survey. *JAMA.* 1998;280(18):1569–1575.

33. Lin KM, Poland RE, Anderson D. Psychopharmacology, ethnicity and culture. *Transcult Psychiatr Res Rev.* 1995;32:1–40.

34. Lin KM, Poland RE, Lau JK, and Rubin RT. Haloperidol and Prolactin Concentrations in Asians and Caucasians. *J Clin Psychopharmacol.* 1988;8:195–201.

35. Lin KM, Poland RE. Ethnicity, culture and psychopharmacology. In: Bloom FE, Kupfer DJ, eds. *Psychopharmacology: The Fourth Generation of Progress.* New York, NY: Raven Press; 1995:1907–1917.

36. Dahl ML, Yue QY, Roh HK, et al. Genetic analysis of the CYP2D locus in relation to debriso-quine hydroxylation capacity in Korean, Japanese and Chinese subjects. *Pharmacogenet.* 1995; 5(3):159–164.

37. Ingelman-Sundberg M. The human genome project and novel aspects of cytochrome P450 research. *Toxicol Appl Pharmacol.* 2005;207(suppl 2):52–56.

38. Ingelman-Sundberg M. Pharmacogenetics of cytochrome P450 and its applications in drug therapy: the past, present and future. *Trends Pharmacol Sci.* 2004;25(4):193–200.

39. Wan YJ, Poland RE, Han G, et al. Analysis of the CYP2D6 gene polymorphism and enzyme activity in African-Americans in southern California. *Pharmacogenet.* 2001;11(6):489–499.

40. Mendoza R, Wan YJ, Poland RE et al. CYP2D6 polymorphism in a Mexican American population. *Clin Pharmacol Ther.* 2001;70(6):552–560.

41. Aklillu E, Persson I, Bertilsson L, et al. Frequent distribution of ultrarapid metabolizers of debriso-quine in an ethiopian population carrying duplicated and multiduplicated functional CYP2D6 alleles. *J Pharmacol Exp Ther.* 1996;278(1):441–446.

42. Correia C, Santos P, Coutinhoet AM, et al. Characterization of pharmacogenetically relevant CYP2D6 and ABCB1 gene polymorphisms in a Portuguese population sample. *Cell Biochem Funct.* 2009;27(4):251–255.

43. Ingelman-Sundberg M. Duplication, multiduplication, and amplification of genes encoding drug-metabolizing enzymes: evolutionary, toxicological, and clinical pharmacological aspects. *Drug Metab Rev.* 1999;31(2):449–459.

44. Luo HR, Aloumanis V, Lin KM, et al. Polymorphisms of CYP2C19 and CYP2D6 in Israeli ethnic groups. *Am J Pharmacogenomics.* 2004;4(6):395–401.

45. Xie HG, Stein CM, Kim RB, Wilkinson GR, Flockhart D A, Wood AJ Allelic, genotypic and pheno-typic distributions of S-mephenytoin 4'-hydroxylase (CYP2C19) in healthy Caucasian populations of European descent throughout the world. *Pharmacogenet.* 1999;9(5):539–549.

46. Goldstein JA, Ishizaki T, Chiba K, de Morais SM, Bell D, Krahn PM Evans D A. Frequencies of the defective CYP2C19 alleles responsible for the mephenytoin poor metabolizer phenotype in various Oriental, Caucasian, Saudi Arabian and American black populations. *Pharmacogenet.* 1997;7(1):59–64.

47. Anderson KE, Kappas A. Dietary regulation of cytochrome P450. *Ann Rev Nutr.* 1991;11:141–167.

48. Allen JJ, Rack PH, Vaddadi KS. Differences in the effects of clomipramine on English and Asian volun-teers. Preliminary report on a pilot study." *Postgraduate Med J.* 1977;53(suppl 4):79–86.

49. Branch RA, Salih SY, Homeida M. Racial differences in drug metabolizing ability: a study with antipy-rine in the Sudan. *Clin Pharmacol Ther.* 1978;24(3):283–286.

50. Okey AB. Enzeme induction in cytochrome P-450 system. In: Kalow W, ed. *Pharmacogenetics of Drug Metabolism.* New York, NY: Pergamon Press; 1992.

51. Schein JR. Cigarette smoking and clinically significant drug interactions. *Ann Pharmacother.* 1995;29 (11):1139–1148.

52. Ahsan CH, Renwick AG, Waller DG, et al. The influence of dose and ethnic origins on the pharmacoki-netics of nifedipine. *Clin Pharmacol Ther.* 1993;54:329–338.

53. Kinirons MT, Lang CC, He HB, et al. Triazolam pharmacokinetics and pharmacodynamics in Caucasians and Southern Asians: ethnicity and CYP3A activity. *Br J Clin Pharmacol.* 1996;41:69–72.

54. Rashid TJ, Martin U, Clarke H, et al. Factors affecting the absolute bioavailability of nifedipine. *Br J Clin Pharmacol.* 1995;40(1):51–58.

55. Ajir K, Smith M, Lin KM, et al. The pharmacokinetics and pharmacodynamics of adinazolam: multi-ethnic comparisons. *Psychopharmacol (Berl).* 1997;129(3):265–270.

56. Lin KM, Lau JK, Smith R, et al. Comparison of alprazolam plasma levels in normal Asian and Caucasian male volunteers. *Psychopharmacol (Berl).* 1988;96(3):365–369.

57. Castaneda-Hernandez G, Hoyo-Vadillo C, Palma-Aguirre JA, Flores-Murrieta FJ. Pharmacokinetics of oral nifedipine in different populations. *J Clin Pharmacol.* 1993;33(2): 140–145.

58. Chavez-Teyes L, Castaneda-Hernandez G, Flores-Murrieta FJ. Pharmacokinetics of midazolam in Mexicans: evidence for interethnic variability. *Clin Drug Invest.* 1999;17:233–239.

59. Hoyo-Vadillo C, Castafieda-Hernandez G, Herrera JE, et al. Pharmacokinetics of nifedipine slow release tablet in Mexican subjects: further evidence for an oxidation polymorphism. *J Clin Pharmacol.* 1989;29(9):816–820.

60. Palma-Aguirre JA, Nava Rangel J, Hoyo Vadillo C, et al. Influence of Mexican diet on nifedipine pharmacodynamics in healthy volunteers. *Proc West Pharmacol Soc.* 1994;37:85–86.

61. Johnson JA. Predictability of the effects of race or ethnicity on pharmacokinetics of drugs. *Int J C Pharmacol Ther.* 2000;38(2):53–60.

62. Sowunmi A, Rashid TJ, Akinyinka OO, et al. Ethnic differences in nifedipine kinetics: comparisons between Nigerians, Caucasians and South Asians. *Br J Clin Pharmacol.* 1995;40(5):489–493.

63. Gonzalez FJ, Nebert DW. Evolution of the P450 gene superfamily: animal-plant 'warfare,' molecular drive and human genetic differences in drug oxidation. *Trends Genet.* 1990;6:182–186.

64. Kliewer SA, Goodwin B, Willson TM. The nuclear pregnane X receptor: a key regulator of xenobiotic metabolism. *Endocr Rev.* 2002;23(5):687–702.

65. Wang Z, Gorski JC, Hamman MA, et al. The effects of St John's wort (Hypericum perforatum) on human cytochrome P450 activity. *Clin Pharmacol Ther.* 2001;70(4):317–326.

66. Piscitelli SC, Burstein AH, Chaitt D, et al. Indinavir concentrations and St John's wort [letter]. *Lancet.* 2000; 355:547–548.

67. Brobst DE, Ding X, Creech KL, et al. Guggulsterone activates multiple nuclear receptors and induces CYP3A gene expression through the pregnane X receptor. *J Pharmacol Exp Ther.* 2004;310(2):528–535.

68. Lichti-Kaiser K, Staudinger JL. The traditional Chinese herbal remedy tian xian activates pregnane X receptor and induces CYP3A gene expression in hepatocytes. *Drug Metab Dispos.* 2008;36(8):1538–1545.

69. Tu JH, He YJ, Chen Y, et al. Effect of glycyrrhizin on the activity of CYP3A enzyme in humans. *Eur J Clin Pharmacol.* 2010;66(8):805–810.

70. Volak LP, Ghirmai S, Cashman JR, et al. Curcuminoids inhibit multiple human cytochromes P450, UDP-glucuronosyltransferase, and sulfotransferase enzymes, whereas piperine is a relatively selective CYP3A4 inhibitor. *Drug Metab Dispos.* 2008;36(8):1594–1605.

71. Agbonon A, Eklu-Gadegbeku K, Aklikokou K, et al. In vitro inhibitory effect of West African medicinal and food plants on human cytochrome P450 3A subfamily. *J Ethnopharmacol.* 2010;128(2):390–394.

72. Blumenthal M. Twenty-seven major botanicals and their uses in the United States. In: Eskinaszi D, ed. *Botanical Medicine: Efficacy, Quality Assurance, and Regulation.* Larchmont, NY: Mary Ann Liebert, Inc.; 1998.

73. Fujita K. Food-drug interactions via human cytochrome P450 3A (CYP3A). *Drug Metabol Drug Interact.* 2004;20(4):195–217.

74. Nielsen SE, Breinholt V, Justesen U, et al. In vitro biotransformation of flavonoids by rat liver microsomes. *Xenobiotica.* 1998;28:389–401.

75. Oesterheld J, Kallepalli BR. Grapefruit juice and clomipramine: shifting metabolic ratios. *J Clin Psychopharmacol.* 1997;17:62–63.

76. Kirchheiner J, Schmidt H, Tzvetkov M, et al. Pharmacokinetics of codeine and its metabolite morphine in ultra-rapid metabolizers due to CYP2D6 duplication. *Pharmacogenomics J.* 2007;7 (4):257–265.

77. Kim H, Lim SW, Kim S, Kim JW, Chang YH, Carroll BJ, Kim DK. "Monoamine transporter gene polymorphisms and antidepressant response in koreans with late-life depression." *JAMA.* 2006;296(13):1609–1618.

78. Noble EP, Zhang X, Ritchie TL, Sparkes RS. Haplotypes at the DRD2 locus and severe alcoholism. *Am J Med Genet.* 2000;96(5):622–631.

79. Barr CL, Kidd KK. Population frequencies of the A1 allele at the dopamine D2 receptor locus. *Biol .Psychiatry.* 1993;34(4):204–209.

80. McLeod HL, Fang L, Luo X, Scott EP, Evans WE. Ethnic differences in erythrocyte catechol-O-methyltransferase activity in black and white Americans. *J Pharmacol Exp Ther.* 1994;270(1):26–29.

81. Rivera-Calimlim L, Reilly DK. Difference in erythrocyte catechol-O-methyltransferase activity between Orientals and Caucasians: difference in levodopa tolerance. *Clin Pharmacol Ther.* 1984;35(6):804–809.

82. Zhou HH, Sheller JR, Nu H, et al. Ethnic differences in response to morphine. *Clin Pharmacol Ther.* 1993;54(5):507–513.

83. Cepeda MS, Farrar JT, Roa JH, et al. Ethnicity influences morphine pharmacokinetics and pharmacodynamics. *Clin Pharmacol Ther.* 2001;70(4):351–361.

84. Stamer UM, Zhang L, Stuber F. Personalized therapy in pain management: Where do we stand? *Pharmacogenomics.* 2010;11(6):843–864.

85. Jannetto PJ, Bratanow NC. Utilization of pharmacogenomics and therapeutic drug monitoring for opioid pain management. *Pharmacogenomics.* 2009;10(7):1157–1167.

86. Werner U, *Werner* D, Rau T, et al. Celecoxib inhibits metabolism of cytochrome P450 2D6 substrate metoprolol in humans. *Clin Pharmacol Ther.* 2003;74(2):130–137.

87. Karjalainen MJ, Neuvonen PJ, Backman JT. Rofecoxib is a potent, metabolism-dependent inhibitor of CYP1A2: implications for in vitro prediction of drug interactions. *Drug Metab Dispos.* 2006;34(12):2091–2096.

88. Rosemary J, Adithan C. The pharmacogenetics of CYP2C9 and CYP2C19: ethnic variation and clinical significance. *Curr Clin Pharmacol.* 2007;2(1):93–109.

89. Kuffner EK, et al. The effect of acetaminophen (four grams a day for three consecutive days) on hepatic tests in alcoholic patients—a multicenter randomized study. *BMC Med.* 2007;5:13.

90. Kang TS, et al. Comparison of genetic polymorphisms of CYP2E1, ADH2, and ALDH2 genes involved in alcohol metabolism in Koreans and four other ethnic groups. *J Clin Pharm Ther.* 2009;34(2):225–230.

91. Lin KM. Integrating theory, practice and economics in psychopharmacology. In: Ng C, Lin KM, Singh B and Chiu E, eds. *Ethno-psychopharmacology: Advances in Current Practice*, Cambridge University Press; 2008:158–168.

92. Ng J, Lin KM, Smith M. Psychopharmacotherapy in the age of accelerating diversity. In: Georgiopoulos AM, Rosenbaum JF, eds. *Perspectives in Cross-Cultural Psychiatry*. Philadelphia, PA: Lippincott Williams & Wilkins; 2005

Contextual Issues in Pain Medicine

28

INTEGRATIVE MEDICINE APPROACH TO CHRONIC PAIN

STEPHEN DAHMER, MD
Integrative Family Medicine Attending, Beth Israel Continuum
Center for Health and Healing, New York, New York, USA

RAYMOND Y. TEETS, MD
Institute for Family Health, Beth Israel Residency in Urban
Family Medicine, Department of Family and Social Medicine,
Albert Einstein College of Medicine of Yeshiva University,
New York, New York, USA

EMILIE SCOTT, MD
Department of Family Medicine, University of California,
Irvine, South Orange, California, USA

Key Points

- An Integrative Medicine approach to pain elicits a broader picture of the patient's situation, provides a wide array of treatment options, and improves the chance to mitigate chronic pain.
- Integrative Medicine combines conventional medicine with the most evidence-based Complementary and Alternative Medicine (CAM) modalities available.
- An anti-inflammatory diet, along with fish oil, and trial of glucosamine sulfate or s-adenosylmethionine may mitigate chronic pain.
- Manual medicine modalities, such as chiropraxy, massage, or osteopathic manipulation offer a novel and safe way to address chronic pain.
- Acupuncture and Yoga offer a means to address chronic pain and also improve functionality for the patient with chronic pain.
- Mind-body therapies can significantly improve the quality of life for a patient with chronic pain.

Chronic pain is a common reason for patients to seek medical care. Its cause is generally complex and multifactorial. Integrative medicine (IM) can offer a means to develop a more comprehensive treatment approach for patients with chronic pain, eliciting a broader picture of the patient's condition and combining conventional medicine with complementary and alternative medicine (CAM). Immediate and complete relief of chronic pain may be an unrealistic goal, and so it is important to establish appropriate goals of care in the treatment of chronic pain. The following three goals are an important starting point when addressing chronic pain:

1. Addressing the patient's pain in the context of the patient's life situation, what Giordano and colleagues[1] refer to as the "patient-specific context"
2. Ameliorating the patient's pain and/or improving quality of life
3. Improving the patient's risk profile by diminishing their need for polypharmacy, invasive interventions, and unproven alternative therapies

THE PROCESS

An IM history includes a conventional history and inquires about nutrition, social support, work, exercise, stress-relieving strategies, a spiritual history, as well as the patient's conception of their clinical situation. CAM use is addressed including dietary supplement intake and the use of CAM practitioners (e.g., acupuncturist, chiropractor, Reiki practitioner). In designing the therapeutic plan, the physician determines what methods the patient might be interested in exploring. The plan can include nutritional and dietary supplements, stress-relieving techniques, exercise, or a referral to CAM providers. An assessment of the patient's social support can identify possible resources for the patient. The literature on the effects of social support on chronic pain is complex, suggesting that not all social support results in improved pain burden or less disability.[2] However, perceived support, type of caregiver responses, and patient-coping style all interact over time to have an effect on the patient's suffering. Assessing these factors is important, and could lead to an intervention such as couples' counseling.[3]

NUTRITION, HERBS, AND SUPPLEMENTS

Dietary modifications

An anti-inflammatory diet is one high in fruits, vegetables, fiber, fish, and mono-unsaturated fats such as olive oil. The Mediterranean diet is a well-known example. Anti-inflammatory diets can favorably influence the biochemical process of inflammation present in pain syndromes.[4] Clinical studies, though limited, do suggest a role for an anti-inflammatory diet in chronic pain. A recent Cochrane review reviewed dietary interventions for rheumatoid arthritis.[5] They found 14 randomized controlled trials, with heterogeneity of interventions and outcomes. Diets that were included in the trials included the Mediterranean diet, vegetarian diets, allergy-elimination diets, elemental diets, and vegan diets. Studies showed improved pain scores with the Mediterranean and vegetarian diets, but not with other diet interventions. Studies were small, and had risk of moderate bias (given that it's difficult to blind food interventions) and drop-out rates were generally higher in the dietary intervention groups than their controls. Doctors should be aware of risks with diet interventions, including unintentional weight loss and nutrient deficiencies.

Some culinary herbs have also been shown to contain anti-inflammatory properties, for instance ginger (Zingiber officinale) and turmeric (Curcuma longa). These herbs have shown to impact inflammation in beneficial ways, via cytokine secretion and lymphocyte proliferation.[6] Studies are examining the concentrated forms of these herbs, but the data is mixed, and not convincing enough to recommend such herbs beyond the use at food doses (i.e., in cooking).[7,8] A trial of the Mediterranean diet can be beneficial for the chronic pain patient, representing a generally safe and overall beneficial diet. Adding in culinary herbs as detailed above also may provide some added benefit.

Omega-3 fatty acids

Omega-3 fatty acids can be taken as supplements, and clinical studies of omega-3 fatty acid supplements have shown that they can improve pain symptoms, mostly with rheumatoid arthritis. Omega-3 fatty acids can improve symptoms such as joint tenderness and morning stiffness, and decrease the amount of medication required by patients with rheumatoid arthritis.[9] A meta-analysis of 17 placebo-controlled studies evaluated the effect of omega-3 fatty acids on joint pain. These studies largely used fish oils (combined DHA + EPA) as therapy rather than alpha-linolenic acid. The joint pains were in the context of rheumatoid arthritis, dysmenorrhea, or inflammatory bowel disease. The quality of the studies was variable, but overall the conclusion was that fish oils can be helpful in the context of inflammatory joint pain syndromes. Doses above 2.7 gm daily, for a period exceeding three months, seemed to insure the greatest effect. Laboratory and animal studies also suggest that diets rich in omega-3 fatty acids may benefit people with osteoarthritis, but no clinical outcome studies have clearly shown benefit in osteoarthritis.[10] Further studies are needed to sort out their role in other inflammatory syndromes such as osteoarthritis.

Glucosamine sulfate and chondroitin

Glucosamine sulfate stimulates the production of glycosaminoglycans (the key structural components of cartilage) as well as the incorporation of sulfur into cartilage. Sulfur is necessary for making and repairing cartilage.[11] Chondroitin is a glucosaminoglycan that may also be beneficial for cartilage. The literature has been mixed in terms of showing efficacy for combined glucosamine and chondroitin in osteoarthritis. There have been some negative studies, but a meta-analysis in 2000 of 15 studies suggested that there was likely some moderate benefit.[12] Vlad et al performed a further analysis of 15 more recent and more rigorous glucosamine trials,[13] showing that the glucosamine *hydrochloride* preparation is not efficacious. Further trials are needed of sufficient rigor to eliminate any industry bias and shed more light on the benefits, but glucosamine sulfate with chondroitin sulfate may be efficacious.

Both glucosamine sulfate and chondroitin are safe and well-tolerated. There is the possible risk of allergy with a patient with known shellfish allergy, given that glucosamine is often produced from marine exoskeletons. The daily dose for treatment of osteoarthritis is 1500 mg/1200 mg of glucosamine sulfate with chondroitin sulfate, respectively.

S-adenosyl-methionine

S-adenosyl-methionine (SAMe) has a role as a methyl donor biochemically, and has been studied as a supplement for osteoarthritis pain. The mechanism for reducing pain is unclear, but may be anti-inflammatory or increasing proteoglycan synthesis in joints.[14] Several meta-analyses have reviewed the clinical data for treatment of osteoarthritis pain, and have generally agreed that is helpful both for pain and function. The Agency for Healthcare Research for Quality reviewed 11 studies, looking at either SAMe versus placebo, or versus a nonsteroidal anti-inflammatory drug (NSAID). Though there was some heterogeneity in the studies, the meta-analysis suggests that SAMe decreased pain relative to placebo, and appeared to be equivalent to NSAID.[15] A more recent small study of 61 patients compared SAMe to celecoxib, finding an equivalent effect, though the onset of pain relief took about one month for the SAMe.[14] A dose of 600–1200 mg has been used in the studies to good relief. Of note, SAMe does also have an antidepressant effect, and so should be used with caution in those patients with risk of mania. Adverse effects from SAMe have been mild.[16]

MANUAL MEDICINE

Manual medicine includes such CAM modalities as chiropraxy, osteopathic manipulation therapy (OMT), and massage. The concept of joint subluxation in chiropraxy proposes a biomechanical model of spinal pain that emphasizes normal function in the active, passive, and neural integration systems of the spine as a prerequisite for stability.[17] The loss of spinal stability occurs when one of the components of the active (musculotendinous), passive (ligamentous), and neural integration (proprioceptors, nociceptors) systems become dysfunctional. Compensations by the other systems may trigger movement impairments, such as pain avoidance, or control impairments, such as pain provocation. Manual therapy interventions also seem to have neurophysiologic effects that can cause pain modulation, similar to acupuncture. These techniques are known to trigger similar populations of proprioceptive afferents (groups I and II) that can gate nociception in the dorsal horn.[18]

Manual medicine can be used as an adjunct to other modes of pain control. Research for chiropraxy alone has been mixed, generally not showing benefits over standard therapy, but showing similar efficacy to conventional therapies. Meeker and Haldeman[19] reviewed 43 randomized controlled trials (RCTs) using chiropraxy for acute, subacute, and chronic low back pain. Thirty of these RCTs favored chiropraxy over the comparison treatment in at least one patient subgroup. The remaining 13 reported no significant differences, and none of the RCTs reported that chiropraxy was less effective than the comparison treatment. Other systematic reviews have confirmed these results.[20–22]

The most recent analysis of 12 systematic reviews including 69 unique trials on efficacy of spinal manipulation concluded that the only nonpharmacologic therapies with evidence of efficacy are superficial heat and spinal manipulation (i.e., chiropraxy), with fair evidence for small to moderate benefits.[23]

Osteopathic manual therapy

In theory, OMT suggests similar benefits as chiropraxy. However, it has not been studied to the same degree. One small study found that patients in an osteopathic treatment group (83 patients) required significantly less medication (analgesics, anti-inflammatory agents, and muscle relaxants, $P<.001$) and used less physical therapy (0.2% vs 2.6%, $P<.05$) than the standard medical therapy group (72 patients).[24] OMT is also successful as an adjunctive therapy but at increased cost. It may also contribute to patients' improved psychological status.[25] Further studies are needed to assess OMT's role in chronic pain.

Massage

Massage therapy is defined as soft-tissue manipulation by trained therapists for therapeutic purposes.[26] Massage typically is used as an adjunctive therapy rather than as the main treatment.[27] It can help relieve muscle tension, reduce stress, and evoke feelings of calmness. Massage induces a variety of positive physiologic effects that may contribute to tissue repair, pain modulation, relaxation, and improved mood.[19] The main theories regarding the analgesic effects of massage include gate theory, the serotonin hypothesis, and the restorative sleep hypothesis.[28] Animal models suggest a role of oxytocin acting in the periaquaductal gray area of the midbrain, influencing descending antinociceptive systems in this area.[29]

In their comprehensive review, the Cochrane Collaboration recently reported that massage alone was superior to relaxation, acupuncture, and self-care education for lower back pain. It was found equal in efficacy to corsets and exercises, but found inferior to spinal manipulation therapy.[18,30–33] The investigators of the Cochrane Review concluded that massage therapy may benefit patients with subacute and chronic nonspecific lower back pain, particularly when combined with exercise and education. Direct plus indirect costs for the massage group were about 40% lower than for acupuncture or self-care groups (although not statistically significant), suggesting that initial costs of massage may be offset by reduced health care utilization. On the other hand, in a randomized controlled trial of 579 patients with chronic or recurrent low back pain, exercise and six lessons in the Alexander technique were compared with massage alone. Massage was found to have moderate effectiveness at three months, but that did not persist to one year. In contrast, the Alexander technique lessons and exercise did show benefits in the Roland Disability Score at three months and one year.[34]

MANUAL MEDICINE SUMMARY

Adverse effects from manual medicine therapy have generally focused on risks from spinal manipulation. These adverse clinical events are rare, making them difficult to evaluate. None of the previously mentioned RCTs or any case series have reported a serious complication, such as worsening lumbar disc herniation or cauda equina syndrome. The risk of a serious adverse event, including data from observational studies, has been estimated at less than one per million patient visits.[35,36] In a Danish series, inclusive of 99% of chiropractors for a ten-year period, five cases of cerebrovascular accident and one death were identified.[37] One of the most comprehensive assessments of the complications of spinal manipulation was conducted in 1996.[38] Relevant case reports, surveys, and review articles were identified using a search of online databases. Estimates of the incidence of cauda equina syndrome following lumbar manipulation range from one case in one million to one in one hundred million.[39]

Considering the evidence supporting the efficacy of chiropraxy in low back pain and the extreme rarity of serious complications from lumbar spinal manipulation, it would be prudent to recommend a trial of chiropraxy for low back pain, especially in the subset of patients who are interested in such an approach, intolerant of nonsteroidal anti-inflammatory drugs, or looking for adjuvant treatments to conventional therapies. Massage therapy is best prescribed in combination with exercise and education, and there is evidence supporting its use for short-term relief of low back pain. Although OMT shares theoretic underpinnings with chiropraxy, it is less well established through studies.

Acupuncture

Acupuncture is part of a larger system of healing within Traditional Chinese Medicine (TCM). According to TCM, acupuncture attempts to influence the life force, or energy, known as qi (pronounced "chee") that flows through energy pathways (meridians) in the body. Achieving the proper flow of this energy is believed to create health and wellness, which can be achieved by stimulating the acupuncture points.[40,41] Modern research has confirmed the physiologic effects created by this needling process, with studies showing that acupuncture may alter brain chemistry by changing the release of neurotransmitters and neurohormones. These biochemical modulators can then affect the central nervous system, further influencing immune reactions and processes that regulate a person's blood pressure, blood flow, and body temperature.[42] Research using functional magnetic resonance imaging (fMRI) has demonstrated the neuromodulatory effect of acupuncture stimulation. Results of unilateral acupuncture needling showed bilateral neural modulation of cortical and subcortical structures in fMRI, causing a signal decrease in the limbic region and other subcortical areas. This was in contrast to fMRI findings with simple tactile stimulation.[43]

Conventional studies support acupuncture's efficacy in providing some clinical improvement in lower back pain. One meta-analysis not only supported the analgesic effect of acupuncture for lower back pain, but also suggested that acupuncture can improve functionality and lead to decreased use of analgesic medications in this population.[44]

Patients who received acupuncture for an eight-week period had a greater reduction in low back pain than those on a waiting list control.[45] In a prospective, randomized, controlled trial of 174 patients and a follow-up of three months, Molsberger and colleagues[46] demonstrated that 12 treatments of acupuncture coupled with conventional orthopedic treatment (COT) was much more effective (P%.02) than COT alone, or sham acupuncture with COT, in relieving chronic low back pain.

Literature evaluating acupuncture's safety shows that major adverse events are exceedingly rare and are usually associated with poorly trained and unlicensed acupuncturists.[47-50] Acupuncture is effective when used alone and as an adjunct therapy, and can contribute to mitigating lower back pain. Acupuncture is likely to be most beneficial in patients who have high expectations of benefit,[51] an effect that could point to some placebo effect.

Research on acupuncture has had some limitations, including incomplete understanding of the physiologic effect, use of standardized treatment regimens rather than the individualized approach that characterizes most acupuncture practice, and blinding of participants; yet, based on published evidence, acupuncture is safe and has been shown to be an effective therapeutic strategy for analgesia, likely to benefit patients with low back pain. It should be discussed with patients amenable to this approach and patients should be referred to competent acupuncturists in their area.

Yoga

Yoga is generally regarded as a CAM approach to health that not only increases flexibility, strength, and stamina but also fosters self-awareness, emotional stability, and peace of mind.[52] Increasing numbers of physicians and patients today are recognizing yoga as a complementary therapy and incorporating it in treatment of diseases and disorders.[23,53]

Recent studies of rheumatic diseases have shown that the use of yoga asanas (postures) positively affected the well-being of study participants.[54,55] Additional studies have shown that yoga can be added as a complementary therapy to the traditional management of arthritis.[55-59] One higher-quality trial (101 patients) found six weeks of Viniyoga (a therapeutically oriented style) to be slightly superior to conventional exercise (mean difference in Roland disability [RD] scores,1.8; confidence interval [CI] 3.5 to 0.1) and moderately superior to a self-care education book (mean difference in RD questionnaire scores, 3.4; CI 5.1 to 1.6) in terms of RD scores at 12 weeks.[60] Yoga was also associated with decreased medication use at week 26 (21% of patients) compared with exercise (50%) and the self-care book (59%), although the rate of provider visits for back pain did not differ.

Preliminary evidence has suggested that Viniyoga is an effective treatment of chronic low back pain and physicians should feel comfortable recommending experienced instructors to interested patients. Other yoga styles (Bikram, Vinyasa, and Iyengar) may be too vigorous or need modification for patients who are unfamiliar with yoga. Future research evaluating yoga for chronic back pain should investigate the effectiveness and safety of other therapeutically oriented styles of yoga and help delineate the therapeutic mechanism of action.

Mind-body therapy

The connection between the mind and the body is particularly significant in the realm of treating chronic pain. Mind-body therapies include cognitive behavioral therapy, hypnosis, biofeedback, and mindfulness-meditation. For many patients, the addition of a mind-body approach to treating chronic pain leads to a significant improvement in quality of life. Lower back pain can persist even in the absence of active local tissue damage[60] suggesting a centrally mediated pain process.[61] Centrally maintained pain has been correlated with cortical plasticity, which refers to the theory that the brain can undergo neurological changes over time, in correlation with sensations of chronic pain.[62,63] Many of the mind-body therapies enlisted in the treatment of chronic pain strive to correct these imbalances.

Cognitive behavioral therapy

The most commonly utilized behavioral treatment approach for chronic pain is cognitive behavioral therapy.[64] Cognitive behavioral therapy alone or within the context of an interdisciplinary pain rehabilitation program has the greatest empiric evidence of all the psychological therapies, including psychodynamic and behavioral therapies, for success in the treatment of chronic pain.[65] A Cochrane review from April 2009 showed that cognitive behavioral therapy had some small positive effects on pain, disability, and mood, whereas other behavioral therapies showed no evidence of benefit. This review was based on 40 studies assessing the success of cognitive behavioral therapy versus usual care in the treatment of pain conditions, excluding headache and pain associated with malignant disease.[66]

Hypnosis

Several hypnotic approaches are commonly utilized in the treatment of chronic pain, including direct suggestion of anesthesia, glove anesthesia, pain displacement, and physical dissociation. Multiple studies comparing hypnosis to a no-treatment intervention have shown that hypnosis interventions consistently produce significant decreases in pain associated with a variety of chronic-pain problems, including low back injuries and arthritis.[67] A review of 13 studies evaluating hypnosis in the treatment of chronic pain, excluding headache, found that hypnosis is generally more effective for pain reduction than nonhypnotic interventions such as attention, physical therapy, and education in the treatment of chronic pain. However, these studies suffered from a lack of standardization of the hypnotic techniques used, low enrollment, and a lack of long-term follow up.[68]

Biofeedback

The goal of biofeedback is to help patients learn to control physiological processes through monitoring and feedback of physiologic variables, such as heart rate or skin temperature. Some researchers suggest pain can be maintained or exacerbated by autonomic nervous system dysregulation and that through training with biofeedback, people can repair the autonomic nervous system.[65] An example is electromyographic feedback in patients with tension headaches, which teaches patients to manipulate the tension in their frontalis muscle. A meta-analysis of 94 studies evaluating the benefit of biofeedback in the treatment of adult migraine and tension headache found a significant decrease in the frequency of headaches, improved perceived self-efficacy, decreased symptoms of anxiety and depression, and decreased medication consumption.[69] Given the established benefit of biofeedback in the treatment of headaches, further studies of biofeedback in the treatment of chronic pain, such as low back pain, are warranted.

Meditation

Meditation has been identified as a widely used mind-body therapy for chronic pain relief.[70] Mindful-meditation is the meditative technique that is most commonly researched and utilized for the treatment of chronic pain.[71] Mindfulness meditation is a detached awareness, in which one allows all thoughts to enter consciousness, and then lets them go without emotional attachment. Kabat-Zinn describes the process of pain reduction with mindfulness meditation as an "uncoupling" of the physical sensation from the emotional and cognitive experience of pain.[72]

Mindful-meditation can be an effective strategy for helping chronic pain patients cope more effectively with their conditions. In a four-year follow-up report, the majority (60%–72%) of 225 chronic pain patients who had completed an eight-week mindful-meditation program reported "moderate to great improvement" in pain status.[73] These findings suggest that meditation programs, especially mindful-meditation, may alleviate both the short- and long-term effects of chronic pain; however, more research needs to be performed to establish meditation as an effective intervention in the treatment of chronic pain in diverse populations.

Mind-body therapy summary

Mind-body therapies show evidence that they can be beneficial for chronic pain from various causes. Though the evidence has shortcomings, given the safety of the therapies, we recommend exploring these modalities with the chronic pain patient.

SUMMARY

An Integrative Medicine (IM) approach to pain therapeutics utilizes multiple strategies to contribute to an improved clinical state. In addition, it can often allow for better understanding of the patient-specific context. A Mediterranean diet can lower pro-inflammatory compounds in the body, and adding fruits, vegetables, and legumes to the diet could in the long term potentially improve the overall pain profile. Fish oil supplements of three grams daily, and a trial of either glucosamine sulfate with chondroitin at 1500 mg/1200 mg or SAMe at 600–1200 mg total daily may also be beneficial. Encouraging exercise, especially yoga and low-impact high-aerobic exercise such as swimming, could be important to mitigate chronic pain. Cognitive behavioral therapy (CBT) or biofeedback could be helpful, and acupuncture could be considered. Regardless of specific modalities chosen, exploration with the patient will allow some control in the matter, and increase commitment to the approach.

Our recommendation is not to throw multiple modalities at chronic pain at one time, but instead to offer two to three therapies as appropriate each visit. The strength of the IM approach is that it allows us to focus more explicitly on the patient's context, both in terms of pain inputs, as well as following the patient's goals in mitigating pain. Certainly, the level of evidence for the therapies is often not as strong as ideal, and more study is needed. However, given our precept to "do no harm," and as the modalities have good safety profiles, the overall net effect to the patient can be beneficial.

REFERENCES

1. Giordano J, Michael ME. A crisis in chronic pain care: an ethical analysis. Part three: toward an integrative, multi-disciplinary pain medicine built around the needs of the patient. *Pain Physician.* 2008;11:775–784.
2. Boothby JL, Thorn BE, Overduin LY, et al. Catastrophizing and perceived partner responses to pain. *Pain.* 2004;109:500–506.
3. Turk DC, Okifuj A, Sharff L. Chronic pain and depression: role of perceived impact and perceived control in different age cohorts. *Pain.* 1995;61:93–101.
4. Seaman DR. The diet-induced proinflammatory state: a cause of chronic pain and other degenerative diseases? *J Manipulative Physiol Ther.* 2002;25(3):168–179.
5. Hagen KB, Byfuglien MG, Flazon L, et al. Dietary interventions for rheumatoid arthritis. *Cochrane Database Syst Rev.* 2009;(1):CD006400.
6. Plaeger SF. Clinical immunology and traditional herbal medicines. *Clin Vaccine Immunol.* 2003;10(3):337–338.
7. Blumenthal M, Goldberg A, Brinckmann J. *Herbal Medicine: Expanded Commission E Monographs.* 2000. Integrative Medicine Communications.
8. Funk JL, Frye JB, Oyarzo JN, et al. Efficacy and mechanism of action of turmeric supplements in the treatment of experimental arthritis. *Arthritis Rheum.* 2006; 54(11):3452–3464.
9. Goldberg RJ, Katz J. A meta-analysis of the analgesic effects of omega-3 polyunsaturated fatty acid supplementation for inflammatory joint pain. *Pain.* 2007;129:210–223.
10. Ameye LG, Chee WS. Osteoarthritis and nutrition. From nutraceuticals to functional foods: a systematic review of the scientific evidence. *Arthritis Res Ther.* 2006;8(4):R127.
11. Leffler CT, Philippi AF, Leffler SG, et al. Glucosamine, chondroitin, and manganese ascorbate for degenerative joint disease of the knee or low back: a randomized, double-blind, placebo-controlled pilot study. *Mil Med.* 1999;164(2):85–91.
12. McAlindon TE, LaValley MP, Gulin JP, et al. Glucosamine and chondroitin for treatment of osteoarthritis: a systematic quality assessment and meta-analysis. *JAMA.* 2000;283(11):1469–1475.
13. Vlad SC, LaValley MP, McAlindon TE, et al. Glucosamine for pain in osteoarthritis: why do trial results differ? *Arthritis Rheum.* 2007;56(7):2267–2277.
14. Najm WI, Reinsch S, Hoehler F, et al. S-adenosyl methionine (SAMe) versus celecoxib for the treatment of osteoarthritis symptoms: A double-blind crossover trial. *BMC Musculoskelet Disord.* 2004;5:6.
15. Hardy M, Coulter I, Morton SC, et al. *S-Adenosyl-L-Methionine for Treatment of Depression, Osteoarthritis, and Liver Disease.* Evidence Report/Technology Assessment Number 64. Agency for Healthcare Research and Quality, US Dept of Health and Human Services. AHRQ publication 02-E033. Rockville, MD; 2002.
16. Soeken KL, Lee WL, Bausell RB, et al. Safety and efficacy of S-adenosylmethionine (SAMe) for osteoarthritis. *J Fam Pract.* 2002;51:425–430.
17. Panjabi MM. A hypothesis of chronic back pain: ligament subfailure injuries lead to muscle control dysfunction. *Eur Spine J.* 2006;15(5):668–676.
18. Melzak R. From the gate to the neuromatrix. *Pain.* 1999 August (suppl 6):S121–S126.
19. Wright A, Sluka KA. Nonpharmacological treatments for musculoskeletal pain. *Clin J Pain.* 2001;17:33–46.
20. Bronfort G, Haas M, Evans RL, et al. Efficacy of spinal manipulation and mobilization for low back pain and neck pain: a systematic review and best evidence synthesis. *Spine J.* 2004;4(3):335–356.

21. Ferreira ML, Ferreira PH, Latimer J, et al. Does spinal manipulative therapy help people with chronic low back pain? *Aust J Physiother.* 2002;48(4):277–284.

22. Ferreira ML, Ferreira PH, Latimer J, et al. Efficacy of spinal manipulative therapy for low back pain of less than three months' duration. *J Manipulative Physiol Ther.* 2003;26(9):593–601.

23. Chou R, Huffman LH. Nonpharmacologic therapies for acute and chronic low back pain: a review of the evidence for an American Pain Society/American College of Physicians clinical practice guideline. *Ann Intern Med.* 2007;147(7):492–504.

24. Andersson GB, Lucente T, Davis AM. A comparison of osteopathic spinal manipulation with standard care for patients with low back pain. *N Engl J Med.* 1999;341(19):1426–1431.

25. Williams NH, Wilkinson C, Russell I. Randomized osteopathic manipulation study (ROMANS): pragmatic trial for spinal pain in primary care. *Fam Pract.* 2003;20(6):662–669.

26. Field TM. Massage therapy effects. *Am Psychol.* 1998;53(12):1270–1281.

27. Furlan AD, Brosseau L, Imamura M, et al. Massage for low back pain [review]. *Cochrane Database Syst Rev.* 2002;(2):CD001929.

28. Ireland M, Olson M. Massage therapy and therapeutic touch in children: state of the science. *Altern Ther Health Med.* 2000;6:54–63.

29. Lund I, Ge Y, Yu LC. Repeated massage-like stimulation induces long-term effects on nociception: contribution of oxytocinergic mechanisms. *Eur J Neurosci.* 2002;16(2):330–338.

30. Hsieh CY, Phillips RB, Adams AH, et al. Functional outcomes of low back pain: comparison of four treatment groups in a randomized controlled trial. *J Manipulative Physiol Ther.* 1992;15(1):4–9.

31. Godfrey CM, Morgan PP, Schatzker J. A randomized trial of manipulation for low-back pain in a medical setting. *Spine.* 1984;9(3):301–304.

32. Pope MH, Phillips RB, Haugh LD, et al. A prospective randomized three week trial of spinal manipulation, transcutaneous muscle stimulation, massage and corset in the treatment of subacute low back pain. *Spine.* 1994;19(22):2571–2577.

33. Cherkin DC, Sherman KJ, Deyo RA, et al. A review of the evidence for the effectiveness, safety, and cost of acupuncture, massage therapy, and spinal manipulation for back pain. *Arch Intern Med.* 2003;138(11):898–906.

34. Little P, Lewith G, Webley F, et al. Randomised controlled trial of Alexander technique lessons, exercise, and massage (ATEAM) for chronic and recurrent back pain. *BMJ.* 2008;337:a884.

35. Oliphant D. Safety of spinal manipulation in the treatment of lumbar disk herniations: a systematic review and risk assessment. *J Manipulative Physiol Ther.* 2004; 27(3):197–210.

36. Stevinson C, Ernst E. Risks associated with spinal manipulation. *Am J Med.* 2002; 112(7):566–571.

37. Klougart N, Leboeuf-Yde C, Rasmussen LR. Safety in chiropractic practice. Part II: treatment to the upper neck and the rate of cerebrovascular incidents. *J Manipulative Physiol Ther.* 1996;19(6):563–569.

38. Koes BW, Assendelft WJ, van der Heijden GJ, et al. Spinal manipulation for low back pain. An updated systematic review of randomized clinical trials. *Spine.* 1996;21(24):2860–2871.

39. Kapral MK, Bondy SJ. Cervical manipulation and risk of stroke. *CMAJ.* 2001; 165(7):907–908.

40. Jing-Nuan W. A short history of acupuncture. *J Altern Complement Med.* 1996;2(1):19–21.

41. The Academy of Traditional Chinese Medicine. *An Outline of Chinese Acupuncture.* Peking: Foreign Languages Press; 1975.

42. National Center for Complementary and Alternative Medicine. Acupuncture: an introduction. http://nccam.nih.gov.elibrary.aecom.yu.edu/health/acupuncture/introduction.htm#. Accessed April 9, 2009.

43. Hui KK, Liu J, Makris N, et al. Acupuncture modulates the limbic system and subcortical gray structures of the human brain: evidence from fMRI studies in normal subjects. *Hum Brain Mapp.* 2000;9(1):13–25.

44. Manheimer E, White A, Berman B, et al. Meta-analysis: acupuncture for low back pain. *Ann Intern Med.* 2005;142:651–663.

45. Brinkhaus B, Becker-Witt C, Jena S, et al. Acupuncture in patients with chronic low back pain. *Arch Intern Med.* 2006;166:450–457.

46. Molsberger AF, Mau J, Pawelec DB, et al. Does acupuncture improve the orthopedic management of chronic low back pain—a randomized, blinded, controlled trial with 3 months follow up. *Pain.* 2002;99(3):579–587.

47. Chung A, Bui L, Mills E. Adverse effects of acupuncture. Which are clinically significant? *Can Fam Physician.* 2003;49:985–989.

48. Ernst G, Strzyz H, Hagmeister H. Incidence of adverse effects during acupuncture therapy—a multicentre survey. *Complement Ther Med.* 2003;11(2):93–97.

49. Filshie J. Safety aspects of acupuncture in palliative care. *Acupunct Med.* 2001; 19(2):117–122.

50. MacPherson H, Thomas K, Walters S, et al. A prospective survey of adverse events and treatment reactions following 34,000 consultations with professional acupuncturists. *Acupunct Med.* 2001;19(2):93–102.

51. Kalauokalani D, Cherkin DC, Sherman KJ, et al. Lessons from a trial of acupuncture and massage for low back pain: patient expectations and treatment effects. *Spine* (Phila Pa 1976). 2001;26(13):1418–1424.

52. Garfinkel M, Schumacher HR Jr. Yoga. *Rheum Dis Clin North Am.* 2000;26(1):125–132, x.

53. Saper RB, Eisenberg DM, Davis RB, et al. Prevalence and patterns of adult yoga use in the United States: results of a national survey. *Altern Ther Health Med.* 2004;10(2):44–49.

54. Garfinkel MS, Singhal A, Katz WA, et al. Yoga-based intervention for carpal tunnel syndrome: a randomized trial. *JAMA.* 1998;280(18):1601–1603.

55. Garfinkel MS, Schumacher HR Jr, Husain A, et al. Evaluation of a yoga based regimen for treatment of osteoarthritis of the hands. *J Rheumatol.* 1994;21(12):2341–2343.

56. Maurer BT, Stern AG, Kinossian B, et al. Osteoarthritis of the knee: isokinetic quadriceps exercise versus an educational intervention. *Arch Phys Med Rehabil.* 1999;80(10):1293–1299.

57. Fisher NM, Gresham G, Pendergast DR. Effects of a quantitative progressive rehabilitation program applied unilaterally to the osteoarthritic knee. *Arch Phys Med Rehabil.* 1993;74(12):1319–1326.

58. Kreindler H, Lewis CB, Rush S. Effect of three exercise protocols on strength of persons with osteoarthritis of the knee. *Top Geriatr Rehabil.* 1989;4:32–39.

59. Sherman KJ, Cherkin DC, Erro J, et al. Comparing yoga, exercise, and a self-care book for chronic low back pain: a randomized, controlled trial. *Ann Intern Med.* 2005;143(12):849–856.

60. Flor H. Cortical reorganization and chronic pain: implications of rehabilitation. *J Rehabil Med.* 2003;41(suppl):66–72.

61. Kerr CE, Wasserman RH, Moore CI. Cortical dynamics as a therapeutic mechanism for touch healing. *J Altern Complement Med.* 2007;13(1):59–66.

62. Flor H, Knost B, Birbaumer N. Processing of pain- and body-related verbal material in chronic pain patients: central and peripheral correlates. *Pain.* 1997;73(3):413–421.

63. Flor H, Elbert T, Knecht S, et al. Phantom-limb pain as a perceptual correlate of cortical reorganization following arm amputation. *Nature.* 1995;375(6531):482–484.

64. Morley S, Eccleston C, Williams A. Systematic review and meta-analysis of randomized controlled trials of cognitive behaviour therapy and behaviour therapy for chronic pain in adults, excluding headache. *Pain.* 1999;80(1–2):1–13.

65. Turk DC, Swanson KS, Tunks ER. Psychological approaches in the treatment of chronic pain patients—when pills, scalpels, and needles are not enough. *Can J Psychiatry.* 2008;53(4):213–223.

66. Eccleston C, Williams AC, Morley S. Psychological therapies for the management of chronic pain (excluding headache) in adults. *Cochrane Database Syst Rev.* 2009;(2):CD007407.

67. Yapko M. *Trancework.* 3rd ed. New York, NY: Brunner-Routledge; 2003.

68. Elkins G, Jensen MP, Patterson DR. Hypnotherapy for the management of chronic pain. *Int J Clin Exp Hypn.* 2007;55(3):275–287.

69. Nestoriuc Y, Martin A, Rief W, et al. Biofeedback treatment for headache disorders: a comprehensive efficacy review. *Appl Psychophysiol Biofeedback.* 2008;33(3):125–140.

70. Wolsko PM, Eisenberg DM, Davis RB, et al. Use of mind-body medical therapies. *J Gen Intern Med.* 2004;19(1):43–50.

71. Teixeira ME. Meditation as an intervention for chronic pain: an integrative review. *Holist Nurs Pract.* 2008;22(4):225–234.

72. Kabat-Zinn J. An outpatient program in behavioral medicine for chronic pain patients based on the practice of mindfulness meditation: theoretical considerations and preliminary results. *Gen Hosp Psychiatry.* 1982;4(1):33–47.

73. Kabat-Zinn J, Lipworth L, Burney R. Four-year follow-up of a meditation-based program for the self-regulation of chronic pain: treatment outcomes and compliance. *Clin J Pain.* 1987;2:159–173.

29

PHYSICIANS' PERCEPTION OF PAIN AS RELATED TO EMPATHY, SYMPATHY AND THE MIRROR-NEURON SYSTEM

MOHAMMADREZA HOJAT, PHD
Research Professor of Psychiatry and Human Behavior,
Director of Jefferson Longitudinal Study, Center for
Research in Medical Education and Health Care, Jefferson
Medical College, Philadelphia, Pennsylvania, USA

MITCHELL J.M. COHEN, MD
Vice Chair for Education, Director, Pain Medicine Program,
Department of Psychiatry, Jefferson Medical College,
Philadelphia, Pennsylvania, USA

Key Points

- Pain is conceptualized as an experience comprising somatosensory, cognitive, and emotional components.
- The physician's understanding of a patient's pain is enhanced through cognitive (empathy), emotional (sympathy), and neurological (mirror-neuron system) activation.
- The link between cognitive, emotional, and somatosensory pain components in patients, and empathy, sympathy, and neurological activation in physicians can be explained by the perception-action model.
- Brain imaging studies suggest that similar brain regions are activated in a person experiencing pain and an observer of the person in pain.
- The distinct cognitive (e.g., empathic engagement) and emotional (e.g., sympathetic involvement) responses to observing others' pain require study with brain imaging to identify brain regions associated with these responses.
- Because empathic understanding contributes to better clinical outcomes, but excessive sympathy can impede objectivity in clinical reasoning and decisions, ample opportunities must be provided in medical education to enhance empathy, and regulate sympathy in physicians-in-training.

*"By far, the most frequently used drug in general practice was the doctor.
It was not only the bottle of medicine or the box of pills that mattered,
but the way doctor gave them."*

Michael Balint[1]

*The baby startled first at the touch of the immunization needle in her tiny thigh,
then came bursts of cries. The mother anxiously rushed to her baby's side, held
her tight in her arms, gently put the baby on her chest, while patting her back
started to talk in a calm motherly voice: "Oh my little girl ... don't cry baby, it's
over ... ." The little girl gazed at her mother's eyes, stopped crying, cuddling in
the security of her mother's arms as if her pain had gone away to the sky. ...
I accompanied my wife and my daughter that day to the pediatrician's office,
observed this event happen between my daughter and my wife, and wondered
"What is in the mother's tender care that soothes her baby's pain?"*

(Personal observation of one of the authors, MH).

EMBARKING ON A JOURNEY

The soothing effect of a mother's tender loving care on her baby's pain, described in the aforementioned observation, is a prototype of the analgesic value of empathic attention by a significant person.[2] A physician, as a significant authority figure, delivers the gift of healing to a patient in pain in a similar manner. It is the human need for affiliation that prompts us to feel soothed in the presence of significant others, and to feel distressed when left behind.[3] In this chapter, we embark on a journey that will attempt to provide explanations for the aforementioned observation.

EXPERIENCE OF PAIN IN THE PATIENT

Pain, according to the International Association for the Study of Pain, is defined as "An unpleasant sensory and emotional experience associated with actual or potential tissue damage."[4] This complex definition sets forth the core elements of human pain: activated sensation, affective reaction, and cognitive appraisal. All three components are subjectively experienced and objectively demonstrated in functional brain imaging. These components exhibit plasticity, the capacity to change dramatically in response to internal and external events. The findings that placebos can alter patients' pain support the notion that perception of pain is a bio-psycho-social experience that "includes cognitive evaluation of the potential for harm and affect as well as sensory components."[5]

PHYSICIAN'S UNDERSTANDING OF PATIENT'S PAIN

A physician's understanding and feeling of a patient's pain is enhanced through three channels: the cognitive account (empathy), affective sharing (sympathy), and activation of the mirror-neuron system (MNS).

1. Cognitive account (empathy)

Effective physicians possess interpersonal skills that facilitate human connection and a treatment relationship, which leads to improved understanding of patients' problems and concerns. According to Goubert and colleagues,[2] a better understanding of others in pain requires an understanding of empathy, which is itself rooted in the human need for affiliation and developed out of evolutionary pressure for survival.[6]

The findings that human beings are capable of reacting to the distress of others at an early age[7-9] and that infants are capable of imitating adults' facial gestures[10] provide support for the notion that the roots of empathy extend beyond social learning. Empathic capacity, anchored in an in-born neural network, demonstrates plasticity similar to human pain, influenced by factors including early attachment experiences, learning, and education.[6]

Despite the importance of empathy in patient care, there is a lingering controversy about its conceptualization and there is no consensus on its definition.[6] Adding to the conceptualization issue is the notion that there are different types of empathy. For example, Davis[11,12] describes two kinds of empathy: "cognitive" and "emotional." Cognitive empathy is described as: "attempts to entertain the perspective of others"[12] and "the capacity for role taking."[12] Emotional empathy, on the other hand is described as: "a tendency to react emotionally to the observed experiences of others."[12] Emotional empathy has also been described in terms of "vicarious empathy."[13] To avoid the conceptualization dilemma, we suggest that: (1) cognitive empathy is more in tune with our adapted definition of empathy in the context of patient care (see below), and is the intended meaning of empathy in this chapter; (2) emotional or vicarious empathy is an entity that we believe is conceptually equivalent to the notion of sympathy (see below).

In the context of patient care we adapted the following definition of empathy as a predominantly *cognitive* (rather than an emotional) attribute that involves an *understanding* of patients' experiences, concerns, and perspectives (rather than shared feelings) combined with a capacity to *communicate* both this understanding and an *intention to help*.[6,14,15] In addition, we propose that a helping behavior that results from an empathic engagement in patient care is likely to emerge from an *altruistic* motivation.[16] This speculation is supported by Batson[17] and Valeriani et al[18] who suggest that it is the intrinsically altruistic nature of empathy that prompts individuals to help others, even if rendering such help could result in personal distress or physical danger. According to Tait,[19] such empathic engagement is a powerful tool in pain management.

Empathy is a nonemotional entity that often requires intentionality,[2] voluntary effort, and active mentalizing.[6,20,21] Empathic understanding has been described within the frame of the theory of mind,[22] which is a capacity to represent the state of mind of others.[23] A special feature of empathy in patient care is that an empathic physician stands in his or her patients' shoes, knowing that self and patient should not be merged into one. Such merging crosses the border between empathy and sympathy, resulting in the clinician and patient sharing emotions and pain. Because of its cognitive nature, empathy always improves understanding. Empathy, even in excess, can lead to personal growth and career satisfaction for the physician, and to optimal clinical outcomes for the patient.[24,25] It is thus reasonable to assume a direct relationship between empathy and clinical outcomes, such that outcomes progressively improve with increasing empathy, reaching a maximum clinical effect but never decreasing.[6,14,15]

2. Emotional sharing (sympathy)

In contrast to empathy, sympathy is an emotional state. Feeling patients' pain and sharing patients' suffering are features of sympathetic involvement. Similar to empathy, there is no agreed upon definition of sympathy in patient care. As a result, empathy and sympathy have often mistakenly been used interchangeably.

In the context of patient care, we adapted the following definition of sympathy as a predominantly *emotional* (as opposed to cognitive) attribute that involves *feeling* (as opposed to understanding) of patients' pain and suffering.[6,15] We also propose that helping behaviors resulting from sympathy are likely to serve *egoistic* motivations, perhaps alleviating the helper's distress that develops when emotions and pain are shared.[6,15,16] Because of its emotional nature, an overabundance of sympathy can impede objectivity, which is central to optimal clinical reasoning and decision making.

Sympathetic involvement, in contrast to empathic engagement, often occurs rapidly, automatically, and involuntarily.[6,20] When we watch a fallen athlete on the stadium floor unable to rise after a severe injury, we feel sympathy. We may gasp, feel intense anxiety, a "pit" in our stomachs, and vicariously feel the pain of the injured competitor.[26] We do not immediately cognitively analyze how to address the injury. This immediate response is akin to what we are calling sympathy. In contrast, empathy is less hamstrung by reactive emotionality and can lead to a plan of action. Frequent sympathetic involvement in patient care can be exhausting for physicians, leading to career burnout, compassion fatigue,[25] and vicarious traumatization.[27] Therefore, we speculate that the relationship between sympathy and clinical outcomes resembles an inverted U shape (similar to that between anxiety and performance), implying that while controlled, limited sympathy may be beneficial; excessive sympathy, however, can be detrimental.[6,15]

Despite their distinguishing features in painful suffering, emotion (the driving force in sympathy) cannot subjectively be fully isolated from cognition (the driving force in empathy). Separately and in their interactions, sympathy and empathy have different consequences in patient care,[6,15] thus it is important to distinguish them.[28] In the context of patient care, an overlap of about 24% has been reported between the two concepts.[6] (This overlap was calculated from a correlation of 0.49 between measures of empathy and sympathy: $r=0.49$, coefficient of determination or $r^2=0.49^2=.24$.) Mindfulness of emotional factors is central to optimal patient care as a point of human connection and an aspect of the medical history. Excessive emotional involvement in patient care, however, benefits neither the physician nor the patient.

3. Mirror-neuron system (MNS)

A third approach to understanding another person in pain is through a neurophysiological mechanism known as the *mirror-neuron system (MNS)*, originally discovered in monkeys at the University of Parma in Italy.[29,30] It was found that a set of neurons in the ventral premotor cortex of the monkeys' brain (known as the F5 area) discharged when the monkey observed others performing hand actions (e.g., grasping, tearing, holding, manipulation).[31] The same set of neuron cells discharged when the monkey actually performed the same hand actions.

It was also found that the brain area F5 contained a population of neurons—audio-visual mirror-neurons—that discharge not just with the execution or observation of a specific action but also when this action was only heard (e.g., tearing paper, breaking nuts).[31,32] At the University of California in Los Angeles, the MNS was demonstrated in humans.[33]

An important finding with regard to the MNS is that observed acts must be goal-directed to recruit mirror-neurons, meaning that random acts or acts performed by robots do not activate the MNS.[34] Goal-directed, non-repetitive robot acts, however, can activate the MNS.[35] These findings imply that the MNS has a mediating role not only in the understanding of others' actions, but also in predicting the goals and consequences of such actions.[31,36,37]

EXPLANATORY MECHANISM: PERCEPTION-ACTION MODEL (PAM)

Over a century ago, Theodore Lipps, who introduced the concept of empathy (*einfühlung* in the German language) into psychology, stated: "When I observe a circus performer walking on a tight rope, I feel I am inside him." (Cited in Carr et al.[38]) He also proposed that seeing someone else's facial expression triggers the observer to automatically adopt a similar facial expression, known as facial mimicry (cited in Jabbi and Keysers).[39] These behaviors can be explained by the perception-action model (PAM) formulated by Preston and de Waal.[40] They suggested that perceptions of another person's cognitive, emotional, and somatosensory states automatically activate representations of those states in the observer, unless inhibited.[40]

The link between the PAM, empathy, and sympathy is supported by findings that nonconscious mimicry of the postures, mannerisms, and facial expressions of others (also known as the chameleon effect)[41] can be observed to a greater extent in more empathic and sympathetic individuals.[38] In general, studies of the MNS, mimicry, imitation of facial expressions, empathy, and sympathy, indicate that all are triggered by mechanisms that transform perception to action.[42] The PAM also helps to understand mechanisms underlying the physician-patient connection in pain experiences. Craig and Weiss[43] proposed that exposure to others in pain has a significant effect on our perception of pain, because, through PAM, such exposure elicits imitation that activates cognitive, emotional, and behavioral representations of the state of the person in pain.

RESEARCH PARADIGMS IN PERCEPTION OF PAIN

Three approaches have often been used in social neuroscience research to study perception of pain: (1) studying pain parameters when the person is experiencing pain (self pain); (2) recording psychological changes and neurological activities (e.g., by functional magnetic resonance imaging, fMRI) when observing another person in pain and imagining one's self as experiencing the other person's pain (self-perspective, or first-person perspective); (3) recording psychological changes and neurological activities when an observer watches another person in pain and imagines how that person experiences pain (other-perspective or third-person perspective).

In one of the earlier experiments on perception of pain in others, conducted by Ezra Stotland,[44] three groups of participants viewed a subject whose hand was strapped in a heat generating machine. One group was instructed just to watch the event nonjudgmentally (neutral observation). The second group was instructed to imagine their own hand strapped in the machine (self-perspective). The third group was told to imagine how the person whose hand was strapped was feeling (other-perspective). It was found that imagining the pain of others could generate empathic and sympathetic connections, and produce tangible physiological responses (e.g., palm sweating, galvanic skin response) that corresponded to perception of pain as predicted by PAM. Data from functional brain imaging studies show that imagining pain in self and others, in the absence of any painful stimulus, activates critical brain areas involved in pain perception.[26] Words evocative of pain in one's self or others can also activate the brain's pain matrix.[45]

Observing someone in pain activates neurons in the observer similar to those that are firing in the person experiencing pain.[46,47] In addition, it was noticed that self-perspective, compared to other-perspective, yielded higher pain ratings and involved greater activation of the limbic, prefrontal, and secondary (versus primary) somatosensory cortex. The primary somatosensory cortex (S1) is involved in precise localization and characterization of pain, which is required to accurately diagnose and treat patients. The primary somatosensory cortex shows relatively less activation in observers adopting the self-perspective. Thus the self-perspective's strong emotional identification with the sufferer reduces activation of analytic-cognitive capacities required for optimal care.

This brain's pain-related network, also referred to as the brain's pain matrix, includes biological correlates for the sensory, emotional, and cognitive components of pain.[48] The ventrolateral thalamus and primary somatosensory cortex are involved in accurate localization, quantification, and description of the sensory component. The dorsomedial thalamus, amygdala, anterior cingulate cortex (ACC), anterior insular cortex (AI), as well as medial prefrontal and orbitofrontal cortex convey emotional aspects of pain and connect new pain to memories of past painful experiences.[49] These emotionally important regions are among those activated when observers adopt the self-pain perspective. The dorsolateral prefrontal cortex, and middle and posterior cingulate cortex are involved in the cognitive appraisal and planning component of pain. These areas are activated when observers adopt the other-pain perspective.[2]

An important issue suffering benign neglect in pain research is the psychological motivation prompting us to help people in pain. Perception of pain via the self-perspective approach is likely to initiate an egoistic motivation to reduce personal distress associated with the activated brain that controls emotional pain response; whereas the other-perspective approach is likely to instigate an altruistic motivation to help,[2,16,17] which at least in part, derives from activation of the cognitive-evaluative regions of the pain matrix. Altruistic motivation is more aligned with our characterization of cognitively focused empathy, which allows planning. Egoistic motivation fits better with our description of emotionally driven sympathy.

Whether observation of pain in others leads to empathic engagement (and altruistic motivation) or to sympathetic distress (and egoistic motivation), depends upon maintaining the self-other differentiation.[50] The self-other separation is blurred in self-perspective, but more distinct and better preserved in the other-perspective. In other words, in the self-perspective observation the clinician and patient merge in one (and ultimately become "*I am you*"), while in the other-perspective they preserve their separate individuality and remain distinct as two individuals ("*I and you*"). Thus, the other-perspective is better matched to the clinical reasoning and action required of physicians.

COMMON NEUROLOGICAL UNDERPINNINGS

Technological advances in functional brain imaging have provided a real-time window into brain events during human pain. Whether pain starts from a blow to the spleen or to the right thumb, the resulting activated pain matrix involves increased neuronal firing in areas throughout the brain. These linked activated brain regions fire bilaterally, sequentially, and hierarchically. The pain matrix demonstrates linked activated regions spanning levels from the medulla to the prefrontal cortex. The matrix is responsive to a wide range of internal and external influences, from the quality of sleep and level of anxiety to ambient temperature, barometric pressure, and stressful events.[51,52]

In prior sections we have attributed components of the pain experience in the sufferer and observer to various brain regions. Our ability to do so is a result of remarkable research findings from studies applying functional brain imaging technology. These studies have included imaging the brains of patients experiencing the pain of chronic illness as well as imaging these patients and normal subjects when given experimentally controlled painful stimuli (e.g., heat, cold, pinch, gastric distention, chest pain). Brain imaging has also been performed when subjects are imagining pain, watching video recordings of sports injuries, and distracted or emotionally aroused during administration of painful stimuli.[26] Functional MRI (fMRI) research[21,46,47,53–55] and neurophysiological studies[56–58] have demonstrated the neurophysiology of the MNS, showing changes in activation of the pain matrix (e.g., ACC and AI) when subjects observe painful stimuli delivered to other individuals[47,53,54,59–61] or when they imagine their partners in a painful situation.[21]

These studies provide evidence for the neurological underpinnings of why we flinch, wince, cringe, or recoil when observing others in pain and almost "feel" the hurt.[18] Affective brain regions (ACC and AI) are activated by observing a loved one receiving a painful electric shock.[21] It is interesting to note that research participants with higher scores on measures of empathy or sympathy (e.g., Interpersonal Reactivity Index,[11,12] and Balanced Emotional Empathy Scale[62]) showed stronger activations in pain-related areas when observing their partners being subjected to painful stimuli.[21]

In a pain study, a series of pictures of hands and feet in painful situations and another series of pictures of hands and feet in nonpainful situations were shown to research participants.[47] The fMRI images showed activation of several brain regions in the observers that are known to play a significant role in pain processing (e.g., ACC, AI, the cerebellum). Brain regions associated with feeling an emotion can be influenced by seeing the facial expression of that emotion, a phenomenon described as emotional contagion or sympathy.[21] For example, the observation of disgust automatically activates neural substrates that are selectively activated during the feeling of disgust.[63]

Several neuroimaging studies have demonstrated commonalities and differences in pain matrix activation when subjects experience pain themselves and when they observe others in pain.[53] Common areas include thalamus, ACC, AI, and prefrontal cortex (PFC). Observers do not show activation of S1, which codes the sensory intensity, location, and quality of pain.[26,51] Specifically, areas involved in emotional and cognitive responses to pain are activated in both experienced and observed pain.

This is especially true when the person in pain is a significant person, such as a family member, friend, or partner.[64] For example, mothers listened to recorded infant cries and white noise control sounds. The fMRI results indicated that the mothers showed significantly greater ACC activity during the infant cries compared to control sounds. The ACC and right medial PFC were the brain regions showing substantial increased activity with the cries compared to white noise. This finding demonstrates the plasticity or reactivity of the pain matrix to internal psychological factors.

In another fMRI study, it was observed that the bilateral AI, rostral ACC, brainstem, and cerebellum were activated when subjects received pain or were signaled that loved ones were experiencing pain. It was noted that activation in brain areas when observing others in pain is correlated with individual empathy scores,[21] suggesting that empathy is one royal road to understanding others in pain.

Evidence also suggests that empathic engagement seems to be more contingent upon the frontocortical brain areas, which have been implicated in mentalization and the theory of mind.[20,22] The medial PFC has also been implicated in the theory of mind,[65] suggesting that this area of the brain may constitute a partial system for empathy.[20] The medial PFC appears to play a role in the ruminative focus on pain and apprehension about pain's implications.

Sympathetic involvement with a person in pain increased activity in the AI and thalamus, which are involved in processing negative or unpleasant emotions.[20] It is also interesting to note that pain-related areas in the ACC have extensive output connections to premotor areas, a brain region observed to contain much of the MNS in macaque monkeys.[53]

Some of the same neural activities in the experience of physical pain are also involved in the experience of social pain (e.g., separation, rejection, social exclusion, losing a significant person).[3] Thus, the expression of being *hurt* by experiencing loneliness, rejection, and separation is not metaphoric only, but real in nature and operates by sharing common neuroanatomical underpinnings with physical pain. Studies have demonstrated that sadness, social exclusion, and physical pain activate similar limbic regions (e.g., ACC, AI).[42] It should also be mentioned that in addition to the somatosensory, cognitive, and emotional factors, other variables such as genetics, gender, and culture contribute to the perception of pain and to the physicians' approach in the treatment of pain.[66–68]

CONCLUDING REMARKS

In this chapter we attempted to explain the perception of patient pain, as observed by the physician through psychosocial and neurological processes such as empathy, sympathy, and a synchronized neurological interaction between patient and physicians, known as the mirror-neuron system.

Our argument that empathy in patient care can always lead to positive outcomes, but sympathy in excess could be detrimental, has important implications for medical education and physician training. We suggest a two-fold training approach to foster empathy and regulate sympathy: (1) Develop targeted programs to enhance physicians' empathic understanding of their patients, and the ability to form therapeutic interpersonal connections with them. (2) Train physicians to regulate their tendency to emotionally "feel" their patients' pain and suffering. Some specific approaches to enhance empathic understanding (but not sympathetic involvement) in patient care have been suggested.[14] It is imperative to specifically remind physicians who treat pain patients to control strong affective responses to patients' symptoms, while at the same time closing gaps in the empathic understanding of patients in pain. Physicians must exert full efforts to understand, but not join, patients' pain and suffering.

Based on our review of the literature on neurological imaging in pain research, no clear distinction has been made between clinician empathy and sympathy (or cognition and emotion) and their differential effects on patients' pain. Thus, current pain research outcomes cannot be specifically attributed to only one of the two concepts. There are, however, a few exceptions in which attempts were made to separate cognitive and emotional empathy[20,69,70] with limited success.

The challenge ahead is to develop research designs that evoke empathic responses on one occasion, and sympathetic reactions on another, and examine similarities and differences in brain activation between those reactions (e.g., using event-related brain imaging). Based on our characterization of empathy and sympathy, in combination with preliminary neurological findings,[19,60,61] we predict distinct brain activation for empathy (e.g., prefrontal cortex) and sympathy (e.g., insular and cingulate cortex). Brain lesion research may also shed light on the detrimental effects of damage to cortical or limbic structures of empathy (cognitive understanding) and sympathy (emotional involvement).

THE END OF THE JOURNEY

How does the observation of a mother soothing her baby after an immunization prick relate to our journey in this chapter? Maternal love includes a good dose of empathy, sympathy, and neurophysiological attunement that foster infant development, and ultimately human survival. These neuro-psycho-social entities serve as strong glue for human affiliation, attachment, and bonding. These features, in the context of patient care, lay the foundation for a compassionate and trusting patient-physician relationship. The combined effects of the neurophysiology, cognition, and emotion in the mother-child interaction affect the plasticity of the pain matrix to reduce the child's pain and suffering. In the process not only the child, but the mother also, feels better. A physician's empathic presence for a patient in pain can similarly reduce symptoms and improve outcomes, offering reciprocity of satisfaction for both.

ACKNOWLEDGMENTS

We would like to thank Joseph S. Gonnella, MD for his critical review of this chapter and valuable suggestions. We would also like to thank Dorissa Bolinski for her editorial assistance.

REFERENCES

1. Balint M. *The doctor, his patient and the illness.* New York: International University Press; 1957.
2. Goubert L, Craig KD, Vervoort T, et al. Facing others in pain: the effects of empathy. *Pain.* 2005;118:285–288
3. Eisenberger N, Lieberman M, Williams K. Does rejection hurt? An fMRI study of social exclusion. *Science.* 2003;302:290–292.
4. Merskey H, Bogduk, N. eds. *Classification of Chronic Pain.* 2nd ed. Seattle, WA: International Association for the Study of Pain Press;1994.
5. Wager T, Rilling JK, Smith EE, et al. Placebo-induced changes in fMRI in the anticipation and experience of pain. *Science.* 2004;303:1162–1167.
6. Hojat M. *Empathy in Patient Care: Antecedents, Development, Measurement, and Outcomes.* New York, NY: Springer; 2007.
7. Zahn-Waxler C. Caregiving, emotion, and concern for others. *Behav Brain Sci.* 2002;25:48–49.
8. Sagi A, Hoffman ML. Empathic distress in newborns. *Dev Psychol.* 1976;12:175–176.
9. Martin GB, Clark RD. Distress crying in neonates: species and peer specificity. *Dev Psychol.* 1982;18:3–9.
10. Meltzoff AN, Moore MK. Newborn infants imitate adult facial gestures. *Child Dev.* 1983;54:702–709.
11. Davis MH. Measuring individual differences in empathy: evidence for a multidimensional approach. *J Pers Soc Psychol.* 1983;44:113–126.
12. Davis MH. *Empathy: a Social Psychological Approach.* Boulder, CO: Westview; 1994.
13. Mehrabian A, Epstein NA. A measure of emotional empathy. *JPers.* 1972;40:525–543.
14. Hojat M. Ten approaches for enhancing empathy in health and human services cultures. *J Health Human Serv Admin.* 2009;31:412–450.
15. Hojat M, Vergare MJ, Maxwell K, et al. The devil is in the third year: A longitudinal study of erosion of empathy in medical school. *Acad Med.* 2009;84:1182–1191.
16. Dovidio JF. The empathy-altruistic hypothesis: paradigm and promise. *Psychol Inq.* 1991;2:126–128.
17. Batson CD. *The Altruism Question: Toward a Social-Psychological Answer.* Hillsdale, NJ: Lawrence Erlbaum Associates; 1991.
18. Valeriani M, Betti V, Le Pera D, et al. Seeing the pain of others while being in pain: A laser-evoked potentials study. *Neuroimage.* 2008;40:1419–1428.
19. Tait RC. Empathy: necessary for effective pain management? *Curr Pain Headache Rep.* 2008;12:108–112.
20. Nummenmaa L, Hirvonen J, Parkkola R, Hietanen J. Is emotional contagion special? An fMRI study on neural systems for affective and cognitive empathy. *Neuroimage.* 2008;43:571–580.
21. Singer T, Seymour B, O'Doherty JP, Kaube H, Dolan RJ, Frith CD. Empathy for pain involves the affective but not sensory components of pain. *Science.* 2004;303:1157–1162.
22. Wellman H. *The Child's Theory of Mind.* Cambridge, MA: Bradford Books/MIT Press; 1991.

23. Premack D, Woodruff G. "Does the chimpanzee have a theory of mind?" *Behav Brain Sci.* 1978;4:515–526.

24. Hojat M, Louis D, Markham FW, Wender R, Rabinowitz C, Gonnella JS. Physicians' empathy and clinical outcomes for diabetic patients: building the evidence-base medicine. *Acad Med.* 2011;86(3):359–364.

25. Figley CR. *Compassion Fatigue: Coping with Secondary Traumatic Stress Disorder in Those who Treat the Traumatized.* New York, NY: Brunner/Mazel; 1995.

26. Ochsner KN, Zaki J, Hanelin J, et al. Your pain or mine? Common and distinct neural systems supporting the perception of pain in self and other. *Soc Cogn Affect Neurosci.* 2008;3:144–160.

27. Linley PA, Joseph S. Therapy work and therapists' positive and negative well-being. *J Soc Clin Psychol.* 2007;26:385–403.

28. Villenmure C, Bushnell C. Mood influences supraspinal pain processing separately from attention. *J Neurosc.* 2009;29:705–715.

29. Gallese V, Fadiga L, Fogassi L, Rizzilatti G. Action cognition in the premotor cortex. *Brain.* 1996;119:593–609.

30. Rizzilatti G, Fadiga L, Gallese V, Fogassi L. Premotor cortex and the recognition of motor action. *Cogn Brain Res.* 1996;3:131–141.

31. Kohler E, Keysers C, Umilta AM, Fogassi L, Gallese V, Rizzolatti G. Hearing sounds, understanding actions: action representation in mirror-neurons. *Science.* 2002;297:846–848.

32. Keysers C, Kohler E, Umilta MA, Nanetti L, Fogassi L, Gallese V. Audiovisual mirror neurons and action recognition. *Exp Brain Res.* 2003;153: 628–636.

33. Iacoboni M, Woods RP, Brass M, Bekkering H, Mazziotta JC, Rizzolatti G. Cortical mechanism of human imitation. *Science.* 1999;286:2526–2528.

34. Tai YF, Scherfler C, Brooks DJ, Sawamoto N, Castiello U. The human premotor cortex is "mirror" only for biological actions. *Curr Biol.* 2004;14:117–120.

35. Gazzola V, Rizzolatti G, Wicker B, Keysers C. The anthropomorphic brain: the mirror neuron system responds to human and robotic actions. *Neuroimage.* 2007;35(4):1674–1684.

36. Di Pellegrino G, Fadiga L. Fogassi L, Gallese V, Rizzolutti G. Understanding motor events: a neurophysiological study. *Exp Brain Res.* 1992;91:176–180.

37. Umilta MA, Kohler E, Gallese V, Fogassi L, Fadiga L, Keysers C, Rizzolatti G. I know what you are doing: a neurophysiological study. *Neuron.* 2001;31:155–165.

38. Carr L, Iacoboni M, Dubeaut MC, Mazziotta JC, Lenzi GL. Neural mechanisms of empathy in humans: A relay from neural systems for imitation to limbic areas. *Proc Natl Acad Sci USA..* 2003;9:5497–5502.

39. Jabbi M, Keysers C. Inferior frontal gyrus activity triggers anterior insula response to emotional facial expression. *Emotion.* 2008;8:775–780.

40. Preston SD, de Waal FB. Empathy: its ultimate and proximate bases. *Behav Brain Sci.* 2002;25:1–20.

41. Chartrand TL, Bargh JA. The chameleon effect: the perception-behavior link and social interaction. *J Pers Soc Psychol.* 1999;76:893–910.

42. Loggia ML, Mogil JS, Bushnell CM. Empathy hurts: Compassion for another increases both sensory and affective components of pain perception. *Pain.* 2008;136:168–176.

43. Craig KD, Weiss SM. Vicarious influences on pain-threshold determinations. *J Pers Soc Psychol.* 1971;19:53–59.

44. Stotland E. *Exploratory investigation of empathy.* In: Berkowitz L, ed. *Advances in Experimental Social Psychology.* New York, NY: Academic Press; 1969:271–314.

45. Richter M, Eck J, Staube T, Miltner WHR, Weiss T. Do words hurt? Brain activation during the processing of pain-related words. *Pain.* 2010;148:198–205.

46. Botvinick M, Jha AP, Bylsma LM, Fabian SA, Solomon PE, Prkachin KM. Viewing facial expression of pain engages cortical areas involved in the direct experience of pain. *Neuroimage.* 2005;25:312–319.

47. Jackson PL, Meltzoff AN, Decety J. How do we perceive the pain of others? A window into the neural processes involved in empathy. *Neuroimage.* 2005;24:771–779.

48. Tracey I. Imaging pain. *Br J Anaesth.* 2008;101:32–39.

49. Apkarian AV, Bushnell MC, Treede RD, Zubieta JK. Human brain mechanisms of pain perception and regulation in health and disease. *Eur J Pain.* 2005;9:463–484.

50. Lamm C, Batson CD, Decety J. The neural substrate of human empathy: effects of perspective-taking and cognitive appraisal. *J Cogn Neurosci.* 2007;19:42–58.

51. Bushnell MC, Duncan GH, Hofbauer RK, Ha B, Chen JI, Carrier B. Pain perception: Is there a role for primary somatosensory cortex? *Proc Natl Acad Sci.* 1999;96:7705–7709.

52. Peyron R, Laurent B, Garcia-Larrea L. Functional imaging of brain responses in pain: A review and meta-analysis. *Clin Neurophysiol.* 2000;30:263–288.

53. Morrison I, Lloyd D, di Pellegrino G, Roberts N. Vicarious responses to pain in anterior cingulate cortex: is empathy a multisensory issue? *Cogn, Affect Behav Neurosci.* 2004;4:270–278.

54. Jackson PL, Brunet E, Meltzoff AN, Decety J. Empathy examined through the neural mechanisms involved in imaging how I feel versus how you feel pain. *Neuropsychologia.* 2006;44:752–761

55. Saarela MV, Hlushchuk Y, Williams AC, Schurmann M, Kalso E, Hari R. The compassion brain: human detect intensity of pain from another's face. *Cereb Cortex.* 2007;17:230–237.

56. Avenanti A, Bueti D, Galati G, Aglioti SM. Transcranial magnetic stimulation highlights the sensorimotor side of empathy for pain. *Nat Neurosci.* 2005;8:955–960.

57. Avenanti A, Paluello IM, Bufalari I, Aglioti SM. Stimulus-driven modulation of motor-evoked potentials during observation of others' pain. *Neuroimage.* 2006;32:316–324.

58. Bufalari I, Aprile T, Avenanti A, Di Russo F, Aglioti SM. Empathy for pain and touch in the human somatosensory cortex. *Cereb Cortex.* 2007;17:2553–2561.

59. Morrison I, Peelen MV, Downing PE. The sight of others' pain modulates motor processing in human cingulate cortex. *Cereb Cortex.* 2007;17:2214–2222.

60. Morrison I, Lloyd D, di Pellegrino G, Roberts N. Vicarious responses to pain in anterior cingulate cortex: is empathy a multisensory issue? *Cogn, Affect Behav Neurosci.* 2004;4:270–278.

61. Jackson PL, Meltzoff AN, Decety J. How do we perceive the pain of others? A window into the neural processes involved in empathy. *Neuroimage.* 2005;24:771–779.

62. The Balanced Emotional Empathy Scale (BEES). Available from: A. Mehrabian, 1130 Alta Mesa Road, Monterey, CA, 93940, USA.

63. Wicker B, Keysers C, Plailly J, Royet JP, Gallese V, Rizzolatti G. Both of us disgusted in my insula: the common neural basis of seeing and feeling disgust. *Neuron.* 2003;40:655–664.

64. Holden C. Imaging studies show how brain thinks about pain. *Science.* 2004;303: 1121.

65. Gallager HL, Frith CD. Functional imaging of "theory of mind." *Trends Cogn Sci.* 2003;7:77–83.

66. Safdar B, Heins A, Homel P, et al. Impact of physician and patient gender on pain management in the emergency department—a multicenter study. *Pain Med.* 2009;10:364–372.

67. Grossman M, Wood W. Sex differences in intensity of emotional experience: a social role interpretation. *J Pers Soc Psychol.* 1993;65:1010–1022.

68. Weisman CS, Teitelbaum MA. Physician gender and the physician–patient relationship: Recent evidence and relevant questions. *Soc Sci Med.* 1985;20(11):1119–1127.

69. Dziobek I, Rogers K, Fleck S, et al. Dissociation of cognitive and emotional empathy in adults with Asperger syndrome using multifaceted empathy test (MET). *J Autism Dev Disord.* 2008;38:464–473.

70. Shamay-Tsoory SG, Tomer R, Goldsher D, Berger BD, Aharon-Peretz J. Impairment in cognitive and affective empathy in patients with brain lesions: anatomical and cognitive correlates. *Neuropsychology.* 2004;26:1113–1127.

30

PAIN, CULTURE, AND PATHWAYS TO CARE

GURVINDER S. KALRA, MD, DPM
Assistant Professor, Department of Psychiatry, Lokmanya Tilak Municipal Medical College & Sion General Hospital, Mumbai, Maharashtra, India

SUSHAM GUPTA, MBBS, MRCPSYCH
Consultant Psychiatrist, East London NHS Foundation Trust, Assertive Outreach Team—City & Hackney, London, UK

DINESH BHUGRA, MA, MSC, MBBS, FRCPSYCH, MPHIL, PHD
Professor of Mental Health and Cultural Diversity, Institute of Psychiatry, King's College London, London, UK

Key Points

- Pain is a universal experience and many languages have more than one expression for pain depending upon its nature and severity.
- Explanatory models of pain will determine where the patient seeks help.
- In socio-centric societies other members of the in-group may play a bigger role in enabling the patient to seek help and determine which pathways into care are followed.
- Factors such as language differences between patients and clinicians, and personality factors are likely to affect pain management.
- The explanatory models and pathways to care that patients follow when in pain, are important determinants when setting up pain management clinics.
- The issues of cultural influences on pain perception and experience gain importance in multi-cultural and multi-ethnic populations.

INTRODUCTION

Pain is a universal experience and part of everyday life in medicine. The word is derived from *poena*—the Latin word associated with punishment or penalty. It is one of the most frequent complaints brought to physicians everywhere. Pain can be both physically and psychologically mediated. It is the physical symptom of underlying pathology of physiological processes that causes the most human suffering in medicine. From an anthropological point, cultural and societal factors dictate expression of emotions, and hence have a learned component.[1] Pain is one of the most common causes of inability to work and also places a great economic burden on society in the form of lost man-power and disability benefits.

Historically, the cruelty suffered by slaves in America was in part due to widely held beliefs that those of African descent (and also Native Americans) were somehow less sensitive to pain. Even a "medical" term—"*Dysaesthesia Aethiopsis*" or "an obtuse sensibility of body," was used to describe the genetic insensitivity to pain in Blacks.[2] However, inadequate analgesia in view of such preconceived beliefs regarding pain can be extremely discriminatory and is a human rights issue. The results of various research studies need proper interpretation as it might be difficult to differentiate among actual pain perception, pain expression, and pain tolerance. This is particularly true for multi-ethnic medical settings. Pain means different things in different cultures and to different people. Furthermore, explanations and perceived locus of control for pain will determine which pathways patients choose to seek help.

SEEKING CARE WHEN IN PAIN: CULTURAL INFLUENCES

The culture one belongs to influences the way one thinks and acts in all kinds of situations[3] and also affects one's expectations of how the world works and how one interacts with it. Pain is a universal perception and experience; however, people respond to it with their own individual emotions and behaviors. Pain sensation may reflect anatomy and physiology, but only the associated sociocultural factors form the foundation for the expression and treatment of pain.[4] It is inevitable that culture will influence how an individual expresses response to painful stimuli and to pain itself,[5,6,7,8] physical or psychological, including help-seeking behavior.[6,9,10] Thus patients from enduring cultures may usually find meaning in their pain and choose to tolerate it without seeking help, something which shows self-efficacy in them.

In order to understand the diverse perceptions and responses to pain, one needs to look at the tremendous cultural diversity found throughout the world. Cultural diversity refers to both overt and covert differences among different groups.[11] Individuals learn appropriate behaviors and emotional responses by watching the actions of others who are similar to themselves, or in other words, members of their own ethnocultural group. Ethnicity distinguishes people based on behavior, ancestry, beliefs, history, biology, and physical characteristics[12] and a combination of these factors is likely responsible for racial and ethnic differences in expression of pain as well as sensitivity to pain.[13] The members of some ethnic groups have a higher tolerance for pain than others and can endure increasing levels of pain.[13] People from certain cultures that value stoicism, may avoid vocalizing with screams, moans, or groans to express pain, sometimes even to the point of denying having any pain when asked. It is possible that these individuals correlate expressing pain with weakness and hence fear projecting a weak image of self to others. Other cultures may be more expressive about pain and may consider crying and moaning appropriate responses when in pain. For example, in Indian culture, when a relative dies, the aggrieved relatives express their psychological pain and grief by crying loudly, sometimes thumping their chests with both hands. Members of such cultural groups may prefer not to be alone when they are in pain[14,15] and, in fact, may be encouraged to have someone with them all the time as they are dealing with their grief. On the other hand, in the considerably more stoic Western cultures, the grieving individual need not express his or her psychological pain in a similar way. The contemporary

North American culture favors a private and virtually invisible mourning process.[16] At this juncture, one can think of the professional mourners who are considered an important part of the ceremony of loss. The *Rudaali* (literally translated as "female weeper") are such professional mourner women in Rajasthan, India who wail for hours and thump their chests at the funeral of someone from the royal families. The bereaved family members are actually capable of grieving themselves, but expression of such grief is considered a sign of weakness especially in the Rajasthani royal families, due to their social status. Also, the splendor and reputation of the person is revealed by the number of people who wailed and cried at the funeral. It is believed that the loud cries of these professional mourners disturb the dead person's soul on its journey to the other world, and can sometimes bring it back. Until relatively recently, public mourning meant public beating of breast and wailing by women if someone from the family died. The closer the relative was to the deceased, the higher the level of wailing. One can understand cultural influences on pain by taking the example of the *Pokot* in Kenya, who honor higher tolerance to pain and denigrate expression of pain as inappropriate. Among them, the cutting of the clitoral area during female circumcision is publicly performed and is regarded as a test of stamina, wherein the female is taught not to show any emotion when in pain during the procedure.[17]

Various researchers have tried studying cultural influences on pain. Woodrow et al.[18] demonstrated that Whites tolerated more pain than Orientals, while Blacks occupy an intermediate position. These racial differences were more marked in men than in women. The researchers had applied mechanical pressure on the Achilles tendon of 41,119 subjects to determine pain tolerance. They clearly differentiated between pain threshold (the level of stimulus at which the subject first recognizes pain or discomfort[19]) and pain tolerance (highest level of stimulus at which the subject requests stimulus cessation[20]), and selected pain tolerance due to its greater clinical utility. Patients seek medical help due to intolerance to pain rather than when they recognize presence of pain.

Zola[21] observed that patients of an Italian ethnic background reported pain more frequently than did patients of Irish or Anglo-Saxon ethnic background. These findings were replicated by Zborowski[22] who reported that patients of Italian and Jewish background expressed pain more intensely. Chin[23] reported that Chinese patients might not complain of pain and might not want to ask for pain medication, while Guarnero[24] reported that Mexicans want pain relief as quickly as possible. However, one has to understand the weaknesses of cross-cultural pain studies, as it is difficult to accurately assess and compare research findings of cultural pain responses because of the diverse methods used to assess and measure the expression of pain. Thus some studies report no significant cultural differences in pain response,[25,26] while others show significant cultural influences on pain.[26,27] Keefe et al[28] had gone to the point of saying that there is no consistent experimental evidence to show cultural differences in pain response.

Cultures that instill a sense of self-efficacy and control in individuals encourage them to tolerate pain and take personal control of their health and well-being.[29] Other cultures may be fatalistic, encouraging individuals to believe that they have little control over their health, well-being, and pain,[30] thus rendering them relatively helpless in times of pain. Any healthcare professional's perception of pain, and the right and wrong ways to respond to it, are bound to be influenced by the cultural milieu in which he or she was born and brought up.[31] Consequently, any deviations from one's cultural norms for dealing with pain may seem wrong to the health professional—a reflection of his or her own *ethnocentricism*.[31,32] The health professional should understand that patients' diverse cultural patterns are not right or wrong but merely different. Along these lines, it would be interesting to know the differences in expression of pain in sociocentric and ego-centric societies.

EXPLANATORY MODELS AND PATHWAYS INTO CARE

Explanatory models direct the patient in one direction or another when seeking care. Once a patient has experienced a symptom, she or he will try and explain it to themselves and those around them, especially family and caregivers. Family and caregivers then will add their own explanations to those of the patient. For example, if the patient and the caregiver believe in a supernatural explanation for pain and illness, they are more likely to seek help from folk healers or shamans; on the other hand, if the causes are seen as spiritual-religious then they will seek help from spiritual or religious healers. If the explanation is perceived as psychological or physical, then a primary care physician may be approached. We know from Zola's work that a vast majority of individuals will seek treatment in the personal or folk sector and only a small proportion will approach the professional sector.[33] This finding needs further exploration in the context of pain treatment, given that pain has differing cultural meanings and significance.

Frijda[34] talks about the concerns patients have—these concerns are described as giving an emotional meaning to an experience. Concerns are also part of the help-seeking pathway. An additional challenge is to determine at what point an individual becomes a patient. Seeing a shaman or faith healer does not make an individual a patient and this underlying emotion may delay help-seeking as it may also be seen as stigmatizing or medicalizing normal human experience. Thus, pathways to care will be determined by the explanation or concern, the support/understanding offered by family and caregivers, and also the resources available. If an individual has to travel miles to seek help, and also pay large amounts, the affordability of care will also play a role in help-seeking. It is likely that in a sociocentric society the advice of others may be more acceptable and also play a bigger role in seeking help in comparison with an ego-centric society. Choice of healers whether they are folk or professional will be determined by resources, ease of access, reputation of the healer, and other factors. Sometimes in order to get better quicker, individuals will consult multiple healers, as if seeking an additive effect. In certain cultures there is no distinction between various schools of thought. In situations where the individual wishes to get back to work sooner, so as to earn money and keep the family together, she or he may well try every possible venue. With increasing globalization, this will continue to change and it is inevitable that more traditional models may give way to more modern views and help-seeking. Pathways can be explored by asking in a step-wise fashion about patient journeys from the onset of symptoms to the point at which clinicians are seeing them. A useful addition is to explore their concerns and explanatory models to see if these also change with each step.

ETHNIC DIFFERENCES IN PAIN PERCEPTION AND RESPONSE

Another aspect of pain assessment is to understand what meaning pain has for the patient and how he or she prefers to get it treated. Although this is linked with explanatory models, it also determines coping strategies as well as help-seeking (allopathic treatment, alternative therapies, home remedies, cultural healers). Culture appears to affect pain threshold and tolerance, along with reactions to pain that may be modulated by psychological and cognitive variables.[35,36] Cognitive processes that are influenced by culture will undoubtedly exert a powerful influence on pain processing,[35] as will psychological factors such as situational and emotional factors. The understanding of the experience of pain will also depend upon whether the individual sees pain as subject to an external locus of control. For example, people who have pain, along with those caring for them, are likely to be more tolerant of pain if it is seen as being caused by an evil eye, some external influence, or some previous incarnation over which a person has no individual control. If the locus of control is seen as internal, then the patient may be held responsible and evince little sympathy, especially in sociocentric societies.

Pain is a universal experience, but reactions to it at both personal and social levels will differ according to a number of factors including personality, past experience, and learning from others. These patterns of pain expression are influenced by the person's total life experience as a member of a certain culture or society. On perceiving pain, it is possible that the individual's past memories and cultural beliefs may influence whether these pain impulses reach the level of awareness and how they are perceived and responded to.[37] Koffman et al[38] found two important meanings of pain in their Black Caribbean patients' accounts: pain as a "test of faith" that strengthened their religious beliefs and pain as a "punishment" that was associated with wrongdoing. These may be seen as religious explanations and such meanings may influence the patient's ability to accommodate their distress.

The bio-cultural model proposed by Bates[39] describes pain perceptions and responses within a cultural context[40] and conceptualizes the complex interaction of biological, cultural, and psychosocial factors in the process of human pain perception. It discusses how various developmental cultural processes (e.g., language, pain-related beliefs) influence verbal and nonverbal pain expression, as well as pain processing at the neurobiological level, which modulates the overall pain experience. Clinicians should recognize that differences in attitudes, beliefs, and emotional and psychological states associated with different ethnic groups[41] will affect when and how help is sought. Social learning and modeling within the family or the kinship group will affect how psychological influences help determine help-seeking pathways.

It is possible that patients who perceive their pain as an indication of disease onset or progression may complain of pain more and be disturbed by it to a higher degree. To support this point, O'Mahony et al[42] documented that patients with cancer pain experience a greater degree of depression and anxiety if they believe their pain is related to a worsening of their condition. Thus cultural attitudes towards disease and health may also influence the meaning of pain.[43]

Laboratory studies have failed to show any consistent relationship between ethnicity and pain threshold or any inter-ethnic differences.[44] However, clinical studies have reported ethnic differences in both pain perception and response. A study found that Vietnamese patients with fixation of femoral fractures received a fraction of morphine compared to their American counterparts over a fifteen-day period (0.9 mg versus 30.2 mg). However, only 8% of the Vietnamese sample complained of inadequate pain relief as opposed to 80% of the American patients.[45] Another study found that Europeans reported less severe postoperative pain than black American or Latino patients.[46] Studies from America suggest that ethnic minorities are at risk of receiving inadequate analgesia in various settings including emergencies and cancer treatment.[47,48] In another study of 250 patients with open reduction and internal fixation, Whites received 22 mg of morphine equivalents per day, Hispanics 13 mg/day, and Blacks 6 mg/day, even after controlling for other variables.[49] (See also Chapters 14,16,17,18.) However, when self-administering opioids, Asian and Caucasian patients did not differ in the amount utilized for postoperative pain.[50]

TREATMENT OF PAIN

Culture often influences attitudes towards treatment,[9,10,51] as well as prevention and what is perceived as good medical care.[3] Indian patients, for instance, may become increasingly apprehensive at routine blood tests and fear losing their "precious" blood during such tests; underneath they may have the belief that retaining one's blood is necessary to assure the wholeness of the body. Associated pain will therefore have specific meanings in such patients. While dealing with a culturally different patient, the health professional may label some of the patient's cultural perceptions about pain as irrational. This cultural conflict may lead to miscommunication, misdiagnosis, and inappropriate care, all of which ultimately cause patient discontent. In some cultures, patients seek more directive interventions, whereas in others they seek equal partnership, hence it is imperative that clinicians are aware of patient expectations.

Each individual carries his or her own culture around with them. It is important that healthcare providers keep this crucial point in mind in order to provide patients with culturally acceptable pain management. At the same time, they should refrain from stereotyping patients by assuming that they will adhere to a particular culture's typical pain patterns. For instance, in some cultures pain may signify a deserved punishment, and so the patient may not be ready to follow any pain medication regimen, which makes his response to pain different from the typical "Western" response. Stereotyping such differing responses as unacceptable is bound to make the patient less satisfied with the health professional's attitude and will further distance the patient from medical services. Finding a midway point to suit everyone is important to being culturally competent and respecting cultural beliefs of the patient. This gives the patient a sense of being valued, which in turn improves communication, increases patient satisfaction, and improves treatment outcomes. To help a patient with pain, health professionals must first assess how the patient thinks and feels about the pain experience.

Depending upon the cultural competence of the clinicians, patients belonging to a minority cultural group may receive suboptimal interventions and therefore be at a high risk for poor pain outcomes. This may be more likely when patients belong to a culture that differs from that of their healthcare provider. This cultural difference poses a challenge for properly assessing and managing the patient's pain.

Sometimes healthcare professionals and therapists may feel inefficient working with individuals from cultures with diverse attitudes to pain, and believe that these patients are not compliant with the pain treatment plan. These beliefs and the behaviors that result from them need to be recognized in the cultural context of the individuals and not necessarily be seen as a lack of willingness to deal with the pain.[52]

Patients in Western biomedical culture would prefer medications as the first line of treatment for their pain, because the explanatory models in these cultures regard pain to be completely organic and hence something that can be cured or controlled only by medicines. On the contrary, in some cultures where models of illness are less dependent upon mind-body dualism, alternative therapies such as acupuncture, yoga,[53] massage, and aromatherapies may be the preferred treatment modalities.[54] Yoga in particular has been found to be effective in chronic pain[55] and low back pain.[56] Some cultures prescribe spiritual rituals or other acts that balance hot and cold or *yin* and *yang* as treatments for pain.[57,58,59]

FACTORS AFFECTING MANAGEMENT

Factors that may affect pain management include:

1. Language differences: Language being a crucial tool for successful communication between individuals is essential for effective healthcare consultation. As is shown in Table 30.1, different languages have varying numbers of words describing pain. One also cannot ignore the fact that cultures may differ within their languages regarding the number of words used to describe pain, with some languages containing more words to describe pain.[60] For instance, the Japanese usually use a single term to describe pain,[61] while the Thai people may use more than a dozen words for pain.[62] This would indicate that like the apocryphal relationship between the number of words that can be used to describe snow and its characteristics, varying prevalence of pain-related words may indicate something about the attitudes and the experience of pain by different cultural groups. Furthermore, if the health professional's language is different than that of the patient, and if no interpreter is used, it could lead to faulty assessment of the condition of the patient and hence to suboptimal pain management.[63,64] One may use nonverbal cues such as facial expression, body posture, etc., to assess pain,[65] but these are as likely as language to vary across cultures and hence lead to misinterpretation.[66]

Use of an interpreter should be encouraged in case of language differences between the patient and the physician.[64,67,68] Both the therapist and the interpreter should see themselves as being involved in a team, with clearly defined roles to play. Therapy with an intermediated communication by an interpreter makes the one-on-one therapy, a "therapy in a triangle." The role of an interpreter in the patient-therapist relationship can vary from being a mere objective translator incapable of processing feelings[69,70] to being a culturally competent co-therapist.[71,72,73] However, one needs to understand that patients can experience problems when answering through an interpreter due to a possible influence on the answers. It is not advisable to use family members as interpreters because it may compromise patients' abilities to understand and be understood.[74]

2. Assessment tools: Pain assessment tools include numeric and visual analog scales, some of which have been translated into different languages. However, the translations may convey different meanings that compromise their validity.[75] (See also Chapter XXXX). As Kleinman (1980)[76] has argued, researchers and clinicians must be aware of the category fallacy where assessment tools developed in one culture should not be blindly employed in other cultures without adequate conceptual equivalence. The wording of these assessment tools is also important not only because words may have different meanings in different cultures, but because meanings may also differ among individuals. Several pain assessment tools have been translated and tested for validity across cultural and linguistic groups, for instance, the Pain Numeric Rating Scale,[77] Brief Pain Inventory,[78] and the McGill Pain Questionnaire.[79, 80, 10]

It may thus be beneficial to include open-ended questions in the pain interview, as that will demonstrate to the patients that the healthcare professionals want to understand them as unique beings with unique pain experiences.[81] In one study on different American ethnic groups—Hispanics, American Indians, American Africans, and Whites using the McGill Pain Questionnaire (MPQ), all the groups distinguished pain from ache or hurt. "Pain" was rated as the most intense term amongst the three terms: pain, ache, and hurt.[82] There is a great need to validate measures of pain for their reliable use across cultures.

3. Patient personality factors: Patients from more pain-tolerant cultures prefer not to complain and therefore may underreport their pain.[53] Many patients may refuse to take opioid pain medications due to cultural taboos[83] or due to genetic differences that make them more likely to experience adverse effects. Some patients may prefer more familiar, local, or culturally accepted remedies, which may include herbs as well as various touch therapies.[61] Patients may have more faith in ancient folk medicine systems, such as religious gurus or astrological predictions, which give them an edge over the newer biomedical systems. In collectivist cultures such as Indian, family choice takes precedence over individual choice. This along with the higher values placed on alternative medicine systems leads to the patient ultimately choosing the latter[84] in the age of medical pluralism. Clinicians trained in Western medicine and others who are not familiar with these alternate therapies,

TABLE 30.1 Pain description in different languages

Language	Different words that refer to pain
Afrikaans	Pyn
Czech	Bolest; otrava; trest; žal; zármutek; hoře
Danish	Smerte
Dutch	Pijn; smart; leed; lijden; zeer; straf; wee
Estonian	Valu; piin; vaev
Filipino	Sakit; kirot; lungkot; kalungkutan; sama ng loob
Finnish	Kipu; tuska; kivut; karsimys; murhe; piina; riesa; kiusankappale
French	Peine (mental distress); douleur (physical pain); souffrance; mal; tristesse; effort; punition
German	Schmerz, leid, Qual, Qualen, Kummer, Muhe
Greek	Ponos
Hindi	Dukh; dard; peera; vedna; vyatha; kasht, klesh; yantrna; takleef
Indonesian	Sakit; rasa sakit; kesakitan; rasa nyeri; penderitaan; kepedihan; perasaan sakit; hukuman
Irish	Pian
Italian	Pena (mental distress); dolore (physical pain); sofferenza; male; fatica; travaglio; castigo; doglie del parto
Korean	Gotong [(go) refers emotional pain, (tong) physical]; guoi-ro-um; aa-pm.
Latin	Dolor; morsus; angor; cruciatus; adflictio; poena; aegrum; cruciamen; afflictio
Norwegian	Smerte
Polish	Ból; cierpienie; bolesność; boleść; przykrość; męka; dolegliwość; strapienie; obolałość
Portuguese	Dor; sofrimento; pena; pesar; trabalho; castigo; dores de parto; abacaxi; aflição; mágoa; esforço; punição
Romanian	Durere; suferinţă; chin; effort; eforturi; pacoste; pedeapsă; necaz; osteneală; durerile facerii; ameninţare cu pedeapsă; calamitate; bătaie de cap; supărare
Spanish	Dolor; pena; sufrimiento
Swedish	Smarta; ont; vark; pina; plaga; kval; angslan; sorg; straff
Turkish	Ağrı; acı; sızı; sancı; eziyet; dert; ızdırap; elem; ceza; azap; emek; zahmet
Welsh	Poen

may discourage patients from using them, which creates a barrier that negatively affects the therapeutic relationship.

CONCLUSIONS

Pain assessment and management pose a challenge for clinicians. The main challenge is the difficulty in cultural interactions between clinicians and patients due to differences in perspective between Western medicine and belief systems held by an increasingly heterogeneous population from diverse ethnic backgrounds. This is especially complicated while setting up appropriate services to deal with assessment and management of pain in a multi-cultural setting. Management of pain is central to most aspects of medicine. It affects how people seek health care and its appropriate management is likely to improve compliance with treatment in general. Knowledge of variations in expression of pain and coping mechanisms to address it, can vastly reduce overall morbidity in clinical settings. Patients may well use pluralistic pathways to relieve pain and therefore thorough enquiry into these pathways and other treatments is crucial to understanding a patient's experience. This is still an evolving field and requires ongoing research to understand not only the cultural concepts of pain, but how this understanding might help reduce the distress that pain causes.

REFERENCES

1. Free MM. Cross-cultural conceptions of pain and pain control. *Proc* (Bayl Univ Med Cent). 2002;15(2):143–145.
2. Clark EB. The sacred rights of the weak: pain, sympathy, and the culture of the individual rights in Antebellum America. *Journal of American History*. 1995; 82(2):463–493.
3. Leininger MM. Essential transcultural nursing care concepts, principles, examples, and policy statements. In: Leininger MM, McFarland MR, eds. *Transcultural Nursing: Concepts, Theories, Research and Practice*. 3rd ed. New York: McGraw Hill; 2002:45–70.
4. Rey R. *The History of Pain*. Cambridge, MA: Harvard University Press; 1998.
5. Zborowski M. Cultural components in response to pain. *J Soc Issues*. 1952; 8:16–30.
6. Lasch KE. Culture, pain and culturally sensitive pain care. *Pain Manag Nurs*. 2000;1(3)(suppl 1):16–22.
7. Mazanac P, Kitzes J. Cultural competences in hospice and palliative care. In: Forman WB, Kitzes JA, Anderson RP, Sheehan DK, eds. *Hospice and Palliative Care: Concepts and Practice*. 2nd ed. Boston, MA: Jones & Bartlett Publishers; 2003:170–188.
8. Fink R, Gates R. Pain assessment. In: Ferrell BR, Coyle N, eds. *Textbook of Palliative Nursing*. 2nd ed. New York, NY: Oxford University Press; 2006:53–75.
9. Joint Commission Resources. *Approaches to Pain Management: An Essential Guide for Clinical Leaders*. Oakbrook Terrace, IL: The Joint Commission; 2003.
10. Melzack R, Katz J. The McGill pain questionnaire: appraisal and current status. In: Turk DC, Melzack R, eds. *Handbook of Pain Assessment*. 2nd ed. New York, NY: Guilford Press; 2001:35–52.
11. Betancourt JR, Green AR, Carrillo JE, Park ER. Cultural competence and health care disparities: key perspectives and trends. *Health Affairs* (Millwood). 2005;24(2):499–505.
12. Edwards CL, Fillingim RB, Keefe F. Race, ethnicity and pain. *Pain*. 2001;94:133–137.
13. Campbell CM, Edwards RR, Fillingim RB. Ethnic differences in responses to multiple experimental pain stimuli. *Pain*. 2005;113(1–2):20–26.
14. Nayak S, Shiflet SC, Eshun S, Levine FM. Culture and gender effects in pain beliefs and the prediction of pain tolerance. *Cross-cultural Research*. 2000;34(2):135–151.
15. Kelley LS, Tripp-Reimer T, Choi E, Enslein J. Ethnogeriatric issues in critical care. In: Fulmer TT, Foreman MD, Walker MK, eds. *Critical Care Nursing of the Elderly*. 2nd ed. New York, NY: Springer Publishing Company; 2001:353–377.
16. Ashenburg K. *The Mourner's Dance: What We Do When People Die*. New York, NY: North Point Press; 2003.
17. Johansen E. Pain as a counterpoint to culture: toward an analysis of pain associated with infibulation among Somali immigrants in Norway. *Med Anthropol Q*. 2002;16:312–340.
18. Woodrow KM, Friedman GD, Siegelaub AB, Collen MF. Pain tolerance: differences according to age, sex and race. *Psychosom Med*. 1972;34(6):548–556.

19. Wolff BB. Factor analysis of human pain responses: pain endurance as a specific pain factor. *J Abnorm Psychol.* 1971;78:292–298.

20. Gelfand S. The relationship of experimental pain tolerance to pain threshold. *Can J Psychol.* 1964;18:36–43.

21. Zola IK. Culture and symptoms: an analysis of patients presenting complaints. *American Sociological Review.* 1966;31:615–630.

22. Zborowski M. *People in Pain.* San Francisco, CA: Jossey-Bass; 1969.

23. Chin P. Chinese. In: Lipson JG, Dibble SL, eds. *Culture & Clinical Care.* San Francisco, CA: UCSF Nursing Press; 2005:98–108.

24. Guarnero PA. Mexicans. In: Lipson JG, Dibble SL, eds. *Culture & Clinical Care.* San Francisco, CA: UCSF Nursing Press; 2005:330–342.

25. Edwards RR, Doleys DM, Fillingim RB, Lowery D. Ethnic differences in pain tolerance: clinical implications in a chronic pain population. *Psychosom Med.* 2001; 63:316–323.

26. Zatzick DF, Dimsdale JE. Cultural variations in response to painful stimuli. *Psychosom Med.* 1990;52:544–557.

27. Green CR, Baker TA, Smith EM, Sato Y. The effect of race in older adults presenting for chronic pain management: a comparative study of black and white Americans. *Pain.* 2003;4:82–90.

28. Keefe FJ, Lumley MA, Buffington ALH, et al. Changing face of pain: evolution of pain research in psychosomatic medicine. *Psychosom Med.* 2002;64:921–938.

29. Marks R, Allegrante JP, Lorig K. A review and synthesis of research evidence for self-efficacy—enhancing interventions for reducing chronic disability: implications for health education practice (part II). *Health Promot Pract.* 2005;6(2):148–156.

30. Purnell LD, Paulanka BJ. *Transcultural Health Care: A Culturally Competent Approach.* 3rd ed. Philadelphia, PA: FA Davis; 2008.

31. Davitz LL, Davitz JR. Culture and nurses' inference of suffering. In: Copp LA. (ed). *Perspectives on pain.* New York: Churchill Livingstone; 1985.

32. Sutherland LL. Ethnocentrism in a pluralistic society: a concept analysis. *J Transcult Nurs.* 2002;13(4):274–281.

33. Zola IK. Pathways to the doctor—from person to patient. *Soc Sci Med.* 1973;7:677–689.

34. Frijda NH. *The Emotions.* Cambridge, UK: Cambridge University Press; 1986.

35. Melzaek R, Wall PD. *The Challenge of Pain.* Harmondsworth, England: Penguin Books; 1982:173.

36. Turk DC, Melzack R. *Handbook of Pain Assessment.* 2nd ed, New York, NY: Guilford Press; 2001:50.

37. Walco GA, Harkins SW. Life-span developmental approaches to pain. In: Gatchel RJ, Turk DC, eds. *Psychological Factors in Pain: Critical Perspectives.* New York, NY: Guilford Publications; 1999:107–170.

38. Koffman J, Morgan M, Edmonds P, Speck P, Higginson IJ. Cultural meanings of pain: a qualitative study of Black Caribbean and White British patients with advanced cancer. *Palliat Med.* 2008;22(4):350–359.

39. Bates MS. Ethnicity and pain: a biocultural model. *Soc Sci Med.* 1987;24(1):47–50.

40. Spires A. Managing cultural diversity in caring. In: Kenworthy N, Snowley G, Gilling C, eds. *Common Foundation Studies in Nursing.* London: Elsevier; 2001:129–145.

41. Bates MS, Edwards WT, Anderson KO. Ethnocultural influences on variation in chronic pain perception. *Pain.* 1993;52(1):101–112.

42. O'Mahony S, Goulet J, Kornblith A, et al. Desire for hastened death, cancer pain and depression: report of a longitudinal observational study. *J Pain Symptom Manage.* 2005;29:446–457.

43. Beach MC, Price E, Gary TL, et al. Cultural competence: a systematic review of health care provider educational interventions. *Med Care.* 2005;43:356–373.

44. Lasch KE. Culture and pain. *Pain: Clinical Updates.* 2002;10(5).

45. Carragee EJ, Vittum D, Truong TP, Burton D. Pain control and cultural norms and expectations after closed femoral shaft fractures. *Am J Orthop.* 1999;28(2):97–102.

46. Faucett J, Gordon N, Levine J. Differences in postoperative pain severity among four ethnic groups. *J Pain Symptom Manage.* 1994;9(6):383–389.

47. Chaturvedi N, Raj H, Ben-Shlomo Y. Lay diagnosis and health-care-seeking behaviour for chest pain in south Asians and Europeans. *Lancet.* 1997;350(9091):1578–1583.

48. Cleeland CS, Gonin R, Hatfield AK, et al. Pain and its treatment in outpatients with metastatic cancer. *N Engl J Med.* 1994;330(9):592–596.

49. Ng B, Dimsdale JE, Shragg GP, Deutsch R. Ethnic differences in analgesic consumption for postoperative pain. *Psychosom Med.* 1996;58(2):125–129.

50. Lee A, Gin T, Oh TE. Opioid requirements and responses in Asians. *Anaesth Intensive Care.* 1997;25(6):665–670.

51. Lasch KE, Wilkes G, Montuori LM, Chew P, Leonard C, Hilton S. Using focus group methods to develop multicultural cancer pain education materials. *Pain Manag Nurs.* 2000;1(4):129–138.

52. Russell S, Daly J, Hughes E, Hoog Co C. Nurses and "difficult" patients: negotiating non-compliance. *J Adv Nurs.* 2003;43(3):281–287.

53. Kalra G, Bhugra D. Mutual learning and research messages: India, UK, and Europe. *Indian J Psychiatry.* 2010;52(7)(suppl 3):S56–S63.

54. Carroll R. Complementary and alternative medicine: history, definitions, and what it is today. In: Snyder L, ed. *Complementary and Alternative Medicine: Ethics, the Patient, and the Physician.* Totowa, NJ: Humana Press; 2007:7–44.

55. Teets RY, Dahmer S, Scott E. Integrative medicine approach to chronic pain. *Primary Care.* 2010;37:407–421.

56. Sherman KJ, Cherkin DC, Erro J, Miglioretti DL, Deyo RA. Comparing yoga, exercise, and a self-care book for chronic low back pain: a randomized, controlled trial. *AnnIntern Med.* 2005;143:849–856.

57. Dunn KS, Horgas AL. Religious and nonreligious coping in older adults experiencing chronic pain. *Pain Manag Nurs.* 2004;5(1):19–28.

58. Unruh AM. Spirituality, religion and pain. *Can J Nurs Res.* 2007;39(2):66–86.

59. Cherniack EP, Ceron-Fuentes J, Florez H, Sandals L, Rodriguez O, Palacios JC. Influence of race and ethnicity on alternative medicine as a self-treatment preference for common medical conditions in a population of multi-ethnic urban elderly. *Complement Ther Clin Pract.* 2008;14(2):116–123.

60. Vlaar AP, ten Klooster PM, Taal E, et al. A cross-cultural study of pain intensity in Egyptian and Dutch women with rheumatoid arthritis. *J Pain.* 2007;8(9):730–736.

61. Hobara M. Beliefs about appropriate pain behavior: cross-cultural and sex differences between Japanese and Euro-Americans. *Eur J Pain.* 2005;9:389–393.

62. Chaudakshetrin P, Prateepavanich P, Chira-Adisai W, et al. Cross-cultural adaptation to the Thai language of the Neuropathic Pain Diagnostic Questionnaire (DN4). *Journal of Medical Association of Thailand.* 2007;90(9):1860–1865.

63. Smedley BD, Stith AY, Nelson AR. *Unequal Treatment: Confronting Racial and Ethnic Disparities in Health Care.* Washington, DC: National Academies Press; 2003.

64. Wilson-Stronks A, Lee KK, Cordero CL, Kopp AL, Galvez E. *One Size Does Not Fit All: Meeting the Health Care Needs of Diverse Populations* [electronic resource]. Oakbrook Terrace, IL: The Joint Commission; 2008. http://www.jointcommission.org/assets/1/6/HLCOneSizeFinal.pdf .Accessed January 13, 2011.

65. McCaffery M, Ferrell BR, Pasero C. Nurses' personal opinions about patients' pain and their effect on recorded assessments and titration of opioid doses. *Pain Manag Nurs.* 2000;1(3):79–87.

66. Brinkus R, Narayan MC. Communication as the fabric of community-based nursing practice. In: Sorrell JM, Redmond GM, eds. *Community-based Nursing Practice: Learning Through Students' Stories.* Philadelphia, PA: FA Davis; 2002:253–276.

67. Joint Commission Resources. *Providing culturally and linguistically competent health care.* Oakbrook Terrace, IL: The Joint Commission; 2006.

68. Office for Civil Rights. *Guidance to Federal Financial Assistance Recipients Regarding Title VI Prohibition Against National Origin Discrimination Affecting Limited English Proficient Persons.* U.S. Department of Health and Human Services. 2003. http://www.hhs.gov/ocr/civilrights/resources/specialtopics/lep/policyguidancedocument.html. AccessedOctober 10, 2010.

69. Acosta FX, Cristo MH. Development of a bilingual interpreter program: An alternative model for Spanish-speaking services. *Prof Psychol.* 1981;12:474–481.

70. Musser-Granski J, Carrillo DF. The use of bilingual, bicultural paraprofessionals in mental health services: issues for hiring, training and supervision. *Community Ment Health J.* 1997;33(1):51–60.

71. Brune M, Akbayir E. Die Macht der Sprache in der Psychotherapie. *Psychotherapie zu Dritt. Fluchtlingsrat, Zeitschrift fur Fluchtlingspolitik in Niedersachsen.* 2008;125:26–36.

72. Mudarikiri MM. Working with interpreters in adult mental health. In: Tribe R, Raval H, eds. *Working with Interpreters in Mental Health.* London & New York: Routledge; 2003.

73. Tribe R. Bridging the gap or damming the flow? Some observations on using interpreters/bicultural workers when working with refugee clients, many of whom have been tortured. *Br J Med Psychol.* 1999;72(4):567–576.

74. Divi C, Koss RG, Schmaltz SP, Loeb JM. Language proficiency and adverse events in US hospitals: a pilot study. *Int J Qual Health Care.* 2007;19(2):60–67.

75. Davidhizar R, Giger JN. A review of the literature on care of clients in pain who are culturally diverse. *Int Nurs Rev.* 2004;51(1):47–55.

76. Kleinman A. *Patients and Healers in the Context of Culture* [master's thesis]. Berkley, CA: University of California Press; 1980.

77. McCaffery M, Pasero CL. *Pain Clinical Manual.* 2nd ed. St. Louis, MO: Mosby; 1999.

78. Cleeland CS, Ryan KM. Pain assessment: global use of the Brief Pain Inventory. *Annals of the Academy of Medicine, Singapore.* 1994;23(2):129–138.

79. Melzack R. The McGill Pain Questionnaire: major properties and scoring methods. *Pain.* 1975;1(3):277–299.

80. Melzack R. The short-form McGill Pain Questionnaire. *Pain.* 1987;30(2):191–197.

81. Beach MC, Saha S, Cooper LA. *The Role and Relationship of Cultural Competence and Patient Centeredness in Health Care Quality* [electronic resource]. New York, NY: Commonwealth Fund; Report No. 960. http://www.commonwealthfund.org/usr_doc/Beach_rolerelationshipcultcomppatient-cent_960.pdf. Published October 2006. Accessed October 10, 2010.

82. Gaston-Johansson F, Albert M, Fagan E, Zimmerman L. Similarities in pain descriptions of four different ethnic-culture groups. *J Pain Symptom Manage.* 1990;5(2):94–100.

83. Lovering S. Cultural attitudes and beliefs about pain. *J Transcult Nurs.* 2006;17(4):389–395.

84. Gambheera H, Williams S. Shared challenges in psychiatric research in India and Sri Lanka. *Indian J Psychiatry.* 2010;52:S80–S82.

The Future of Analgesia in Diverse Populations

/// 31 /// CULTURE, PHARMACOGENOMICS, AND PERSONALIZED ANALGESIA

MARIO INCAYAWAR, MD, MSC, DESS
Director, Runajambi–Institute for the Study of Quichua Culture and Health, Otavalo, Ecuador *and* Former Henry R. Luce Professor in Brain, Mind and Medicine, Cross-Cultural Perspectives, Claremont Colleges, Claremont, California, USA

KNOX H. TODD, MD, MPH
Professor and Chair, Department of Emergency Medicine, The University of Texas MD Anderson Cancer Center, Houston, Texas, USA

The world population has recently reached the impressive figure of seven billion. This population, far from homogeneous, is richly diverse. With globalization and increased migration, countries around the world are more multi-ethnic and multi-cultural than ever before. Given this demographic background, the ability to understand human pain experience and managing it competently becomes increasingly difficult. Despite pain being a universal and common human experience, it is neglected worldwide.[1,2] Fortunately, in the last two decades, interest in pain is growing among social and biomedical researchers, clinicians, educators, and health policy makers.

In wealthy countries, when doctors face patients with complex pain symptoms, they usually refer them to pain specialists and pain clinics. In poor and remote communities such as the Andes in South America, Indigenous Peoples rely almost exclusively on family and traditional healers to control their pain.[3] When pain practitioners are working in urban areas, they rely on other specialized health professionals to co-manage and better treat their patients' pain. Furthermore, modern pain clinics have developed an original clinical strategy to work as a multidisciplinary team. A psychologist deals with any psychological issues the patient may have. A psychiatrist is expected to deal with the patient's comorbid serious mental disorders that often accompany chronic pain. The anesthesiologist will help the pain team with technical medical procedures such as inserting spinal pumps or stimulators. And the social worker is expected to manage economic and social barriers preventing patients from receiving good medical care and achieving general wellbeing. Sometimes, the pain team benefits from the input of anthropologists and linguists, as well as the assistance of translators. However laudable the goal of this collaborative approach, it often remains fragmented because each specialist will dutifully focus on one single dimension of pain affecting a given patient. What is lacking today in well-resourced pain treatment centers is not the valuable contribution of more disciplines and specialists. What is missing are broadly educated clinicians who understand the multiple dimensions of pain. There is an urgent need for clinicians trained in multiple disciplines who are able to use integrative approaches to pain diagnosis and treatment. There is a need for health professionals who are skilled in understanding the dynamically intertwined social, cultural, psychological, and biological dimensions of pain.

Pain practitioners who are attempting to provide a better quality of care in an increasingly diverse population should focus their attention on both their patients' cultural characteristics, which can be predicted to modulate the pain experience, and on the individuality of each patient, which explains observed variations in suffering and responses to pain treatment.

In this chapter, we discuss how a multidisciplinary and integrative approach to pain should be considered. Some familiarity with the cultural background of our patients and awareness of the provider's own cultural characteristics will allow us to better understand our patients' values, attitudes, and preferences. Knowledge of patients' cultural practices will allow us to determine the impact of culture on biological processes, including the origin and development of pain-related disease, and the patients' response to pharmacological and nonpharmacological treatments. This understanding could eventually lead us to the practice of a person-centered or personalized medicine.

CULTURE AND PAIN

Cultures shape the belief system, attitudes, and behaviors of patients and healthcare providers, as well as their interactions in the medical encounter. It makes sense that our respective cultures provide us with useful theories about illness and pain causation, estimates about how long it will last, how it will affect our lives and those of our relatives, whom we should consult, and ultimately what we prefer as a treatment. Interestingly, one's culture could render difficult the understanding and appreciation of another's worldview. As the philosopher Sandra Hardings at UCLA put it, culture is both a useful toolbox for an individual and at the same time it is a prison.[4]

How patients perceive illness is paramount in their decision-making related to health. If they feel that a proposed diagnosis or treatment does not fit with their beliefs, even if it occurs in the best medical center, the patients' frustration will emerge. They will subsequently not adhere to the therapeutic plan and the latter will most probably fail. A careful consideration of patients' belief systems and attitudes could facilitate a fruitful negotiation of explanatory models[5] of illness or allow for recognition of inaccurate or erroneous beliefs. A culturally sensitive approach to medical care will translate into better health outcomes.[6]

Prejudice, stereotyping, and lack of empathy towards people who are different are phenomena deeply entrenched in our psychology and biology. Although most scholars assume beliefs, attitudes, and preferences are learned and thus modifiable, recent neuroscience research highlights the complexity of these human behaviors and suggests it may not be that simple. The chapters of Drs Alexander Green on implicit and explicit bias among physicians and Mohammadreza Hojat on empathy, sympathy, and the mirror neurons provide some glimpses into the intricate biological underpinnings of racial prejudice and empathy. The anterior cingulate cortex, implicated in pain processing and empathy towards people in pain, is more active if the person in pain is of the same ethnic group.[7] Face processing (visual scanning, face memory, and facial emotion recognition) abilities of healthy individuals appear to be less accurate when they are evaluating faces and emotions in other ethnic groups: the "other-race effect." What is striking is that the "other-race effect" appears early in life and is present even in infants.[8] In a recent psychiatric study the "other-race effect" was studied among patients suffering from schizophrenia, a condition that affects the ability to recognize emotions and severely impairs the thought process. This study reveals that even patients suffering from a severe mental disorder such as schizophrenia exhibited a strong "other-race effect." These patients were able to evaluate accurately the faces and emotions of people of the same ethnic group.[9] Pinkham and his team explain that the "other-race effect" exhibited by individuals with schizophrenia in this study "may reflect normative developmental experience with faces and perhaps even normative development of the neural mechanisms of face processing." In addition, the noradrenergic system appears to mediate the implicit "outgroup" racial bias. According to a recent study conducted by Terbeck and her team at University of Oxford, propranolol, a beta adrenoreceptor antagonist, effectively abolished implicit racial bias.[10] By extension, ethnicity could be a sort of biological prison that makes it difficult for us to place ourselves in the position of others.

Cross-cultural interactions can cause serious miscommunication with important clinical consequences. In a study in the New England region of the United States, Bates found high expressiveness of pain among Latino patients, even among those who were adjusting well to their pain and considered they had a happy life despite the pain. Bates found that many American staff nurses believed this expressiveness to be inappropriate, especially in men. Referring to a patient, one nurse said "He starts to yell when I apply the alcohol swab— even before I put in the needle for the I.V. He looks so macho but he acts like a baby."[11]

When interactions between ethnically or culturally discordant doctors and patients unfold well they are treated as "good" patients. In the United States and the United Kingdom, doctors appear to expect low expression of emotions and pain in their patients. In an interesting observation made in Britain by Bond, he says "Any observant visitor to a hospital ward in Britain will become aware, sooner or later, that ability to endure pain with little or no complaint is admired and regarded as highly desirable behavior."[12] "Stoicism in a pain sufferer is rewarded with admiration, sympathy, and more material expressions of approval, notably administration of pain relieving medicines." In contrast, when patients are found "overexpressive" they will be viewed as complainers. Those patients who whine in pain, "especially if regarded as excessive or unnecessary are punished by expressions of disapproval, both verbal and practical, in the form of withholding analgesics or the administration of placebo substances."[12]

Thus, understanding not only patients' culture but also being aware of the pain practitioner's values, beliefs, and attitudes related to pain and its treatment is useful in the clinical setting.

PHARMACOGENOMICS AND ANALGESIA

The remarkable advances of genetics in the last two decades are contributing to better understanding of the mechanisms and causes of diseases and pain at the molecular level.[13,14,15] In line with these developments, pharmacogenomics allows us to explore how patients in certain countries or from certain ethnic groups respond differently to a wide range of medicines, including pain medicines.[16–18] As stated by Stamer, pharmacogenomics have the potential to be used as a diagnostic tool[19] and eventually as a screening and preventive resource. Dr. Keh-Ming Lin, one of the leading figures in this field, provides a fascinating discussion of the topic elsewhere in this book. Pharmacogenomic research indicates that individuals can respond differently to a given medicine, experience different side effects, or have different interactions with other medicines or food. The pharmacogenomic information gained in this area is so robust that the U.S. Food and Drug Administration (FDA), recently decided to launch a website and post the pharmacogenetic information on many drugs. It is named Table of Pharmacogenomic Biomarkers in Drug Labels available at http://www.fda.gov/Drugs/ScienceResearch/ResearchAreas/Pharmacogenetics/ucm083378.htm. The FDA considers that this information could be very useful for clinicians and must play an important role in identifying responders and nonresponders to medications, avoiding adverse events, and optimizing drug dosage. Several analgesics, anti-inflammatory drugs, and psychotropics used in pain management are included.

The phenotype of being fast or poor metabolizers of a given drug is dependent on genes that control the drug metabolizing isoenzymes of cytochrome P450. Several isoenzymes appear to be distributed differently among different human groups.[16] Below are examples of the prevalence of certain isoenzymes among different ethnic groups and nationalities and their clinical implications.

PHARMACOGENOMIC MARKERS OF SELECTED ANALGESICS

The following is taken and summarized from the U.S. Food and Drug Administration website listed above.

Codeine and CYP2D6 genomic biomarker	People who are ultra-rapid metabolizers (UM) of codeine due to a specific CYP2D6*2x2 genotype convert codeine into its active metabolite, morphine, more rapidly and completely than people who are poor metabolizers. The rapid conversion results in higher serum morphine levels. Patients who are ultra-rapid metabolizers of codeine may experience overdose symptoms such as extreme sleepiness, confusion, or shallow breathing, even at usual dosages. The prevalence of CYP2D6 (UM) phenotype varies widely according to ethnicity. Estimates are 0.5% to 1% in Chinese and Japanese, 0.5% to 1% in Hispanics, 1% to 10% in Caucasians, 3% in African Americans, and 16% to 28% in North Africans, Ethiopians, and Arabs. Physicians prescribing codeine-containing drugs should choose the lowest effective dose for the shortest period of time and inform their patients about these risks and the signs of morphine overdose.
Celecoxib and CYP2C9	Patients who are known or suspected to be poor CYP2C9 metabolizers or have previous history/experience with other CYP2C9-related compounds such as warfarin or phenytoin should be given celecoxib with caution. Physicians should consider starting treatment at half the lowest recommended dose in poor metabolizers.
Tramadol and Acetaminophen are linked to CYP2D6	Approximately 7% of the Caucasian populations have reduced activity of the CYP2D6 isoenzyme of cytochrome P450. These individuals are poor metabolizers of debrisoquine, dextromethorphan, and tricyclic antidepressants, among other drugs. On healthy subjects, concentrations of tramadol are approximately 20% higher in poor metabolizers versus rapid metabolizers.

In vitro drug interaction studies in human liver microsomes indicate that inhibitors of CYP2D6 such as fluoxetine and its metabolite norfluoxetine, amitriptyline, and quinidine inhibit the metabolism of tramadol to various degrees. The full pharmacological impact of these alterations in terms of either efficacy or safety is unknown. Concomitant use of serotonin re-uptake inhibitors and MAO inhibitors may enhance the risk of adverse events, including seizure and serotonin syndrome.

It is worth noting that diet is capable of influencing CYP2D6 enzyme activity as well. Several other drug-metabolizing enzymes are also known to be influenced by diet. For example, CYP3A4 appears to be inhibited by grapefruit juice or corn, and probably CYP1A2 by coffee. Cultural practices such as consuming large quantities of coffee daily as occurs in many Western countries and corn among the Indigenous Peoples of the Americas could have an effect on how patients respond to pharmacotherapy. Therefore, pain clinicians should consider their patients' cultural practices in order to deliver more person-centered medical care. Without overgeneralizing pharmacogenomic information and stereotyping patients, clinicians should use the maxim "Start low and go slow." This is a wise message coming from pharmacogenomics that could help health professionals when they are working to control pain in a multicultural society.

EPIGENETICS AND PAIN

Another cornerstone development of the last decade that may influence enormously the field of pain and analgesia is epigenetics. It is generally accepted that health and disease, including pain, are the result of interactions between genes and the environment. These interactions are mediated by the DNA sequence and by modifications that affect the transcriptional capacity of genes. Epigenetic processes such as DNA methylation, micro RNAs, or histone tail modification affect gene expression through direct modifications to the DNA or the way it is packaged into chromatin.[20–22]

Epigenetics is a kind of missing link for understanding how external environmental factors (physical, psychosocial, such as early experiences in life, or prenatal exposures[23]) could affect the inner workings of genes and ultimately the emergence of disease, pathology, and treatment responses through effects on the pharmacodynamics and pharmacokinetics of drugs used to control pain.[22,24,25]

Bees provide us a wonderful example of the powerful influence of epigenetics. Genetically identical *Apis mellifera* larvae will develop into a fertile queen or sterile honeybee worker following feeding with royal jelly. Diet based on royal jelly induces DNA methylation that shifts the expression of genes towards the development of a queen.[26] Furthermore, the social environment in the hive appears to trigger neural epigenetic changes among the worker bees determining who will become a forager or a nurse.[27]

Important epigenetic influences have been proposed to explain the development of cardiovascular diseases among African Americans,[28] cancer,[29] psychiatric disorders,[30,31] autoimmune diseases,[32] neurological diseases,[33] diabetes,[34] and pain and analgesia.[25,35,36] Recently, Zhan showed that inflammatory acute pain in rats is able to epigenetically impair GABA synaptic inhibition in the brainstem nucleus raphe magnus. It shed light on how acute pain could transition to chronic pain.[37] In these medical conditions, epigenetic changes seem to occur by psychosocial and physical environmental influences while the genome sequence remains intact. It provides explanations for the possibility of transmission of a recently acquired trait or vulnerability from one generation to another. Social adversity in early life, such as difficulties in school or child abuse, have the potential to cause epigenetic changes that in turn influence gene expression and therefore cause profound neurobiological changes later during adolescence or adult life.[30,38] It would not be a surprise to see that other psychosocial stressors that entire human groups experience such as wars, colonization, social rejection following racial discrimination, bullying, and what is called historical trauma (due to colonization) suffered by the Indigenous Peoples of the Americas also play a role in epigenetic changes and human disease. It is safe to anticipate that epigenetic studies of pain and analgesia will be fostered in the foreseeable future. It will be instrumental in individualizing therapy with conventional analgesics and in the development of the new generation epigenetic analgesic treatments based on small RNA molecules.[25]

PERSONALIZED PAIN MEDICINE

Patient care and treatment outcomes could be improved with the inclusion of cultural and pharmacogenomic input in the diagnosis and management of pain. Pain practitioners working in a multicultural setting should learn and develop skills for interacting with their patients in a way that is respectful of a patient's values and preferences, taking into account their personal histories, past life events, and lifestyle, as well as their genetic makeup. They should seek to provide the patient with physical and emotional comfort and allow the participation of patients' relatives and significant others in the medical encounter. This is one core message of *Culture, Brain, and Medicine*.

In psychiatry and other clinical disciplines, attempts are made to formulate and adopt a patient-centered humanistic medicine.[39,40] Advances in genetics, pharmacogenomics, epigenetics, brain imaging, and identification of biomarkers are bringing us a step closer to screening, genetic counseling, and finely tailored pain treatments. These developments are pointing to the establishment of what could be called "personalized medicine."[41,42] The "one-drug-fits-all" approach to treatment may finally be replaced by more targeted, person-centered therapeutics. The Institute of Medicine of the National Academies in the United States is urging pain practitioners to adhere to this new integrative approach in its groundbreaking report titled "Relieving Pain in America—A Blueprint for Transforming Prevention, Care, Education, and Research," published in 2011.[43] It is agreed that our understanding of molecular, genomic, and epigenetic processes is incomplete without considering cultural, social, psychological, and behavioral influences on health and disease.

We propose a new synthesis for understanding and controlling pain; that is, an integrative approach that aims to personalize care by not only considering the genomic profile of our patients, but by taking into account their cultural characteristics as well. Acknowledging the interactions of molecules, genes, and culture could yield a more appropriate and effective personalized pain medicine. Furthermore, this approach has the potential to transform the way pain medicine is taught to young students and future pain professionals, and in so doing meets the need for trained clinicians who are versed in multiple disciplines and are able to use an integrative approach to diagnose and treat pain. A personalized medicine will have non-negligible positive effects in improving doctor-patient relationships, patient satisfaction, adherence to treatment plans, and health outcomes and inequities.

In this book, we have placed culture in the forefront of our approach to study pain in an integrative manner. Culture should not be considered solely for knowing more about our patients' values, beliefs, and practices. It should be studied with the purpose of unveiling its effects upon biological systems and the pain neuromatrix. Intriguing recent research on pharmacogenetics, social neuroscience, cultural neuroscience, and epigenetics demonstrates how the social and physical environment together strongly modulate the individual's biological responses. Diet regimens shaped by culture directly affect individual patient responses to medicines including analgesics. Early social, family, and personal and group experiences also seem to affect brain development and susceptibility to physical and mental disorders, including acute and chronic pain. A person-centered pain medicine could offer patients culturally sensitive and genomics-wise medical care. Culture allows us to appreciate the inner workings of the encultured and environmentally embedded brain.

REFERENCES

1. U.S. Department of Health and Human Services, Management of Cancer Pain Guideline Panel. *Management of Cancer Pain*. Rockville, MD: U.S. Dept. of Health and Human Services, Public Health Service, Agency for Health Care Policy and Research; 1994. No. 94–0592.
2. Gureje O, Von Korff M, Simon GE, Gater R. Persistent pain and well-being: a World Health Organization study in primary care. *JAMA*. Jul 1998;8;280(2):147–151.
3. Incayawar M, Saucier JF. Pain in remote Andean communities—learning from Quichua (Inca) experience. *Rural Remote Health*. Apr 2010;10(3):1379.
4. Harding SG. Cultures as toolboxes for science and technologies. In: Harding SG, ed. *Is Science Multicultural? Postcolonialisms, Feminisms, and Epistemologies*. Bloomington: Indiana University Press; 1998.
5. Kleinman A. *Patients and Healers in the Context of Culture—An Exploration of the Borderland Between Anthropology, Medicine, and Psychiatry*. Berkeley: University of California Press; 1980.
6. Petrie KJ, Jago LA, Devcich DA. The role of illness perceptions in patients with medical conditions. *Curr Opin Psychiatry*. Mar 2007;20(2):163–167.
7. Xu X, Zuo X, Wang X, Han S. Do you feel my pain? Racial group membership modulates empathic neural responses. *J Neurosci*. Jul 1 2009;29(26):8525–8529.
8. Sangrigoli S, De Schonen S. Recognition of own-race and other-race faces by three-month-old infants. *J Child Psychol Psychiatry*. Oct 2004;45(7):1219–1227.
9. Pinkham AE, Sasson NJ, Calkins ME, et al. The other-race effect in face processing among African American and Caucasian individuals with schizophrenia. *Am J Psychiatry*. May 2008;165(5):639–645.
10. Terbeck S, Kahane G, McTavish S, Savulescu J, Cowen PJ, Hewstone M. Propranolol reduces implicit negative racial bias [published online ahead of print Feb 28, 2012]. *Psychopharmacology (Berl)*. doi:10.1007/s00213-012-2657-5.
11. Bates MS. *Biocultural Dimensions of Chronic Pain—Implications for Treatment of Multi-ethnic Populations*. Albany: State University of New York Press; 1996.
12. Bond MR. The suffering of severe intractable pain. In: Kosterlitz HW, Terenius LY, Merskey H, Dahlam K, eds. *Pain and Society—Report of the Dahlem Workshop on Pain and Society, Berlin 1979, November 26–30*. Weinheim: Verlag Chemie; 1980:53–62.
13. Young EE, Lariviere WR, Belfer I. Genetic basis of pain variability: recent advances. *J Med Genet*. Jan 2012;49(1):1–9.
14. Cox JJ, Reimann F, Nicholas AK, et al. An SCN9A channelopathy causes congenital inability to experience pain. *Nature*. Dec 14 2006; 444(7121):894–898.
15. Schwedt TJ, Dodick DW. Third gene identified for hereditary headache. *Lancet Neurol*. Sep 2005;4(9):519–520.
16. Ng CH, Lin KM. *Ethno-Psychopharmacology—Advances in Current Practice*. Cambridge, England: Cambridge University Press; 2008.

17. Lin KM, Poland RE. Ethnicity, culture, and psychopharmacology. In: Bloom FE, Kupfer DJ, eds. *Psychopharmacology: The Fourth Generation of Progress*. New York, NY: Raven Press, Ltd.; 1995:1907–1917.

18. Lin KM, Poland RE, Nakasaki G. *Psychopharmacology and Psychobiology of Ethnicity*. Washington, DC: American Psychiatric Press; 1993.

19. Stamer UM, Stuber F. The pharmacogenetics of analgesia. *Expert Opin Pharmacother.* Oct 2007;8(14):2235–2245.

20. Meaney MJ, Szyf M. Environmental programming of stress responses through DNA methylation: life at the interface between a dynamic environment and a fixed genome. *Dialogues Clin Neurosci.* 2005;7(2):103–123.

21. Szyf M. The early life environment and the epigenome. *Biochim Biophys Acta.* Sep 2009; 1790(9):878–885.

22. Allis CD, Jenuwein T, Reinberg D. *Epigenetics*. Cold Spring Harbor, N.Y: Cold Spring Harbor Laboratory Press; 2007.

23. Oberlander TF, Weinberg J, Papsdorf M, Grunau R, Misri S, Devlin AM. Prenatal exposure to maternal depression, neonatal methylation of human glucocorticoid receptor gene (NR3C1) and infant cortisol stress responses. *Epigenetics.* Mar 2008;3(2):97–106.

24. Gluckman PD, Hanson MA, Cooper C, Thornburg KL. Effect of in utero and early-life conditions on adult health and disease. *N Engl J Med.* Jul 3 2008;359(1):61–73.

25. Doehring A, Geisslinger G, Lotsch J. Epigenetics in pain and analgesia: an imminent research field. *Eur J Pain.* Jan 2011;15(1):11–16.

26. Kucharski R, Maleszka J, Foret S, Maleszka R. Nutritional control of reproductive status in honeybees via DNA methylation. *Science.* Mar 28 2008;319(5871):1827–1830.

27. Lockett GA, Kucharski R, Maleszka R. DNA methylation changes elicited by social stimuli in the brains of worker honey bees. *Genes Brain Behav.* Mar 2012;11(2):235–242.

28. Kuzawa CW, Sweet E. Epigenetics and the embodiment of race: Developmental origins of US racial disparities in cardiovascular health. *Am J Hum Biol.* Jan 2009;21(1):2–15.

29. Jovanovic J, Ronneberg JA, Tost J, Kristensen V. The epigenetics of breast cancer. *Mol Oncol.* Jun 2010;4(3):242–254.

30. McGowan PO, Szyf M. The epigenetics of social adversity in early life: Implications for mental health outcomes. *Neurobiol Dis.* Jul 2010;39(1):66–72.

31. Murgatroyd C, Spengler D. Genetic variation in the epigenetic machinery and mental health. *Curr Psychiatry Rep.* Feb 4 2012;

32. Javierre BM, Hernando H, Ballestar E. Environmental triggers and epigenetic deregulation in autoimmune disease. *Discov Med.* Dec 2011;12(67):535–545.

33. Gray SG. Epigenetic treatment of neurological disease. *Epigenomics.* Aug 2011;3(4):431–450.

34. Slomko H, Heo HJ, Einstein FH. Minireview: Epigenetics of obesity and diabetes in humans. *Endocrinology.* Mar 2012;153(3):1025–1030

35. Géranton SM. Targeting epigenetic mechanisms for pain relief. *Curr Opin Pharmacol.* Feb 2012;12(1):35–41.

36. Low LA, Schweinhardt P. Early life adversity as a risk factor for fibromyalgia in later life. *Pain Res Treat.* [published online Oct 12, 2011]. Doi: 10.1155/2012/140832.

37. Zhang Z, Cai YQ, Zou F, Bie B, Pan ZZ. Epigenetic suppression of GAD65 expression mediates persistent pain. *Nat Med.* 2011;17(11):1448–1455.

38. Essex MJ, Thomas BW, Hertzman C, et al. Epigenetic vestiges of early developmental adversity: childhood stress exposure and DNA methylation in adolescence. *Child Dev.* Sep 2 2011;

39. Carrillo JE, Green AR, Betancourt JR. Cross-cultural primary care: a patient-based approach. *Ann Intern Med.* May 18 1999;130(10):829–834.

40. Mezzich J, Snaedal J, van Weel C, Heath I. Toward person-centered medicine: from disease to patient to person. *Mt Sinai J Med.* May 2010;77(3):304–306.

41. Stamer UM, Zhang L, Stuber F. Personalized therapy in pain management: where do we stand? *Pharmacogenomics.* Jun 2010;11(6):843–864.
42. Gordon E, Koslow SH. *Integrative Neuroscience and Personalized Medicine.* New York, NY: Oxford University Press; 2011.
43. Institute of Medicine. *Relieving Pain in America—A Blueprint for Transforming Prevention, Care, Education, and Research.* Washington, DC: The National Academies Press; 2011.

INDEX